Predictive Algorithms for Rehabilitation and Assistive Systems

V. Rajesh Kumar Korupalli
Woxsen University, India

Padmini Ranasinghe
Johns Hopkins University School of Medicine, USA

Dorianne Feldman
Johns Hopkins University School of Medicine, USA

IGI Global
Scientific Publishing
Publishing Tomorrow's Research Today

Vice President of Editorial Melissa Wagner
Director of Acquisitions Mikaela Felty
Director of Book Development Jocelynn Hessler
Production Manager Mike Brehm
Cover Design Jose Rosado

Published in the United States of America by
IGI Global Scientific Publishing
701 East Chocolate Avenue
Hershey, PA, 17033, USA
Tel: 717-533-8845
Fax: 717-533-7115
Website: https://www.igi-global.com E-mail: cust@igi-global.com

Library of Congress Cataloging-in-Publication Data

Names: Kumar, Korupalli V. Rajesh, 1989- editor. | Ranasinghe, Padmini, editor. | Feldman, Dorianne Rachelle, 1975- editor.
Title: Predictive algorithms for rehabilitation and assistive systems / edited by Rajesh Kumar K V, Padmini Ranasinghe, Dorianne Feldman.
Description: Hershey, PA : IGI Global Scientific Publishing, 2025. | Includes bibliographical references and index. | Summary: "The objective of the book is to explore how advanced predictive algorithms can be applied in developing and optimizing rehabilitation and assistive technologies"-- Provided by publisher.
Identifiers: LCCN 2024058325 (print) | LCCN 2024058326 (ebook) | ISBN 9798337301945 (hardcover) | ISBN 9798337301952 (paperback) | ISBN 9798337301969 (ebook)
Subjects: LCSH: Artificial intelligence--Medical applications--Case studies. | Self-help devices for people with disabilities--Case studies. | Self-help devices for older people--Case studies.
Classification: LCC R859.7.A78 P73 2025 (print) | LCC R859.7.A78 (ebook) | DDC 610.285/63--dc23/eng/20250211
LC record available at https://lccn.loc.gov/2024058325
LC ebook record available at https://lccn.loc.gov/2024058326

British Cataloguing in Publication Data
A Cataloguing in Publication record for this book is available from the British Library.

Table of Contents

Detailed Table of Contents

Algorithms play a major role in understanding and quantifying survival or time-to-event data. There are three main areas where algorithms are at work with survival analysis data. It is used in estimation of survival probability and estimating impact of covariates on the survival function. Secondly, algorithms can extract pseudo-individual patient level data from a survival curve plot with the aid of some event and censoring details. Finally, the most important area where algorithms play a vital role is in rehabilitation of patients from a diverse setting of healthcare needs. From managing diabetes patients to optimizing the time-to-recovery for patients post stroke or knee surgery, self-learning or supervised algorithms are increasingly playing an important role in the medical field. This chapter deals with these diverse aspects of algorithms in the clinical sector with a basic introduction and few snippets of case-studies as examples.

Rehabilitation is undergoing a revolution with machine learning (ML) enabling personalized solutions based on patient-specific data. Unlike current rehabilitation practices that lack adaptability, ML optimizes physical, cognitive, and psychological aspects through real-time monitoring, modeling, and intervention. Computer vision enhances movement analysis, NLP supports psychological assessments,

therapy, regenerative therapies, and personalized medicine approaches, informed by machine learning, can transform pain management paradigms.

This chapter examines the transformative role of predictive algorithms in assistive technologies, showcasing their ability to enhance accessibility and independence for individuals with disabilities. Leveraging advancements in artificial intelligence and machine learning, these algorithms enable devices to adapt to users' unique needs, improving mobility, communication, health monitoring, and home automation. Applications such as smart wheelchairs with terrain adaptation, context-aware communication tools, wearable health monitors with proactive alerts, and personalized smart home systems are explored. The chapter addresses current gaps, including limited contextual understanding and real-time learning, while discussing ethical concerns like data privacy and security. Future directions emphasize interconnected ecosystems that integrate multiple devices for holistic support. This chapter underscores how predictive algorithms drive innovation, fostering inclusivity and improving the quality of life for users.

Liver disease is one of the most prominent causes of the increase in the death rate worldwide. Early detection can help in better management and treatment of the disease. Machine learning can help in accurate and efficient diagnosis of Liver disease. This paper aims to develop a machine learning model for the detection of Liver disease. The main focus is to predict liver disease based on a software engineering approach using classification and feature selection techniques. The model has a good accuracy and can be used for early detection of Liver disease. This proposed methodology has the potential to contribute to improved patient outcomes and quality of life. In this paper, different machine learning algorithms such as Logistic Regression, Multi-Layer Perceptron, Decision Tree Random Forest, Support Vector Machine, Extreme Gradient Boosting and K-Nearest Neighbours have been used to detect the liver disease. In this proposed work, the accuracy of the algorithms is compared

the benefits of such innovations while, at the same time, maintaining patient and doctor autonomy as well as the principles of the practicing ethics in the medical field.

Preface

INTRODUCTION

The integration of predictive algorithms into rehabilitation and assistive systems represents a profound transformation in modern healthcare and patient care. As the global population ages and the prevalence of chronic and neurodegenerative conditions increases, there is a pressing need for scalable, adaptive, and intelligent solutions. Technologies such as artificial intelligence (AI), machine learning (ML), natural language processing (NLP), and wearable sensors are revolutionizing how medical professionals assess, treat, and support individuals through recovery and daily living. This book emerges from this landscape as a curated exploration of cutting-edge research and applications designed to improve patient outcomes, promote autonomy, and redefine the future of assistive systems.

This volume addresses the confluence of data science and biomedical innovation. It brings together interdisciplinary contributions that cover diverse aspects—ranging from prosthetics and orthotics to neurorehabilitation and senior citizen support. Each chapter contributes unique insights into the design, implementation, and potential of predictive algorithms in clinical environments. Emphasizing personalization, real-time decision-making, and seamless integration with current technologies, the chapters illuminate how computational intelligence can meet real-world rehabilitation challenges in adaptive and ethical ways.

Moreover, the book serves as a bridge between academic research and practical application. It not only informs healthcare practitioners and researchers but also invites policymakers, technologists, and designers to reflect on how predictive tools can be scaled responsibly. This preface aims to provide a roadmap for the reader, highlighting each chapter's relevance and contextualizing the broader significance of predictive algorithms in assistive technologies today.

CHAPTER OVERVIEW

Chapter 1: Algorithms for Evidence Synthesis in Clinical Domain

This chapter explores how survival analysis algorithms facilitate the estimation of survival probability, the influence of covariates, and the extraction of individual patient-level data. The role of these algorithms in personalized patient rehabilitation across varied clinical conditions is discussed through examples and case studies.

Chapter 2: Data-Driven Rehabilitation Using Machine Learning Approaches for Adaptive Recovery and Treatment

Focusing on machine learning's role in real-time rehabilitation, this chapter discusses personalized treatment through computer vision, natural language processing, and ML-powered robotics. The integration of wearable tech, VR, and IoT enhances remote and adaptable recovery systems.

Chapter 3: Enhancing Recovery—Statistical Approaches for Personalized Rehabilitation

The shift to patient-centered rehabilitation is underscored by statistical modeling and machine learning. By employing regression, clustering, and survival analysis, this chapter illustrates how recovery paths can be accurately predicted and therapies customized to the individual.

Chapter 4: AI-Driven Predictive Models for Personalized Rehabilitation and Assistive Systems

This chapter focuses on AI models driven by reinforcement learning and deep learning that enable data-based rehabilitation planning. It also covers federated learning and IoMT, exploring challenges like data privacy and ethical considerations in intelligent healthcare systems.

Chapter 5: AI-Driven Prosthetics and Orthotics

Examining AI's transformative role in prosthetic and orthotic design, this chapter reviews technologies such as gait analysis, brain-computer interfaces, and IoT-enabled components. It highlights both innovation and limitations—particularly ethical, financial, and regulatory challenges.

Chapter 6: Natural Language Processing for Assistive Communication Devices

This chapter addresses the integration of NLP into communication aids for individuals with physical impairments. By using AI to interpret speech, text, or gestures, assistive technologies become more intuitive and personalized, improving daily interaction and autonomy.

Chapter 7: Smart Assistive Technology for Senior Citizens

An analysis of assistive technologies geared toward aging populations, this chapter examines mobility tools, sensory enhancements, and emergency systems. It evaluates obstacles like affordability and acceptance, along with the need for human-centered technology design.

Chapter 8: Wearable Technology and Sensor Data in Neurorehabilitation

Here, the authors explore how wearable devices provide continuous monitoring and feedback in neurorehabilitation. Predictive models tailor therapy to the user in real-time, demonstrating measurable gains in patient-specific outcomes and therapy effectiveness.

Chapter 9: Machine Learning Techniques for Personalized Rehabilitation

This chapter outlines machine learning methods, such as neural networks and decision trees, applied to individualized recovery strategies. It emphasizes how ML, combined with wearable data, offers precision in rehabilitation planning and execution.

Chapter 10: Enhancing Rehabilitation Through Predictive Analytics in Wearable Technology

Delving deeper into biomechanical sensing and computational intelligence, this chapter showcases how data from medical-grade wearables transforms raw data into clinical insights for treating stroke, cardiovascular, and neurological impairments.

Chapter 11: Predictive Medicine in Pain Management and Assistive Systems

Pain relief through exoskeletons, sensor fusion, and neuromorphic computing is central in this chapter. Combining predictive modeling with pharmacological and gene-based approaches, the chapter proposes new directions for real-time, personalized pain management.

Chapter 12: Enhancing Daily Living for Individuals With Disabilities

This chapter evaluates AI-based predictive systems that optimize mobility, communication, and home automation. By tailoring environments to user needs, these technologies foster greater independence and challenge traditional models of disability support.

Chapter 13: Liver Disease Prediction Using Classification and Feature Selection

A focused exploration of disease prediction, this chapter demonstrates how ML can enhance early diagnosis and management of liver disease using feature selection and classification techniques, offering broader implications for algorithm-based health screening.

Chapter 14: Intelligent Cognitive Interfaces for Rehabilitation

This chapter explores the use of brain-computer interfaces and AI-driven cognitive tools in rehabilitation for individuals with cognitive impairments. Predictive models help track patient engagement and recovery trajectories in mental and neurological health.

Chapter 15: Deep Learning for Mobility Assistance Devices

Advanced deep learning models enable responsive, user-adaptive mobility aids. This chapter discusses gait pattern recognition, terrain classification, and predictive obstacle avoidance as core functionalities in AI-empowered assistive devices.

Chapter 16: Integrating Emotional AI in Assistive Robotics

With a focus on emotional intelligence, this chapter investigates how affective computing enhances human-robot interaction. Predictive emotional models are shown to improve engagement and therapeutic outcomes in emotionally-aware rehabilitation systems.

Chapter 17: Ethics and Responsible AI in Assistive Rehabilitation Technologies

Concluding the technical arc, this chapter reflects on data governance, algorithmic bias, consent, and transparency. It calls for regulatory frameworks and ethical design principles that ensure assistive AI systems remain trustworthy and inclusive.

CONCLUSION

The research presented in this volume confirms that predictive algorithms are no longer just theoretical tools—they are being actively integrated into systems that restore movement, communication, and quality of life for patients around the world. As the healthcare landscape continues to evolve, the role of computational intelligence in rehabilitation and assistive systems will only become more central. By focusing on personalization, real-time feedback, and scalable deployment, these technologies are setting new benchmarks in care delivery and patient empowerment.

However, this advancement brings with it a complex array of technical, ethical, and practical challenges. Data privacy, affordability, user diversity, and algorithmic transparency must be navigated thoughtfully. The chapters in this book do not shy away from these concerns—instead, they engage with them head-on, offering both caution and optimism. By highlighting success stories and addressing current limitations, the book serves as both a celebration of progress and a guide for future innovation.

Looking forward, collaboration will be essential. Engineers, clinicians, data scientists, policymakers, and patients must work together to shape a future where predictive algorithms truly serve the diverse and dynamic needs of humanity. This book aims to inspire such collaboration and spark continued research in building assistive and rehabilitative technologies that are not only intelligent but also inclusive and human-centered.

V. Rajesh Kumar Korupalli
Woxsen University, India

Padmini Ranasinghe
Johns Hopkins University School of Medicine, USA

Dorianne Feldman
Johns Hopkins University School of Medicine, USA

Chapter 1
Algorithms for Evidence Synthesis in Clinical Domain

Amritendu Bhattacharya
https://orcid.org/0000-0001-6237-7290
Woxsen University, India

Ravilisetty Revathi
https://orcid.org/0000-0003-4988-2158
Woxsen University, India

Boya Venkatesu
https://orcid.org/0000-0003-1280-7525
Woxsen University, India

ABSTRACT

Algorithms play a major role in understanding and quantifying survival or time-to-event data. There are three main areas where algorithms are at work with survival analysis data. It is used in estimation of survival probability and estimating impact of covariates on the survival function. Secondly, algorithms can extract pseudo-individual patient level data from a survival curve plot with the aid of some event and censoring details. Finally, the most important area where algorithms play a vital role is in rehabilitation of patients from a diverse setting of healthcare needs. From managing diabetes patients to optimizing the time-to-recovery for patients post stroke or knee surgery, self-learning or supervised algorithms are increasingly playing an important role in the medical field. This chapter deals with these diverse aspects of algorithms in the clinical sector with a basic introduction and few snippets of case-studies as examples.

DOI: 10.4018/979-8-3373-0194-5.ch001

1. INTRODUCTION

Time-to-event or Survival analysis is a critical method in areas related to clinical or health economic evaluation of oncology domains. In this space predicting time to death or time to recovery is of utmost importance. Meta-Analysis is critical to synthesize evidence for a wide range of decision making in healthcare but since it requires time and a lot of manual effort, continuous monitoring of body parameters can aid in decision making along with the utilization of historic data.

Just imagine a critically ill patient with multi-organ failure is admitted in order to prevent sepsis, a potentially life-threatening condition where the immune system goes into a hyperactive mode leading to massive inflammation across the body causing organ damage. What should be the first line of treatment. Depending on degree of lymphopenia, several studies have predicted that if lymphopenia persists up to Day 4 post, the sepsis-related immunosuppression could be predicted by the level of lymphocytes. Hence continual monitoring of lymphocyte levels along with few other potential biomarkers could help clinicians decide on ventilation and introduction of required medicines at the correct timepoint.

Similarly continuous glucose monitoring technologies have evolved that control and add insulin as per the body's requirement. Such continuous tracking with historical knowledge of cut-off points is very useful in areas such as diabetes management and in oncology, just to name a few.

Algorithms play a vital role in understanding the time-to-event data and in managing its downstream processes. Algorithms can be used to model the survival data. Algorithms can also be used to estimate the impact of factors impacting the outcome. Finally, a different set of algorithms can be used for continual evidence synthesis and continuous monitoring of human health and play a vital role in rehabilitation from several diseases.

The chapter is structured into the following sections. Firstly, we deal with Survival analysis and censoring. Secondly, we deal with semi-parametric Cox regression and introduce the concept of covariate impact on the outcome. Thirdly we highlight the alternate measures to hazard ratio in the survival data analysis. Fourthly we discuss the concept of data extraction from historic Kaplan Meier Curves and how algorithms can help in better data extraction. Finally, we deal with automation of data collection for conducting Meta-Analysis and Network Meta-Analysis. Then few algorithms for Survival Prediction are highlighted. Some Machine Learning algorithms and their application in healthcare is provided as snippets of case-studies. A note on the application of artificial intelligence (AI)-driven survival analysis is provided and its potential is highlighted with an example from a case study.

2. SURVIVAL ANALYSIS AND CENSORING

How long does it take an electric bulb to fuse? How do companies ensure that their car battery at least lasts more than 2 years without a replacement? These are questions answered by reliability engineering. Rare events are modelled by poison distribution. Some more frequent events-based scenarios follow exponential distribution. Such questions in the medical field become a question of survival.

Survival analysis helps us find out how long it may take for a patient with third degree burn to stay in a hospital bed before recovery. For that we need to start collecting data once subjects with third degree gets admitted to the hospital. They are discharged once they have reached a level of recovery. Let's say we collect data of 100 patients' data over a period of 6 months. If all the patients recover and get discharged and we have the data recorded for each of them, then the average length of stay in hospital can be obtained by a simple arithmetic mean.

But rarely can we be so lucky to get such data, especially when dealing with patients that have third degree burn. Some of them unfortunately die and hence they never have a recovery date. They get censored with respect to our objective of recovery. There could also be cases where families of patients cannot afford the medical cost and opt for early discharge before complete recovery. This also is a case of censoring. Rare still is a scenario where patient has to be in hospital for long term of few years. For calculation purpose we have to set a deadline of study duration and any subject exceeding that timeframe need to be censored at the point of cut-off. This last case is a case of right censoring.

Th above scenario can be considered as a typical example of what a survival analysis entails.

Survival analysis is a statistical method for analysing the time-to-event data: the duration of time until the target event takes place, such as time from knee-replacement surgery till the time the patient can again walk independently. It is known by different names such as reliability engineering. In economics it is called as duration analysis and event history analysis in sociology. In telecom industry and human resource arena, they go by the name of Churn data analysis. For example, in the telecom industry it is crucial to know at what rate the customer is likely to end their association with the telecom network and switch to a rival network. In healthcare it is important to estimate how quickly a patient can recover. Survival analysis helps us to know the proportion of events and the rate of occurrence of such events. They also point out significant co-variates that impact the outcome. There could be competing risks. For example, a subject with a heart disease under study may die of malaria, which is an unrelated cause of death. There are ways to take such factors into account.

In order to frame and answer time-to-event data, we first need to define lifetime for every specific issue under analysis. In clinical survival, death is ultimate reliability measure. In survival analysis terminology such outcomes are defined as overall survival. However, it is more important to have surrogate endpoints that can indicate the health of a subject. We cannot wait for subjects to die. Progression Free Survival and Disease-Free Survival are examples of surrogate endpoints. The endpoints are scaled in terms of complete recovery, partial recovery, progressive disease etc. Competing risks attempt to remove ambiguity.

In the basic step, survival analysis is about modelling the time to first event data. For example, if the endpoint under study is case of death, the event can occur only once. Recurring data models can have events repeated. For example, fever can relapse. Recurrent event modelling is another important analysis method in medical research.

The following terms need to be specified in survival analyses:

> Event: Death, disease occurrence, disease recurrence, recovery, or other experience of interest
> Time: Time duration is from start of entry to study till occurrence of event or dropout or end of the study duration if the event does not take place till then.
> Censoring: If any subject drops out of the study due to any reason such as lost to follow-up or wilful withdrawal of consent, such subjects are counted till that timepoint and marked as censored. Also, in situations where trial study comes to an end and still the event of interest hasn't occurred, such subjects are considered as censored at the end of trial.

The below Figure 1 depicts the time-to-event graph with individual subjects either having event or censoring.

Figure 1. Time-to-event plot of individual subjects with event/censoring

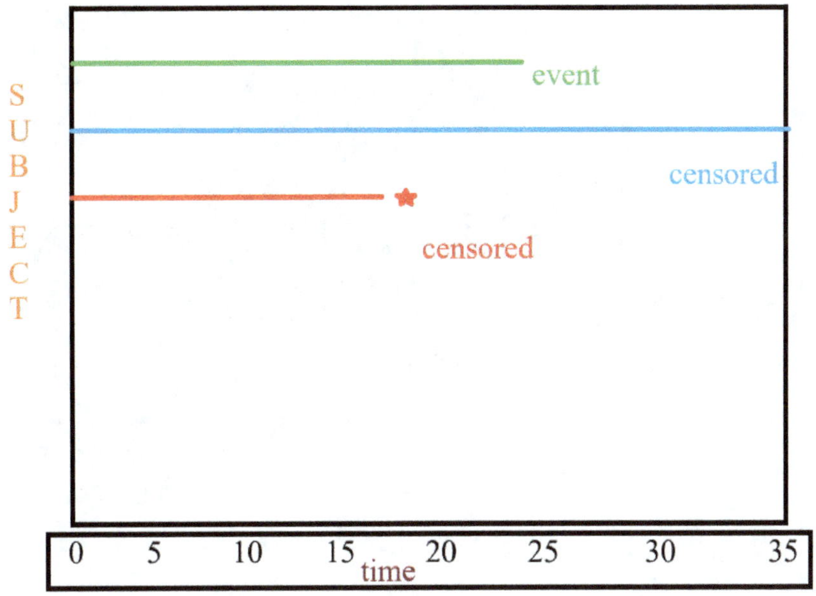

Survival curve is generally depicted by S(t) which refers to the probability of survival for longer time than time t

The obtained survival curve is referred as Kaplan-Meier curve and looks like a non-standard staircase as depicted in Figure 2. The example dataset has 5 subjects with one event occurring at equally spaced timepoints of 1,2,3,4 and 5.

The dataset structure for this is provided in the table 1 below.

Table 1. Data of 5 subjects with event at equally spaced interval at 1,2,3,4 and 5

time	status	treat
1	1	trt_Arm
2	1	trt_Arm
3	1	trt_Arm
4	1	trt_Arm
5	1	trt_Arm

Figure 2. 5 subjects with 1 event each at equally spaced timepoints of 1,2,3,4 and 5.

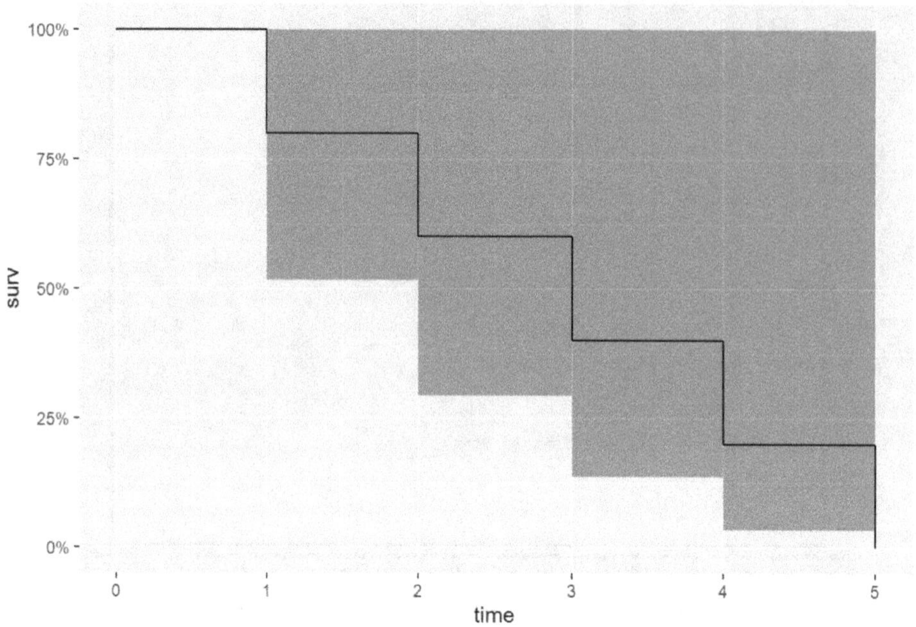

Next let's contrast the Kaplan Meier plot if we have a total of 5 subjects and 5 equally spaced timepoints and there is only 1 event, but in one scenario at first timepoint 1 and in another scenario a timepoint 5 at last. This is provided in Figure 3.

The dataset for this is provided for reference here in table 2.

Table 2. Data of two sets of 5 subjects with 1 event each (at first timepoint in group 1 and at last timepoint in group 2

time	status	treat
1	1	one event at first timepoint
2	0	one event at first timepoint
3	0	one event at first timepoint
4	0	one event at first timepoint
5	0	one event at first timepoint
1	0	one event at last timepoint
2	0	one event at last timepoint
3	0	one event at last timepoint
4	0	one event at last timepoint
5	1	one event at last timepoint

Figure 3. 5 subjects with 2 scenarios: 1 early event versus 1 late event

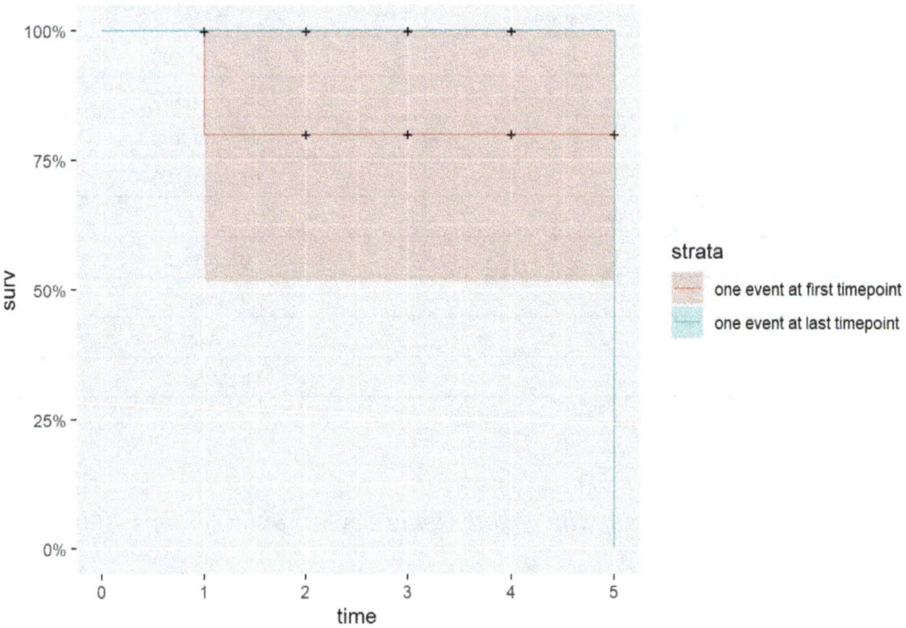

Let us also put a contrasting figure to see the drop in survival percentage over time with one scenario with just 5 subjects with another scenario of 100 subjects. Let one events occur at each timepoint from 1 to 100 in the 100 subject-dataset. Let one event in the 5 subject group occur at an interval of 20 timepoints each. The contrasting Kaplan Meier plot of the two groups below in Figure 4 helps us get an idea of the survival probability drop in terms of study size and event occurrences.

A snapshot of the data is provided below in table 3.

Table 3. One group with 100 subjects in arm with 1 event each from time 1 to 100 and another group of 5 subjects in another arm with 1 event in every interval of 20.

time	status	treat
1	1	trt_Arm_100
2	1	trt_Arm_100
3	1	trt_Arm_100
Cont..	Cont..	Cont..
Cont..	Cont..	Cont..
Cont..	Cont..	Cont..

continued on following page

Table 3. Continued

time	status	treat
97	1	trt_Arm_100
98	1	trt_Arm_100
99	1	trt_Arm_100
100	1	trt_Arm_100
20	1	trt_Arm_5
40	1	trt_Arm_5
60	1	trt_Arm_5
80	1	trt_Arm_5
100	1	trt_Arm_5

Figure 4. Kaplan Meier plot with equally spaced events in two groups: 100 subject group and 5 subject group.

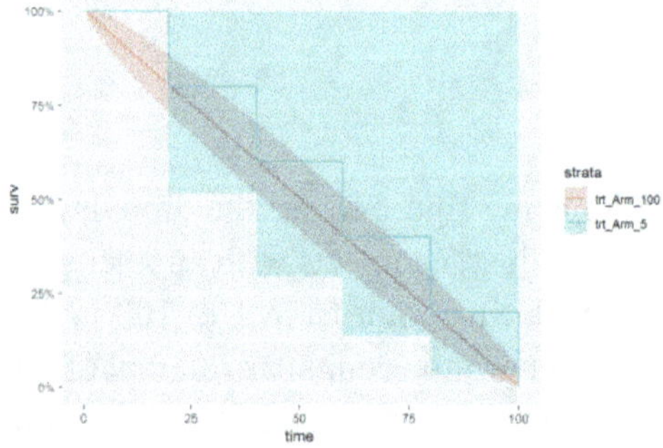

The survival probability is dependent on 3 things, namely, the count of subjects at risk, the censoring timepoints and event count.

Most survival analyses face the censoring issue. In fact, it is preferred over logistic regression because it takes care of censoring better. Subjects with no information on events are not modelled in logistic regression. However, in survival analysis, all data of subjects are utilised in modelling till they have an event or are censored. Censoring happens when information of the outcome in some subjects are unknown either because of missed follow up or consent withdrawal or simply because the study closure and the endpoint under study has not yet taken place. The three main reasons of censoring are: At the study closure, event doesn't occur, or when a subject absconds from the study follow-up, or if there is withdrawal for any reason including removal of consent. The Censoring can be right, left or interval based. Right censoring is commonly observed. In Left censoring, survival time is unknown on the left side of the follow-up period. Interval censored data comes when we do not know the exact timepoint when censoring has taken place between 2 timepoints.

The hazard function is a measure of instantaneous probability per unit time for the event to take place, provided the subject survival up to time t. Between the probability of survival in the miniscule small time period between y and y + Δ y post time y. The magnitude of hazard estimate in that interval quantifies the risk during that time. The hazard functions are all about conditional failure.

Hazard ratio can be considered as a kind of relative risk. If Hazard ratio between two groups is 1.5 then the risk in the group in numerator is 1.5 times that of the other group in the denominator.

It is important to note that as the number of subjects in the study increases and given a drop in survival probability at any instance, it is a factor or several combinations of the number of events and censoring that may take place in that interval.

3. COX REGRESSION

Before we come to Cox regression, let us first discuss the need for it and its related or alternate methods. Suppose we have a survival outcome and we obtain the Kaplan Meier plot. It is also very important to understand some of the important factors that drive these outcomes. In a continuous or categorical endpoint-based regression model, predictors impact on outcomes are estimated in terms of the coefficient. In survival models, there is a time component in addition to status (event or censored). The regression methods in modelling survival data similarly estimates the impact of predictors on the outcome.

In clinical trials the time from start till event occurrence or censoring is recorded for the different competing treatment arms. Then once the data is collected, they are summarized in Kaplan-Meier curves along with a table of median estimates. The 25th and 75th percentiles are also provided. The two or more treatment arms are then statistically compared using the log rank or Wilcoxon two sample tests. There are several other test statistics based on Frequentist and Bayesian frameworks that can be used as an alternative.

The Cox proportional hazards model was developed by Sir David Cox. It is the de-facto model for survival analysis, especially for analysing medical data. The model is a semi-parametric model and assumes no distribution of the outcome being modelled but its predictors can follow specific distribution. It also expects the proportionality assumption. There are different ways to check if the proportionality has been met. The basic way to check is by a quick visualisation of the obtained graph. There are formal statistical methods to check, for example by the Martingale's residuals-based approach, to point one of the available options. We find in real medical data or in data from other domains, the proportionality assumption does not hold or have deviations. In spite of such drawbacks, the popularity of this model has not been impacted and continues to dominate the analysis space.

The log rank test is a modified Chi-square test to check if the hypothesis that the survival curves are the same for 2 or more groups. There are several other tests for survival data such as the Peta method. In the new Bayesian framework, new testing methods have evolved.

4. ALTERNATE ENDPOINTS OF ANALYSIS IN SURVIVAL DATA

While Cox Proportional Hazard model is popular, we do face the proportionality assumption violation as a major concern.

However, it is common knowledge that clinical data is such that the proportionality assumption is most often violated. The Cox-proportional hazard ratio is still the most popular survival analysis estimate due to its ease of derivation and also the legacy issues.

There are many alternate models that have emerged. The parametric survival models are a great alternate.

There are several alternate statistical estimates. Some existed since a long time such as the parametric hazard ratio based on Weibull distribution. Others are relatively new such as the Restricted Mean Survival Time estimates developed by Parmar et al.

Weibull regression models are also frequently used in survival analysis. Various variants of these models also exist in literature.

4.1. Parametric Hazard Ratio

Parametric models for time-to-event have been in existence since long. Usually pharmacokinetic data follows Weibull or exponential distribution or a variant of those family of distribution. If we plot a time-to-event data, they tend to suggest a tentative distribution. If the data follows a known distribution, its details and parameters can be used to have a better generalization of the data and its moments.

Using parametric model, we can decipher the acceleration/deceleration as well as hazard ratio.

Some of the parametric models are: Exponential, Weibull, Gamma, Gompertz, Exponential and log-logistic survival model.

Bayesian parametric models have also emerged as an option that have proven to be equally good while requiring less hyper-parameter tuning.

A parametric modelling approach has the benefits of parametric estimate derivation. The disadvantage associated with the parametric model starts when there are local deviations from the assumptions. More the deviation, more difficult it is to interpret.

4.2. Restricted Mean Survival Time (RMST)

Restricted mean survival time (RMST) is one approach that does not need the proportionality assumption. Over that it provides the benefit of ease of interpretation. The estimation of difference between two groups can be understood intuitively. That is a definite advantage over the Cox proportional regression method.

It is the combined area of the survival up to a given time. It has advantages over the mean and median based approaches.

Let us delve briefly into the basic difference between the mean, median follow-up and survival duration-based approach and the approach based on RMST. In median follow-up, the censoring is not considered. In RMST, the follow-up is up to a restricted point and censoring is factored in.

The mean survival time is area under the curve of the survival function up to defined point. The mean survival time is best suited to be used when the censoring is missing or at very negligible level. Without having knowledge of the distribution, one cannot predict the future events if the last remaining subject at risk gets censored. Skewness in data also is a factor where median should be used preferentially over the mean.

Unless there is at least drop till 50% survival probability, one cannot estimate the duration of median survival.

RMST is akin to mean survival but is up to by a certain defined time point. And that verily, is its advantage over the mean or median based approach.

To compare two arms in survival analysis, the log-rank test is utilised. It does not give a treatment effect measure.

The main ease in operating with RMST is ability to provide results in absolute or relative. The difference between 2 survival curves can be easily interpreted using RMST. Royston and Parmar initially developed the RMST based approach. Other methods such bootstrapping can be used. RMST and log-rank test almost give comparable results when the assumption of proportionality holds. RMST has also been used in analysis of data on rehabilitation of stroke patients.

4.3. Other Measures: Restricted Mean Time Lost (RMTL)

In data involving competing risk, Restricted mean time lost (RMTL) is has emerged as a good option. RMTL based differences can used as an outcome in scenarios where proportional hazards assumption is not met. Bayesian estimates of RMLT and RMST have added a new layer of stability in these measures.

By no means are the above-mentioned list of measures an exhaustive list. It is an active area of research and new methodologies are evolving.

Table 4. Comparison of different methods of survival data analysis

Method	Details	Advantages	Disadvantages
Cox-Proportional models	Uses proportionality assumption	Simple and most well-known model	Deviation from proportionality assumption weakens the results
Parametric Regression Models	Uses distributions such as Weibull, gamma	Theoretically grounded and easier to interpret	Deviation from assumed distribution can impact results
RMST	Mean survival time (restricted)	Easier to interpret. Good for assessing impact of short duration studies	Difficulty in handling data from heterogeneous designs.

5. INDIVIDUAL PATIENT DATA EXTRACTION FROM KAPLAN MEIER CURVE

Data is central to any kind of analysis. The notion that data is considered the new oil, is true when decisions worth billions hinge on the input data. Models can be varied and some may be optimal in certain situations but all of them are limited by the quality of data.

Data is scarce, and a highly protected resource. The very reason for conducting meta-analysis for evidence synthesis based on overall meta level estimates is because the individual patient level data is not easily available. Most data are protected and dissemination in public domain is highly restricted. In the other industries such as marketing and sales, the data-driven decisions are based on collected data variables to identify the most lucrative products and their target customers and models to optimize their sales and profits.

In the clinical field, what the randomized controlled trials reveal are usually overall demographics, summary of baseline and post-baseline characteristics in terms of means and standard deviation for continuous data and frequency for categorical data. The binary outcomes like odds ratio, risk ratio or risk difference are common but for researchers outside of the study team do not have access to subject level data.

In the trials that deal with survival data, we only get aware of the hazard ratio between the intervention and control but the details of censoring and event time-points remain out of access.

Usually, every trial provides the Kaplan Meier plot. Here lies the opportunity to derive pseudo individual patient data (IPD) based on digital tools that extract the x-y axis co-ordinates of the data points and algorithms that can then generate a probabilistic patient level data.

There are subtle differences in which different publications and research papers provide the Kaplan Meier plots. Some provide the numbers of subjects at risk and events at certain time intervals between the starting and ending timepoints. A subset of such studies also provides the censoring numbers in those intervals. Some highlight the location of an event by a dot or circle while in few studies the censoring timepoints are also highlighted by a perpendicular line at the corresponding locations.

The data extraction process could be done via software such as DigitizeIT and Webplotter through a graphical technique. One needs to upload the Kaplan Meier plot and define the X- (minimum- to -maximum) and Y- (minimum- to -maximum) co-ordinates. The defining or highlighting of the survival curve line differs between software. However, to generalise, they allow the user to mark the events manually or highlight the survival line automatically. Once the x-y co-ordinated are extracted, some checks are done to see that there is an orderly decrease in survival probability with time.

Once this step is done, there are several other softwares such as the IPDfrom KM hosted at the *MD Anderson Cancer Center.* They use algorithms to utilize the available information on risk count, event count at defined intervals and the x-y co-ordinate data to simulate and get us a pseudo individual patient data. If the censoring data is available, then that is also utilized. Else the censoring data is assumed and their distribution is also assumed. For example, one easy assumption is to consider equal distribution of censoring over the entire timepoint.

In survival analysis related trials, usually only the Hazard Ratio and its corresponding 95% confidence intervals are reported. The demographics section also provide the details of subjects in each arm at the beginning of analysis. The Kaplan Meier plot sometimes provides a glimpse of the numbers at risk at certain intervals along the way from start to end of trial. However, this information from the plot or research paper cannot conclusively help us extract the data at patient level. A framework needs to be developed so that every related publication should provide a meaningful data to derive such detailed data from a plot. It should at least be of a level that the extracted data can be further used for meta-analysis.

It should be recommended that a corresponding table of events, censoring and subject at risk at fixed time intervals should be provided by every research publication on clinical trial involving survival analysis.

Guyot et al (2012) were one the first teams to develop an algorithm that could generate the pseudo individual patient level data from digitised Kaplan Meier plots based on mathematical solutions. The reproducibility was an issue due to a great degree of manual intervention in preparing the data extraction. However, with time, there have been standardisations on how to prepare for the data extraction and subsequent individual patient level data creation. Note that the final outcome is a de-identified patient level data that is very similar in nature to the original data. Now the question is, how can, we be sure. One way is to re-compute the hazard ratio and it should match the originally published hazard ratio. In no way is this the only way to check. But it is definitely the first step on the right direction.

Several research groups have tested and validated the extraction process developed by Guyot et al (2020) and have reported good level or stability and reproducibility by multiple different extractors.

Many variants and alternate approaches have emerged. Liu et al. (2014) used PostScript file and vector image method to obtain the data coordinate. They claimed 200 times better resolution.

IPDfromKM by Liu et al (2021) developed the iterative algorithm based on Kaplan Meier and is referred as the "iKM" in their research publication.

Rogula et al in 2022 took an additional approach by using the censoring points if available on the Kaplan Meier plot and obtained good results. They validated their results using simulations.

Modified versions of each of the above-mentioned extraction software and algorithm are available in literature.

6. AUTOMATION OF META-ANALYSIS AND NETWORK META-ANALYSIS

6.1. Meta-Analysis

Suppose we come across as a research publication that reports one new drug for healing skin wound to be better than another drug that has been in the market for over a decade. How do we decide if the new drug is indeed better. To find solutions for questions, we need to accumulate data from many more studies and then make a combined evaluation based on an accepted framework. This is the essence of meta-analysis.

Let's assume we want to know if a newly approved drug for a dermatological scar is better or heals the wound quicker in comparison to the current market leading drug. We scan through the Phase 2 and Phase 3 trial results that have compared the efficacy of the two drugs head-to-head. We find about 12 studies conducted over the past 5 years, each in different countries or geographical regions. Out of them 2 are conducted on paediatric patients below the age of 18. The remaining 10 are conducted on adults with the age range between 18 to 48. Do all studies show similar trends? We find that in 8 of the 10 studies, both the drugs show equivalence in terms of efficacy. In 2 studies the new drugs show significantly better results. In both the paediatric studies, the two drugs were again found to be equivalent.

Can we simply combine all the 12 studies? Should we leave the 2 paediatric studies out and combine the remaining 10 because they are similar in terms of the subject age. When we delve deeper, we find that framing the rules for combining studies for a meta-analysis itself is a big task. If involves checking several aspects such as baseline characteristics of subjects, inclusion and exclusion criteria in each of the studies to see any common factors and also if the endpoints are similar. We can combine studies if they report the same endpoint, however we also need to be careful to note if the definition of the endpoint is also same. Some studies have different cut-off points for defining endpoints such as clinical remission. In skin wound related endpoints, there could be several related disease or wound indices which must be carefully checked.

Once we check all such aspects, we broadly define the design of included studies for meta-analysis based on the PICOT rule. The initials of the 5 terms: Population characteristics, Interventional group, Comparison group, Outcome and Timeframe of the study or endpoint under evaluation together form the acronym.

Meta-analysis is a rule-based aggregation of contrast estimates between two comparison groups. Let us think of a scenario when we need to decide if we should one drug over another for treating a skin allergy, especially if the price category similar for both the drugs. We search for published results from clinical trials to see if there is data. We decide that we will opt for the drug that has a better recovery rate or a quick recovery time. From the scientific databases we find 15 trial that have results with similar patient profile, with the same endpoint of our interest and include both the potential drugs between which we need to choose. Once our inclusion, exclusion criteria is met, we conduct a meta-analysis to know the winner. Sometimes the result is not clear as the confidence interval signals no difference. However, it helps us inform in a better way to help us take a decision. Now suppose a new trial result is published in future which alters the overall result. This meta-analysis therefore a never-ending update. To do this on regular intervals, we need to work toward automating meta-analysis that would need minimal manual intervention.

Pouliopoulou et al (2023) studied whether respiratory exercise-based rehabilitation interventions helped adults with post–COVID-19 condition. A meta-analysis was conducted. Before that, most rehabilitation guidelines were based on expert panel opinions.

A systematic review followed by meta-analysis was done They searched reputed such as Clinical Trials Registry. Certain Mesh terms and keywords were used related to COVID-19

They used a Bayesian approach for analysis and estimates along with 95% credible intervals were reported. Risk of bias analysis were conducted and reported.

6.2. Network Meta-Analysis

Now let's take the complexity level to another dimension. Suppose there exists several alternate drugs to treat the same category of wound. Two new drugs have gained regulatory approval based on equivalence of one of the already existing drugs. How do we know the relative effectiveness of each drug relative to each other? Can we have a framework to rank the treatments in terms of their relative efficacy. This is where Network Meta-Analysis comes to our aid. Not only does it use the direct comparison, it also estimates the indirect estimates via the connecting nodes.

As part of the Network Meta-Analysis, we also need to check for transitivity and consistency. Transitivity refers to the check that in the individual included studies, the covariates do not have a differential impact. Consistency is in terms of similarity between direct and indirect comparison estimates.

Network Meta-Analysis has become a valuable tool not just for indirect comparison in terms of efficacy, but for in health economics for relative cost-effectiveness.

NMA is definitely an indispensable tool, but the plethora of methodologies and differences in frameworks present a challenge in taking medical decisions. Therefore, results of different frameworks must be evaluated before coming to any conclusion. Since the Bayesian framework is more flexible and the probabilistic nature of the questions answered by NMA tend to be based on conditional probabilities, it is the do-to methodology by many health technology assessment bodies and tend to do better in presence of complex data with hierarchical structures.

Further such comparisons need to be done with more complicated data networks to understand the methodological aspects better.

Table 5. Comparison for Frequentist and Bayesian Framework in NMA

Framework	Details	Comments
Frequentist	Based on graph theoretical approach and large data sampling	Easier to interpret but limited by availability of data
Bayesian	Based on Conditional probability	More suitable for answering the survival and meta-analysis questions

6.3. Problems in Automating Meta Analysis and Network Meta Analysis

The input data required for meta-analysis and NMA are varied such as inclusion, exclusion criteria, population, disease details, treatment groups and results. There is no one standard of reporting these details. This non-structured data is the biggest hurdle in automating meta-analysis and NMA.

Current approaches require a lot of human intervention in terms of manually curating data from several research papers and data repositories and then re-creating a dataset with required variables. The concept of a repository of conducted and planned meta-analysis and NMA is also new and there are several overlapping evidence syntheses as different timepoints. There is also no easy way to add results of any new study of trial results that meet the inclusion criteria of any given meta-analysis. Hence there could be a potential new and contradictory finding or even a confirmative result from a large trial but there could be a large potential delay in adding its results that could have a huge bearing on the conclusion of the results.

6.4. Automation in Evidence Synthesis

The automation process includes several steps and the two most important steps are highlighted below:

First is extraction of data from repositories and published articles written in natural language, which is quite heterogeneous and from trials that did not envisage that its results will also be used for meta-analysis by other researchers

Secondly to model meta-analysis, from a causal inference approach.

One long term solution is to standardise the way the input variables and results are provided by researchers via databases or publications. Standardized reporting is a more robust solution, but it may take a long time to realise.

The short-term solution should optimize the level of automation in both the data acquiring phase as well as the analysis model. Another area of improvement should be the automated addition of new study results as and when available.

Improvement in natural language processing and scanning for potential research papers at the title, abstract and full text level should aid the curation process. Software such as easySLR and Nested Knowledge have used Artificial Intelligence (AI) and Machine Learning in systematic review and further innovation in this area will increase automation. Large language models (LLM) and other AI techniques have been employed to conduct automated data extraction, data curation and meta-analysis. With advances in LLM and generative AI technology, the field of evidence synthesis will be greatly transformed. The major impact of that would be the speed at which meta-analysis and NMA results will be obtained and updated.

Living systematic reviews with coding and machine learning techniques are being employed towards continuous updates in meta-analysis and NMA.

Based on the NMA results and taking into account the population characteristics, new adjusted estimates can be generated using population adjusted indirect comparison (PAIC). The PAIC has several categories such as Matched adjusted indirect comparison (MAIC) and Simulated treatment comparisons (STC).

Another potential development that will help this field is the advances in graphical and statistical tools that would ultimately help in interpretation of results and the uncertainty around the results.

Two major steps are needed that will aid such automation. There should be a broad standardization in the collection of clinical data endpoints so that every unique clinical trial in every therapeutic area collects data of relevant important endpoints. The potential timelines of important endpoints should also be encouraged. For example, every clinical trial should be encouraged to report short term (say week 12 or week 24) endpoints as well as long term endpoints such as week 52 or week 104. This will enable the automated system to have good enough volume of data that can increase the precision of estimates. This becomes more critical in the case of rare diseases. For example, in case of a disease like paroxysmal nocturnal haemoglobinuria (PNH), which is a rare disease, there are very few clinical trials available with results. Rare still is the consistency of the endpoints for which results are available. In different clinical trials there are different endpoints related to elevated lactate dehydrogenase (LDH). Some trials report descriptive details such as mean levels while other trials report the ration of LDH/ Upper limit of normal levels. This kind of situation is not ideal for automation because we cannot collate and obtain meta-level information. Hence the primary requirement for automation is consistency of data timepoints and endpoints. Scale based endpoints cause additional challenges. The second major challenge is automating evidence synthesis is the access to data. If NMA is conducted with only the publicly available data, then there is a definitive chance of bias creeping in. Hence there has to be some concession given to provide access to trial data results for conducting automated NMA. This can only happen with formation of global policies and nodal agencies from governmental and non-governmental organizations. Obviously, guidelines will evolve to take care new aspects like digitized or generated pseudo data into account. A lot of research is ongoing to understand the best way to integrate real world data with data from randomized clinical trials.

7. ALGORITHMS AND PREDICTION METHODS IN SURVIVAL ANALYSIS

It is one thing to generate the Kaplan Meier Survival curve from a given data. It is another major task to be then able to predict future events if the trial or study had not stopped at the pre-determined timepoint. Predicting the future events or occurrence of events among subjects that drop out early from the study due to other reasons such as lost to follow-up is of great importance.

Predictive events in survival data could also be linked to recurrent event occurrence as well as to prediction of long-term remission.

A related predictive work is about the progression of the disease based on biomarkers or significant co-variate levels.

The importance of accurate prediction in healthcare outcomes cannot be quantified. Every life saved or any increase in quality of life is the ultimate goal of medical science.

Semi-Parametric models of survival are associated with modest predictive power. Often, parametric distribution-based models such as those based on Weibull or Gompertz distribution have been used to augment the predictive ability of survival algorithms. There are new methods based on Dirichlet process as well as Fractional Polynomial based approaches that have shown tremendous potential and are increasing in popularity.

Here we briefly compile a list of algorithms that are popular in predicting survival function.

7.1. Kaplan-Meier: It is a non-parametric method based on the product limit estimate as described in earlier sections. While it is simple and easy to understand, its predictive probability of future events is modest.

7.2. Cox-Regression Model: It is a semi-parametric regression model which takes into account the co-variates impact on the survival.

7.3. Random Survival Forest: This is a Machine learning a machine learning algorithm and an extension of the Random Forest approach in the survival data settings with right-censored data. Some of the recent applications of Random survival forest are 1. Analysis of biomarkers for heart related risk assessment in chronic renal disease and 2. Risk assessment after transplantation at short and long-term duration (Cambray et al, 2020), 3. Assessment of heart related risk assessment in subjects with chronic renal ailments.

7.4. Neural Networks: A well-known regression method that can be used to predict survival outcomes. Neural networks have been used to train and develop survival models in healthcare with a focus on cancer and cardiology. Kantidakis et al., (2022) used Neural network in survival prediction in 2022

7.5. Convolution Neural Networks (CNN): Convolutional neural network (CNN) is a popular deep learning technique and a specialized form of artificial neural network (ARR). There are convoluted layers that extract features for input data to extract data features. CNN models enable us to get meaningful hierarchical features to characterize data from oncology subtype and also from prognosis endpoints. They have been employed in high-dimensional data space, especially in genomics and specifically in genome wide association studies. A simple diagram of an example CNN is shown below in Figure 5. It contains a network of unseen layers that connect the first and final layers

Figure 5. Structure of a convoluted neural network

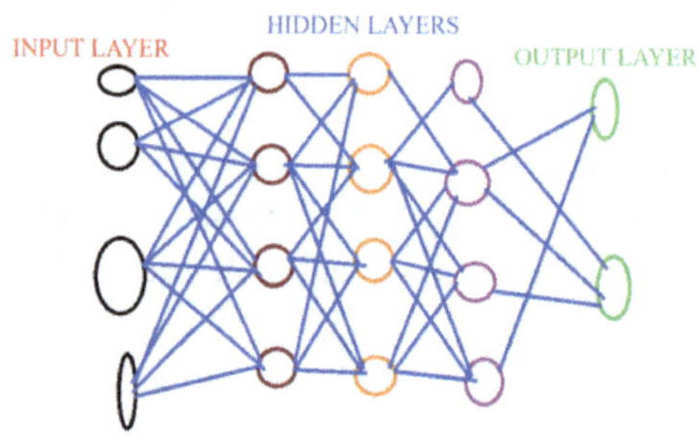

7.6. Dirichlet Process based Survival Prediction: Dirichlet distribution is multivariate beta distribution while Dirichlet process is a distribution over Dirichlet distribution. Mangili et al (2015) have present a robust Dirichlet process-based survival prediction applying a prior near-ignorance approach that does not assume any particular distribution and also does not need to consider any infinite dimensional parameter when we do not have knowledge of prior.

7.7. Fractional polynomial based survival prediction: Researchers have found that fractional polynomials-based approaches perform better than ordinary integer-ordered dynamics. In Network Meta Analysis with survival data, the application of fractional polynomials has provided good results.

7.8. Support Vector Machines: This approach was first proposed by Vapnik in 1995 to predict binary outcomes. They are grounded in theoretical predictions of separating high dimensional data and mathematically prove the existence of a hyperplane that can partitional the data for the two outcomes. By 2000, Vapnik had extended the application of Support Vector Machines to continuous outcomes. Generally, two approaches of Support Vector Machines have been taken for survival prediction. One is regression based and the other is based on ranking. A combination of both the approaches have also been in application. A Support Vector Machines based regression has also evolved.
7.9. Gradient Boost and XGBoost: Gradient Boost and XGBoost are popular machine learning algorithms for for classification and regression tasks based on decision trees. In Gradient boost method, a model is built to predict the outcome and a second model is built to rectify the error of the first model. Both the frameworks work based on optimization of loss function. FPBoost: a Fully Parametric Gradient Boosting for Survival Analysis is an algorithm developed by Alberto Archetti et al (2024)
7.10. AI-driven survival analysis-There are several AI- driven approaches for predicting survival based on histological sample images, which is a part of 'digital patahology'. One example is a work by Parvaiz et al (2024) where their team has generated AI-driven cancer survival prediction using digital histology data.

Please note that the list and categories of survival prediction algorithms are techniques are just a sample of the methods that have and are evolving in this field. There are several algorithms that combine 2 or more of the above techniques such as combining deep learning with Cox Proportional models.

8. SOME CASE STUDIES OF APPLICATION OF SURVIVAL PREDICTION METHODS IN CLINICAL DATA

With so many different techniques and choices to conduct a survival analysis and build a predictive model, it is important to compare and rank the different methods. Several studies use an ensemble of methods to come to any conclusion. However, depending of the collected data and details of co-variates as well as the depth of used models, different scenarios have indicated that one size does not fit all. The ranking of different methods is also prone to bias. There are several published research articles that compare two or more Machine Learning techniques and discuss the merits and demerits of using each one of them. There are also research publications that inform the users about which technique is most suitable in different scenarios and ways to improve predictive models. We discuss few case studies based on research publications to give a flavour of this research and application area.

Tizi and Barrado (2023) conducted a comparative study of 5 different machine learning algorithms in a oncological data setting with diversified sub-categories such as Pancreatic and Gastric cancer, to name a few out of the 10 cancer data that was used. The 5 different methods that they selected were 1. The standard Hazards model with Ridge penalty, 2. Gradient Boosting, 3. Random Survival Forests, along with a loss function, 4. linear Support Vector Machine and 5. kernel Support Vector Machine. All the 5 techniques gave comparable results.

Now let us look at some recent application and methods in this area that hold lot of promise. There are lot of radiological and imaging data of oncology sample, both from biopsy and via scanning. If Machine Learning models could be integrated with high-resolution imaging techniques, could be end up with better diagnosis and prognosis. The answer is 'Yes'. Self-Learning and Assisted-Learning algorithms can scan images of pathological samples and guide medical practitioners.

For example, Degan Hao and team have proposed a deep learning-based approach for gastric carcinoma survival prediction using SurvivalCNN. This technique radiology scans and other pathological covariates as input data. For Breast cancer prediction, Othman et al have proposed a one Hybrid Deep Learning model with Decision-Level Fusion. Many attempts have been made to study which of the three popular classifiers namely the Convoluted Neural Network, Artificial Neural Network or Naïve Bayesian predict lung cancer based on biopsy data. The result is also dependent on the accuracy and detail of the biopsy data used as input for the models.

Koyoma et al proposed an "Artificial intelligence-based personalized survival prediction using clinical and radiomics features in patients with advanced non-small cell lung cancer" and work such as these will herald a new era in personalized medicine.

In patients with Pancreatic Carcinoma, the overall survival is very low. Personalized therapy could better help individual patients. Buwei Teng et al, 2024 used Recursive Feature Elimination method based on 6 different Machine Learning methods for feature selection. This has the potential to improve personalized healthcare.

Another example is the use of 4-layer graph convolutional neural network (GCN) by Xu Yan et al (2024) in survival prediction in diverse cancer subgroups such as gastric and colon cancer. Such leveraging of imaging based artificial techniques is a big boost to the area of diagnostics. It also highlights the fact that along with the improvements in modelling techniques, the need for advances in hardware and imaging technologies can augment the predictive power as there are lot of hidden layers of information.

Another area where predictive algorithms are used frequently are in meta-analysis and network analysis and has been discussed in previous sections based on statistical approaches. However, the role of Machine Learning and Artificial Intelligence in this area of evidence synthesis is wide open.

Sepsis is a condition that many patients face with multi organ failure that triggers an immunological response that can be potentially fatal. Early clinical detection of sepsis is crucial but difficult to achieve. Real time prediction using Machine Learning is promising approach to predict sepsis and thereby, facilitate rehabilitation of the affected patient.

In a non-oncology setting, Machine Learning have been used in the rehabilitation of stroke affected patients. Rehabilitation based on robotics has emerged as an option. This robotics-based methods are intensive and very precise to match the expected level of physical function. Machine learning algorithms can make the robotics-based methods of rehabilitation super effective. They can self-learn and chart their own course of future actions, thereby requiring minimal human intervention. The drawback of caregiver-based approach is substantially reduced. Qingsong Ai and team, in 2021 conducted a review on the use of for robot-assisted rehabilitation of limb augmented by Machine Learning. As these methods stabilise, they have the potential to revolutionise this healthcare industry and the way patients can be rehabilitated post-surgery. The field of physiotherapy of patients suffering from diseases such as Parkinson's disease or Dystonia will be completely transformed and the time to recovery of rehabilitation will get shorter.

In the area of sports such as soccer, any sport related injury can jeopardise careers of players and have immense psychological and economic bearing. Machine learning techniques have been used to help players recover faster and get back into the sports arena. It's an expanding area and has huge scope for further application. A big advantage of machine learning in sports is the huge amount of money involved. There is a huge volume of data being collected right from the diet to physical fitness and laboratory samples. Hence a lot of factors can be analysed to understand what factors can lead to quicker recovery of players. As data starts emerging, predictive models can suggest what more data to collect for even better prediction. Both generalised and personalised recovery paths can be implemented using a mixture of statistics, medicine and augmented machine learning.

We can finally conclude that this is a very active area of research which has two major components. One is the clinical data part which includes techniques and methods for extracting accurate data from images, scans and written records. The other is the advances in algorithms via Artificial Intelligence and Machine Learning. With advances in computational research and increasing use of stabilized Bayesian techniques, this area will continue to evolve and make a real difference to patient care.

9. ETHICAL CONSIDERATIONS OF ALGORITHMS USED FOR SURVIVAL ANALYSIS AND NMA

Ethical considerations are important due to the impact of the results on medical decisions that have a direct bearing on the patients. Any misleading results or estimates can have critical consequence on patients. Researchers need to ensure that the data is collected in a planned manner and the methodology is published in public domain. The interpretation of results and the uncertainty around them must be explained clearly. While it is easier to explain the survival estimates being dependent on the collected data, greater care must be made in interpreting the treatment rankings provided by NMA. Usually, undue importance is given to treatment rankings instead of understanding the methodology. The Guideline set by agencies such as the Cochrane network or PRISMA guidelines must be strictly followed while conducting NMA. Risk of bias analysis should be presented. Similar care must be taken to explain the generated IPD and the uncertainty levels in order to give a proper context.

A practical example of the importance of transparency and ethical consideration can be explained with the example of the NMA using living systematics reviews of COVID-19 related data using MetaInsight which is a web based NMA tool.

To summarize, transparent reporting of methodology and results is a vital and ethical way of disseminating information.

10. LIMITATIONS

The general outline of algorithms used in survival prediction, meta-analysis and NMA is presented. An overview of the pseudo-IPD generation is given. However, a comparison of the competing algorithms and methods is not done using a common dataset. Hence a comparative analysis of the different methods is limited. AI- driven approaches for both survival prediction and NMA is a huge topic of interest. Reason et al (2024) have published the use of Large Language models (LLM) and Generative pre-trained transformer (GPT) for automation of NMA. However, detailed AI-driven approaches are out-of-scope for this chapter.

While different software such as DigitizeIT that help generate pseudo-IPD are briefly mentioned, the details of the actual process is not described. Interested readers are urged to check details of each mentioned tool of software in the websites of individual tools.

R and Python are some of the programming and statistical languages and knowledge of these are a pre-requisite for algorithm development in this space. Specific R packages such as netmeta and gemtc are popular packages for conducting frequentist and Bayesian NMA respectively and need a separate chapter to be described in detail.

Further methodological developments are occurring in all the three mentioned areas of survival prediction, NMA and pseudo-IPD generation and this is an active research area. Some techniques used currently have the potential to become obsolete in a short span of time.

11. RECAP AND CONCLUSION

Survival Analysis is a well establishes method and both the popular Cox model as well as the alternate methods such as RMST are well recognised. Both Frequentist and Bayesian frameworks for analysis have a proven track record. There are three distinct areas in which algorithms can help. One is use of computational power to generate the most accurate hazard ratios and related or alternate estimates. The second is to predict and re-create a patient level dataset from Kaplan Meier plots especially when the original dataset is needed but unavailable in public domain. To do these more accurate graphical techniques and machine learning algorithms need to be developed. The third and the most important are for algorithm development in the field of survival analysis is in the area of real healthcare settings. If machine learning algorithms can self-learn the best recovery path for rehabilitating stroke or cancer patients, it will revolutionise the field of healthcare. Optimising and improving accuracy remain key to achieving these goals. With the advent of AI revolution, there will be a major shift in the automation in this field. Historic trends can get consolidated over time. It can also help a lot of real time analysis for diseases such as COVID and Ebola. Therefore, the development of the right algorithms and continuous improvements in algorithms along with the data flow and analysis will remain a very important subject in healthcare.

REFERENCES

Abbade, L. P., Wang, M., Sriganesh, K., Jin, Y., Mbuagbaw, L., & Thabane, L. (2017). The framing of research questions using the PICOT format in randomized controlled trials of venous ulcer disease is suboptimal: A systematic survey. *Wound Repair and Regeneration, 25*(5), 892–900. DOI: 10.1111/wrr.12592 PMID: 29080311

Ai, Q., Liu, Z., Meng, W., Liu, Q., & Xie, S. Q. (2021). Machine learning in robot assisted upper limb rehabilitation: A focused review. *IEEE Transactions on Cognitive and Developmental Systems.*

Archetti, A., Lomurno, E., Piccinotti, D., & Matteucci, M. (2024). FPBoost: Fully Parametric Gradient Boosting for Survival Analysis. *arXiv preprint arXiv:2409.13363.*

Balduzzi, S., Rücker, G., Nikolakopoulou, A., Papakonstantinou, T., Salanti, G., Efthimiou, O., & Schwarzer, G. (2023). netmeta: An R package for network meta-analysis using frequentist methods. *Journal of Statistical Software, 106*(2), 1–40. DOI: 10.18637/jss.v106.i02

de Vries, E., Houterman, S., Janssen-Heijnen, M. L. G., Nijsten, T., van de Schans, S. A. M., Eggermont, A. M. M., & Coebergh, J. W. W. (2007). Up-to-date survival estimates and historical trends of cutaneous malignant melanoma in the south-east of The Netherlands. *Annals of Oncology : Official Journal of the European Society for Medical Oncology, 18*(6), 1110–1116. DOI: 10.1093/annonc/mdm087 PMID: 17434898

Diallo, A., Carlos-Bolumbu, M., Cervantes-Gonzalez, M., Wozniak, V., Diallo, M. H., Diallo, B. D., Delamou, A., & Galtier, F. (2021). Immunogenicity and safety of Ebola virus vaccines in healthy adults: A systematic review and network meta-analysis. *Human Vaccines & Immunotherapeutics, 17*(10), 3771–3783. DOI: 10.1080/21645515.2021.1932214 PMID: 34270366

DR, C. (1972). Regression models and life tables. *Journal of the Royal Statistical Society. Series A (General), 34*, 248–275.

Elias, B. L., Polancich, S., Jones, C., & Colvin, S. (2015). Evolving the PICOT method for the digital age: The PICOT-D. *The Journal of Nursing Education, 54*(10), 594–599. DOI: 10.3928/01484834-20150916-09 PMID: 26431521

Forne, C., Cambray, S., Bermudez-Lopez, M., Fernandez, E., Bozic, M., & Valdivielso, J. M. (2020). Machine learning analysis of serum biomarkers for cardiovascular risk assessment in chronic kidney disease. *Clinical Kidney Journal, 13*(4), 631–639. PMID: 32905292

Gahlot, D. S., Krieder, S., & Raicu, I. Accelerating Simulation Codes through the GeMTC Framework.

Guyot, P., Ades, A. E., Ouwens, M. J., & Welton, N. J. (2012). Enhanced secondary analysis of survival data: Reconstructing the data from published Kaplan-Meier survival curves. *BMC Medical Research Methodology*, *12*(1), 1–13. DOI: 10.1186/1471-2288-12-9 PMID: 22297116

Hao, D., Li, Q., Feng, Q. X., Qi, L., Liu, X. S., Arefan, D., Zhang, Y.-D., & Wu, S. (2022). SurvivalCNN: A deep learning-based method for gastric cancer survival prediction using radiological imaging data and clinicopathological variables. *Artificial Intelligence in Medicine*, *134*, 102424. DOI: 10.1016/j.artmed.2022.102424 PMID: 36462894

Hutton, B., Catala-Lopez, F., & Moher, D. (2016). The PRISMA statement extension for systematic reviews incorporating network meta-analysis: PRISMA-NMA. *Medicina Clínica (English Ed.)*, *147*(6), 262–266. DOI: 10.1016/j.medcle.2016.10.003 PMID: 27040178

Kantidakis, G., Hazewinkel, A. D., & Fiocco, M. (2022). Neural networks for survival prediction in medicine using prognostic factors: A review and critical appraisal. *Computational and Mathematical Methods in Medicine*, *2022*(1), 1176060. DOI: 10.1155/2022/1176060 PMID: 36238497

Koyama, J., Morise, M., Furukawa, T., Oyama, S., Matsuzawa, R., Tanaka, I., Wakahara, K., Yokota, H., Kimura, T., Shiratori, Y., Kondoh, Y., Hashimoto, N., & Ishii, M. (2024). Artificial intelligence-based personalized survival prediction using clinical and radiomics features in patients with advanced non-small cell lung cancer. *BMC Cancer*, *24*(1), 1417. DOI: 10.1186/s12885-024-13190-w PMID: 39558311

Lerner, I., Créquit, P., Ravaud, P., & Atal, I. (2019). Automatic screening using word embeddings achieved high sensitivity and workload reduction for updating living network meta-analyses. *Journal of Clinical Epidemiology*, *108*, 86–94. DOI: 10.1016/j.jclinepi.2018.12.001 PMID: 30528791

Liu, N., Zhou, Y., & Lee, J. J. (2021). IPDfromKM: Reconstruct individual patient data from published Kaplan-Meier survival curves. *BMC Medical Research Methodology*, *21*(1), 111. DOI: 10.1186/s12874-021-01308-8 PMID: 34074267

Liu, Z., Rich, B., & Hanley, J. A. (2014). Recovering the raw data behind a non-parametric survival curve. *Systematic Reviews*, *3*(1), 1–10. DOI: 10.1186/2046-4053-3-151 PMID: 25551437

Mangili, F., Benavoli, A., de Campos, C. P., & Zaffalon, M. (2015). Reliable survival analysis based on the Dirichlet Process. *Biometrical Journal. Biometrische Zeitschrift*, *57*(6), 1002–1019. DOI: 10.1002/bimj.201500062 PMID: 26296502

Othman, N. A., Abdel-Fattah, M. A., & Ali, A. T. (2023). A hybrid deep learning framework with decision-level fusion for breast cancer survival prediction. *Big Data and Cognitive Computing*, *7*(1), 50. DOI: 10.3390/bdcc7010050

Parvaiz, A., Nasir, E. S., & Fraz, M. M. (2024). From Pixels to Prognosis: A Survey on AI-Driven Cancer Patient Survival Prediction Using Digital Histology Images. *Journal of Imaging Informatics in Medicine*, *37*(4), 1–24. DOI: 10.1007/s10278-024-01049-2 PMID: 38429563

Pouliopoulou, D. V., Macdermid, J. C., Saunders, E., Peters, S., Brunton, L., Miller, E., Quinn, K. L., Pereira, T. V., & Bobos, P. (2023). Rehabilitation interventions for physical capacity and quality of life in adults with post–COVID-19 condition: A systematic review and meta-analysis. *JAMA Network Open*, *6*(9), e2333838–e2333838. DOI: 10.1001/jamanetworkopen.2023.33838 PMID: 37725376

Reason, T., Benbow, E., Langham, J., Gimblett, A., Klijn, S. L., & Malcolm, B. (2024). Artificial Intelligence to Automate Network Meta-Analyses: Four Case Studies to Evaluate the Potential Application of Large Language Models. *PharmacoEconomics Open*, *8*(2), 205–220. DOI: 10.1007/s41669-024-00476-9 PMID: 38340277

Rogula, B., Lozano-Ortega, G., & Johnston, K. M. (2022). A method for reconstructing individual patient data from Kaplan-Meier survival curves that incorporate marked censoring times. *MDM Policy & Practice*, *7*(1), 23814683221077643. DOI: 10.1177/23814683221077643 PMID: 35128059

Royston, P., & Parmar, M. K. (2011). The use of restricted mean survival time to estimate the treatment effect in randomized clinical trials when the proportional hazards assumption is in doubt. *Statistics in Medicine*, *30*(19), 2409–2421. DOI: 10.1002/sim.4274 PMID: 21611958

Sarkis-Onofre, R., Catalá-López, F., Aromataris, E., & Lockwood, C. (2021). How to properly use the PRISMA Statement. *Systematic Reviews*, *10*(1), 1–3. DOI: 10.1186/s13643-021-01671-z PMID: 33875004

Teng, B., Zhang, X., Ge, M., Miao, M., Li, W., & Ma, J. (2024). Personalized three-year survival prediction and prognosis forecast by interpretable machine learning for pancreatic cancer patients: A population-based study and an external validation. *Frontiers in Oncology*, *14*, 1488118. DOI: 10.3389/fonc.2024.1488118 PMID: 39497722

Tizi, W., & Berrado, A. (2023). Machine learning for survival analysis in cancer research: A comparative study. *Scientific African*, *21*, e01880. DOI: 10.1016/j.sciaf.2023.e01880

van Valkenhoef, G., Kuiper, J., & van Valkenhoef, M. G. (2016). Package 'gemtc'.

Vapnik, V. (1995). Support-vector networks. *Machine Learning*, *20*(3), 273–297. DOI: 10.1007/BF00994018

Vapnik, V., & Chapelle, O. (2000). Bounds on error expectation for support vector machines. *Neural Computation*, *12*(9), 2013–2036. DOI: 10.1162/089976600300015042 PMID: 10976137

Wang, P., Li, Y., & Reddy, C. K. (2019). Machine learning for survival analysis: A survey. *ACM Computing Surveys*, *51*(6), 1–36. DOI: 10.1145/3214306

Xin, Y., Owen, R., Bradbury, N., Cooper, N., & Sutton, A. MetaInsight. https://crsu.shinyapps.io/MetaInsight/. Accessed 05 February 2025.

Yan, X., Wang, W., Xiao, M., Li, Y., & Gao, M. (2024, March). Survival prediction across diverse cancer types using neural networks. In *Proceedings of the 2024 7th International Conference on Machine Vision and Applications* (pp. 134-138). DOI: 10.1145/3653946.3653966

Chapter 2
Data-Driven Rehabilitation Using Machine Learning Approaches for Adaptive Recovery and Treatment

Ramakrishna Gandi
https://orcid.org/0000-0001-7213-5789
Geethanjali College of Engineering and Technology, India

G. Suseela
https://orcid.org/0000-0002-9162-7444
SRM Institute of Science and Technology, India

Swati Singh
https://orcid.org/0009-0004-7702-2504
Vardhaman College of Engineering, India

LNC. Prakash K
https://orcid.org/0000-0002-0084-1331
CVR College of Engineering, India

V. Kishen Ajay Kumar
https://orcid.org/0000-0002-1965-8924
Institute of Aeronautical Engineering, Hyderabad, India

Malla Sudhakara
https://orcid.org/0000-0002-2559-4074
Chistats Labs Private Limited, India

ABSTRACT

Rehabilitation is undergoing a revolution with machine learning (ML) enabling personalized solutions based on patient-specific data. Unlike current rehabilitation practices that lack adaptability, ML optimizes physical, cognitive, and psychological aspects through real-time monitoring, modeling, and intervention. Computer vision enhances movement analysis, NLP supports psychological assessments, and predictive models optimize treatment plans. Applications such as wearable tech-

DOI: 10.4018/979-8-3373-0194-5.ch002

nology, telerehabilitation, and ML-driven robotics improve patient interaction and supervision, offering flexible and remote care. Integrating ML with technologies like VR and IoT creates patient-centric, accessible solutions with superior prognostic value. These advancements usher in a new era of algorithms designed for better patient care, safety, and personalized therapeutic processes.

1. INTRODUCTION

Machine learning (ML) is transforming the area of rehabilitation by providing data-driven insights and customized treatment strategies. While effective, traditional rehabilitation approaches primarily rely on uniform methods that might not fully explain personal variations in recovery trajectories. ML provides a robust toolkit for tracking patient development in real-time, project results and customizing rehabilitation strategies.

Figure 1. ML's roles in enhancing rehabilitation

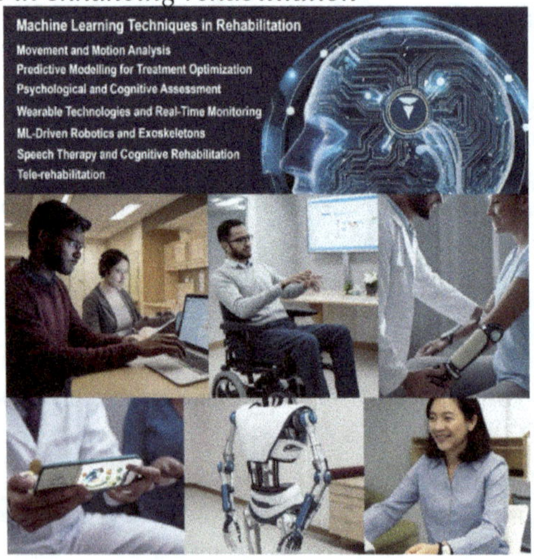

1.1 Overview of Rehabilitation Needs: Physical, Cognitive, and Psychological Rehabilitation

Using massive databases including clinical assessments, sensor data, and patient comments, ML presents a means to significantly increase rehabilitation efficacy (Takacs and Barnabas, 2006).

- Physical Rehabilitation: Often by focused physical therapy, physical rehabilitation seeks to recover movement, strength, and function. This covers handling musculoskeletal problems, enhancing balance, and avoiding re-injury.
- Cognitive Rehabilitation: For people with brain injuries, stroke, or neurological illnesses, cognitive rehabilitation enhances memory, attention, and problem-solving abilities.
- Psychological Rehabilitation: Mental and emotional wellness, which psychological rehabilitation encourages is absolutely vital for a patient's entire recovery. Usually, it addresses stress, anxiety, or motivation issues influencing rehabilitation program adherence.

Understanding these different demands will help ML to provide particular treatments aimed at each region, therefore facilitating a more complete approach to rehabilitation.

1.2 Role of ML in Enhancing Rehabilitation: How ML Addresses Limitations in Traditional Rehabilitation

Machine learning helps to bridge some of the challenges and constraints of traditional rehabilitation methods. ML enhances every major emphasis of rehabilitation in the following ways:

1. *Movement and Motion Analysis:* Conventional approaches of evaluating posture and movement depend on visual observation or basic motion-capture technologies, which would not fully represent the complexity of human movement. Computer vision and position estimate offer precise, automated analysis of gait, posture, and gesture detection among other machine learning approaches. Reliable, objective data lets therapists design tailored treatment plans, monitor progress over time, and spot minor problems.
2. *Predictive Modeling for Treatment Optimization:* Many times motivated by a generic strategy, rehabilitation ignores patient-specific recovery times. To project recovery times and most likely results, ML-driven prediction models consider individual elements like health history, demographics, and treatment progress. This predictive tool helps doctors to allocate resources and change therapies based on expected recovery criteria, therefore facilitating individual planning.
3. *NLP in Psychological and Cognitive Assessment:* Standardized tests or self-reported data have long been the basis of psychological and cognitive rehabilitation assessments; this can overlook continuous changes in mental or emotional condition. NLP improves this by sentiment, cognitive, and psychological well-being analysis of a patient's voice, text, or social media data. This ongoing

observation allows quick interventions and more dynamically tracks therapy development.

4. *Wearable Technologies and Real-Time Monitoring:* Periodic, conventional rehabilitation assessments are often carried out between therapy sessions rather than happening in real-time. On the other hand, wearable devices driven by ML continuously track physiological signals including heart rate, steps, or balance, therefore offering real-time data on a patient's functional state. When evaluating this time-series data, ML systems find trends, track development, and provide real-time alarms for quick intervention.
5. *ML-Driven Robotics and Exoskeletons for Assisted Therapy:* Often demanding and time-consuming, physical therapy in traditional settings lacks the flexibility to satisfy the demands of patients. Using reinforcement learning, ML-powered robotics, and exoskeletons, motions, and forces are changed in response to patient capabilities, hence providing tailored support. This technology not only makes the therapist more capable but also gives patients more freedom on their road to recovery.
6. *Speech Therapy and Cognitive Rehabilitation:* Conventional therapy methods in cognitive rehabilitation could not be able to sufficiently include the patient or change their needs. By use of adaptive, tailored exercises, ML techniques—particularly in speech and language models like RNNs—help in language recovery and cognitive enhancement. For illnesses like aphasia, ML-based speech treatment dynamically adapts to meet the patient's progress, therefore improving language abilities more precisely than more passive treatments.
7. *Tele-rehabilitation and Remote ML Applications:* Location, resources, or patient mobility usually define access to rehabilitation. Supported by ML, tele-rehabilitation increases therapy accessibility by means of virtual, remote sessions and continuous home monitoring. This method not only improves accessibility but also offers real-time comments, therefore enhancing the effectiveness and interaction of remote meetings.

1.3 Current Trends and Applications: Emerging ML Trends in Healthcare and Rehabilitation

Major advancements in personalized treatment, predictive outcome modeling, and real-time monitoring changing rehabilitation are driven by fast expanding relevance of machine learning in healthcare. By allowing continuous tracking via wearables and smart devices and adapting treatment to specific patient data, ML enhances a more responsive and efficient rehabilitation process. Moreover, little knowledge given by ML-driven instruments in psychological and cognitive tests enhances patient recovery and treatment. The impact of ML in healthcare is becoming more and more as many new elements significantly influence rehabilitation as following:

- Predictive Modeling for Recovery: Predicting recovery timeframes, likelihood of problems, and treatment plan adherence is increasingly done using machine learning algorithms. Planning resources and patient expectations depend much on these forecasts.
- Integration of Wearable Technology: Wearable sensors detect a patient's physical activity and physiological responses, much as accelerometers and gyroscopes do. Using this data, ML methods offer automatic, continual insights that enable treatment to be modified.
- Natural Language Processing (NLP) in Cognitive Rehabilitation: Cognitive ability increases with NLP making use of language understanding, memory testing, and speech pattern analysis. This holds the most promise for patients who are unable to formulate words due to cognitive problems caused by large strokes or significant brain damage.
- Virtual and Augmented Reality (VR/AR): VR/AR technologies are enabling new ways physical and cognitive rehabilitation can take place by providing interactive environments where patients may safely practice motions or cognitive tasks (driven by ML) resulting in increased engagement and motivation.

These trends highlight how innovative ML is for rehabilitation; it is more patient-oriented, accurate, and effective.

2. MACHINE LEARNING TECHNIQUES IN MOVEMENT AND MOTION ANALYSIS

Machine learning (ML) presents interesting developments in movement and motion analysis with automated and consistent monitoring, categorization, and interpretation of human movement data. Techniques of vision-based motion analysis aim to detect, track, identify, and generally understand the behavior of objects in image sequences (L. Wang et al., 2011). Important outcomes of this evolution are biomechanics, physical therapy, and rehabilitation. Among other methods of machine learning, convolutional neural networks (CNNs) let one study movement and create customized rehabilitation programs.

Motion and action research find tremendous value in gait measurement, posture evaluation, and gesture identification. Fundamental disciplines such human-computer interface, therapeutic rehabilitation, and sports science, provide whole understanding of human biomechanics. Three main fields computer vision for gait and posture assessment, pose estimation models, and motion tracking and gesture identification where machine learning assists movement analysis are investigated in this part.

These actual examples of machine learning methods used in several domains demonstrate different approaches to investigate motion and movement.

- *Gait Analysis for Clinical Rehabilitation*: Examines patient gait patterns to provide individualized rehabilitation strategies and efficient progress tracking for those with mobility problems.
- *Posture Assessment in Workplace Ergonomics*: Examines workers' positions to prevent injuries, therefore enhancing their well-being and lowering the occupational-related health hazards.
- *Sports Performance and Injury Prevention*: Breaks down sportsmen's motions to maximize talents, therefore enhancing performance and reducing the likelihood of injury.
- *Human-Computer Interface (HCI):* Gesture detection allows touchless control of devices, therefore providing a fundamental and practical solution in hands-free environments.
- *Fall Detection*: Monitoring elderly patients for falls or unusual motions guarantees patient safety in elder care and helps to enable rapid emergency responses.
- *Dancing and Ballet Analysis*: Assesses dancers' motions to improve form and accuracy, therefore enhancing technique and customized coaching built in biomechanics.

2.1. Computer Vision for Gait and Posture Evaluation: Movement Tracking with CNNs

Combining computer vision with deep learning approaches including convolutional neural networks (CNNs) results in successful analysis of human gait and posture. These techniques allow one to evaluate bodily movement patterns in great precision covering walking forms, balance, and postural alignment. Researchers and practitioners can find minute variations in gait and posture that are important for medical, athletic, and ergonomic reasons by aggregating movement via video or sensor data and CNNs processing it.

Figure 2. Yoga pose estimation used in machine learning

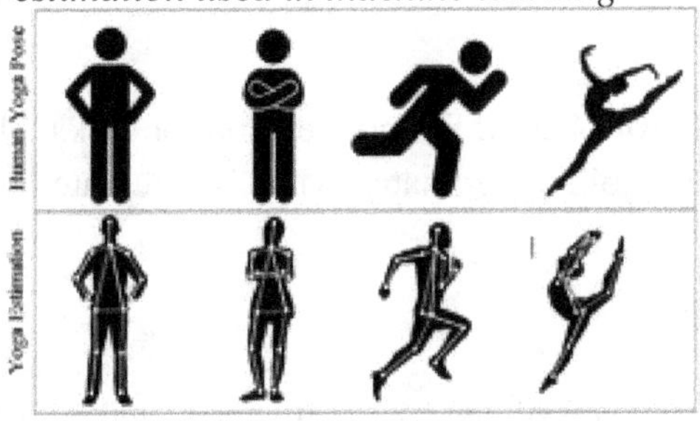

In the data collection phase, video cameras capture continuous images of movement from numerous angles, periodically enhanced by wearable sensors including gyroscopes and accelerometers. Normalizing data, identifying significant joints (such as elbows, knees, ankles), and enhancing image quality helps preprocessing to guarantee consistent input for the CNN.The CNN architecture—which may use ResNet or VGGNet—learns spatial patterns in joint position while pose estimation models—e.g., OpenPose track joint angles and positions over frames. By merging CNNs with RNNs or LSTMs, temporal models investigate movement sequences, therefore providing whole gait cycle and posture analysis. Through gait analysis, quantification of measurable information of gait, and its interpretation frailty and dementia syndromes can be diagnosed (M. Nieto-Hidalgo, 2018).

2.2 Example of CNN Usage in Gait Analysis

The CNN architecture which may use ResNet or VGGNetlearns spatial patterns in joint position while pose estimation models e.g., OpenPose track joint angles and positions over frames. By merging CNNs with RNNs or LSTMs, temporal models investigate movement sequences, therefore providing whole gait cycle and posture analysis.

Equations and Models: Usually, optimizing loss functions and training procedures helps to increase model accuracy using gait and posture data, thus influencing CNN performance.

1. ***Cross-Entropy Loss:*** Used for classification tasks, Cross-Entropy Loss minimizes the difference between the predicted and actual classifications of gait or posture. The loss function is defined as

$$Loss = -\sum_i y_i \cdot \log(\hat{y}_i)$$

where y_i represents the true label, and $\hat{y}_i$ denotes the predicted probability of the model.

2. ***Mean Squared Error (MSE):*** For pose estimation tasks, MSE is used to reduce errors in predicting joint coordinates. MSE is calculated as:

$$MSE = \frac{1}{N}\sum_{i=1}^{N}(y_i - \hat{y}_i)^2$$

where y_i is the actual coordinate, and is the predicted coordinate for each joint.

Powerful tools in gait and posture analysis, these loss functions enable CNNs efficiently identify movement patterns or forecast joint locations..

2.3 Pose Estimation Models: Analyzing Human Body Poses and Applications in Physical Therapy

The discipline of physical therapy has been completely transformed with the introduction of posture estimate models as essential instruments for the study of human body forms. Markerless human pose estimation relies on recent advances in computer vision to automatically track anatomical landmarks so-called keypoints of the human body from digital videos (J. Stenum et al., 2021). They teach you about how to measure joint alignment, muscle activation patterns, and movement efficiency. Pose estimation evaluations of rehabilitation progress based on differences in key human body landmarks that demonstrate posture abnormalities.

Deep learning models are the key instruments used in pose estimation, enabling accurate real-time detection of anatomical landmarks such as joints. Among these areas, OpenPose, PoseNet and MediaPipe are relatively popular models. These models analyze the visual input with Convolutional Neural Networks (CNNs) and hence, acquire substantial pose information.

Usually, the optimal performance of loss functions in training provides the best evidence of the correctness of posture evaluation. The mean squared error (MSE), which computes the variance between the expected and actual key point coordinates, is one widely used statistic.

$$MSE = \frac{1}{N}\sum_{i=1}^{N}(y_i - \hat{y}_i)^2$$

where y_i is the actual coordinate is the predicted coordinate for each joint.

In more complex applications, the total error can be computed by summing the individual joint errors across all key points:

$$Total\ Error = \sum_{j=1}^{j}\left(\left(x_j - \hat{x}_j\right)^2 + \left(y_j - \hat{y}_j\right)^2\right)$$

In this equation, j signifies the total number of joints, while x_j, y_j and $\hat{x}_j$, $\hat{y}_j$ correspond to the actual and predicted coordinates of each joint, respectively.

There are numerous advantages of pose estimation methods in the domain of the physical therapy span. These models help therapists to accurately supervise patient exercises, which ensure patients follow proper movement patterns. And most important, real-time input of their joint angle is effective for injury prevention. Stance estimates also allow the therapists to monitor rehabilitation and modify therapy interventions based on the response of patients as they progress or present ongoing postural difficulties.

2.4 Motion Tracking and Gesture Recognition: Techniques for Tracking Body Movement Accurately

Motion tracking and gesture detection is the application that often relies on from rehabilitation to human computer interface (HCI) and virtual. The machine learning methods, such as real time detection, body motion and gesture analysis, improve user experience and interaction through these technologies.

Techniques and Process: Usually, motion tracking and gesture recognition consist in three main phases:

1. ***Detection***: The system is first in motion tracking and gesture recognition, detecting inside any frame's main body parts or particular motions. This method, which usually identifies human movements by cameras or depth sensors, extracts from the backdrop areas of interest, such as hands, arms or face characteristics, thanks to image processing.
2. ***Tracking***: The system then runs continuously over each video frame after the first motions are found. By means of small characteristics and motion changes, the system is creating an accurate sequential motion record of a continuous tracking. The program analyzes the frame by frame perturbations and using this can create a full, complete dataset of every aspect of the action or posture. The result of this full monitoring method can unveil complex motions and use in later research like gesture recognition accuracy improvement, movement pattern detection, and anomaly detection.
3. ***Recognition***: After the first set of the discovered motions, the system is run continuously across every video frame. This continuous tracking is accomplished by the use of little features and motion changes, leading to an accurate sequential record of motion. By means of analysis of frame-by-frame

variations, the program can build a complete dataset that includes every element of a motion or posture. One can understand complicated motions and support later studies such as gesture recognition accuracy improvement, motion pattern identification, or anomaly detection based on this complete monitoring approach.

Applications and Impact: Technologies in motion tracking and gesture recognition find extensive use in several domains:

1. ***Healthcare and Rehabilitation:*** These instruments record patients' activities and offer personalized treatment during physical therapy, so that therapists are able to understand how healing 'feels.' For example, as a sensor tracks a patient's range of motion by ensuring that the right therapy is being given to the joints but not going beyond that, that prevents damage.
2. ***Human-Computer Interaction (HCI):*** Gesture detection for touchless interfaces naturally foments basis motions for user-object interaction. This makes it particularly helpful in places like hospitals where hygiene is extremely important as it reduces direct contact with surfaces.
3. ***Entertainment and Gaming:*** In gaming, the motion tracking helps to move characters with body motions so that players can be more involved. VR provides immersion as well because the VR takes you on how and where to maneuver within virtual environments so they need to move around physically.

3. PREDICTIVE MODELING FOR TREATMENT OPTIMIZATION

Predictive modeling aims to modify rehabilitation's projection paths of recovery and treatment strategies to thus enhance patient outcomes. Strong tools offered by machine learning (ML) assist one in analyzing patient data, project recuperation times, and treatment modification techniques, thus optimizing clinical decision-making. Emphasizing patient recovery and evaluating the mathematical bases of numerous treatments, this part explores how predictive modeling supports therapeutic optimization in rehabilitation.

3.1 Predicting Patient Recovery: Using ML for Outcome Predictions in Recovery Time

Effective estimation of recovery times drives customized therapy most of the time. ML methods are used to identify trends and patterns in a patient's medical records, allowing accurate prediction of recovery time–therefore helping clinicians to modify their treatment regime. Having this expected timeline allows patients and their families to more appropriately prepare for each phase of rehabilitation, thus helping them participate in the recovery process with greater meaning. However, from data sources to challenges, we summarize here the main concepts of predictive modeling in rehabilitation in order to provide a holistic overview of their influence on therapeutic optimization.

1. *Data Sources in Predictive Modeling:* Various data sources are used in predictive modeling in rehabilitation. Basic patient data including demographic information, past medical history, and relevant clinical metrics (including a patient's concurrent disease history) can substantially influence recovery outcomes when placed in Electronic Health Records (EHRs). Wearable gadgets, including sensors designed for rehabilitation and fitness trackers, record vital indicator (e.g. heart rate, blood pressure) and activity metric (e.g., steps taken, range of motion) data in real time and provide progress and recovery benchmarks for functional measures. Although subjective emotions are reflected by self reported variables such as pain, tiredness, and motivation for adherence to treatment plans, clinical evaluations with pain scales and mobility tests lead to objective data of recovery outcomes. By tracking instantaneous intervention effects using treatment-specific factors such as workout length, session frequency, and therapeutic response, tying treatment characteristics to recovery outcomes for patients undergoing certain treatments, it is possible to characterize the role of treatment specific factors on instantaneous intervention effects.
2. *Outcome Metrics in Rehabilitation:* Time-to-recovery is one of the many outcome factors which provide feedback on predictive modeling success. This will approximate how long a patient can take to become functionally independent a and models of treatment intensity can provide range or definite schedules. Models also assess functional independence, or the ability to start at least some of the basic chores in daily life in an independent fashion, and so expect to see an increased mobility, cognitive capacity and performance of own care. Additionally, for patients with challenging conditions, knowing the probability of future consequences such as re-injury or hospitalization is important and permits the development of anticipative changes to the treatment plan to promote safety and recovery.

Figure 3. Framework for predictive modeling in rehabilitation

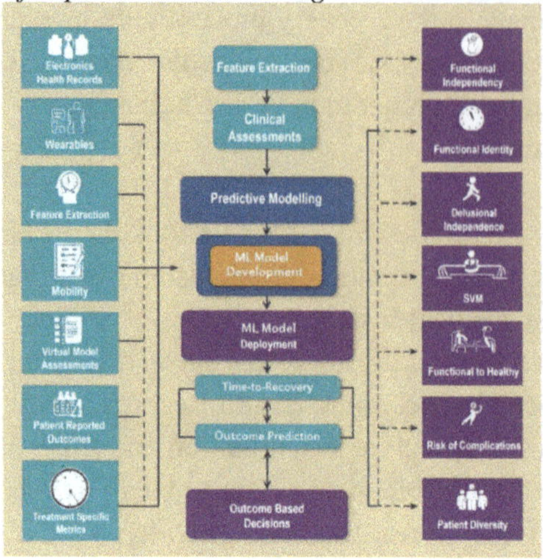

3. *Challenges in Predictive Modeling:* The time-to-recovery value plays a preponderant role when evaluating the effectiveness of the predictive modeling. This number is how long it takes one patient to reach functional independence, which is case specific, and can range from being an exact timing or create a range based on individual characteristics and treatment intensity. The evaluation of functional independence shapes by projecting the changes in mobility, cognitive ability, and self care practice in order to allow patients to achieve the independence in doing daily chores. Also, patients with difficult conditions need to be able to anticipate the danger of risk of re-injury, or hospitalization, and it helps to allow the change proactive changes in treatment regimens to improve safety and recovery.

Predictive models enable doctors to better understand patient demands, therefore guiding more efficient general treatment success rates, patient participation, and resource allocation. These models allow rehabilitation treatments to be improved in ways that were not possible before, therefore offering a more tailored, data-driven method of patient therapy.

3.2 Models and Algorithms: Regression, Decision Trees, SVM, and Other Algorithms in Predictive Modeling

Many ML models are applied in rehabilitation to project directions of therapy and recovery outcomes. Every model has different advantages and disadvantages depending on the particular objectives of the prediction task, the degree of data complexity, and the necessity of model interpretability. Mostly used for basic models like Logistic Regression and Decision Trees (Zhang et al., 2022), simple predictions in rehabilitation find application.

1. ***Logistic Regression:*** Binary classification problems, including those involving patient functional independence prediction, call for logistic regression. It forecasts, from independence to dependency, the probability p of an outcome, as follows:

$$p = \frac{1}{e^{-\left(\beta_0 + \sum_{i=1}^{n} \beta_i x_i\right)}}$$

where the log-odds of the outcome show a linear pattern of the input variables. Logistic regression is effective for interpretable binary classification since it helps one to clearly see how each feature affects the possibility of recovery.

2. ***Decision Trees:*** By partitioning data into subsets depending on feature values, decision trees produce an easily understandable tree-like model. At every node, decision trees divide the data according to the feature that best lowers the impurity. Impurity can be quantified for classification problems using entropy or the Gini index:

$$Gini(t) = 1 - \sum_{i=1}^{C} p_i^2$$

$$Entropy(t) = -\sum_{i=1}^{C} p_i log\left(p_i\right)$$

where, at node t, p_i is the likelihood that a sample fits class i.

Complex tasks, such as predicting outcomes from continuous wearable data, frequently employ Ensemble Models, Support Vector Machines (SVMs) or Neural Networks to enhance accuracy and adaptability.

3. ***Random Forest:*** Random Forests predict rehabilitation patient outcomes by aggregating data from many clinical, demographic, and sensor-based sources. This integrated technique is rather useful when patient histories, therapy responses,

and real-time monitoring data differ substantially in complicated and dynamic data—typical in rehabilitation. Through aggregating several decision trees to represent a range of aspects influencing recovery, Random Forests lower the danger of overfitting and hence improve forecast accuracy and reliability.

Random Forests, for instance, can estimate recovery times, evaluate the probability of particular milestones (e.g., regaining mobility), and even project possible difficulties depending on the aggregating of individual tree projections. This method guarantees that forecasts are grounded on a "forest" of several points of view, therefore offering a fair picture of the restoration process. Random Forests follows this formula for prediction:

$$\hat{y} = \frac{1}{T}\sum_{t=1}^{T} f_t(x)$$

where T is the overall count of trees and $f_t(x)$ shows the t-th tree's prediction.

Every tree in rehabilitation picks trends from subsets of data including patient demographics, wearable sensor data, and therapy-specific metrics, therefore generating a powerful and full prediction model for patient recovery.

4. ***Support Vector Machine (SVM):*** SVMs identify the best hyperplane to divide classes with a maximum margin. Given a dataset with N samples (x_i, y_i), where $y_i \in \{-1,1\}$, SVM finds the hyperplane w·x+b=0 that maximizes the margin between classes. The objective is to minimize:

$$\min_{w,b} \frac{1}{2} \| w \|^2 \text{ subject to } y_i(w.\,x_i - b) > 1, \forall i$$

SVM can thus be extended to handle non-linear data by means of kernel functions, which translate input data into higher dimensions where a separating hyperplane can be found. Since SVM can manage high-dimensional data and thereby has efficiency, it is useful for complex rehabilitation datasets. Its resistance to overfitting especially helps in binary classification tasks to enhance its prediction performance.

5. ***Long Short-Term Memory (LSTM):*** Considered a type of recurrent neural network (RNN), the Long Short-Term Memory (LSTM) model is meant to record long-term dependencies in sequential input. Its unique gating methods allow it to faithfully reproduce time-series patterns, so it is rather fitting for tracking patient development over time in applications for rehabilitation. Long-term dependencies in patient progress and time-series data analysis assist the LSTM model to be rather successful in rehabilitation. Using their gating systems—forget, input,

and output gates—LSTMs selectively retain or discard information over time, therefore allowing exact forecasts of recovery milestones and possible failures. The following are the basic formulae for every gate:

(i) *Forget Gate:* Decides what to throw away from knowledge:

$$f_t = \sigma\left(W_f \cdot \left[h_{t-1}, x_t\right] + b_f\right)$$

(ii) *Input Gate:* Decides which up-to-date information to add:

$$i_t = \sigma\left(W_i \cdot \left[h_{t-1}, x_t\right] + b_i\right)$$

$$C_t = tanh\left(W_C \cdot \left[h_{t-1}, x_t\right] + b_C\right)$$

(iii) *Output Gate:* Generates the revised concealed state:

$$o_t = \sigma\left(W_o \cdot \left[h_{t-1}, x_t\right] + b_o\right)$$

$$h_t = o_t \, . \tanh\left(C_t\right)$$

4. NATURAL LANGUAGE PROCESSING IN PSYCHOLOGICAL AND COGNITIVE ASSESSMENT

Natural Language Processing (NLP) is indispensable in psychological and cognitive assessment when someone analyses language to find patterns linked to mental and cognitive health. By use of language element analysis, NLP models may detect minute signals linked with mental health problems, cognitive decline, and personality traits, therefore offering important support in both clinical and research environments. NLP techniques search text and speech data in mental health tests for symptoms of diseases including depression, anxiety, and schizophrenia. Regular unpleasant emotions, strong frequency of first-person pronouns, or limited language use have been associated with depression symptoms and other mental health disorders.

4.1. Sentiment Analysis for Mental Health Monitoring: Assessing Psychological Well-Being Through Language

Sentiment analysis is applied increasingly in mental health monitoring to assess psychological well-being by means of written or spoken language in an area of natural language processing (NLP). This approach provides insights into an individual's emotional state by evaluating textual signals, tone, and context in their communication, so helping early detection of mental health problems including depression, anxiety, and stress.

Key Techniques and Components:

1. ***Natural Language Processing Models:*** The textual emotional cues based, sentiment analysis depends on what Natural Language Programming models are designed to detect. Common, but generally outrun by more sophisticated methods are Term Frequency-Inverse Document Frequency (TF-IDF) and Bag of Words (BoW). Sentiment is examined in the context of full phrases or paragraphs by deep learning techniques such as LSTM networks and CNNs, as opposed to words, as used by typical approaches.
2. ***Lexicon-Based and Machine Learning Approaches***: ML techniques are combined with lexicon-based approaches, and this is performed for the purpose of sentiment analysis. Not only do they provide a simple rule-based approach to sentiment recognition, but leveraging pre-defined word lists for certain emotions helps make lexicon-based algorithms effective. This approach might miss additional more complex verbal features that are important to sentiment interpretation, including sarcasm and context-specific cases.
3. ***Contextual and Temporal Analysis***: From basic positive or negative classification, sentiment analysis for mental health monitoring integrates context and temporal trends. For instance, monitoring such changes over time enables one to see the relation of better or worse mental health. Contextual and temporal analysis are very beneficial, especially to those who will utilize this knowledge to help prevent declining mental health early on.

Applications and Impact:

1. ***Depression and Anxiety Detection:*** Sentiment analysis searches in personal notebooks, treatment notes, and social media posts for indicators of anxiety and depression. If you regularly feel tired, sad, or helpless, for example, this could be a sign that you are depressed and need to see a mental health professional.
2. ***Stress Monitoring:*** In areas of great concern, such as offices or schools, sentiment analysis can monitor stress signals across time. Real-time comments enable businesses to respond fast to assist staff members, therefore preventing stress and promoting overall wellness.
3. ***Therapeutic Feedback and Support:*** In therapeutic environments, sentiment analysis is also applied to monitor patient development. Therapists can evaluate the effects of treatment and make necessary changes to therapy procedures by looking at changes in language used over time, therefore offering a quantitative assessment of therapeutic results.

4.2. LSTM (Long Short-Term Memory) Networks in Sentiment Analysis

LSTM networks, a type of recurrent neural network (RNN), are advantageous in sentiment analysis because of their ability to identify long-term dependencies in textual data. LSTMs possess characteristics that enable them to maintain information across extended sequences, rendering them particularly suitable for understanding context in language-based data, in contrast to conventional RNNs (M. Dua et al., 2024). In sentiment analysis especially, this function is quite helpful since effective assessment of sentiment depends on an awareness of the context of words and phrases across time. The mechanism of LST is already discussed in 3.2.

Figure 4. Long short-term memory (LSTM) architecture

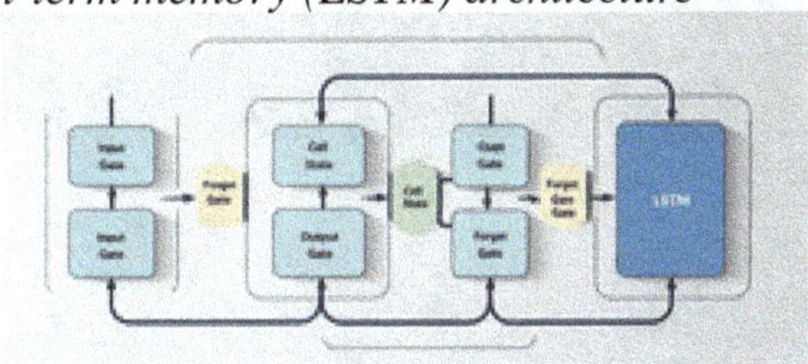

Application of LSTM in Sentiment Analysis

LSTMs use these gating mechanisms to manage the flow of information. Which makes it possible to remember relevant sentiments across long passages of text. In sentiment analysis, this architecture is applied to classify text sentiment, even in cases where sentiment may shift or involve complex language structures. For instance, in analyzing the sentence "The movie started off slow but ended up being fantastic," an LSTM model would retain the context from "slow" to "fantastic" to infer a positive sentiment.

5. WEARABLE TECHNOLOGIES AND REAL-TIME MONITORING IN REHABILITATION

Wearable devices allow constant monitoring of patient activity and physiological reactions, thereby enhancing rehabilitation. Real-time feedback from devices including exoskeletons, smart clothes, and sensor-equipped bands helps to assist in the exact tracking of rehabilitative measurements including mobility, heart rate, and muscle activity. This instant information gives doctors and patients practical insights to modify routines and activities, therefore promoting adherence and optimizing therapeutic results. Furthermore, the gathered data provides vital information for changing treatment strategies, which results in a more dynamic, patient-oriented approach to rehabilitation.

Figure 5. The Gait smart device

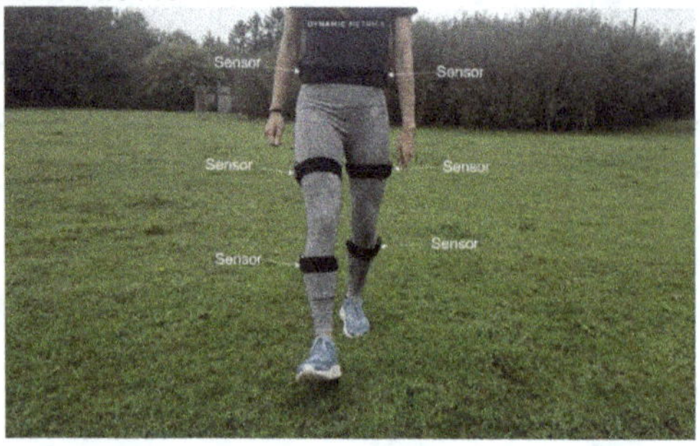

Source: NNUH

5.2 Wearable Devices and Data Collection: Sensors and Wearables Used in Rehabilitation

Particularly for real-time data on patient movement, muscular activity, and responses to stimulation, wearable devices have been invaluable in rehabilitation. Among other technologies, accelerometers, gyroscopes, electromyography (EMG) sensors, and heart rate monitors allow one to constantly monitor measures associated with recovery. Often found in wearable bands or clothing, accelerometers and gyroscopes give entire body posture, motion, and balance information—all of which are vital for evaluating mobility changes and spotting abnormalities (M. Chan et al., 2012). EMG sensors particularly in settings for muscle rehabilitation aid to collect muscle activity, thereby enabling one to assess training adherence and intensity.

Data gathered outside hospitals is among the most important benefits wearable sensors have in rehabilitation because of accessibility. Wearable devices gather data and send it back to doctors for ongoing monitoring; comfort in their homes allows patients to follow advised activity. Furthermore, the data acquired allows pertinent data to be used to adapt therapy plans accordingly in order to generate a more dynamic, patient-centered approach to rehabilitation.

Table 1. Overview of wearable devices in rehabilitation: Data collection, sensors, and medical applications

Name of Wearable Device	Process of Data Collection	Sensors Used	Medical Applications
Smartwatch	Continuous monitoring and real-time data transfer	Accelerometer, Heart Rate Sensor	Monitoring cardiovascular health, activity tracking
Smart Clothing	Embedded sensors collect physiological data	Electromyography (EMG) sensors	Muscle activity analysis, rehabilitation exercises
Exoskeleton	Sensor data collected to assist movement	Pressure and Motion Sensors	Support for mobility and gait training
Fitness Band	Tracks daily physical activity and vital signs	Heart Rate Sensor, Pedometer	Tracking steps, calories, heart rate monitoring
Smart Insoles	Real-time foot pressure and gait analysis	Pressure Sensors	Gait analysis and fall risk assessment
Wearable EEG Headbands	Collects brainwave activity to monitor cognitive states and mental workload	EEG (Electroencephalography) Sensors	Cognitive rehabilitation, monitoring mental fatigue and stress levels
Respiration Monitors	Tracks breathing patterns and respiratory rate by detecting chest or abdomen movements	Respiratory Sensors	Useful in pulmonary rehab, tracking conditions like COPD or asthma
Knee Braces with Sensors	Records joint motion and load distribution to assess knee health post-injury or surgery	Flex Sensors, Force Sensors	Knee rehabilitation, joint load analysis, and injury prevention

5.3 Fall Detection and Vital Monitoring in Rehabilitation Settings

System evolution in fall detection and vital monitoring systems tends to primarily deliver improvements in safety for at-risk patients in rehabilitation. Body motions and health are continually recorded in the form of sensors which include accelerometers, gyroscopes, and heart rate monitors. Fall detection systems differentiate between normal movement and events that are suggestive of a fall in order to detect unusual patterns of activity such as an abrupt change in motion speed or direction (P. Vallabh et al., 2017). When a fall or irregularity is found, the device immediately tells medical professionals or caretakers, therefore providing quick help and maybe preventing more serious injuries.

Vital monitoring in rehabilitation tracks many health signs, including heart rate, blood pressure, and respiratory rate, so exceeding basic fall detection. This enables medical professionals to evaluate a patient's physiological reaction to rehabilitative activities and therapies, therefore guaranteeing that treatments are safe and suitably modified to the patient's tolerance capacity. Data from these devices helps doctors create patient-centered recovery programs that fit real-time physical input, therefore enabling consistent, quantifiable advancement in rehabilitation.

Figure 6. Wearable sensors and systems with application in rehabilitation.

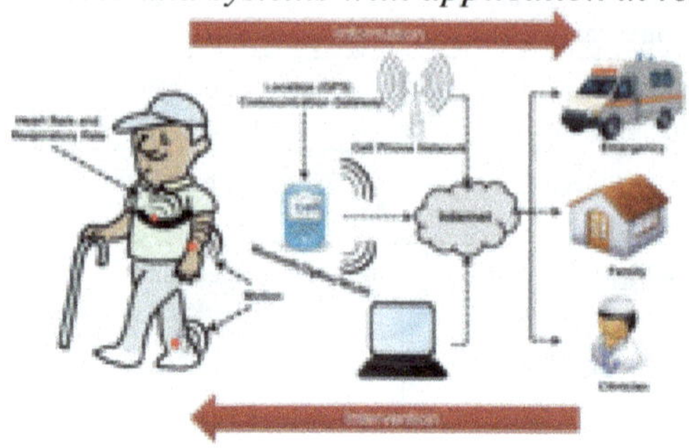

Source: https://jneuroengrehab.biomedcentral.com/articles/10.1186/1743-0003-9-21/figures/1

Patient safety and independence are much enhanced by constant observation of health statistics and falls. For example, these devices help patients participate in therapeutic activities near their doctors in outpatient rehabilitation or home care settings. By allowing early intervention in response to significant medical changes, and helping to reduce hospital readmission rates, this approach makes rehabilitation safer and more efficient overall.

6. ML-DRIVEN ROBOTICS AND EXOSKELETONS FOR ASSISTED THERAPY

Exoskeletons driven by machine learning (ML) and enhanced support in motor rehabilitation and mobility augmentation are transforming aided therapy. An important component of motor skill retraining for those with disabilities or injuries, these devices enable patients to complete controlled, repeating motions by combining adaptive learning algorithms with robotic hardware. By analyzing real-time data including the patient's movement patterns, strength, and range of motion, ML algorithms modify the robotic help level, so offering tailored support that varies with the patient's development (G. Chen et al., 2013).

Exoskeletons are wearable robotic systems that provide external mechanical support to wreaked and paralyzed body parts. In assisted therapy, exoskeletons help patients through specific movements, walking practices, arms lifting, or even finer motor skills with precision. ML algorithms continuously process sensor data from these exoskeletons and based on the data they make real-time adjustments to adopt patients changing capabilities. Thus, doctors can change treatment procedures after each session which can be very effective and customized for the patients. This adaptability improves patient safety and a more personalized therapy experience.

6.1 Types of Robotic Devices for Physical Therapy

Rehabilitation robotics transforms the conventional approach in physical therapy with innovative solutions that support patients recovering from various disease, such as stroke, traumatic brain injuries and even neurodegenerative disorders. These robotic systems enable precise and repetitive movements essential for regaining motor control, strength, and functional abilities. The primary types of robotic devices are:

1. ***End-Effector Robots***: Designed to interact with patients' extremities, including hands or feet, this kind of robot uses one point of contact. Often mimicking natural movement patterns by guiding the limb through controlled, pre-set trajectories, these are extensively employed in rehabilitation exercises of both upper and lower limbs. It helps patients in stroke treatment to conduct controlled arm or hand motions required for recovering functional motor ability. These instruments let therapists change resistance, range, and movement speed based on patient development, therefore fulfilling the particular needs of every patient.
2. ***Exoskeletons:*** Exoskeletons are outer robotic frames worn over certain body parts—like the arms, legs, or torso. Matching exoskeletons with the natural mobility of joints provides motorized support and resistance to assist or oppose patient movement. These devices are rather useful for those with spinal cord injuries or other severe motor impairments in gait training since they offer safe and under control walking motions. With their adjustable settings, exoskeletons let patients continuously improve strength and coordination, therefore allowing endurance and mobility over time.
3. ***Wearable Robotic Systems:*** Usually, compact, lightweight wearable robotic devices are designed to be exactly situated on specific joints—that of the wrist, elbow, knee, or ankle. These devices let users assess their therapy and training program in real-time by combining integrated sensors tracking muscle activity and movement patterns. By allowing technique changes and hence increasing compliance with recommended rehabilitative activities, this quick responsiveness increases therapeutic advantages. Wearable robots let patients freely continue their therapy either in a clinical setting or at home. For exercises involving stretching and bending, for example, a knee-worn wearable gadget can enable patients to ensure proper motion and reduce their risk of injury.

Figure 7. Exoskeletons in assisted therapy

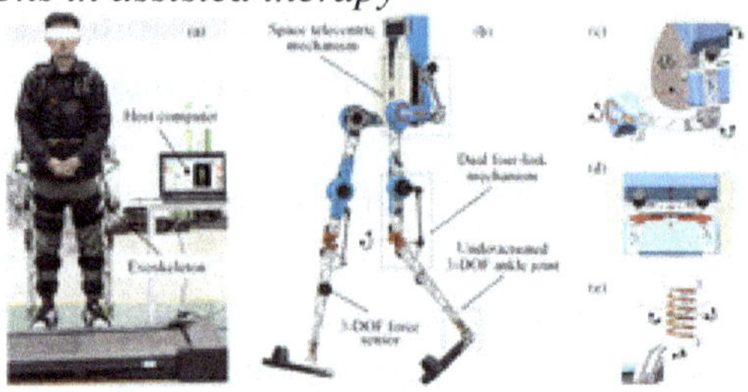

Source: https://cjme.springeropen.com/articles/10.1186/s10033-024-01113-6

4. ***Assistive Robotics for Functional Training:*** Many robotic tools are made especially for daily tasks like acquiring, grasping, and other functional requirements. Especially for those with upper limb issues, these assistive robots aim to increase fine motor skills and agility. Through task-specific motions—such as object picking or tool control—these robots assist in improving functional independence and quality of life.
5. ***Virtual Reality-Integrated Robots:*** Rehabilitation robotics employ virtual reality (VR) to provide a fascinating and energizing treatment environment. By use of VR-integrated robots, patients can engage in therapeutic activities in virtual environments such as virtual city exploration or virtual kitchen item selection. This combination offers ideal conditions for mobility exercise, hence increasing patient involvement and therapeutic adherence.

Mostly reliant on these robotic technologies are rehabilitation and physical therapy. It guarantees that patients get regular, efficient training, and measurable feedback, and maximize their mobility potential. As technology advances in line with related patient development and specific therapeutic needs, these robots find more and more applications. Rehabilitation robots maximize the outcomes of physical treatment using continuous monitoring.

6.2 Adaptive Control and Feedback Systems: Real-Time Adjustment in Therapy Devices

Therapeutic device capability has been transformed by tailored, data-driven support that changes in real time from adaptive control and feedback systems. These systems interact with many embedded sensors including those tracking movement, muscular activity, and biofeedback signals like heart rate using sophisticated algorithms and control loops. This continuous data stream allows a device to almost immediately change its behavior and follow a patient's bodily response to treatment sessions. In gait training, for instance, sensors in an exoskeleton know when the patient is ready to bear weight and then automatically modify resistance or assistance with movement exactly as needed. Patients relearning in motor skills depend on this degree of reactivity since it aids in lowering gadget dependency and misuse issues.

Predictive modeling which allows devices to track a patient's motions and change them—is fundamental in adaptive systems. Predictive control systems in robotic-assisted rehabilitation may look at past data from a patient's sessions and modify current surroundings depending on trends, therefore producing a learning effect enabling simpler, promising therapy. The tool can, for example, gently change a patient's movement patterns showing muscular weakness or a growing imbalance over time, therefore promoting balanced recovery.

Furthermore, motivating patients with their fast performance results are adaptive feedback systems. Visual and aural feedback presents patients with real-time measurements of range of motion, repetition accuracy, and strength on connected screens or mobile devices. This feedback helps doctors to more rapidly identify and fix any therapeutic problems as well as motivates adherence by increasing patient knowledge of their development. This therefore sharpens the patient's learning curve and increases the efficacy of rehabilitation programs. Here are some instances of real-time modification in therapeutic equipment:

1. ***EksoGT Exoskeleton for Gait Training:*** Designed for physical rehabilitation for those recovering from spinal cord injuries, strokes, and other mobility-impairing conditions, the EksoGT is a robotic exoskeleton. It responds in real-time to a patient's weight distribution and gait to provide necessary support just when needed. This helps patients to actively contribute to the re-acquisition of walking patterns since the device reduces support gradually over time, therefore promoting independence and strengthening muscles.
2. ***Hand Therapy Glove for Stroke Rehabilitation:*** The SaeboGloves and other handheld devices are meant for hand and arm rehabilitation in patients with stroke. With sensors tracking hand and finger motions, the gadget changes resistance depending on the patient's abilities. When a patient exhibits improvement, the glove reduces support; it increases aid when the patient is having trouble moving. Using fine motor training with increasing obstacles, this instantaneous feedback and modification enable patients to achieve functional recovery of hand movements.

Figure 8. High-tech stroke rehab product for hand - Neofect Smart Glove

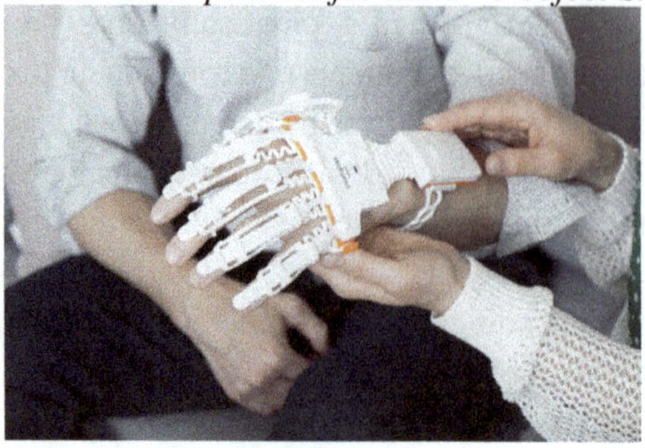

Source: https://www.neofect.com/us/smart-glove

3. ***ReWalk Exoskeleton for Paraplegic Support:*** ReWalk allows persons with lower-limb issues to stand, walk, and climb stairs using a motorized exoskeleton. The device modulates its steps in response to minute changes in the user's upper body, therefore enabling real-time adaptation. Since the gadget responds to variations in force and balance, therefore enables users to negotiate different environments boost muscle memory for improved stability, and helps users to have a more natural walking pattern.

Depending on clinical accuracy, adaptive control, and feedback systems expose a great stride toward a responsive, customized treatment paradigm that accords great relevance along with patient involvement. These technologies provide a more holistic approach to rehabilitation that helps to optimize recovery paths and thereby produce better long-term functional outcomes by combining real-time analysis with dynamic reaction capabilities.

7. SPEECH THERAPY AND COGNITIVE REHABILITATION USING MACHINE LEARNING

Machine learning (ML) has become a great tool in cognitive rehabilitation and voice therapy when providing novel approaches for tailored therapy. ML techniques enable patients undergoing speech therapy to acquire voice power, fluency, and pronunciation by allowing the development of sophisticated systems able to identify and analyze speech patterns (A. Ghosh et al., 2022). These devices provide focused training and detect specific speech defects including stuttering or articulation problems using voice recognition technologies. ML-driven solutions ensure that everyone follows a tailored treatment route addressing their particular demands depending on user success through real-time customization of workouts.

Figure 9. Classification of normal and pathological voices.

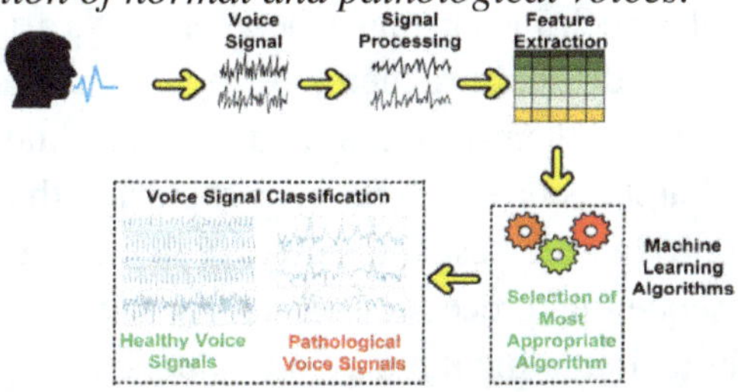

Source: https://www.sciencedirect.com/science/article/pii/S0952197624002057

ML models considerably assist patients with neurological disorders including traumatic brain injury (TBI) or dementia in cognitive rehabilitation to improve memory, attention, and problem-solving ability. Predictive modeling and pattern recognition let ML systems study patient development and modify the difficulty of cognitive activities. Usually comprising logical problem-solving activities, pattern recognition, and memory recall exercises, these activities are aimed at activating brain areas needing restoration. ML systems enable therapists to track particular indicators of improvement by assisting in the evaluation of changes over time and necessary modification of their treatment programs.

Deep learning and natural language processing (NLP) can be used in speech therapy apps to replicate conversational practice and help patients improve their verbal interaction abilities. Analogous to this, cognitive rehabilitation programs might employ ML to dynamically change the complexity of activities depending on daily patient performance. Good rehabilitation results depend on patients who practice regularly; so, these ML-powered devices provide ongoing support and inspiration to help them to do so.

In cognitive rehabilitation and speech therapy, ML is enabling treatment programs to become more effective and accurate. ML generates a more complex and dynamic approach to therapy using personal data and adaptive learning that perhaps accelerates recovery and improves the general quality of life for patients.

7.1 ML Models for Speech and Language Therapy

Recurrent Neural Networks (RNNs) are a subset of neural networks particularly well-suited for tasks involving sequential data, such as speech and language processing.

In the framework of speech and language therapy, RNNs offer innovative options for patients with language difficulties, therefore allowing coordinated and effective rehabilitation. RNNs allow them to retain and evaluate knowledge across time, therefore their natural architecture is perfect for capturing the subtleties of spoken and written language. RNNs are best at identifying speech patterns like flow, tone, and rhythm by their sequential processing capability. One could consider inputs in light of context rather than treating them as individual data pieces. Recovering linguistically is crucial. It lets the model develop words in line with common sense and discourse. The most often used RNNs in language recovery are conventional RNNs, long short-term memory (LSTM), and gated recurrent units (GRU). Particularly LSTMs address a basic difficulty in language processing known as the "vanishing gradient" problem, which could cause traditional RNNs in extended sequences of data processing to be hampered. Long sequences of strong information retention by LSTMs and GRUs help them to effectively handle challenging language patterns, sensitive intonations, and contextual phrases. Since language mostly relies on the background and past conversational flow, speech treatment relies on this ability.

Real-time voice recognition systems enable RNNs developed for therapy to aid in language rehabilitation. These tools dissect patient speech into words, syllables, and phonemes. After looking over this data, RNN models then provide changes to identify speech errors including mispronunciations or hesitations. Real-time comments provide patients with quick reinforcement, therefore promoting learning and allowing them to improve speech accuracy and fluency by means of overtime.

RNNs also rather successfully produce synthetic speech meant for patient emulation. An RNN model taught on normal speech patterns, for instance, can generate sample sentences with suitable intonation and pronunciation, therefore giving patients a goal model to work with. These models also let users replicate speech interactions to participate in virtual reality sessions. Patients who have to keep regular practice at home and limited access to therapy sessions could find this virtual connection rather helpful. Features of natural language processing (NLP) in RNNs in language recovery also examine and assess text-based data for patients engaged in writing or reading rehabilitation. These models can assist patients in learning grammar, replicating sentences, and increasing vocabulary by using NLP techniques applied within RNN systems. An RNN-based therapy tool might ask patients to finish partial phrases and fill in missing words, hence improving language comprehension and production capacity.

7.2 Application in Aphasia and Cognitive Impairments: Use of ML in Speech Therapy

Particularly for patients with aphasia and other cognitive diseases, speech therapy makes increasing use of machine learning (ML). These illnesses affect knowledge and language output. Therefore, ML-driven solutions aimed to tackle particular patient needs assist such patients. Using speech pattern analysis, ML models may identify mistakes, assess development, and allocate specific duties.

ML systems, for instance, provide real-time feedback on vocabulary use, grammar, and pronunciation in aphasia rehabilitation therefore enabling patients to develop language abilities (N. Azevedo, 2024). Moreover, these instruments for cognitive recovery help memory, attention, and problem-solving. ML systems are rather useful for customized treatment since they can learn and adapt, hence allowing slow development in language and cognitive skills.

Aphasia Therapy: Integrative Methods for Language Recovery

Aphasia treatment seeks to help persons with aphasia a disorder of language ability brought on by brain damage to recover communication abilities. The type and degree of aphasia will greatly affect the available treatment choices; they can call for adaptive technology, speech-language pathologists, family members, and others (J. Fridrksson et al., 2021). Usually, aphasia treatment proceeds in this same manner.:

1. Assessment and Diagnosis
    - **Initial Evaluation:** First assessing the type and degree of aphasia, speech-language pathologists (SLPs) then Tests measuring the patient's comprehension, speaking, reading, and writing abilities abound in this procedure.
    - **Cognitive Screening:** Beyond language, the SLP could search for executive ability, memory, and attention among cognitive skills.

Figure 10. Aphasia group therapy

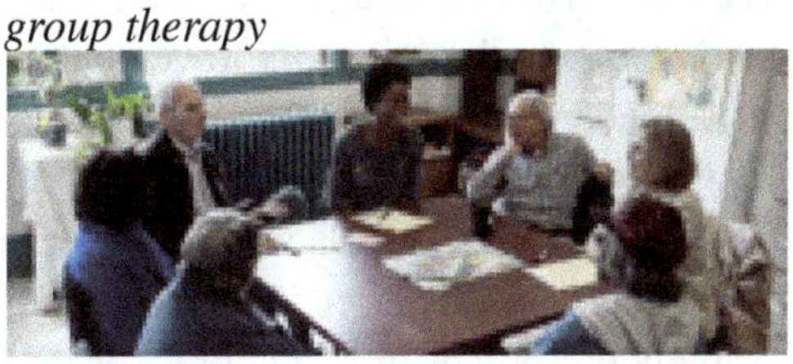

Source: https://tactustherapy.com/aphasia-group-therapy-apps

2. Goal Setting and Personalized Treatment Plan
    - **Collaborative Goal Setting:** The evaluation drives the SLP to work with the patient and their family to create particular, reasonable objectives. These goals cover both long-term (such as having talks) and current communication needs (like asking for help).
    - **Customized Therapy Plan:** The therapy strategy is tailored to the person considering age, kind of aphasia, motivation, and past degree of language proficiency. Plans can call for both ML-based therapeutic devices and traditional approaches.
3. Core Therapy Techniques
    - **Language-Based Exercises:** These are designed to improve specific language skills like word retrieval, sentence formation, and comprehension.
        - *Naming Exercises*: Patients practice seeing objects, people, or ideas to aid in word retrieval. Often employed are cueing, that is, suggestions, or semantic mapping—that which links words by meaning.
        - *Repetition and Drills:* Common phrases or tasks repeated help to improve language processing. The activities get ever more difficult as the patient recovers.
    - **Use of Technology:** Treatments for aphasia involve increased use of computer programs and smartphone apps letting individuals practice language outside of scheduled meetings. Applications rooted in machine learning could provide various degrees of difficulty, tracking of development, and tailored exercises.
4. ML-Based Therapy Tools
    - **Speech Recognition and Feedback Systems:** Crucially for rapid correction and learning, some ML applications provide real-time feedback and employ speech recognition to identify accurate or erroneous pronunciations.
    - **Natural Language Processing (NLP) Models**: These models help to evaluate patients' responses' coherence and syntactic correctness. They let patients imitate speech to allow them practice more naturally.
    - **Data-Driven Adaptive Learning:** The therapy is dynamic and customized since ML tools track patient improvement over time and change exercise difficulty depending on performance.
5. Multimodal Therapy Approaches
    - **Gesture and Visual Aids:** Patients with aphasia may find it challenging to express themselves vocally, hence extra instruments of communication in therapy could be gestures, pictures, or drawing. Together with

language exercises, these instruments provide a multimodal method for recovery.
- **Group Therapy:** Group sessions allow patients to improve their communication skills in a motivating environment. It also encourages social interaction, which would assist in the decrease of isolation and emotional rehabilitation.

6. Family Involvement and Training
   - **Educating Family Members:** Families are often involved in therapy sessions to learn effective ways to communicate with the patient. This helps the patient use their skills in daily life and gives family members tools to support recovery
   - **Home Practice:** Family members can help with home practice activities, therefore strengthening the therapeutic abilities acquired. Many ML products provide home-based activities so that patients may keep practicing either alone or under guidance.
7. Progress Monitoring and Adjustments
   - **Regular Evaluations:** Throughout therapy, SLPs monitor progress through standardized assessments or ML-generated performance data.
   - **Therapy Adjustments:** Based on progress, goals may be updated and new exercises introduced. For patients using ML-based tools, the system may automatically adjust the complexity of tasks based on performance.
8. Long-Term Support and Maintenance
   - **Ongoing Therapy and Practice:** Often long-term, aphasia treatment calls for ongoing practice even once official therapy stops. Either in sessions or with technology-based tools, maintenance therapy helps patients keep and grow in their abilities.
   - **Community Resources:** Some patients join aphasia support groups, employ adapted equipment to help with daily communication or volunteer in local projects. These materials offer continuous assistance even outside of official therapy sessions.

Aphasia therapy is a multifarious, individualized procedure depending more and more on ML and technology to offer adaptive, patient-centered treatment. Every patient's path is different since the therapy develops to satisfy evolving demands and maximize healing possibilities.

8. TELE-REHABILITATION: EXTENDING ACCESS THROUGH REMOTE ML APPLICATIONS

Driven by machine learning, tele-rehabilitation is revolutionizing the way rehabilitation therapies are delivered and allowing patients to get very customized, data-driven treatment right from their homes. Eliminating the need for regular in-person visits helps patients with mobility restrictions, those with chronic medical conditions, and those who live in remote or undeveloped areas especially. Virtual therapy sessions allow ML models to real-time track patient motions, progress, and treatment plan adherence. Designed especially for their needs for rehabilitation, both physical and cognitive activities help patients minimize logistical issues and promote regular involvement in the healing process.

Using wearable sensors and remote monitoring devices, ML systems assemble and evaluate continuous streams of physiological and movement data, therefore providing patients with instantaneous feedback on their posture, form, and general performance. A fast, data rich feedback loop allows patient to rapidly and effectively change their actions, with a minimum chance of injury to themselves. Additionally, ML informs doctors in real time of any anomalies, regressions, or odd events so that they can intervene quickly appropriate for changing patient recovery criteria.

Beyond just offering convenience, telerehabilitation with ML takes technique far beyond that, crafting a custom user experience around each patient's ever-changing, physical and mental health state, thereby turning remote care into a dynamic activity (Mulfari et al., 2022). Healthcare providers have the advantage of close control and the patients select from a rich range of choices determining their own rehabilitation path, resulting in the ability to offer high-quality, effective, and impactful treatment to a much larger population.

9. FUTURE DIRECTIONS AND INNOVATIONS IN ML FOR REHABILITATION

Rehabilitation seems to have seen remarkable progress in recent years, particularly with regard to machine learning (ML). For as long as technology continues to advance, the combination of next-generation algorithms blended with ML mixed with other creative technologies will revolutionize rehabilitation. In this part, the future opportunities of these developments and their consequences on the path of rehabilitation strategies are studied (Brunetti et al., 2023).

9.1 Next-Generation Algorithms: How Future Advancements Might Shape Rehabilitation

Big datasets and increasing processing capability drive the next generation of ML algorithms in rehabilitation; these factors give great relevance to accuracy, adaptability, and scalability. Simulating the recovery of a patient allows Deep Reinforcement Learning (DRL) to change therapeutic plans and provide real-time intervention freedom. Although data privacy and data collecting from far-off sources should be maintained, federated learning helps one to create customized solutions. Transfer Learning especially for uncommon conditions uses knowledge from larger datasets to adapt to specific circumstances. By giving doctors clear, unambiguous reasoning for model judgments, explainable artificial intelligence (XAI) can assist build openness and confidence and hence encourage greater adoption in healthcare environments.

9.2 Integration with Other Technologies: Combining ML with VR, AR, and IoT

New technology including machine learning (ML) will be included into future rehabilitation to enhance patient results (Das et al., 2022). While Virtual Reality (VR) and Augmented Reality (AR) will create customised rehabilitation environments, changing to patient performance in real-time, ML assesses interactions to offer insights on development. Based on movement patterns, ML's prediction of likely problems including falls could help real-time patient monitoring made possible by the Internet of Things (IoT). Combining data from IoT, VR/AR, and clinical sources will also allow more customized therapy recommendations, thereby providing a complete approach to rehabilitation optimizing healing, and improving patient experiences.

Figure 11. Emerging technologies for rehabilitation management using ML

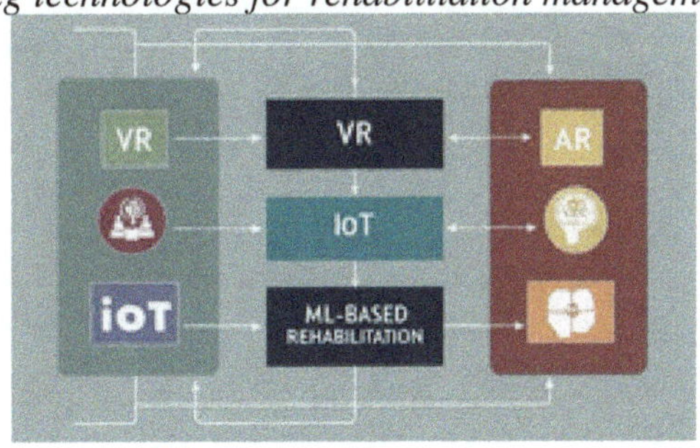

CONCLUSION

Emphasizing how ML approaches might improve patient recovery and support varied rehabilitation treatments, this chapter studied the importance of machine learning (ML) in rehabilitation. Exact assessments in physical treatment are provided utilizing computer vision, posture estimate, and motion tracking techniques thereby enabling motion analysis. While predictive modeling helps build customized treatment plans, natural language processing (NLP) supports cognitive and psychological assessment. Although wearable technologies allow real-time patient monitoring by sensors and fall-detection systems, therefore offering continuous care, improvements in rehabilitation robots improve physical treatment with responsive, adaptive feedback mechanisms. For those with speech or cognitive issues, ML-based speech treatment models provide excellent assistance in order to enable cognitive strengthening and language rehabilitation. Tele-rehabilitation also allows remote access and instantaneous feedback, thereby bridging the distance between patients and experts and so extending the reach of rehabilitation treatments.

As ML continues to evolve, its integration with virtual reality (VR), augmented reality (AR), and the Internet of Things (IoT) suggests a future of even more innovative and accessible rehabilitation solutions. The chapter underscores ML's capacity to address both the physical and psychological needs of rehabilitation, offering a glimpse into the promising future of personalized, technology-driven patient care.

REFERENCES

Azevedo, N., Kehayia, E., Jarema, G., Le Dorze, G., Beaujard, C., & Yvon, M. (2024). How artificial intelligence (AI) is used in aphasia rehabilitation: A scoping review. *Aphasiology*, *38*(2), 305–336. DOI: 10.1080/02687038.2023.2189513

Brunetti, A., Buongiorno, D., Altini, N., & Bevilacqua, V. (2023). Enabling technologies for optimized diagnosis, therapy, and rehabilitation: Obtained results and future works. In Italian Forum of Ambient Assisted Living (pp. 206–223). Springer.

Chan, M., Estève, D., Fourniols, J.-Y., Escriba, C., & Campo, E. (2012). Smart wearable systems: Current status and future challenges. *Artificial Intelligence in Medicine*, *56*(3), 137–156. DOI: 10.1016/j.artmed.2012.09.003 PMID: 23122689

Chen, G., Chan, C. K., Guo, Z., & Yu, H. (2013). A review of lower extremity assistive robotic exoskeletons in rehabilitation therapy. Critical Reviews™ in Biomedical Engineering, 41(4-5).

Das, A., Day, T. W., Kulkarni, V., Buchanan, A., Cottrell, K., John, N. W., & Chatterjee, K. (2022). Towards intelligent extended reality in stroke rehabilitation: Application of machine learning and artificial intelligence in rehabilitation. In *Augmenting Neurological Disorder Prediction and Rehabilitation Using Artificial Intelligence* (pp. 309–329). Elsevier. DOI: 10.1016/B978-0-323-90037-9.00006-0

Dua, M., Bhagat, B., Dua, S., & Chakravarty, N. (2024). A review on Gujarati language based automatic speech recognition (ASR) systems. *International Journal of Speech Technology*, *27*(1), 133–156. DOI: 10.1007/s10772-024-10087-8

Ghosh, A., Chatterjee, S., De, S., & Maji, A. K. (2022, July). Towards data-driven cognitive rehabilitation for speech disorder in hybrid sensor architecture. In *2022 IEEE International Conference on Electronics, Computing and Communication Technologies (CONECCT)* (pp. 1-6). IEEE.

He, J., Guo, Z., Shao, Z., Zhao, J., & Dan, G. (2020). An LSTM-based prediction method for lower limb intention perception by integrative analysis of Kinect visual signal. [Wiley Online Library.]. *Journal of Healthcare Engineering*, *2020*(1), 8024789. DOI: 10.1155/2020/8024789 PMID: 32774824

Jackson, J. C., Ely, E. W., Morey, M. C., Anderson, V. M., Denne, L. B., Clune, J., Siebert, C. S., Archer, K. R., Torres, R., Janz, D., Schiro, E., Jones, J., Shintani, A. K., Levine, B., Pun, B. T., Thompson, J., Brummel, N. E., & Hoenig, H. (2012). Cognitive and physical rehabilitation of intensive care unit survivors: Results of the RETURN randomized controlled pilot investigation. [). LWW.]. *Critical Care Medicine*, *40*(4), 1088–1097. DOI: 10.1097/CCM.0b013e3182373115 PMID: 22080631

Mulfari, D., La Placa, D., Rovito, C., Celesti, A., & Villari, M. (2022). Deep learning applications in telerehabilitation speech therapy scenarios. [Elsevier.]. *Computers in Biology and Medicine, 148*, 105864. DOI: 10.1016/j.compbiomed.2022.105864 PMID: 35853398

Nieto-Hidalgo, M., Ferrández-Pastor, F. J., Valdivieso-Sarabia, R. J., Mora-Pascual, J., & García-Chamizo, J. M. (2018). Gait analysis using computer vision based on cloud platform and mobile device. *Mobile Information Systems, 2018*(1), 7381264.

Shao, Y., Li, T., Shi, W., Liu, Y., & Yang, D. (2024). *PrivacyLens: Evaluating Privacy Norm Awareness of Language Models in Action*

Shtar, G., Rokach, L., Shapira, B., Nissan, R., & Hershkovitz, A. (2021). Using machine learning to predict rehabilitation outcomes in postacute hip fracture patients. [Elsevier.]. *Archives of Physical Medicine and Rehabilitation, 102*(3), 386–394. DOI: 10.1016/j.apmr.2020.08.011 PMID: 32949551

Stenum, J., Cherry-Allen, K. M., Pyles, C. O., Reetzke, R. D., Vignos, M. F., & Roemmich, R. T. (2021). Applications of pose estimation in human health and performance across the lifespan. *Sensors (Basel), 21*(21), 7315.

Takacs, B. (2006). Cognitive, mental, and physical rehabilitation using a configurable virtual reality system. [Citeseer.]. *The International Journal of Virtual Reality : a Multimedia Publication for Professionals, 5*(4), 1–12.

Vallabh, P., & Malekian, R. (2018). Fall detection monitoring systems: A comprehensive review. *Journal of Ambient Intelligence and Humanized Computing, 9*(6), 1809–1833. DOI: 10.1007/s12652-017-0592-3

Wang, L. (Eds.). (2010). *Machine learning for vision-based motion analysis: Theory and techniques*. Springer Science & Business Media. DOI: 10.4018/978-1-60566-900-7

Zhang, Q., Zhang, Z., Huang, X., Zhou, C., & Xu, J. (2022). Application of logistic regression and decision tree models in the prediction of activities of daily living in patients with stroke. [Wiley Online Library.]. *Neural Plasticity, 2022*(1), 9662630. DOI: 10.1155/2022/9662630 PMID: 35126507

ADDITIONAL READING

Fridriksson, J., & Hillis, A. E. (2021). Current approaches to the treatment of post-stroke aphasia. *Journal of Stroke*, *23*(2), 183–201. DOI: 10.5853/jos.2020.05015 PMID: 34102754

Jaramillo-Isaza, S., Delis, A. L., Herrera, E. P., & Ruiz-Olaya, A. F. (2024). Enhancing Telerehabilitation Using Wearable Sensors and AI-Based Machine Learning Methods. In Computational Approaches in Biomaterials and Biomedical Engineering Applications (pp. 266-298). CRC Press.

Sauciuc, G. A., Persson, T., & Madsen, E. (2022). The natural history of musical rhythm: functional and mechanistic theories on the evolution of human rhythm cognition and the relevance of rhythmic animal behaviors.

Chapter 3
Enhancing Recovery:
Statistical Approaches for Personalized Rehabilitation

Ravilisetty Revathi
https://orcid.org/0000-0003-4988-2158
School of Sciences, Woxsen University, India

Amritendu Bhattacharya
https://orcid.org/0000-0001-6237-7290
School of Sciences, Woxsen University, India

Bhanu Prakash Saripalli
School of Sciences, Woxsen University, India

Hanuma Bheemeswara Sai Teja Sathiraju
School of Sciences, Woxsen University, India

G. Shirisha
https://orcid.org/0000-0002-2404-9189
Stanley College of Engineering and Technology for Women, India

ABSTRACT

The shift from traditional, one-size-fits-all rehabilitation approaches to personalized, data-driven models represents a significant advancement in the field of rehabilitation science. Traditional rehabilitation protocols often follow generic treatment regimens that may not fully accommodate the varied needs, progress rates, and individual characteristics of patients. This chapter examines how statistical models and advanced computational techniques can enhance the personalization of rehabilitation, leading to more effective and efficient outcomes. It discusses the application of a range of statistical tools, such as regression analysis, clustering, survival analysis,

DOI: 10.4018/979-8-3373-0194-5.ch003

and machine learning algorithms, to predict patient recovery trajectories and tailor interventions accordingly.

1. INTRODUCTION

An increase in the development of individualized rehabilitation programs has been brought about by the changes in social care delivery systems from the mass production of therapies and treatments to custom-made ones. Rehabilitation which includes physical therapy, occupational therapy, and other treatments helps patients regain their ability to perform respective activities of daily life after the injury, surgery, or illness. In contrast, current forms of rehabilitation deliver multiple therapeutic services that are based on standardized protocols and fail to entail individual alterations to improve results, lengthen the healing process, and dissatisfied patients. Personalized as a type of rehabilitation delivery, is focused to every patient and is based on the needs, capabilities, and overall improvement goals of the patient in need. There are possible improvements in generating complex models of rehabilitation due to innovative wearable technology, digital health applications, and data analysis. One sign of this transformation is the emphasis on statistical methods: quantitative analysis replacing qualitative decision-making, mathematical prediction replacing anecdotal experience. A variety of statistical approaches enables therapists and clinicians to estimate patients' needs, analyze the determinates of recovery, and optimize treatment processes. For instance, survival analysis can provide probability of when a particular patient will reach certain recovery levels, and regression models relate the magnitude of the treatment effort to results achieved. Through the integration of these models with surveillance data from the patients' wearable devices or electronic medical record, clinicians can deliver concrete, respectively, and empirically grounded interventions. It is within this context that the scope of the present chapter is set introducing the statistical principles and methods employed in patient-tailored rehabilitation. We will outline the basic notions in probability and statistics, comment on previously proposed data-based rehabilitation paradigms, and describe how statistical tools can be effectively used by showing a case study. It also emphasizes on the ethical nature of the chapter, discusses privacy concerns and lastly, presents a vision for future development of the field.

2. BACKGROUND AND MOTIVATION

For this reason, the drawbacks of usual rehabilitation programs constructively unfold when healthcare facilities attempt to provide individual patient-oriented care. Traditional methods of rehabilitation involve fixed treatment plans where, necessarily, details can be overlooked such as the nature of the patient's injury, the patient's desire or willingness to work and recover, and their healing rates. For example, an occupational therapy protocol might mandate that all patients participate in 20 sessions of physical therapy within six weeks regardless of patients' needs. This approach means that the clinics may not efficiently deploy the clinical resources necessary for practice or, even worse, provide less than optimum patient care. The provision of wearable devices, EHR, and others have enabled the tracking of patient's progress in real-time. It means that these technologies produce significant amounts of data on individual patients and will allow for the prescription of individual rehabilitation programs. Decisions made regarding treatment plans must be made with statistical help and vary from patient to patient. Patients are expected to exhibit specific recovery degree patterns, and other forecasting models can also predict the rates at which they would recover. Thus, the information given will help to understand the type of interventions that will help the client most of the time. The rationale behind this chapter sprung from the possibility of rehab solution enhancement through statistical models. When recovery is made individualized patients get a treatment program that suits their needs hence increasing patients' compliance and hastening their recovery period than when they receive a generalized treatment plan hence cutting down the health costs. Other predictive models for health care like the readmission/early discharge predictive model make a sound basis for the use of such techniques in rehabilitation. About the statistical models, the therapists can offer directions of use in the distribution of clinical resources, identification of high-risk Service users, and prevention of harm.

3. LITERATURE REVIEW

Such models play a crucial role in determining factors related exclusively to a patient that may affect subsequent recovery, for further therapy to be minutely planned (Tousignant-Laflamme et al., 2022) also highlighted the need for accurate prediction instruments to favorize patients' individualization and best clinical outcomes. In this study, the focus was made on the fact that the use of prediction models can positively impact the patients' involvement and compliance with the rehabilitation programs aimed at presenting a clear and scientifically grounded prognosis for the recovery period. Partitioning methods including k-means as well as hierarchical clustering are useful to group patients according to their time to recovery. For instance, (Liao et al. 2020) provided a survey of methods to assess patient performance and Christian (Williams et al. 2019) used dimensionality reduction and statistical modeling for rehabilitation movements. These approaches enable the independence of therapy plans to those needed and have devised the means of having interventions corresponding to an individual's capabilities and or recovery possibility. Cluster analysis as a method of segmenting patients has been discussed in detail in the literature of rehabilitation science as well. For instance, such grouping as clustering patients based on the progress that they make can assist the therapists in the identification of target intervention for groups that patients that seem to be making slow progress. This approach of segmentation is useful for the allocation of resources and improves the effectiveness of rehabilitation activities. Advanced technologies such as wearable sensors and artificial intelligence in machine learning have highly transformed the concept of minced and timed rehabilitation (Adans-Dester et al. 2020) described that wearable technology and machine learning approaches allow for to monitoring motor recovery and deliver individualized interventions. These technologies provide information on the patient's progress during the therapy hence providing the opportunity to change the therapy modality and intensity as the patient progresses. The study also explored how data from wearable sensors can be incorporated into risk models thus creating more personalized rehabilitation plans. Similar sentiments were expressed by (Campagnini et al., 2022) in a paper about Machine learning methods for predicting Functional Recovery in Post Stroke Rehabilitation to demonstrate their effectiveness. Statistical tools, including random formation trees and support vector machines, are used more often to anticipate recovery results using multiple value sets.

Such developments demonstrate the potential where statistical modeling with the provision of artificial intelligence is likely to define the future of individual rehabilitation. Robot-aided rehabilitation is also highly important to patient-tailored treatments (Sedda et al., 2018) in his work proposed a computational model for recovery dynamics to adapt the therapy process and use a robot for exercising. They are in tandem with the general drift towards the incorporation of technological advancements in the spine of rehabilitation science. Robots enable delivering of therapy that is traditional and controlled depending on the patient's status at the moment and thus present a possibility for developing a large-scale individual therapy approach. Multiple manuscripts explore the nature of central mechanisms in motor recovery and disinhibition of injured pathways. (Braun et al., 2021) discussed the approaches and tools that developed neuroplasticity to stress the received treatment. The study described techniques like task-specific training and repetitive transcranial magnetic stimulation, which facilitate the reorganization of the brain and rehabilitation. Studies of motor learning relevant to stroke published by (Krakauer 2006) helped to determine what is important in terms of feedback, the given tasks, and motivation. These principles serve as a framework when devising proper rehabilitation strategies that utilize neuroplastic processes in their framework. Furthermore, Tran and colleagues have recently compared the integration of different brain stimulation techniques with robotic rehabilitation, showing the benefits of combining neurostimulation strategies with task-related practice. Collectively, it may well point to a potential strategy to augment and optimize recovery in stroke patients. So, the identification and utilization of patient heterogeneity are essential for recovery management. Employing variability in cases of traumatic brain injury, (Covington et al., 2021) promoted the use of sophisticated statistical techniques. Treatment-failures analysis with disease progression modelling was supported by (Forsyth et al. 2010), who also called for a more targeted approach to the design of rehabilitation trials.

This patient heterogeneity characteristic represents both a challenge and a potential opportunity for the rehabilitation science. There are elements of patient variability in responding to therapy that have been addressed using elaborate methods such as mixed-effects and Bayesian hierarchical models. They can assist the researchers and clinicians in applying this knowledge pattern that exists within the various population groups that provide potential for non-generalized, but easily reproducible, mass treatment and prevention approaches. The ethical concerns of applying statistical models in the personal rehabilitation processes are a sensitive issue. In 2015, Winstein and Kay explained ways of incorporating psychological needs into rehabilitation programs focusing on patient-centered strategies (Winstein and Kay, 2005). The study concluded with the need to integrate technocare services with people care by focusing on patients' values in defining interventions (Johnston et al. 2012) responded to issues with practice standards regarding the enhancement of evidential analysis while calling for clarity and fairness regarding application of such models. They also encompass issues to do with privacy and security of personal data collected from the participants. Wearable devices and electronic health records keep increasing concerning the need for proper structures to protect the information. Techniques like differential privacy and federated learning are being developed to maintain that rehabilitative personalization remains privacy-preserving and regulatory compliant. The current chapter greatly benefits from this line of work to examine how statistical models can enhance individualized rehabilitation. Through regression, clustering, event history analysis, Bayesian Statistical analysis, and the combination methodologies of the above models, this chapter evaluates how ailments can be modeled using statistical methods to make science-based rehabilitation programs. In contrast to the previous research, which mainly concentrated on the separate models, this chapter is devoted to an attempt to substantiate the synergy of these approaches toward enhancing patient recovery outcomes. Moreover, this chapter also clarifies the most important ethical issues, privacy policy, and the place of wearable technology in PT with the potential of expanding the global vision of patient-focused PT approaches. By so doing the researchers and the healthcare providers are in a better position to plan and develop fair, efficient, and targeted rehabilitation interventions.

4. STATISTICAL FOUNDATIONS FOR REHABILITATION

It examines the statistical base of individualized rehabilitation planning from models and methods of creating individualized rehabilitation programs. These include probability distribution, conditional probability, and Bayesian inference which form the basis of theoretical frameworks of the predictive models applied in rehabilitation. By learning these fundamentals, the therapist can anticipate the client's performance and determine whether certain therapy changes are advisable.

4.1. Key Probability Concepts

i. **Random Variables**:

Random variables in rehabilitation include "recovery time," "number of therapy sessions," and "change in mobility score" patient outcomes. These are random but they behave probabilistically. For example, the time for recovery for patients may be normally distributed, and a majority of patients will recover in a certain duration, while a few may recover faster or later than this period.

ii. **Conditional Probability**:

Conditional probability discusses the probability of occurrence of an event upon the previous occurrence of another event. For instance, the odds of a patient arising from a wheelchair without assistance later, in the sixth week of therapy may be conditional on the improvement that was made in the early three-week period. In notation, conditional probability is written as $P(A/B)$, where A stands for "walks unassisted" while B stands for 'satisfactory progress after three weeks. It is especially important when the rehabilitation plans require constant updating in response to new information.

iii. **Bayes' Theorem**:

Bayesian analysis is a way of changing a priori probability estimates in light of new data Assuming we have. In rehabilitation it can used to update the forecast of the patient's progress monitor after every therapy session. For instance, if it is estimated that a given number of patients will be mobile after the first three weeks out of 60% of the patient after estimate eight weeks, but Bayes' theorem of a new patient is rushing her through early mobility, then, the current patient will realize a form of early mobility probability. This flexibility is most advantageous with real time rehabilitation applications as the patient's progress is frequently evaluated.

4.2. Probability Distributions

i. **Normal Distribution**:

Patients' recovery also normally distributes, which means most of them will recover in a particular period (for example, 6-8 weeks), very few will recover in a shorter time period and also very few will take longer to recover. In this distribution possibility, therapists are 'able to identify average patterns of recovery and [learn] whether the patient is within this frame or not'.

ii. **Poisson Distribution**:

Poisson distribution is also applied for estimating the number of values of the parameter achieved in a particular period in the case of recovery milestones. For instance, to make the straightforward patient centered objective of 'three improvements in mobility within six weeks,' the Poisson distribution can predict the probability of achieving this goal within the six-week time-frame.

iii. **Markov Models**:

The Markov models are most helpful to monitor the patient's course throughout the various 'stages' like 'phase 1,' 'phase 2,' 'phase 3,' and so forth, relating to the degree of the recovery. In contrast with other models, Markov models presuppose that the future status of a patient is dependent only on the current status, not on the previous one. For example, if in week two this patient progressed from the "initial phase" to the "intermediate phase," their probability of reaching the "full recovery" in week six is considered according to the "intermediate phase" and not the "initial phase." Through these probabilistic concepts, the constructs and derivation of predictive or probabilistic models for individualized rehabilitation are established. By using the concepts of uncertainty and randomness as predictors of patient outcome, therapists can make better predictions and provide better treatments.

5. STATISTICAL MODELS FOR PERSONALIZATION

The most significant role performed by statistical models is to develop well-coordinated strategies for rehabilitation programs dependent on a man's individuality. Enhanced decision makings as compared to model-based rehabilitation programs where judgment can be changed from time to time in new processes based on statistical models. In this section, the author examines statistical models in details that have been most useful in personalizing rehabilitation.

5.1. Regression Models

In rehabilitation, regression models may well be the most employed statistical models. These models show how one dependent variable (last recovery point result, for instance) depends on one or more independent variables (such as therapy sessions, patient's age, severity of the injury).

i. **Linear Regression**:

The dependent variable is usually a continuous measure, while the independent variable is discrete; for example, number of therapy sessions predicting mobility score.: The model takes the form:

$$Y = \beta_0 + \beta_1 X_1 + \beta_2 X_2 + \ldots + \varepsilon$$

Here, Y denote the total score of the patient, and X_1, X_2,.. denote independent variables such as age, severity of the injury, and number of therapy sessions, among others. Multiple linear regression analysis can determine the direction and extent of impact of each factor on patients' status.

ii. Logistic Regression:

For instances whereby the dependent variable is binary, they include, but are not limited to, "able to walk unassisted" = yes/no logistic regression is applicable. It models the probability that an event Y occurs as:

$$P(Y = 1) = \frac{1}{1 + e^{-(\beta_0 + \beta_1 X_1 + \beta_2 X_2 + \ldots)}}$$

It has been possible to predict whether a particular patient will achieve certain milestones such as independent walking using logistic regression considering initial conditions of the patient. For instance, patients who had higher value of initial independence score and younger age can gain early independence.

5.2. Clustering for Patient Segmentation

Clustering algorithms permit the classification of similar patients into clusters where therapists can develop reform programs for each cluster.

i. **K-means Clustering**:

Another method is K-means clustering, where patients are split into *k* bowls depending on such features as age, type of injury, and state of rehabilitation. The results of this study showed that patients who belong to one cluster have similar patterns of recovery and therefore it is more appropriate to group them when administering therapy. For instance, young patients with high mobility ratings at admission could be classified as fast- recovering group whereas patients who postgres low ratings will be placed in slow-recovering group.

ii. **Hierarchical Clustering**:

While K-means works in the transformational way, hierarchical clustering provides the tree-like structure of successively nested clustering. This type of structure is particularly helpful if the patient groups lend themselves to ranking, such as, 'low,' 'moderate,' and 'high' support. It is important to note that therapists can generalize these interventions for the each of the hierarchical groups.

5.3. Survival Analysis

In Survival analysis, the endpoints of interest are the time taken by patients to get to some defined measure of recovery. It is most useful in terms of the probability of the complete recovery in each period of time.

i. **Kaplan-Meier Survival Curve**:

The Kaplan-Meier estimator follows the incidence of surviving the "recovery" phase at any given time with the patient. It produces survival curves, which represents the probability of the patients still on treatment at each time point. For instance, if an organization adopts an assessment curve where 80% of the patient achieves mobility independence in 6 weeks, then the therapists dealing with a new patient group in the same organization can plan for the same.

ii. **Cox Proportional Hazards Model**:

The Cox model determines the factors that are at play in the timing to recovery. The function $h(t)$,means the probability density of recovery failure at the moment time t. One includes age, kind of injury, frequency of therapy and the other to find how each influences the rate of recovery.

5.4. Time Series Analysis

Patients' data is plotted over the time series to analyze the changes or trends, fluctuations, or seasonality in the data being collected.

i. **ARIMA Models**:

Information about patients' recovery is used in predictive patient progress which is done with the help of the Auto-Regressive Integrated Moving Average (ARIMA) model. When the progress of the patient is modeled (e.g. linear with weekly variation) ARIMA can identify the likely time the patient will achieve certain goals. This model makes it possible to flexibly schedule the sessions of the therapy.

ii. **Exponential Smoothing**:

For short term forecasting of the trends in the improvement of the patients exponential smoothing is used because of its ability to put more weight on the most current figures. This method is suitable especially for short-term changes in the therapy density. For instance, if a particular patient has not made much progress in one week the therapists may decide to restrain the next week's session's intensity based on this data.

All these statistical models help to create individual rehabilitation programs. Some of the regression models used were to forecast the effects of these factors on the recovery. The clustering algorithms put together patients with similar recovery progression. Survival analysis quantifies the amount of time necessary to accomplish goals, while time series models forecast performance. These models give the statistical basis for adaptive, patient-centered rehabilitation in conjunction.

6. CASE STUDY: APPLYING STATISTICAL METHODS TO PERSONALIZE REHABILITATION

The following case study shows how statistical models can be used to individuate rehabilitation programs. A synthetic dataset is created based on real-life PT scenarios and it is used for the analysis in this paper. The purpose of this case study is to explain, how one can use regression analysis, survival analysis and clustering to implement patient specific rehabilitation plans.

6.1. Data Collection and Preparation

The data used in this case study consist of data on one hundred patients who are under rehabilitation after lower limb injuries. The following key variables are included:

- **Patient Demographics:** Age, gender, and baseline mobility score.
- **Therapy Data:** Number of therapy sessions, modality of therapy such as physiotherapy, robotic therapy, and attendance rate (ratio of achieved therapy sessions to the sessions advised).
- **Outcome Variables:** Final mobility score and recovery time (number of weeks to achieve a specific milestone, such as walking unaided).

Missing values in the data were addressed and all continuous variables were scaled to have similar ranges for easy comparison. Outliers were removed with Winsorization in order not to heavily bias regression or clustering models.

6.2. Regression Analysis

A linear regression model was developed to predict the patient's final mobility score based on key independent variables:

- Number of therapy sessions (X_1)
- Age (X_2)
- Baseline mobility score (X_3)

The resulting regression equation took the form:

$$\textit{Final Score} = 12.5 + 1.75 \cdot (\textit{Sessions}) - 0.15 \cdot (\textit{Age}) + 0.8 \cdot (\textit{Baseline Score}) + \epsilon$$

Figure 1. Regression fit: Comparison of actual and predicted scores

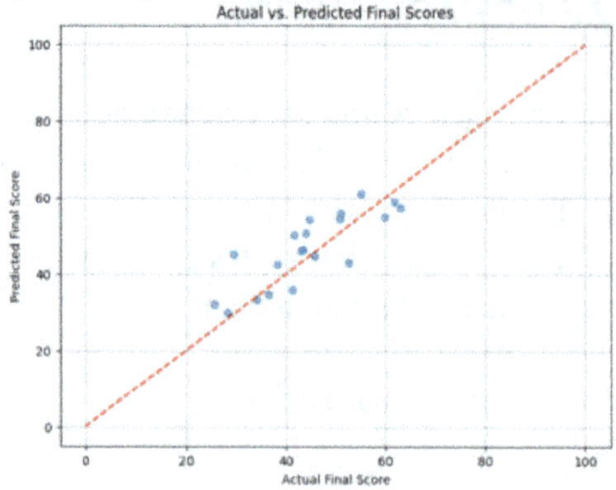

The key findings included:

- Every additional session of the therapy resulted in the gain in the final mobility scale by an average of 1.75 points.
- Older patients had slightly slower rates of improvement and for every year of life beyond 60, the final score was reduced by 0.15.
- We found that patients with higher baseline mobility scores exhibited higher final mobility scores.

The tests showed that the model had an R^2 value of 0.78, indicating that 78% of the variation in the final mobility score could be explained by the model's predictors. This knowledge assists the therapists in determining the degree of significance of different components in the customers' experiences.

6.3. Clustering Analysis

K-means clustering was used to segment patients into distinct groups with similar recovery trajectories.

Figure 2. Cluster analysis of patient recovery time and initial scores

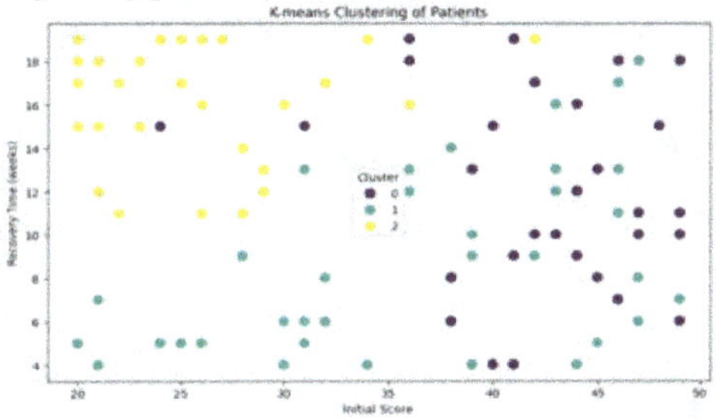

Using three clusters ($k = 3$), The following patient groups emerged:

1. Fast Responders: Patients with high baseline scores, younger age, and high adherence rates.
2. Moderate Responders: Patients with moderate baseline scores, middle age, and average adherence rates.
3. Slow Responders: Patients with low baseline scores, older age, and low adherence rates.

The approaches, in which segmentation was used, are important to be described by therapists. For example, "Slow Responders" were prescribed to get more encouragement, daily feedback, and feedback over the telephone." Therefore, to reach a 'true' longer-term outcome for this group, the "Fast Responders" were offered more difficult tasks to push their recovery even further back.

6.4. Survival Analysis

To estimate the time required for patients to achieve full mobility (defined as walking unaided), a Kaplan-Meier survival curve was generated.

Figure 3. Recovery time survival analysis: Kaplan-Meier curve

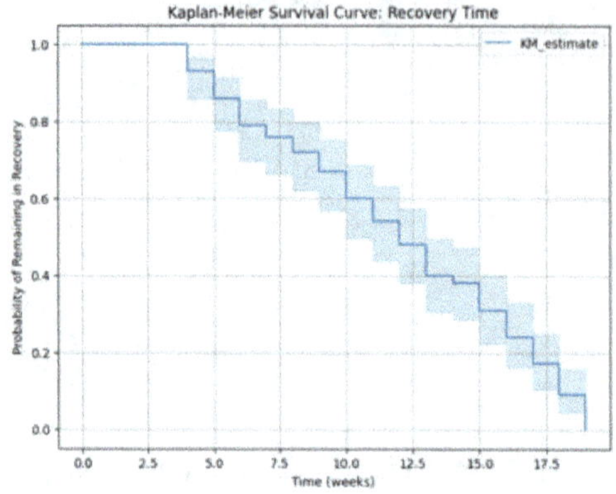

The survival curve showed that:

- 50% of patients reached full mobility by week 8.
- 75% of patients reached full mobility by week 12.

A Cox proportional hazards model was used to identify factors that influence recovery time.

Figure 4. Cox model coefficients

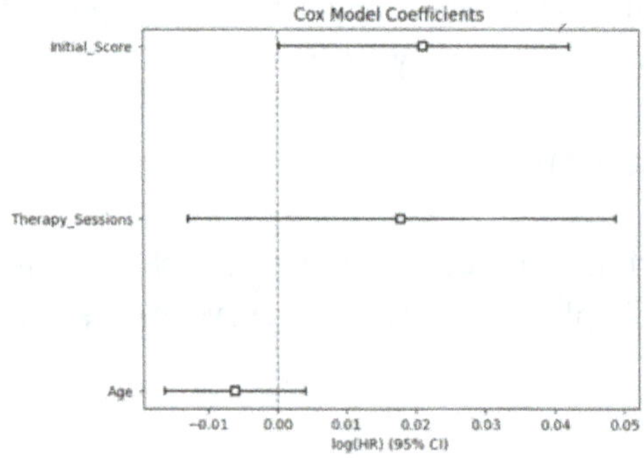

The key findings included:

- Therapy adherence significantly reduced recovery time, with patients attending at least 90% of their scheduled sessions achieving mobility 20% faster than those with lower adherence.

- Age was also a significant predictor, with older patients taking longer to recover.

This analysis allowed the rehabilitation team to prioritize interventions for patients at risk of slow recovery. By identifying at-risk patients early, therapists could modify treatment plans accordingly.

6.5. Key Insights from the Case Study

i. **Predictive Power of Regression Models**:

Through regression analysis, recovery data was evaluated with the patient demographics and therapy intensity ensuring that the therapists adapted when providing the therapy.

ii. **Clustering for Patient Segmentation**:

Using K-means clustering more significant and homogenous subgroups of patients with similar patterns of recover were established and therapists could then develop unique care plans for each of the identified subgroups.

iii. **Survival Analysis for Milestone Prediction**:

Cox models and Kaplan-Meier probability estimates of time to event were used to give therapists a better idea of what to expect and to frame the conversation with the patient and their caregivers.

This particular case demonstrates the effectiveness of statistical approaches in rehabilitation because it elaborates how precise and individual decisions foster a better future for patients.

7. ETHICAL CONSIDERATIONS

The application of such statistical models along with patient records generates issues regarding privacy and bias in patient data, and the will fullness, or otherwise, of predictive models. Active individualized regimens are based on huge volumes of patient information, which must be processed and stored per privacy laws and ethics. The stakeholders in healthcare organizations need to adhere to the privacy regulations like the HIPAA and the GDPR. These regulations require that patient data should not be used with identifiers or that the patient identifiers should be removed from the data set before analysis can commence. Some strategies like differential privacy help retain the patients' anonymity even when there is the creation of statistical models. Two cores are utilized in differential privacy: adding small amounts of noise to the data so that identifiable information cannot be linked back to individual patients. This is the case because predictive models have been shown to perform poorly if some patient groups are excluded from the training data. For example, a trained model based on young patients can give very low efficiency when it is used with elderly patients. Bias is the woe, or set of factors, that gives an unfair advantage in the procurement process: bias is the issue or the problem, and fairness auditing is a means of identifying these biases. Auditing tools compare the model's predictions to the demographic treatment fairness standards. This paper has highlighted the areas where transparency will help to build clinician trust in predictive models. The principles behind EAA enable therapists to comprehend analytical determinations. For example, decision trees display decision routes in a tree format which assists clinicians in appreciating the factors behind each prediction. This enhances the assurance of the therapists in the model's suggestions to the patients.

8. FUTURE DIRECTIONS

Smartwatches with motion sensors help continuously monitor the client's mobility, joint flexibility, and mobility. These can be used to develop individualized rehab programs at the same time with daily changes. Through IoT, wearables can be connected to other web interfaces where statistical computations of real-time data are performed. A combination of the statistical approach, for instance, Cox models with the machine learning approach, for instance, Random forest models has a higher predictive value. While Cox models offer easy-to-interpret estimates in the form of hazard ratios, subsequently, it is possible to model non-linear associations with Machine Learning models. It is possible to achieve better predictions regarding multiple recovery trajectories by combining these approaches in ensemble models. Hence for some applications, Bayesian methods allow for real-time updates on the predictions required and hence possibilities of constructing adaptive therapy systems. These systems apply the feedback collected from the sensors to vary the therapy accomplished. For instance, if a patient develops fatigue the system is in a position to lower the level of exercise. Adaptive systems introduce flexibility and patient patient-orientated approach in the process of rehabilitation.

9. CONCLUSION

Mathematical techniques have revolutionized the practice of rehabilitation through the development of individual patient diagrams. Starting from the predictive models of the final recovery score up to the usage of the survival analysis which estimates milestones achievement, these techniques help the therapists to make the right decisions. Clustering and time series analysis further extend the possibility of developing individualized rehabilitation regimens. When more of its devices become wearable, or longer sequences of data begin to be generated, rehabilitation will grow more flexible. Patients will be given therapy regimens that adapt to the patient's recovery trends to reach the molecular level of optimization. Nevertheless, for predictive models to be used fairly, other issues like data privacy, fairness, and accountability must be captured within such models. The future of personalized rehabilitation is accurately described by the elements of both statistical approaches enriched by the use of machine learning as a hybrid model. Over time, models will continue to evolve, and the therapists themselves will have real-time, empirically driven suggestions on patient approach. This change appears to deliver better patient outcomes while at the same time improving the utilization of clinical resources.

REFERENCES

Adans-Dester, C., Hankov, N., O'Brien, A., Vergara-Diaz, G., Black-Schaffer, R., Zafonte, R., Dy, J., Lee, S. I., & Bonato, P. (2020). Enabling precision rehabilitation interventions using wearable sensors and machine learning to track motor recovery. *NPJ Digital Medicine*, *3*(1), 121. DOI: 10.1038/s41746-020-00328-w PMID: 33024831

Braun, R. G., & Wittenberg, G. F. (2021, April). Motor recovery: How rehabilitation techniques and technologies can enhance recovery and neuroplasticity. [). Thieme Medical Publishers, Inc.]. *Seminars in Neurology*, *41*(02), 167–176. DOI: 10.1055/s-0041-1725138 PMID: 33663001

Campagnini, S., Arienti, C., Patrini, M., Liuzzi, P., Mannini, A., & Carrozza, M. C. (2022). Machine learning methods for functional recovery prediction and prognosis in post-stroke rehabilitation: A systematic review. *Journal of Neuroengineering and Rehabilitation*, *19*(1), 54. DOI: 10.1186/s12984-022-01032-4 PMID: 35659246

Covington, N. V., & Duff, M. C. (2021). Heterogeneity is a hallmark of traumatic brain injury, not a limitation: A new perspective on study design in rehabilitation research. *American Journal of Speech-Language Pathology*, *30*(2S), 974–985. DOI: 10.1044/2020_AJSLP-20-00081 PMID: 33556261

Forsyth, R., Vu, T., Salorio, C., Christensen, J., & Holford, N. (2010). Efficient rehabilitation trial designs using disease progress modeling: A pediatric traumatic brain injury example. *Neurorehabilitation and Neural Repair*, *24*(3), 225–234. DOI: 10.1177/1545968309354534 PMID: 19959829

Johnston, M. V., & Dijkers, M. P. (2012). Toward improved evidence standards and methods for rehabilitation: Recommendations and challenges. *Archives of Physical Medicine and Rehabilitation*, *93*(8), S185–S199. DOI: 10.1016/j.apmr.2011.12.011 PMID: 22840883

Krakauer, J. W. (2006). Motor learning: Its relevance to stroke recovery and neurorehabilitation. *Current Opinion in Neurology*, *19*(1), 84–90. DOI: 10.1097/01.wco.0000200544.29915.cc PMID: 16415682

Liao, Y., Vakanski, A., Xian, M., Paul, D., & Baker, R. (2020). A review of computational approaches for evaluation of rehabilitation exercises. *Computers in Biology and Medicine*, *119*, 103687. DOI: 10.1016/j.compbiomed.2020.103687 PMID: 32339122

Lubetzky-Vilnai, A., Ciol, M., & McCoy, S. W. (2014). Statistical analysis of clinical prediction rules for rehabilitation interventions: Current state of the literature. *Archives of Physical Medicine and Rehabilitation*, *95*(1), 188–196. DOI: 10.1016/j.apmr.2013.08.242 PMID: 24036159

Ma, J., Hobbs, B. P., & Stingo, F. C. (2015). Statistical methods for establishing personalized treatment rules in oncology. *BioMed Research International*, *2015*(1), 670691. DOI: 10.1155/2015/670691 PMID: 26446492

Sartori, M., Llyod, D. G., & Farina, D. (2016). Neural data-driven musculoskeletal modeling for personalized neurorehabilitation technologies. *IEEE Transactions on Biomedical Engineering*, *63*(5), 879–893. DOI: 10.1109/TBME.2016.2538296 PMID: 27046865

Sedda, G., Franzosi, R., Mazzone, A., Sanguineti, V., & Colombo, R. (2019). Robot Assisted Exercise: Modelling the Recovery Process to Personalise Therapy. In Converging Clinical and Engineering Research on Neurorehabilitation III: Proceedings of the 4th International Conference on NeuroRehabilitation (ICNR2018), October 16-20, 2018, Pisa, Italy 5 (pp. 236-240). Springer International Publishing.

Tousignant-Laflamme, Y., Houle, C., Cook, C., Naye, F., LeBlanc, A., & Décary, S. (2022). Mastering prognostic tools: An opportunity to enhance personalized care and to optimize clinical outcomes in physical therapy. *Physical Therapy*, *102*(5), pzac023. DOI: 10.1093/ptj/pzac023 PMID: 35202464

Tran, D. A., Pajaro-Blazquez, M., Daneault, J. F., Gallegos, J. G., Pons, J., Fregni, F., Bonato, P., & Zafonte, R. (2016). Combining dopaminergic facilitation with robot-assisted upper limb therapy in stroke survivors: A focused review. *American Journal of Physical Medicine & Rehabilitation*, *95*(6), 459–474. DOI: 10.1097/PHM.0000000000000438 PMID: 26829074

Williams, C., Vakanski, A., Lee, S., & Paul, D. (2019). Assessment of physical rehabilitation movements through dimensionality reduction and statistical modeling. *Medical Engineering & Physics*, *74*, 13–22. DOI: 10.1016/j.medengphy.2019.10.003 PMID: 31668858

Winstein, C. J., & Kay, D. B. (2015). Translating the science into practice: Shaping rehabilitation practice to enhance recovery after brain damage. *Progress in Brain Research*, *218*, 331–360. DOI: 10.1016/bs.pbr.2015.01.004 PMID: 25890145

ADDITIONAL READING

Pierella, C., Giang, C., Pirondini, E., Kinany, N., Coscia, M., Miehlbradt, J., . . . Micera, S. (2019). Personalizing exoskeleton-based upper limb rehabilitation using a statistical model: A pilot study. In Converging Clinical and Engineering Research on Neurorehabilitation III: Proceedings of the 4th International Conference on NeuroRehabilitation (ICNR2018), October 16-20, 2018, Pisa, Italy 5 (pp. 117-121). Springer International Publishing. DOI: 10.1007/978-3-030-01845-0_23

Seel, R. T., Steyerberg, E. W., Malec, J. F., Sherer, M., & Macciocchi, S. N. (2012). Developing and evaluating prediction models in rehabilitation populations. *Archives of Physical Medicine and Rehabilitation*, *93*(8), S138–S153. DOI: 10.1016/j.apmr.2012.04.021 PMID: 22840880

Chapter 4
AI-Driven Predictive Models for Personalized Rehabilitation and Assistive Systems

B. Rupa Devi
https://orcid.org/0009-0005-1298-737X
Annamacharya Institute of Technology and Sciences, India

V. Neela
REVA University, India

A. Ashwitha
https://orcid.org/0009-0002-9264-2328
Manipal Institute of Technology Bengaluru, Manipal Academy of Higher Education, India

C. Sateesh Kumar Reddy
Vignan's Foundation for Science, Technology, and Research, India

Penubaka Balaji
https://orcid.org/0000-0002-8263-0326
Koneru Lakshmaiah Education Foundation, India

Malla Sudhakara
https://orcid.org/0000-0002-2559-4074
Chistats Labs Private Limited, India

ABSTRACT

The role of artificial intelligence (AI) during rehabilitation and assistive systems is to facilitate AI modeling, real-time environment monitoring, and personalized therapy solutions. Machine learning, deep learning, and reinforcement learning are used for AI-driven predictive models such as prediction of treatment plan optimization, timeline of recovery, and better patient outcomes. They are adaptive and intelligent rehabilitation using data from wearable sensors as well, medical imaging, and assistive robotics in an integrated fashion. Additionally, federated learning and the Internet of Medical Things (IoMT) also aid in providing privacy and security of data in a scalable and trustworthy rehabilitation solution. While decisions faced

DOI: 10.4018/979-8-3373-0194-5.ch004

in the acquisition of data, security, or ethical issues can hinder the realization of a future with highly personalized, efficient, and accessible rehabilitation and assistive systems, AI is nevertheless advancing towards this type of system.

1. INTRODUCTION

Health care benefits from rehabilitation and assistive systems, as these systems are most useful to those who are suffering from an injury, that has recovered to an extent that it can no longer sustain itself, individuals who have fallen into a disability, and or those with a chronic condition. These systems are established to restore mobility, increase functional abilities, and improve the overall quality of life. Previous studies have shown that rehabilitation is traditionally performed following the standardized approach, where patients receive similar therapies according to general medical guidelines. Now these conventional methods are effective to some extent but they ignore individual patient conditions, recovery rates, and how a patient reacts to the drug. The only downside to this however has been that it has paved the way for a far more personalized and technology-first approach to the beverage and something where AI really does make a difference.

The goal of this chapter is to explore the wide application of rehabilitative and assistive systems in which predictive models are run and driven by AI. The objectives include:

Understanding of the fundamental role of AI in the transformation of rehabilitation practices.
Understanding how different AI techniques are used in predictive modeling.
Describing real-world applications and successful case studies.Thinking about the problems and ethical dilemmas of a rehabilitation that leverages AI.
Future and emerging inquiries into the trends and technologies of the personalized rehabilitation and assistive system.

1.1 Understanding Rehabilitation and Assistive Systems

Rehabilitation systems are designed to assist patients in developing lost abilities that include both physical, cognitive, as well as speech-related, after injury, surgery, or neurological disorder (H. Zhang et al. 2024). Devices and technologies that support people with disabilities in their daily lives, unlike assistive systems, are not considered to be assistive systems. These systems include both simple mobility aids such as walkers and advanced robotic exoskeletons that restore movement.

Though medicinal science has advanced, standard therapies for rehabilitation employ the method of trial-and-error adjustments with little flexibility in meeting each patient's individual needs. As a result, there is an increasing demand for intelligent data-driven solutions to offer personalized rehabilitation plans and optimize therapy sessions as well as track progress in real-time.

1.2 How AI is Transforming Personalized Healthcare

Healthcare has been dramatically influenced by AI and can be operated through system-related ways. It affects personalized healthcare in numerous ways including:

1. *Personalized treatment plans:* AI looks at a patient's medical history, mobility patterns, and therapy progress and finds its treatment plan specially tailored for patients.
2. *Real-Time Monitoring:* The pace of the patient's movement, therapy adherence, and response to the treatment is tracked continuously by wearable sensors and AI-powered devices.
3. *Adaptive Learning:* Dynamic therapy recommendations from AI algorithms adapt the treatments beginning from the very start to the patient's progress and individual needs.
4. *Automation and Efficiency:* AI relieves healthcare professionals from the burden of repeating regular assessments and making accurate predictions of the adjustments in treatment.

1.3 The Role of Predictive Models in Improving Patient Outcomes

AI's most powerful application in rehabilitation and assistive systems is predictive modeling. These models leverage historical and real-time patient data to:

1. *Forecast Recovery Trajectories:* AI can predict the period of time a patient will have to spend recovering from an injury or surgery based on the previous cases and certain health parameters of an individual.
2. *Identify Potential Complications:* Risks such as muscle atrophy, therapy non-adherence or neurological decline can be early detected and corresponding interventions are possible.

3. *Optimize Therapy Sessions:* AI makes suggestions on how to change the drug protocol in relation to the patient's response so that the rehabilitation becomes better and faster.
4. *Enhance Decision-Making:* Data-based decisions are made by doctors and therapists with the help of predictive models that remove the uncertainties about the rehabilitation outcome.

2. FOUNDATIONS OF AI IN REHABILITATION AND ASSISTIVE SYSTEMS

Artificial Intelligence in rehabilitation and assistive systems has seen great advancement in modern healthcare. By leveraging AI, more personalized, adaptive, and efficient rehabilitation that not only involves well-known physical rehabilitation exercises but also includes the emotional rehabilitation of patients recovering from stroke, sight or hearing loss, and similar illnesses, is also possible. Due to considerable development in this field of AI, it is important to have insight into the history of AI development, and techniques that are being used in the AI-driven healthcare systems to have better knowledge of this phenomenon.

2.1 Brief History of AI Applications in Healthcare

AI has taken place at the pace and at the same domain as healthcare. From the early rule-based systems to the deep learning model-driven personalized medicine and rehabilitation. During the period of 1950s to 1970s, the main use of AI in healthcare was using expert systems, like MYCIN (Rai, Sahu, and Sawant 2018), which were based on defined rules to assist in diagnosing bacterial infections. In these systems, which constituted an early type of intelligent decision-making, adaptability, and dealing with complex, dynamic medical cases were absent. In the 1980s and 1990s, as computational power increased, ML increasingly provided a stronger replacement for rule-based systems. Medical diagnosis, treatment planning, and patient monitoring were introduced as statistical models that would yield data-driven insights and improve the decision-making process of healthcare.

In medical imaging and robotics, AI made big strides by the 2000s. It became instrumental for detecting diseases like cancers at their early stages through improving diagnostic accuracy and efficiency, which is due to AI-driven image analysis. Other than robotic-assisted surgical systems, such as da Vinci Surgical System (Surgical 2013), the surgeries have become more precise, and less invasive which leads to better patient outcomes. On the other hand, deep learning and personalized healthcare experienced a great rise in applications during the 2010s that changed

AI applications in diverse domains. Naturally, this ushered in the development of AI-powered wearables, smart prosthetics, and assistive speech recognition systems by means of neural networks and their capacity for real-time patient monitoring predictive analytics, and automated rehabilitation.

AI is at the point today where it sits at the very cutting edge of healthcare innovation — making tailored rehabilitation solutions, and providing real-time health monitoring, as well as predictive insights of how to optimize care for a patient. Rehabilitation and assistive systems are being revolutionized by the continuous advancement of AI-driven technologies that bring adaptiveness, efficiency, and patient-centricity to treatment plans.

2.2 Key AI Techniques Used in Rehabilitation

Multiple techniques are used in AI-driven rehabilitation to enhance patient recovery and assistive technologies as displayed in Figure 1. The most significant approaches include:

Figure 1. Key techniques of ML, DL, and RL in Rehabilitation

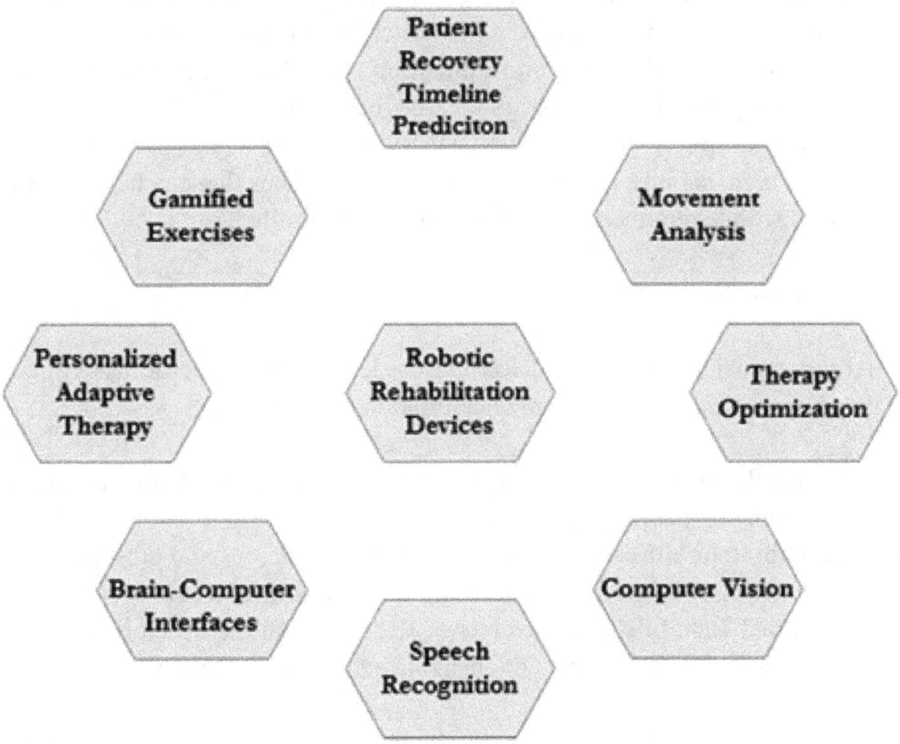

1. Machine Learning (ML)

In Machine learning, algorithms are trained on large amounts of patient data and they learn to find patterns to predict data accordingly. In rehabilitation, ML is used for:

- **Predicting Patient Recovery Timelines:** Patient history and recovery duration are analyzed by AI models.
- **Movement Analysis:** Movement patterns are assessed by ML algorithms to determine abnormality in post-stroke or injury recovery.
- **Therapy Optimization:** ML models suggest modifications in the patient's physical therapy sessions based on the real-time performance data.

2. Deep Learning (DL)

Deep learning, which is a subset of ML, processes complex medical data through artificial neural networks. Applications in rehabilitation include:

- **Computer Vision for Posture and Gait Analysis:** Rehabilitation progress is tracked by AI-powered cameras that watch movement patterns.
- **Speech Recognition for Communication Disorders:** Deep learning models assist people with speech issues to speak out loud.
- **Brain-Computer Interfaces (BCI):** By exploiting neural networks decoding in brain signals, prosthetics and assistive devices that can help move patients with severe mobility impairments are controlled.

3. Reinforcement Learning (RL)

AI systems using reinforcement learning can learn patient-specific needs through trial and error. Key applications in rehabilitation include:

- **Personalized Adaptive Therapy:** AI changes therapy difficulty accordingly depending on the patient's progress.
- **Robotic Rehabilitation Devices:** Robotic exoskeletons and prosthetic limbs are assisted by reinforcement learning for better movement patterns.
- **Gamified Rehabilitation Exercises:** RL is used in the development of AI-driven virtual environments of engaging and adaptive therapy exercises.

Based on these AI techniques, each one helps create more effective and more personalized, as well as more scalable rehabilitation solutions.

3. PERSONALIZATION IN REHABILITATION AND THE ROLE OF AI

Rehabilitation is vital for helping people recover their general health and mobility following an injury or chronic illness (Winstein et al. 2016). It is becoming increasingly effective because personalized rehabilitation tailors treatment to a patient's medical history, developmental stage, and lifestyle. Artificial intelligence (AI)- enabled rehabilitation methods that are more sensitive and adaptive can improve recovery outcomes (Khalid et al. 2024).

3.1 Defining Personalized Rehabilitation

The foundation of personalized rehabilitation is the idea that every patient's road to recovery is unique. It abandons strict, one-size-fits-all treatment methods and uses real-time data to develop customized treatment programs:

- **Adaptive Therapy Plans:** Rehabilitation programs present progress and are dynamically modified based on the patient's reaction.
- **Integration of Multiple Data Sources:** Medical imaging, electronic health records (EHRs), and wearable sensors can supply helpful information for improving treatment.
- **Predictive Insights:** AI-driven analytics can predict possible recovery challenges that present required transformations.
- **Patient-Centric Engagement:** Interactive tools such as digital platforms, and virtual reality (VR) advance participation and motivation.

3.2 Limitations of Traditional Rehabilitation

Despite its benefits, traditional rehabilitation meets several challenges:

Generic Approaches to Treatment: Individual therapy needs standardized rehabilitation programs that may not account for recovery timelines.
Absence of Real-Time Monitoring: Traditional rehabilitation relies on recurring estimates, which postpone changes that could accelerate advancement.
Restricted Resources: Patients in rural regions may not have access to qualified specialized rehabilitation facilities.
Low Patient Adherence: Because many rehabilitation programs lack interesting components, patients become disobedient and cannot fully recover.

3.3 AI's Role in Personalized Rehabilitation

AI-driven rehabilitation has several advantages, including:

Autonomous Patient Evaluation: AI examines a patient's medical background, way of life, and therapeutic development to provide targeted treatment plans. **Continuous Monitoring:** AI systems can identify problems in real-time thanks to wearable technology that tracks muscle activity, movement patterns, and therapy compliance.
Early Risk Detection: Timely predictive algorithms allow for prompt interventions made possible by predictive models that detect problems for Remote Rehabilitation. AI-powered systems enable patients to receive treatment from the comfort of their homes under the watchful eye of medical professionals.

Figure 2. Revolutionizing treatment planning through AI

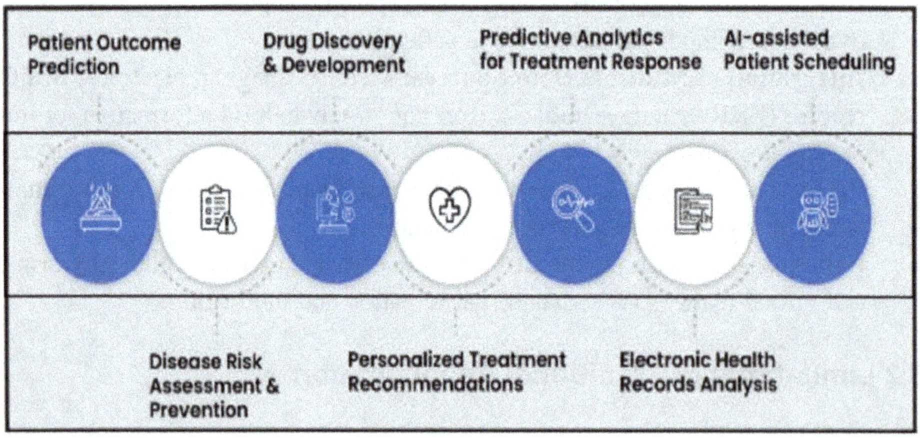

4. AI-POWERED PREDICTIVE MODELS IN REHABILITATION

Rehabilitation and assistive systems have been revolutionized by Artificial Intelligence (AI) which allows predictive modeling, monitoring in real-time, and customized treatment plans. However, these advancements depend on ML and DL techniques of patient progress assessment, therapy session optimization, and assistive solutions that are tailored to individual needs. They use AI-powered predictive models that use a lot of patient data including medical history, sensor readings the therapy outcomes to improve rehab effectiveness. ML-based models, deep learning for assistive technologies, and AI-driven wearable solutions are discussed in this section with the particular algorithms and models that power them. Figure 3 depicts the key roles of predictive analytics in rehabilitation.

Figure 3. Revolutionizing treatment planning through AI

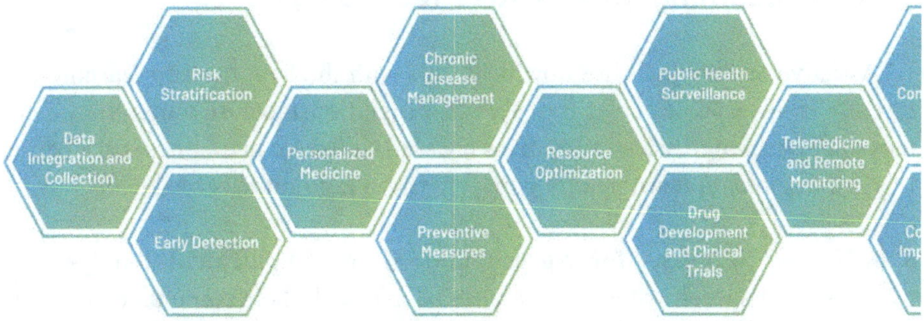

Source: https://copperdigital.com/blog/predictive-analytics-disease-detection-prevention-insights/

4.1 Machine Learning-Based Models

Rehabilitation relies on machine leaning for predicting the time of recovery; optimizing therapy plans and; assessing the patient's progress. AI increases rehabilitation effectiveness by means of supervised learning, reinforcement learning, and ensemble models.

- **Predicting Recovery Timelines Based on Patient History:** AI models that use historical data, patient demographics, and past treatment outcomes are predicted to help as the first step in predicting how long a patient will take to recover. Structured medical records are used as input to such models as Random Forest, XGBoost, and Support Vector Machines (SVM) in an attempt to estimate the recovery duration. For instance, GBDT analyses the patterns of recovery by assessing several clinical parameters and provides more predictable outcomes than traditional statistical methods (Zhou et al. 2021).
- **AI-Driven Assessment of Physical Therapy Effectiveness:** Using wear sensors, AI models like Hidden Markov Models (HMM), Long Short-Term Memory (LSTM) networks, as well as Temporal Convolutional Networks (TCN), do not just analyze the motion data but track the patient progress over time. Among other things, these models detect deviations in movement, mon-

itor therapy adherence, and suggest how rehabilitation programs can be modified. Continuous replay of exercise schedules to each patient is performed with reinforcement learning (RL) algorithms like Deep Q-Networks (DQN) (Talaat 2022) and Proximal Policy Optimization (PPO) (Kalusivalingam et al. 2020).

4.2 Deep Learning for Assistive Technologies

Assistive technologies are now better off with the help of deep learning (DL) recently, being capable of real-time speech recognition, motor function analysis, and movement tracking. Assistive systems are well suited for neural networks because it is instrumental in learning complex patterns in high-dimensional data.

- **Neural Networks for Speech and Motor Impairment Analysis:** AI-powered speech recognition assists people with their communication disorders by adapting to their speech patterns. People with dysarthria or aphasia have their speech processing helped by Convolutional Neural Networks (CNNs), Recurrent Neural Networks (RNNs), and Wav2Vec 2.0 (X. Zhang et al. 2024) transformer-based models. In much the same way, Gated Recurrent Units (GRU), and BiLSTM, analyze motor function by monitoring muscle signals and EMG sensor-derived movement data for rehabilitation planning.
- **Computer Vision in Movement Tracking and Posture Correction:** Computer vision models, driven by AI, interpret a patient's posture and gait from the subject during therapy sessions. These computer vision models include: OpenPose (Sun et al. 2022), DensePose (Güler, Neverova, and Kokkinos 2018), and 3D CNNs. MediaPipe (Kim et al. 2023) and HRNet (Huang, Zhu, and Huang 2019) are pose estimation algorithms that estimate the movement of limbs so that exercises are performed correctly in real-time without risk of injury. GNNs and ST-CNNs also aid in measuring complex motion patterns and giving out automated feedback on posture correction.

4.3 AI and Wearable Technologies

Rehabilitation has been changed to wearable AI devices that provide continuous health monitoring, real-time feedback, and adaptive assistance. The new technologies are powered by AI algorithms to offer personalized assistance to these people with mobility impairments.

- **Smart Prosthetics and Exoskeletons:** Prosthetics and exoskeletons equipped with AI are becoming more and more capable of predicting and moving in real-time, based on the user intent and the adaptation of movement patterns. The robot arms can adapt their behavior to that of the user using Reinforcement Learning models such as Soft Actor-Critic (SAC) (Haarnoja et al. 2018) and Deep Deterministic Policy Gradient (DDPG) (Dankwa and Zheng 2019). Electrically, a set of hybrid CNN-RNN architectures and Adaptive Neural Networks are used to further improve motor control by analyzing kinematic data and EMG signals respectively. Companies like Open Bionics and BrainRobotics inject Bayesian Optimization and Gaussian Processes into prosthetic movement in order to ensure that movement is as close to the real world as possible.

- **Wearable AI for Real-Time Patient Monitoring:** AI-based models like LSTMs, Autoencoders, and Transformer-based models are being used in wearable devices like smartwatches, biosensors, and smart textiles to analyze physiological data. Heart rate, oxygen level, and movement irregularities can be detected by anomaly detection models such as Variational Autoencoders (VAE) (Felius et al. 2024) and Isolation Forests and thus a health deterioration can be intervened as early as possible. Real-time monitoring accuracy in large-scale applications can be improved by the usage of Federated Learning (FL) techniques which ensures that wearable AI system is able to learn from multiple users continuously without compromising data privacy.

Table 1. AI models and algorithms for rehabilitation and assistive systems

Application Area	AI Models & Algorithms	Use Cases
Predicting Recovery Timelines	Random Forest, XGBoost, Support Vector Machine (SVM), Gradient Boosting Decision Trees (GBDT)	Forecasting patient recovery duration based on historical data
AI-Driven Physical Therapy Assessment	Long Short-Term Memory (LSTM), Hidden Markov Models (HMM), Temporal Convolutional Networks (TCN)	Tracking patient progress, therapy effectiveness, and adherence
Optimizing Rehabilitation Schedules	Deep Q-Networks (DQN), Proximal Policy Optimization (PPO), Actor-Critic RL	Adapting therapy plans dynamically based on patient response
Speech Impairment Analysis	Wav2Vec 2.0, BiLSTM, Transformer-based ASR models (e.g., Whisper, DeepSpeech)	Improving speech recognition for patients with neurological conditions
Motor Function Analysis	Gated Recurrent Units (GRU), CNN-LSTM Hybrid, Electromyography (EMG) Signal Processing Networks	Assessing muscle activity for stroke or spinal injury rehabilitation
Computer Vision for Movement Tracking	OpenPose, DensePose, 3D CNNs, HRNet, Spatiotemporal CNNs (ST-CNN)	Monitoring patient movements, posture correction, and gait analysis
Smart Prosthetics and Exoskeletons	Reinforcement Learning (Soft Actor-Critic, Deep Deterministic Policy Gradient), Adaptive Neural Networks	Enhancing prosthetic limb control, optimizing robotic exoskeletons
Wearable AI for Health Monitoring	Autoencoders, LSTMs, Transformer-based models, Variational Autoencoders (VAE)	Real-time monitoring of heart rate, oxygen levels, and movement patterns
Anomaly Detection in Patient Data	Isolation Forest, One-Class SVM, Bayesian Optimization, Gaussian Processes	Detecting abnormal health conditions, alerting caregivers in emergencies
Federated Learning for Personalized Models	Federated Averaging (FedAvg), Split Learning, Secure Multi-Party Computation	Enabling AI-powered health monitoring while maintaining patient data privacy

5. REAL-WORLD APPLICATIONS OF PREDICTIVE MODELS IN PERSONALIZED REHABILITATION AND ASSISTIVE SYSTEMS

When predictive models are incorporated into assistive and rehabilitation systems, personalized support, improved cognitive function, and mobility are transformed (Mahmoudi-Dehaki, Nasr-Esfahani, and Vasan 2025). These cutting-edge technologies provide therapies designed to fit each person's recovery path.

- **Adaptive Prosthetics and Orthotics**

Intelligent learning systems make modern prosthetic limbs and orthotic devices more responsive than ever. These devices analyze movement patterns and adapt in real-time, improving balance, stability, and user comfort. Personalized adjustments help individuals regain mobility with greater precision.

- **Smart Exoskeletons for Mobility Support**

Wearable robotic exoskeletons assist individuals with mobility impairments by providing powered support for walking and movement. Predictive models analyze muscle engagement and gait patterns, adjusting assistance levels dynamically to enhance rehabilitation and independence.

- **Speech and Cognitive Recovery Tools**

Intelligent speech and cognitive therapy treatments provide focused rehabilitation for those recuperating from strokes or other neurological conditions. These technologies optimize exercises, maintain consistent engagement, and tailor them based on ongoing patient progress analysis, which improves long-term results.

- **Stroke Rehabilitation with Predictive Insights**

Individual differences in stroke recovery make it crucial to forecast rehabilitation results precisely. Cutting-edge models evaluate neurological information, physiological reactions, and treatment outcomes to customize recovery regimens, minimizing setbacks and optimizing development.

- **Assistive Robotics for Elderly Care**

Because stroke recovery differs significantly from person to person, it is crucial to forecast rehabilitation results precisely. Advanced models customize recovery strategies to minimize setbacks and maximize development by evaluating neurological data, physical reactions, and therapeutic progress.

5.1 Impact of AI on the Rehabilitation Process

This is the main section of this study, where we analyze the diverse applications of AI-powered techniques in Rehabilitation, as indicated in Figure 4.

Figure 4. AI-powered techniques in rehabilitation process

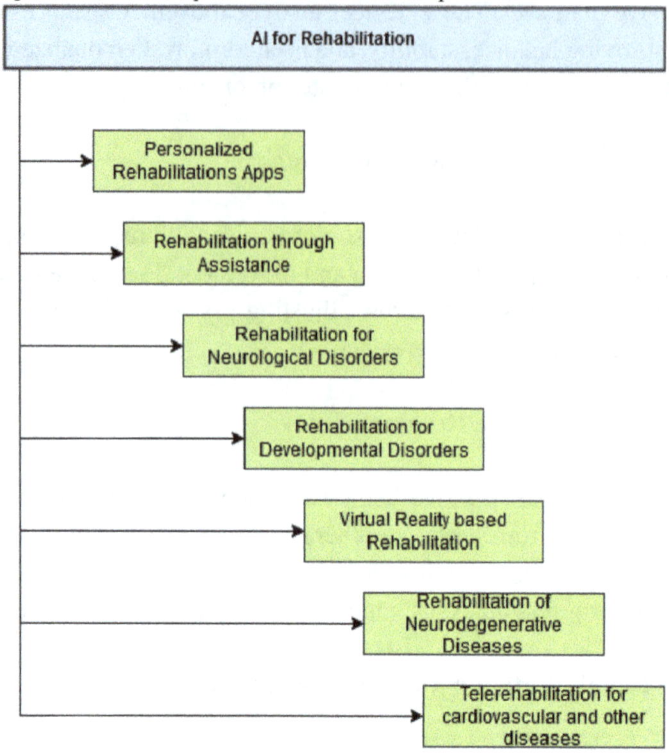

- **Personalized Rehabilitation with Smart and Adaptive Solutions**

Web and mobile apps are crucial in personalized rehabilitation, addressing cognitive and physical impairments through interactive solutions. A dementia-focused Android app enhances memory, concentration, and language skills, with reinforcement learning (RL) showing superior results (Zini, Le Piane, and Gaspari 2022) . Similarly, RL-powered cognitive training benefits multiple sclerosis (MS) patients, while an AI-driven speech model aids in early MCI diagnosis. Smartphone-based interventions lower anxiety in college students, and digital cognitive behavioural therapy is helpful for depression. Customized apps enhance numeracy and communication skills for kids with ASD, and game-based cognitive training aids in recovering from ADHD (L. Chen et al. 2020). These creative approaches promise to improve assistive care.

- **Assisted Rehabilitation: Enhancing Daily Living**

Professional caring is expensive because patients with Down syndrome, brain stroke, and severe dementia frequently struggle with everyday tasks. Adequate Assistive rehabilitation provides adequate substitutes, such as AI-based conversation systems and robotic assistance.

Taleb et al. (Taleb et al. 2022) introduced an assistive system for Alzheimer's patients, using body joint tracking and reinforcement learning to monitor activities and alert caregivers in case of anomalies. Another system combined human activity recognition (HAR) with CNN and transformers, evaluating 2D and 3D skeleton data for task support. AI-powered food assistance helped Alzheimer's patients manage meal times, preventing malnutrition and overeating.

Robotic intervention, such as the LOLA2 assistive robot, provided real-time monitoring for individuals with neurodevelopmental disorders, proving effective in daily task assistance. The M3Rob rehabilitation platform integrated haptic robotics, neurofeedback, and augmented reality, utilizing EMG and EEG signals for personalized stroke rehabilitation (Munteanu et al. 2022).

- **Rehabilitation for Neurological Disorders**

Neurological conditions such as epilepsy, brain tumours, head trauma, and syndromes frequently call for specific rehabilitation techniques.

A study (Brown et al. 2021) improves cognitive behavioural therapy (CBT) by examining patterns of brain activity linked to depression, which aids in the improvement of treatment approaches. A meta-analysis is used in another study (Pike and Robinson 2022) to evaluate reinforcement learning (RL) parameters between control groups and people with anxiety or depression, highlighting essential differences.

Research (Lampit et al. 2022) examines the impact of Computerized Cognitive Training (CCT) on psychosocial, cognitive, and daily functioning in adults with depression, assessing design factors that may influence its effectiveness. Meanwhile, a study (Rodriguez-Villa, Camacho, and Torous 2021) evaluates mobile-based psychiatric rehabilitation tools that aid individuals with serious mental illnesses in improving social and cognitive functions.

Focusing on neurodevelopmental disorders, a study (Nissan et al. 2023) investigated corticostriatal dysfunction in learning and attention disorders using RL techniques to identify cognitive processing differences. Another research study (Vaia et al. 2022) assessed a computer-aided cognitive training program for significant vascular neurocognitive disorder, evaluating its effects on depressive symptoms, cognition, and behavioural patterns.

A study (Gual et al. 2020) also examines the relationship between delirium, motor function, and rehabilitation and highlights the need for exercise for cognitive recovery. AKL-T03 is used in a digital intervention (Keefe et al. 2022) for major depressive illness that improves sustained attention; nevertheless, more research is required to evaluate its wider therapeutic benefit.

- **Rehabilitation for Developmental Disorders**

Developmental disorders encompass conditions that impair cognitive, behavioral, and language development, such as autism spectrum disorder (ASD) and various learning disabilities.

One study used the BEHAVE application to analyze manding repertoire in children with ASD and agenesis of the corpus callosum, demonstrating its utility in data collection and independent behavior evaluation (Merlo et al. 2023a).

A study on Computerized Cognitive Training (CCT) evaluated its impact on intellectual and adaptive functioning in children with intellectual developmental disabilities (IDD), showing improvements in learning, reasoning, working memory, and visual perception (Khalid et al. 2024).

A randomized controlled trial compared neurofeedback, CCT, and a combined approach in 121 children with ADHD. After three months, all three groups exhibited improved life skills, memory, learning, inhibition and reduced inattentive and hyperactive symptoms (Luo et al. 2023).

Children with ASD often face challenges in memory and learning. The RELETAS intelligent tutoring system, integrating Artificial Neural Networks (ANN) and Reinforcement Learning (RL), aimed to enhance working memory and the Zone of Proximal Development (ZPD). Its evaluation showed that the RL agent was rewarded with 1,000 correct answers out of 10,000 questions (Milani et al. 2020).

- **Rehabilitation for Developmental Disorders**

Developmental disorders like autism and learning disabilities affect behavior, cognition, and language. Early intervention through cognitive and behavioral therapy is crucial for independence.

Single-case experimental designs (SCEDs) using tools like BEHAVE have effectively studied neurodevelopmental disorders (Merlo et al. 2023b). Cognitive training (CCT) improves intellectual and adaptive functions in children with intellectual developmental disabilities. RALF, an adaptive framework for dyslexia, enhanced reading skills.

RELETAS, an AI tutoring system for children with autism, showed the potential to enhance cognitive abilities but needs further evaluation (Milani et al. 2020). The COGENT program improved reading speed and comprehension in children with learning disabilities (95). Telerehabilitation during COVID-19 significantly improved cognitive functions in adolescents with learning disabilities and reading skills in children with specific learning disabilities (Capodieci et al. 2023). These findings highlight the value of remote interventions.

- **Virtual Reality-Based Rehabilitation**

Virtual reality (VR) therapies transform cognitive rehabilitation for senior citizens by providing individualized interventions, lifelike simulations, attention enhancement, and at-home exergaming. VR is beneficial for chronic stroke patients in both clinical and home settings. An on-body feedback system for home use, developed in (Schättin et al. 2022) evaluates exergame feasibility and user experience.

VR has also been applied in mental health, especially for schizophrenia and Alzheimer's disease, enhancing rehabilitation outcomes through immersive experiences. Biofeedback-based VR environments assist in treating anxiety and insomnia. In mental and behavioural disorders, programs like Reh@City and Task Generator have shown significant improvements in depression, memory, and social behaviour (66).

Telerehabilitation, particularly during the COVID-19 pandemic, promotes physical activity and cognitive function. Studies on VR gaming, like MoveHero for children with ASD and non-immersive VR for neurocognitive disorders, highlight significant improvements in motor skills and daily activities. VR platforms like VIRTUE have helped stroke survivors regain daily functional abilities with positive outcomes.

- **Rehabilitation of Neurodegenerative Diseases**

Neurodegenerative diseases like Alzheimer's and Parkinson's cause progressive brain decline, but AI interventions have shown potential in slowing progression. Cognitive rehabilitation, such as telephone-based reality orientation therapy (ROT), enhances understanding in dementia patients and reduces caregiver stress (Sanchez-Luengos et al. 2021). Wearable devices, especially sensor-based insoles, help monitor and improve outcomes in Parkinson's and neurocognitive patients.

Cognitive telerehabilitation has proven effective in mild cognitive impairment (MCI), improving cognition and reducing symptoms. AI models, like the RNN framework, help personalize treatment for dementia, while programs like "GRADIOR" maintain cognitive functions in MCI patients. Exergaming also improves physical and mental outcomes in neurocognitive disorders.

Technologies like the VIRTRAEL platform target cognitive skills in older adults with MCI, and mental stimulation programs enhance independence in dementia patients. More research is needed for consistent evidence and integration into treatment guidelines.

- **Telerehabilitation of Cardiovascular and Other Diseases**

Telerehabilitation (TR) has gained prominence in delivering rehabilitation services remotely, aided by advances in AI and telemedicine. For cancer survivors, TR interventions have been assessed for feasibility, effectiveness, and patient satisfaction, showing that physical exercises via telehealth can manage issues like obesity, depression, and smoking (Filakova et al. 2023). A home-based cardio-oncology rehabilitation (CORE) program, integrating sensors, internet platforms, and remote supervision, has improved cardiorespiratory fitness in haematological cancer survivors.

During the COVID-19 pandemic, the need for telerehabilitation platforms grew, with studies showing the positive impact of real-time tracking for range of motion (ROM) exercises. Machine learning-based TR systems for stroke survivors have been developed to improve ROM using smartwatches. Platforms like ArmAssist and MediaPipe focus on rehabilitation through games and exercises, offering home-based solutions for stroke patients and knee fracture monitoring.

6. DATA SOURCES AND CHALLENGES IN AI-DRIVEN REHABILITATION

AI rehabilitation systems need extensive patient records to improve recovery methods and generate individualized care alongside time-sensitive support functions. Healing systems that rely on AI encounter difficulties when obtaining diverse and high-end data due to privacy limitations shortage of medical data and interoperability hurdles. This part examines the main data resources used in AI-driven rehabilitation starting with medical imaging techniques and wearable technology and real-time tracking procedures and details essential concerns around data protection and system security as well as domain transition requirements.

6.1 Medical Imaging and Sensor-Based Datasets

Medical imaging along with sensor data plays a vital role in both condition diagnosis and treatment effectiveness evaluation and patient recovery assessment. The datasets serve AI models to accomplish functions like motion analysis, neuromuscular assessment, and posture correction tasks. Some common data sources are:

1. *Medical Imaging (MRI, CT scans, X-rays, Ultrasound):* The medical imaging tools including MRI and CT scans and X-rays as well as Ultrasound serve to evaluate both functional abnormalities and injuries and degenerative conditions. Complex AI segmentation models such as U-Net and DeepLabV3+ (Yu et al. 2022) assist medical professionals in examining the images.

2. *Motion Capture Systems (e.g., Vicon, OptiTrack):* Motion capture systems like Vicon (Merriaux et al. 2017) and OptiTrack (C. Chen and Kia 2024) monitor body movements for rehabilitation exercises to help in both gait analysis and therapy adaptation.
3. *Electromyography (EMG) and Electroencephalography (EEG) Sensors:* The use of EMG and EEG sensors simultaneously measures muscle activity together with brain signals to help patients improve their motor function abilities.
4. *Smart Cameras and Depth Sensors (e.g., Microsoft Kinect, LiDAR):* These technologies support both gesture recognition and posture correction processes in physiotherapy practice.

Data standardization among medical imaging devices and healthcare centers represents a major challenge when trying to achieve interoperability across the field.

6.2 Wearable Devices and Real-Time Monitoring

AI-driven rehabilitation significantly depends on wearable technology because it delivers live physiological together with movement data. The devices track patients through real-time monitoring while they are outside clinical settings thus enabling continuous assessment along with early intervention. There are various types of wearable devices such as:

1. *Smartwatches and Fitness Bands (e.g., Apple Watch, Fitbit, Garmin):* The health assessment includes regular observations of heart rate together with oxygen saturation (SpO2), activity amounts, and sleep conditions.
2. *Smart Prosthetics and Exoskeletons (e.g., Open Bionics, Ekso Bionics):* The system acquires live sensor data which helps the system modify movements according to user intentions.
3. *Pressure Sensors in Smart Insoles and Mats:* The walking pattern along with body posture receives assistance from monitoring.
4. *Wireless ECG, EMG, and EEG Sensors:* The therapist helps stroke patients and patients with neuromuscular disorders through rehabilitation.

Wearable technology operates well in general but struggles with several problems which include charging capacity restrictions as well as sensor accuracy requirements and user adherence to using the devices dependably.

6.3 Privacy, Security, and Ethical Concerns

The processing of sensitive medical and biometric data by rehabilitation AI systems requires healthcare professionals to solve privacy security and ethical issues to meet healthcare regulation requirements such as GDPR and HIPAA. The key privacy and security issues are:

1. *Data Breaches and Cybersecurity Threats:* Patient health records become vulnerable to unauthorized access because AI systems face hacking threats.
2. *Patient Consent and Data Ownership:* Users must maintain complete authority for both data collection processes and model data usage.
3. *Bias and Fairness in AI Models:* An absence of diversity in training datasets causes artificial intelligence systems to display biases which generates healthcare decisions that create inequality.

FL and Secure Multi-Party Computation methods enable AI models to extract insights from data spread across various medical centers without sharing sensitive information thus improving rehabilitation system privacy.

7. TRANSFORMING REHABILITATION: TRUSTWORTHY SOLUTIONS THROUGH EXPLAINABILITY, SECURITY, AND PERSONALIZATION

In health, the importance of trustworthy rehabilitation solutions has never been greater. Explainable models must be used to foster confidence. Health practitioners can comprehend the reasoning behind AI-driven suggestions because of these models' transparency and explicit information regarding judgments. This transparency is vital to making sure that patients and suppliers can rely on rehabilitation solutions.

- Federated learning is an effective way to analyze patient data and Figure 5 depicts its general architecture. Federated learning improves data security and privacy by allowing many health organizations to train models together without sharing exposed data. This decentralized approach is a promising answer for rehabilitation scenarios since it guarantees that AI models stay strong and efficient while protecting patient anonymity.

Figure 5. Graphical representation of the federated learning model architecture

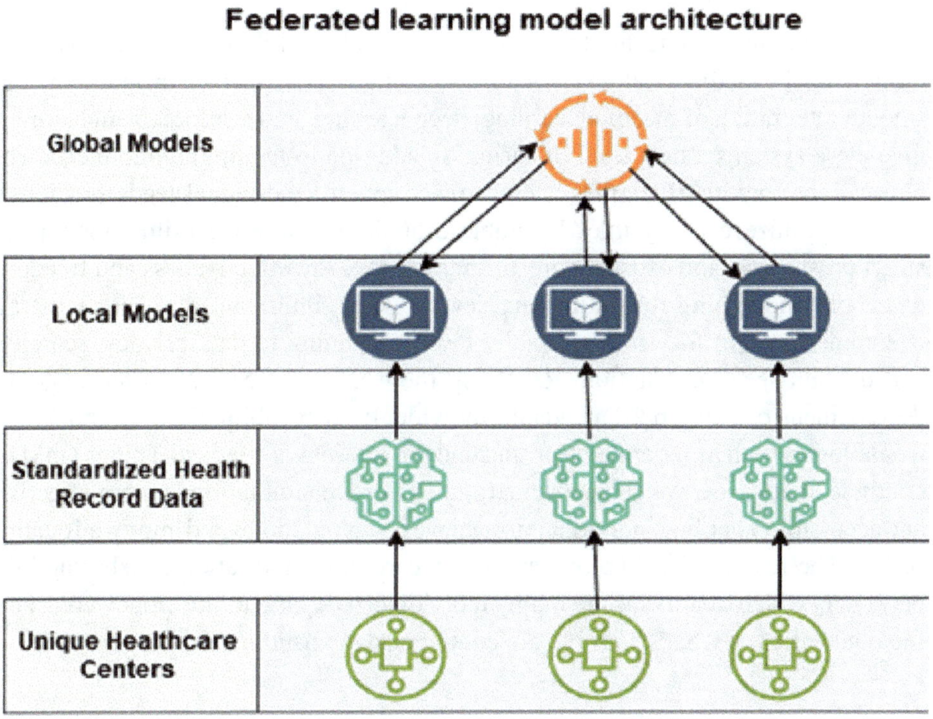

- The Internet of Medical Things (IoMT) is vital in advancing AI-driven rehabilitation. IoMT enables continuous patient health monitoring in real-time by connecting a network of medical devices and sensors. With the help of this enormous amount of data, AI models may be improved to provide individualized, flexible rehabilitation that meets the demands of each patient. The accuracy and effectiveness of rehabilitation procedures are increased by the combination of IoMT and AI.

AI is also revolutionizing mental health and cognitive rehabilitation. Through individualized treatments and specially designed cognitive workouts, AI systems can assist people with mental health issues and cognitive disabilities. These systems provide a continuous, dynamic approach to rehabilitation that improves recovery and well-being by monitoring progress and adjusting to the patient's changing demands.

CONCLUSION

Using cutting-edge technologies in assistive and rehabilitation systems is revolutionizing the medical field. Personalized techniques, data-driven insights, and the smooth integration of machine learning, deep learning, and reinforcement learning give these systems a new level of caring. In addition to facilitating more efficient physical and cognitive therapies catered to each patient's individual needs, predictive models optimize recovery times. Wearable technology-assisted real-time monitoring, smart prosthetics, and exoskeletons further improve the effectiveness and freedom of people undergoing rehabilitation. Nevertheless, significant obstacles must be overcome to move forward, especially those pertaining to data privacy, scarcity, and domain-specific adaption. Resolving these issues is crucial to the ongoing development of safe and dependable individualized rehabilitation programs. As technologies such as federated learning and the Internet of Medical Things (IoMT) continue to advance, we can expect a future where rehabilitation is more effective and accessible, enabling individuals to achieve better outcomes and improved quality of life. The fusion of technology and healthcare in rehabilitation is ushering in a new era in which treatments are highly individualized, patients are empowered, and the boundaries of what's possible are continuously expanding.

REFERENCES

Brown, V. M., Zhu, L., Solway, A., Wang, J. M., McCurry, K. L., King-Casas, B., & Chiu, P. H. (2021). Reinforcement Learning Disruptions in Individuals with Depression and Sensitivity to Symptom Change Following Cognitive Behavioral Therapy. *JAMA Psychiatry*, *78*(10), 1113–1122. DOI: 10.1001/jamapsychiatry.2021.1844 PMID: 34319349

Capodieci, A., Graziani, D., Scali, V., Giaccherini, S., Luccherino, L., & Pecini, C. (2023). Telerehabilitation Pathways in Specific Learning Disorders: Improving Reading and Writing. *Brain Sciences*, *13*(3), 479. DOI: 10.3390/brainsci13030479 PMID: 36979289

Chen, C., & Kia, S. S. (2024). OptiTrack-Aided Supervised Learning for Neural Network Based Ultra-Wideband Ranging Bias Correction. *IEEE Sensors Journal*, *24*(6), 8484–8492. DOI: 10.1109/JSEN.2024.3360187

Chen, L., Lin, L., Weizhou, J., Lin, S., & Lin, W. (2020). "The Research of Cognitive Rehabilitation Training System for ADHD Children." In *Proceedings of the 2020 11th International Conference on E-Education, E-Business, E-Management, and E-Learning*, 422–25. DOI: 10.1145/3377571.3377617

Dankwa, S., & Zheng, W. (2019). "Twin-Delayed Ddpg: A Deep Reinforcement Learning Technique to Model a Continuous Movement of an Intelligent Robot Agent." In *Proceedings of the 3rd International Conference on Vision, Image and Signal Processing*, 1–5. DOI: 10.1145/3387168.3387199

Felius, R., Punt, M., Geerars, M., Wouda, N., Rutgers, R., Bruijn, S., David, S., & van Dieën, J. (2024). Exploring Unsupervised Feature Extraction of IMU-Based Gait Data in Stroke Rehabilitation Using a Variational Autoencoder. *PLoS One*, *19*(10), e0304558. DOI: 10.1371/journal.pone.0304558 PMID: 39365773

Filakova, K., Janikova, A., Felsoci, M., Dosbaba, F., Jing, J. S., Pepera, G., & Batalik, L. (2023). Home-Based Cardio-Oncology Rehabilitation Using a Telerehabilitation Platform in Hematological Cancer Survivors: A Feasibility Study. *BMC Sports Science, Medicine and Rehabilitation*, *15*(1), 38. DOI: 10.1186/s13102-023-00650-2 PMID: 36959613

Gual, N., García-Salmones, M., Brítez, L., Crespo, N., Udina, C., Pérez, L. M., & Inzitari, M. (2020). The Role of Physical Exercise and Rehabilitation in Delirium. *European Geriatric Medicine*, *11*(1), 83–93. DOI: 10.1007/s41999-020-00290-6 PMID: 32297245

Güler, R. A., Neverova, N., & Kokkinos, I. (2018). "Densepose: Dense Human Pose Estimation in the Wild." In *Proceedings of the IEEE Conference on Computer Vision and Pattern Recognition*, 7297–7306. DOI: 10.1109/CVPR.2018.00762

Haarnoja, T., Zhou, A., Hartikainen, K., Tucker, G., Ha, S., Tan, J., Kumar, V., Zhu, H., Gupta, A., & Abbeel, P. (2018). "Soft Actor-Critic Algorithms and Applications." *ArXiv Preprint ArXiv:1812.05905.*

Huang, J., Zhu, Z., & Huang, G. (2019). "Multi-Stage HRNet: Multiple Stage High-Resolution Network for Human Pose Estimation." *ArXiv Preprint ArXiv:1910.05901.*

Kalusivalingam, A. K., Sharma, A., Patel, N., & Singh, V. (2020). Optimizing Industrial Systems Through Deep Q-Networks and Proximal Policy Optimization in Reinforcement Learning. *International Journal of Artificial Intelligence and Machine Learning, 1*(3).

Keefe, R. S., Cañadas, E., Farlow, D., & Etkin, A. (2022). Digital intervention for cognitive deficits in major depression: A randomized controlled trial to assess efficacy and safety in adults. *The American Journal of Psychiatry, 179*(7), 482–489.

Khalid, U. B., Naeem, M., Stasolla, F., Syed, M. H., Abbas, M., & Coronato, A. (2024). Impact of AI-powered solutions in rehabilitation process: Recent improvements and future trends. *International Journal of General Medicine*, •••, 943–969.

Kim, J.-W., Choi, J.-Y., Ha, E.-J., & Choi, J.-H. (2023). Human Pose Estimation Using Mediapipe Pose and Optimization Method Based on a Humanoid Model. *Applied Sciences (Basel, Switzerland), 13*(4), 2700. DOI: 10.3390/app13042700

Lampit, A., Launder, N. H., Minkov, R., Rollini, A., Davey, C. G., Finke, C., Lautenschlager, N. T., & Gavelin, H. M. (2022). Computerized Cognitive Training in People with Depression: A Protocol for a Systematic Review and Meta-Analysis. *Systematic Reviews, 11*(1), 6. DOI: 10.1186/s13643-021-01872-6 PMID: 34991698

Luo, X., Guo, X., Zhao, Q., Zhu, Y., Chen, Y., Zhang, D., Jiang, H., Wang, Y., Johnstone, S., & Sun, L. (2023). A Randomized Controlled Study of Remote Computerized Cognitive, Neurofeedback, and Combined Training in the Treatment of Children with Attention-Deficit/Hyperactivity Disorder. *European Child & Adolescent Psychiatry, 32*(8), 1475–1486. DOI: 10.1007/s00787-022-01956-1 PMID: 35182242

Mahmoudi-Dehaki, M., Nasr-Esfahani, N., & Vasan, S. (2025). The Transformative Role of Assistive Technology in Enhancing Quality of Life for Individuals With Disabilities. In *Assistive Technology Solutions for Aging Adults and Individuals With Disabilities* (pp. 45–72). IGI Global Scientific Publishing.

Merlo, G., Chifari, A., Chiazzese, G., Denaro, P., Firrera, N., Lo Savio, N., Patti, S., Palmegiano, L., Taibi, D., & Seta, L. (2023a). The BEHAVE Application as a Tool to Monitor Inclusive Interventions for Subjects with Neurodevelopmental Disorders. *Frontiers in Psychology, 13*, 943370. DOI: 10.3389/fpsyg.2022.943370 PMID: 36743629

Merlo, G., Chifari, A., Chiazzese, G., Denaro, P., Firrera, N., Savio, N. L., Patti, S., Palmegiano, L., Taibi, D., & Seta, L. (2023b). The behave application as a tool to monitor inclusive interventions for subjects with neurodevelopmental disorders. *Frontiers in Psychology, 13*, 943370. DOI: 10.3389/fpsyg.2022.943370 PMID: 36743629

Merriaux, P., Dupuis, Y., Boutteau, R., Vasseur, P., & Savatier, X. (2017). A Study of Vicon System Positioning Performance. *Sensors (Basel), 17*(7), 1591. DOI: 10.3390/s17071591 PMID: 28686213

Milani, S., Fan, Z., Gulati, S., Nguyen, T., Fang, F., & Yadav, A. 2020. "Intelligent Tutoring Strategies for Students with Autism Spectrum Disorder: A Reinforcement Learning Approach." In *The 2020 CMU Symposium on Artificial Intelligence and Social Good.*

Munteanu, D., Bejan, C., Munteanu, N., Zamfir, C., Vasić, M., Petrea, S.-M., & Cristea, D. (2022). Deep-Learning-Based System for Assisting People with Alzheimer's Disease. *Electronics (Basel), 11*(19), 3229. DOI: 10.3390/electronics11193229

Nissan, N., Hertz, U., Shahar, N., & Gabay, Y. (2023). Distinct Reinforcement Learning Profiles Distinguish between Language and Attentional Neurodevelopmental Disorders. *Behavioral and Brain Functions : BBF, 19*(1), 6. DOI: 10.1186/s12993-023-00207-w PMID: 36941632

Pike, A. C., & Robinson, O. J. (2022). Reinforcement Learning in Patients with Mood and Anxiety Disorders vs Control Individuals: A Systematic Review and Meta-Analysis. *JAMA Psychiatry, 79*(4), 313–322. DOI: 10.1001/jamapsychiatry.2022.0051 PMID: 35234834

Rai, R.B., Sahu, S. & Sawant, S. (2018). "An Analysis on MYCIN Expert System." *MGMCET, International Journal of Research in Engineering, Science and Management.*

Rodriguez-Villa, E., Camacho, E., & Torous, J. (2021). Psychiatric Rehabilitation through Teaching Smartphone Skills to Improve Functional Outcomes in Serious Mental Illness. *Internet Interventions : the Application of Information Technology in Mental and Behavioural Health, 23*, 100366. DOI: 10.1016/j.invent.2021.100366 PMID: 33532245

Sanchez-Luengos, I., Balboa-Bandeira, Y., Lucas-Jimenez, O., Ojeda, N., Pena, J., & Ibarretxe-Bilbao, N. (2021). Effectiveness of Cognitive Rehabilitation in Parkinson's Disease: A Systematic Review and Meta-Analysis. *Journal of Personalized Medicine*, *11*(5), 429. DOI: 10.3390/jpm11050429 PMID: 34069980

Schättin, A., Pickles, J., Flagmeier, D., Schärer, B., Riederer, Y., Niedecken, S., Villiger, S., Jurt, R., Kind, N., Scott, S. N., Stettler, C., & Martin-Niedecken, A. L. (2022). Development of a Novel Home-Based Exergame with on-Body Feedback: Usability Study. *JMIR Serious Games*, *10*(4), e38703. DOI: 10.2196/38703 PMID: 36472900

Sun, J., Wang, Z., Zhang, S., He, X., Zhao, H., Zhang, G., & Zhou, X. (2022). "One-pose: One-Shot Object Pose Estimation without Cad Models." In *Proceedings of the IEEE/CVF Conference on Computer Vision and Pattern Recognition*, 6825–34. DOI: 10.1109/CVPR52688.2022.00670

Surgical, I. (2013). da Vinci. Surgical System. http://www. intusurg. com/html/ davinci. html

Talaat, F. M. (2022). Effective Deep Q-Networks (EDQN) Strategy for Resource Allocation Based on Optimized Reinforcement Learning Algorithm. *Multimedia Tools and Applications*, *81*(28), 39945–39961. DOI: 10.1007/s11042-022-13000-0

Taleb, W. B., Snoun, A., Bouchrika, T., & Jemai, O. (2022). "Reinforcement Learning for Assistance of Alzheimer's Disease Patients." In *2022 8th International Conference on Control, Decision and Information Technologies (CoDIT)*, 1:274–79. IEEE.

Vaia, S., Iavarone, A., Moschiano, F., Strube, C., Gamboz, N., De Pietro, G., Gentile, S., Garofalo, E., Sannino, M., & Mazzi, M. C. (2022). Computer-Aided Cognitive Training in Patients with Neurocognitive Vascular Impairment: Effects on Cognition, Depression and Behavior. *JOURNAL OF GERONTOLOGY AND GERIATRICS*, *70*(2), 99–104. DOI: 10.36150/2499-6564-N357

Winstein, C. J., Stein, J., Arena, R., Bates, B., Cherney, L. R., Cramer, S. C., Deruyter, F., Eng, J. J., Fisher, B., Harvey, R. L., Lang, C. E., MacKay-Lyons, M., Ottenbacher, K. J., Pugh, S., Reeves, M. J., Richards, L. G., Stiers, W., & Zorowitz, R. D. (2016). Guidelines for Adult Stroke Rehabilitation and Recovery: A Guideline for Healthcare Professionals from the American Heart Association/American Stroke Association. *Stroke*, *47*(6), e98–e169. DOI: 10.1161/STR.0000000000000098 PMID: 27145936

Yu, L., Zeng, Z., Liu, A., Xie, X., Wang, H., Xu, F., & Hong, W. (2022). A Light-weight Complex-Valued DeepLabv3+ for Semantic Segmentation of PolSAR Image. *IEEE Journal of Selected Topics in Applied Earth Observations and Remote Sensing*, *15*, 930–943. DOI: 10.1109/JSTARS.2021.3140101

Zhang, H., Le Jiao, S. Y., Li, H., Jiang, X., Feng, J., Zou, S., Xu, Q., Gu, J., & Wang, X. (2024). Brain–Computer Interfaces: The Innovative Key to Unlocking Neurological Conditions. *International Journal of Surgery, 110*(9), 5745–5762. DOI: 10.1097/JS9.0000000000002022 PMID: 39166947

Zhang, X., Zhang, X., Chen, W., Li, C., & Yu, C. (2024). Improving Speech Depression Detection Using Transfer Learning with Wav2vec 2.0 in Low-Resource Environments. *Scientific Reports, 14*(1), 9543. DOI: 10.1038/s41598-024-60278-1 PMID: 38664511

Zhou, S., Ma, Q., Lou, Y., Lv, X., Tian, H., Wei, J., Zhang, K., Zhu, G., Chen, Q., Si, T., Wang, G., Wang, X., Zhang, N., Huang, Y., Liu, Q., & Yu, X. (2021). Machine Learning to Predict Clinical Remission in Depressed Patients after Acute Phase Selective Serotonin Reuptake Inhibitor Treatment. *Journal of Affective Disorders, 287*, 372–379. DOI: 10.1016/j.jad.2021.03.079 PMID: 33836365

Zini, F., Le Piane, F., & Gaspari, M. (2022). Adaptive Cognitive Training with Reinforcement Learning. [TiiS]. *ACM Transactions on Interactive Intelligent Systems, 12*(1), 1–29. DOI: 10.1145/3476777

Chapter 5
AI-Driven Prosthetics and Orthotics

J. Jeyaranjani
SRM Madurai College for Engineering and Technology, India

G. Aninthitha
SRM Madurai College for Engineering and Technology, India

N. Divyashree
REVA University, India

T. Harikala
Annamacharya University, India

S. Z. Parveen
Annamacharya Institute of Technology and Sciences, India

Malla Sudhakara
https://orcid.org/0000-0002-2559-4074
ChiStats Labs Private Limited, India

ABSTRACT

Artificial intelligence (AI) is transforming the field of prostheses and orthotics, enhancing adjustability, functionality, and user comfort. Traditional devices often lack the dynamic responsiveness necessary for optimal user interaction, but AI-driven technologies are changing this by integrating advanced robotics, sensor feedback, and machine learning. This chapter explores the development of AI in prosthetics and orthotics, focusing on rule-based automation, machine learning, and neural interfaces. It highlights key innovations like real-time gait analysis, brain-computer interfaces for thought-controlled limbs, and IoT-enabled devices for remote monitoring. Despite the promise, challenges such as ethical concerns, regulatory compliance, and cost remain. Solutions include government subsidies, open-source models, and enhanced data security. The future of this field lies in overcoming these barriers to improve life quality for individuals with mobility disabilities through innovative, multidisciplinary approaches.

DOI: 10.4018/979-8-3373-0194-5.ch005

1. INTRODUCTION

Artificial intelligence (AI) has found another front of integration for the advancement of healthcare practice: assistive technologies, namely in prosthetics and orthotics. While orthotic and prosthetic devices of traditional nature are effective in supporting structural support and mobility, their lack of adaptability and timeliness responsiveness make it difficult to meet these demands. Nevertheless, intelligent orthotic devices have risen into the field of rehabilitation and support of mobility, based on dynamic adjustments, which are adapted to the requirements of each user.

The intelligent orthotic devices use Artificial Intelligence and machine learning along with sensor-based feedback mechanisms to improve their performance. As AI-driven orthotics have recently advanced, there are recently developed intelligent rehabilitation devices to encourage and recover mobility and support for people with musculoskeletal impairments. As shown in Figure 1, modern orthotic systems incorporate adjustable components like pelvic frames, aluminum alloy hinges, and ankle braces to provide a personalized fit with a better biomechanical alignment. With this, combined with AI-assisted gait analysis and real-time feedback, we achieve optimized rehabilitation outcomes and user comfort.

Figure 1. Intelligent orthotic devices for rehabilitation, featuring an adjustable exoskeleton with advanced support mechanisms

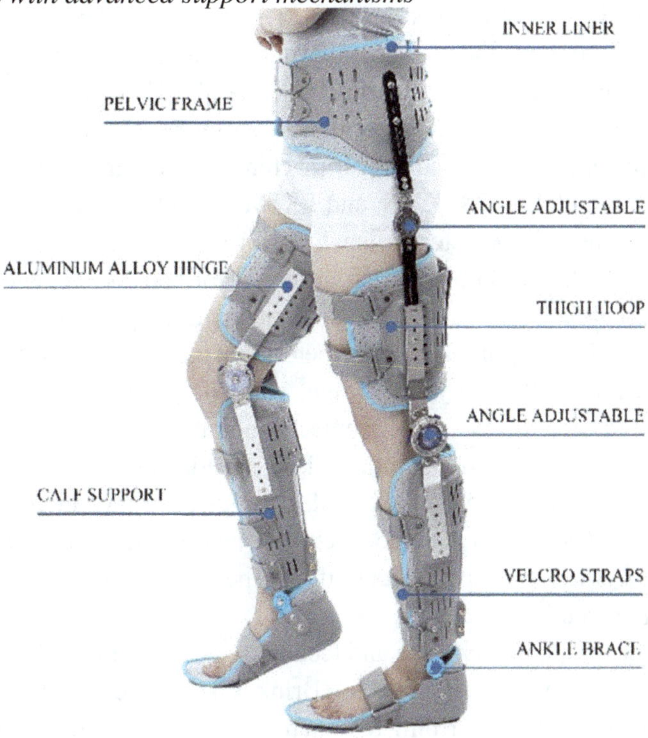

Source: https://s.alicdn.com/@sc04/kf/H0dc0bb1d235b4a15b2ed6e6f841740f1o.jpg

1.1 Background and Motivation

For many years, prosthetics and orthotics have served as an important piece in improving the quality of life for people, living with limb loss, musculoskeletal disorders, and disabilities to mobility (Chui et al. 2019). While the devices are good at supporting, they fail to adapt, respond in real-time, and be comfortable for the users. Although conventional prosthetic limbs and orthotic supports are limited in Dynamic adaptability, control mechanisms are limited, and most have to be fiddled with all the time. As a result of these challenges, there is a strong demand for emerging solutions that build mobility as well as user independence and user experience.

In this field, artificial intelligence (AI) has evolved to be a transformative force, reconfiguring the means of assistive devices operating. AI has enabled prosthetic limbs to also learn how to behave from user behavior, have the ability to adjust to all different terrains, and even help people who have lost sensory functions. Similarly, real-time corrective support through gait disorder is offered for individuals by AI-powered orthotic systems which strengthen a person's posture as well as reduce stress on the body (Seiça et al. 2024). These assistive devices are becoming more intelligent, efficient, and user-friendly, due to the convergence of AI, machine learning, and biomechanical engineering. Chen et al. (Chen et al. 2022) used the Kinect® Motion system to capture gait data of seven healthy subjects performing different gait patterns and compared four machine learning methods used for classification such as CNN, SVM, KNN, and LSTM. Results suggested the use of AI and machine learning in remote gait analysis for clinical decision-making as the CNN (87.6%) and LSTM (83.6%) classifiers outperformed (94.0%) and (94.9%) the SVM (94.9%) and KNN on accurately distinguishing the gait patterns. Noh et al. (Noh et al. 2021) found optimal gait parameters that can predict fall risk. The study included 746 subjects (63–89 years of age) who completed gait tests at multiple speeds while recording the data on the subjects' shoe-type inertial measurement unit sensors. Features such as stride length, walking speed, and stance phase were used to predict fall risk using the XGBoost model. Sensitivity ranged from 43-53% and specificity from 77-84%, and the model achieved an accuracy of 67-70% indicating that these gait features can assist in classifying the level of fall risk in older adults and aid in fall prevention strategies.

In recent decades, biomechanics and technology have been used to integrate AI into prosthetics and orthotics. Brink et al. (Brink, Likens, and Stergiou 2023) established the foundations for describing human movement using kinematic and kinetic descriptions. Recently, these have been upgraded to include artificial intelligence for real-time gait analysis and assistance device adaptation. According to Zou et al. (Zou et al. 2024), CNNs and LSTM networks outperform SVMs in dynamic situations in gait phase classification using multi-sensory data. Using IMU data, Young et al. (Young et al. 2023) used machine learning to predict risk factors of falls in older persons, providing efficient and reliable predictions on how AI might prevent diseases. Kim et al. (Kim, Simon, and Hargrove 2022) discuss neural interfacing for powered transfemoral prostheses, and Vu et al. (Vu et al. 2023) use deep learning for EMG signal decoding to improve prosthetic control. Comparing current biomechanics, including inverse dynamics, with contemporary AI applications, would improve its use as a more sophisticated generation based on conventional research.

There are biomechanics involved in AI-based prosthetics and orthotics as previously mentioned so that joint kinematics, force distribution, and musculoskeletal adaptation can be governed. Real-time gait analysis, sensor fusion, and adaptive control algorithms are used to make artificial limbs as close to real as possible. Likewise, kinesiology is fundamental to motor control, posture control, and gait relearning, which presents real-time corrective feedback through AI-driven orthotic devices to patients with neuromuscular disorders. The manuscript should also discuss neuromechanics of AI integration, both brain-computer interface (BCI), myoelectric control, and neuroplasticity. Deep learning-based neural decoding, haptic feedback for sensory reintegration, and pattern recognition for accurate control of movement are now features of AI-powered prosthetics. Additionally, real-world applications of BCI-controlled exoskeletons and AI-aided gait correction systems can be added to enhance the manuscript's manuscript by adding a combined more comprehensive literature review on computational biomechanics, motor learning, and AI-enhanced rehabilitation. The argument would also strengthen if a comparative analysis of traditional biomechanical models with AI-driven adaptive systems is undertaken. If we address these aspects, it will make the discussion about how AI uses human movement much more comprehensive and solid, providing a better theoretical basis for the research.

1.2 The Evolution of AI in Assistive Technology

The path of AI in prosthetics and orthotics may be followed through a number of significant milestones:

- ***Rule-Based Automation (Early 2000s):*** The early smart prosthetic limbs that were used relied on pre-programmed responses to certain movement patterns, and thus, they were not flexible.
- ***Machine Learning Integration (2010s):*** AI-powered devices started learning from user input to become more accurate in movement and respond quickly.
- ***Neural Interfaces and Deep Learning (2020s-Present):*** Brain-computer interfaces (BCI) and deep learning algorithms make such devices perceive neural signals and give effortless control and real-time adjustments.
- ***Future Prospects (2030s and Beyond):*** The next frontier is AI-powered bio-hybrid prosthetics that can communicate directly with the nervous system and enable near-natural movement and sensory feedback from the synthetic limb (Yoo and Shoaran 2021).

Rule-based automation and machine learning underpin AI-driven prostheses, but their evolution and interaction deserve study. In the early 2000s, rule-based systems used fixed logic to activate specified responses, such as prosthetic knee dampening depending on speed thresholds. While effective for simple activities, their rigidity hampered flexibility to sophisticated user needs. Machine learning (ML) changed the game in the 2010s by letting devices learn from user data. The Touch Bionics i-Limb Ultra uses Reinforcement Learning (RL) to improve grip strength through trial-and-error feedback. Emerging hybrid techniques combine rule-based stability and ML adaptability. The Össur Proprio Foot, for instance, employs rule-based triggers for stability and ML to adjust ankle flexion based on user habits. Discussing these transitions and synergies would illuminate AI's role in improving adaptability and responsiveness.

1.3 AI's Role in Revolutionizing Prosthetics and Orthotics

The future of prosthetics and orthotics is changing with the arrival of advanced technologies that enable more convenient, effective, and life-redeeming ways. Undoubtedly, AI makes one of its key contributions in bringing adaptive learning. With machine learning applied to gait patterns, as well as through the prediction of user's intent, and real-time changes, modern prosthetic limbs are seamless in terms of movement. Also, computer vision through AI makes prosthetic devices recognize and react to environmental changes, for example, picking up when the environment is not even and adjusting foot placement according to it. One of the biggest breakthroughs through the use of AI is the brain-computer interface (BCI), which allows to control of prosthetic limbs without the intervention of nerves (Islam, Vashishat, and Kumar 2024). The systems interpret electrical signals of the brain and allow the users to control artificial limbs with thoughts. This is especially useful for those who have had high-level amputations that would normally exclude them from most artificial limbs.

Additionally, there are AI-driven orthosis solutions improving the rehabilitation of stroke patients, spinal injury patients, and those with neuromuscular disorders. Wearable AI-powered devices with continuous movement detection, an automatic normalization of abnormalities, and real-time corrective feedback enhance users' recovery and improve user mobility. Furthermore, the AI is used to provide timely interventions and adjustments as the orthotic device is monitored remotely.

The development of assistive technology that is more intuitive, responsive, and tailored to the needs of individuals, has been assisted by the introduction of AI into prosthetics and orthotics. This transformation not only makes the mobility of users better but also reflects on the overall quality of life.

This chapter gives a comprehensive view of the current state of the art of AI-driven prosthetics, but it must be recognized that these new technologies also need to be applied in ways that benefit clinicians, engineers, patients, and other users of prosthetic rigs. With the aim of improving prosthetic usability for users, experiencing the practical integration of AI, examining challenges of user adaptation, clinical implementation, and long-term device performance is critical. This chapter discusses not only the current research trends but also creates the connection between technological progress and user-oriented solutions, which are possible with the use of these innovations in clinical settings.

2. CORE TECHNOLOGIES ENABLING AI-DRIVEN PROSTHETICS AND ORTHOTICS

Artificial intelligence (AI) integration into prosthesis and orthotics has revolutionized the profession by allowing more flexible, intuitive, and responsive to user needs devices. The fundamental technologies driving this change machine learning, sensors, robotics, and computer vision are thoroughly explored in this part. Technical knowledge, applications, and examples abound throughout every area to give a whole picture of how these technologies cooperate to produce modern prosthetic and orthotic solutions.

AI-driven prosthetics and orthotics use device- and user-specific algorithms and sensors. CNNs interpret visual data from integrated cameras to enable gesture recognition and object interaction in upper-limb prosthetics, like the Open Bionics Hero Arm, which uses myoelectric sensors and CNNs for intuitive hand control. In contrast, Recurrent Neural Networks (RNNs) and Long Short-Term Memory (LSTM) networks are suited for lower-limb prosthetics, predicting consecutive gait patterns using IMU data to enable smooth terrain transitions. Ottobock's C-Leg uses RNN-based algorithms to adjust knee stiffness in real time using IMU sensor inputs. EMG sensors dominate upper-limb myoelectric control, decoding muscle data with SVMs for accurate finger movements, while pressure sensors in prosthetic feet enhance weight distribution, as shown in the Fillauer AllPro foot. CNN-RNN hybrid models improve performance by incorporating visual ambient signals with sequential movement data. Using CNN and RNN, a prosthetic arm could detect a cup and alter grip strength over time, enhancing adaptability in a busy kitchen. Real-world usefulness requires low latency and responsiveness from hybrid techniques.

2.1 Machine Learning and Neural Networks

Machine learning (ML) and neural networks (Choo and Chang 2023) provide roots for artificial intelligence driven prosthetic and orthotics. These technologies enable objects learn from data, adapt with human activity, and over time develop increasing value. Modern techniques and big datasets let ML models predict user intent, decode challenging signals, and increase device performance.

Key Roles of Machine Learning in Prosthetics & Orthotics:

1. ***Adaptive Learning***: Prosthetic limbs equipped with ML can quickly change their responses and analyze user movement patterns. For example, neural networks can predict the desired motion dependent on muscle signals (via electromyography or EMG) and run it smoothly.

For example, an adaptive learning prosthetic arm may detect when a user is trying to pick up a delicate object and change the grip strength. This means the ML model always learns from user muscle signals and enhances its forecasts to provide a grip neither too tight nor too loose.

2. ***Personalization:*** By training ML models on specific user data, one may design customized control systems. This guarantees that the prosthetic or orthotic instrument fits the personal preferences and biomechanics.

For walking or jogging, for example, a lower-limb prosthetic can pick up the user's stride pattern and adjust the joint stiffness to give ideal support. Data on the user's walking speed, stride length, and ground response forces then enables a model able to dynamically change the behavior of the prosthetic.

3. ***Predictive Maintenance***: ML systems help to reduce downtime and improve reliability by tracking device performance and predicting probable faults.

An artificial intelligence system can, for example, look at sensor data to spot actuator wear and tear, therefore alerting the user or medical practitioner before a failure. Using time-series data from sensors, this creates a model able to identify trends suggestive of either higher or lower vibration or worse efficiency, therefore indicating imminent failure.

Technical Insights

- ***Neural Networks:*** For applications including gesture recognition and gait analysis, deep learning models (Triwiyanto et al. 2023) such convolutional neural networks (CNNs) and recurrent neural networks (RNNs) are routinely used. While RNNs are appropriate for sequential data, including time-series data from sensors, CNNs are especially excellent for processing spatial data, such images from cameras integrated in prosthesis.
- ***Reinforcement Learning:*** Reinforcement learning enables the gadget learn and thereby improves its performance over time relying on user feedback by means of trial and error. Using reinforcement learning, a prosthetic limb could maximize its control strategy for different activities, such as holding objects or ascending stairs.

Table 1 gives a summary of the several artificial intelligence techniques applied in prosthesis and orthotics, stressing their particular uses in improving control, flexibility, and user experience. Real-time decision-making, motion prediction, and adaptive learning all of which depend on these algorithms make artificial intelligence-driven prosthetic and orthotic devices more effective, simple, and sensitive to user needs.

Table 1. Types of AI algorithms used in prosthetics & orthotics

Algorithm	Application
Support Vector Machines (SVM)	Classifies EMG signals to control limb movements.
Artificial Neural Networks (ANNs)	Enables real-time movement prediction.
Convolutional Neural Networks (CNNs)	Used in vision-based prosthetic systems to process images for gesture recognition.
Recurrent Neural Networks (RNNs) & LSTMs	Predicts sequential movement patterns for more fluid motion.
Reinforcement Learning (RL)	Allows prosthetic joints to adapt to different terrains

Practical Applications of AI in Prosthetics

1. ***Myoelectric Control***-AI decodes muscle signals and converts them into exact finger, hand, or limb motions in myoelectric control.
2. ***Personalized Gait Analysis***-ML techniques learn from the walking style of the user and modify the motion of the prosthetic.
3. ***Automated Fall Detection***-Artificial intelligence (AI) picks out unusual walking patterns and warns the user to stop falls.
4. ***Brain-Computer Interface (BCI) Prosthetics***-Neural networks decode brain data to enable thought-directed prosthetic movement in Brain-Computer Interface (BCI) Prostheses.

2.2 Sensors and IoT Integration

To offer exact, intelligent mobility assistance, artificial intelligence-driven prosthesis and orthotics depend on real-time data collecting from embedded sensors. These smart sensors gather motion, muscle activity, pressure, and temperature data so that artificial intelligence models may maximize user experience and refine movement control. Table 2 lists the several sensor kinds employed in artificial intelligence-driven prosthesis and orthotics together with their particular purposes in improving motion control, sensory feedback, and adaptability. Detecting muscle activity, pressure, location, and environmental factors these sensors are essential for prosthetic and orthotic devices to dynamically react to user motions and external conditions for enhanced functionality and user experience.

Table 2. Types of sensors used in AI-driven prosthetics & orthotics

Sensor Type	Functionality	Example Application
Electromyography (EMG) Sensors	Detects muscle contractions and sends signals for movement control	Controlling a prosthetic hand based on muscle activity
Inertial Measurement Units (IMU)	Tracks acceleration, orientation, and angular velocity for stability	Adjusting a prosthetic leg's balance during walking
Pressure Sensors	Measures foot pressure to optimize gait patterns	Detecting uneven weight distribution in a prosthetic foot
Biosensors	Monitors physiological responses (e.g., temperature, hydration) to prevent discomfort	Alerting the user if skin temperature rises due to prolonged use
Optical Sensors	Used for computer vision-based motion tracking	Enabling a prosthetic arm to detect and grasp objects

How IoT Enhances Prosthetics and Orthotics

IoT gadgets' intelligence and adaptability are transforming prosthesis and orthoses. Cloud-based data analysis helps to offer tailored adaptations by letting artificial intelligence models learn from enormous user data. For better mobility, for instance, gait information from hundreds of users supports perfect prosthetic performance.

Remote monitoring allows clinicians track patient development and provide recommendations for changes without in-person visits. Examination of doctor's remote prosthesis use can help to provide recommendations for suitable comfort-oriented modifications.

Real-time data transmission becomes even more crucial since sensors feed artificial intelligence systems motion data constantly. For example, a prosthetic limb guarantees more natural exercise by quick change in stride length based on IMU sensor data (Asgarabad et al. 2023). By enabling prosthesis to become more responsive, IoT is helping users to gain mobility, comfort, and independence.

Showcasing the combination of smart sensors, cloud computing, and artificial intelligence algorithms to improve prosthetic capability, Figure 2 shows an IoT-enabled prosthetic system By means of real-time data collecting, remote monitoring, and adaptive control, this system helps users to gain from customized modifications, predictive maintenance, and seamless interaction with mobile devices and healthcare providers.

Figure 2. IoT-enabled prosthetic system

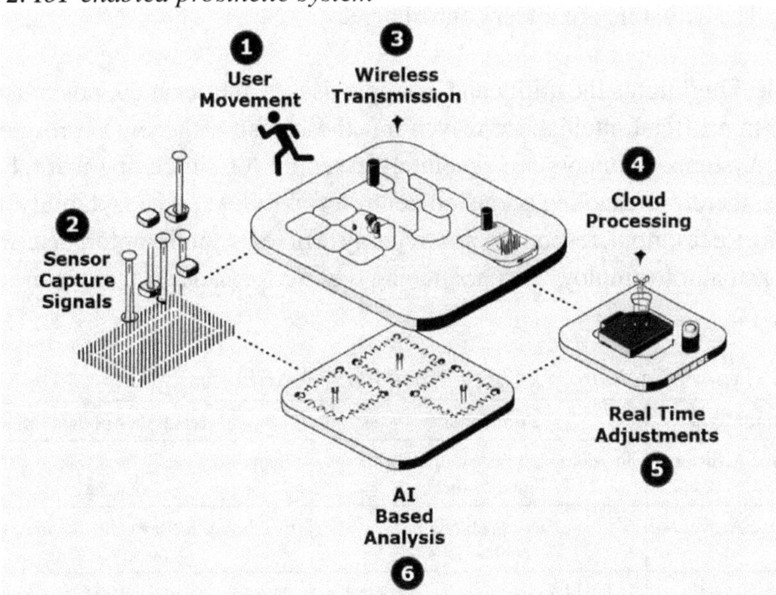

2.3 Robotics and Actuators

Advanced robotics and actuators transfer neural and machine learning signals into physical motion, therefore facilitating the mechanical movement of AI-driven prosthesis and orthoses. These parts guarantee exact, natural, smooth control of manmade limbs (Sanfilippo et al. 2024).

Actuators

1. ***Electric Actuators:*** Perfect for upper-limb prosthesis, offer smooth and silence operation. Highly controlled, these actuators can be tweaked for sensitive jobs. For instance, a prosthetic hand with electric actuators can replicate exact motions for typing on a keyboard or pen gripping. An ML model interprets human muscle impulses and converts them into certain motions, hence controlling the actuators.
2. ***Pneumatic Actuators***: Ideal for lower-limb prostheses, offer high power-to---weight ratios. For activities like running or walking, these actuators are perfect since they can provide notable force. A prosthetic limb incorporating pneumatic actuators, for instance, can change its joint stiffness to offer support throughout various activities. Combining sensor data with

ML techniques lets the prosthetic change to fit the user's gait and terrain. The actuators are under control here.

Table 3 highlights the utility and example uses of the several kinds of actuators utilized in artificial intelligence-driven prostheses and orthoses. In prosthetic and orthotic systems, actuators are absolutely essential for simulating natural muscle motions, therefore enabling precision control, flexibility, and adaptability. Factors including force output, responsiveness, energy efficiency, and comfort determine the type of actuator to employ, so guaranteeing best performance catered to user needs.

Table 3. Types of actuators used in prosthetics & orthotics

Actuator Type	Functionality	Example Application
Hydraulic Actuators	Provides high force output for lower-limb prosthetics	Supporting heavy loads during walking or running
Pneumatic Actuators	Simulates natural muscle contractions	Enabling smooth and lifelike movements in a prosthetic arm
Electromagnetic Actuators	Enables rapid movement control	Allowing quick adjustments in a prosthetic hand for delicate tasks
Soft Actuators	Offers biomimetic motion for enhanced comfort	Providing gentle and flexible movements in a prosthetic finger

Robotic Control Systems

Artificial intelligence systems enable robotic prosthesis made feasible by them to perform challenging tasks such varied force item gripping and real-time gait adjustment. By assessing topography and adjusting joint stiffness, a robotic knee prosthesis, for example, allows the user walk smoothly on uneven ground. The artificial intelligence system uses force sensors and IMUs among other sensors to determine the appropriate degree of stiffness for the knee joint.

Key Advantages of AI-Driven Robotic Prosthetics:

1. ***Real-Time Adaptability:*** Dynamic movement adjustment by AI models depends on sensor inputs. For instance, a prosthetic knee instantly changes its stiffness to suit various surfaces.
2. ***Precision & Stability:*** For more fluid mobility, sensors measure posture and balance. A prosthetic limb, for instance, keeps balance during quick stops or rotations.

3. ***Reduced Cognitive Load:*** Users don't have to work especially hard to regulate motion. For instance, a prosthetic arm changes its grip strength depending on the thing it is handling automatically.

2.4 Computer Vision and Gesture Recognition

Technologies for gesture detection and computer vision improve user-prosthetic or orthotic device interaction (Deshmukh, Khatik, and Saxena 2023). These technologies give gadgets simple, context-aware capabilities and let them "see" and comprehend their surroundings.

Computer Vision

Integration of cameras into prosthesis allows for environmental analysis and contextual information provision. For jobs requiring item recognition and spatial awareness especially, this is quite helpful. For instance, a prosthetic arm featuring a camera can help one to precisely grab objects. The camera records scenes of the surroundings, which a computer vision system subsequently analyzes to locate items. The prosthetic's movements are under control using this data, so guaranteeing proper grip of the object.

Gesture Recognition

Combining computer vision with machine learning allows prosthesis to identify hand gestures or body movements, therefore facilitating simple control. For upper-limb prosthesis especially, this is quite helpful. For instance, a prosthetic arm can smoothly interact with things by sensing a user's gesture to open or close its hand (Jiang et al. 2021). Combining camera data with ML techniques, the gesture recognition system labels user motions and converts them into certain actions. Figure 3 shows how computer vision, machine learning, and sensor-based inputs let prosthetic devices read and react to hand gestures and muscular motions in AI-driven prosthesis. As well as Table 4 compares and contrasts several gesture detection methods applied in artificial intelligence-driven prostheses, therefore highlighting their benefits and constraints.

Figure 3. Gesture recognition in AI prosthetics

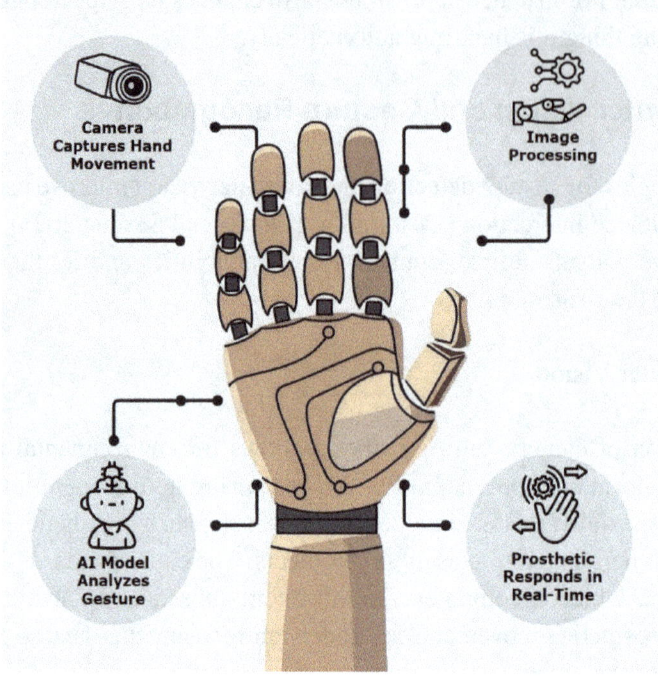

Table 4. Comparison of gesture recognition techniques

Technique	Pros	Cons
Camera-Based	High accuracy, non-invasive	Sensitive to lighting conditions
EMG-Based	Direct muscle signal interpretation	Requires precise sensor placement
Hybrid (Camera + EMG)	Combines strengths of both approaches	Higher cost and complexity

2.5 Ethical Design Considerations

Although the chapter's framework follows the technical foundations, applications, challenges, and trends trajectory, there is a possibility of enhancing the flow of the material by introducing ethical aspects at an earlier stage. At present, ethical considerations (e.g. equity, bias) are only presented in Section 5 while they have a direct relation with technical proposals (Section 2) and use cases (Sections 3-4). For instance, bias in AI models creates an initial problem with the accuracy of analyzing gait data for patients. It would be more appropriate to include the subsection in Section 2, "Ethical Design Considerations" where different types of datasets reduce bias in the CNNs. In the same manner, improving the equity in IoT access within Section 3.4 would improve flow by relating technical feasibility to its ethical implications smoothly

3. APPLICATIONS OF AI IN PROSTHETICS

The integration of AI in orthotics has contributed greatly to the design, customization, and functionality of assistive devices. All of these systems, as shown in Figure 4, use a range of technologies including EEG systems as well as electromyography (EMG) sensors and exoskeletons to achieve a seamless form factor between humans and machines. This integration allows changes to be made in real-time and adds to individual support that leads to improved overall functionality and user experience. Static molds and pre-defined structures are what previous orthotic solutions usually offered, but they were not adaptable to individual's needs. But AI-driven innovations bestowed us the development of smart, adaptive, and personalized orthotic devices for mobility, and comfort, as well as improved outcomes of rehabilitation.

Figure 4. Integration of AI-driven systems in prosthetics and orthotics for enhanced rehabilitation and assistance

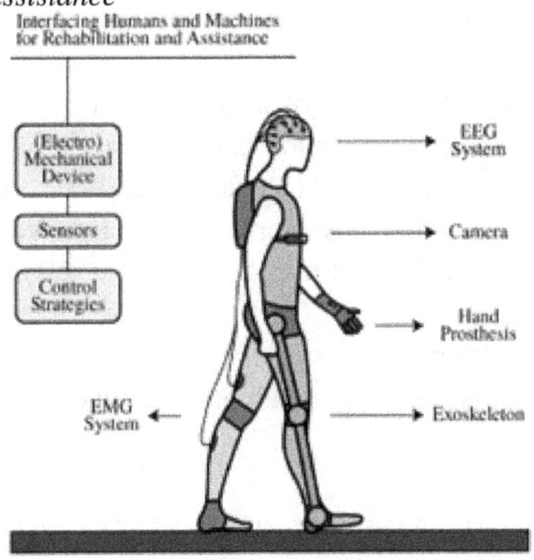

Source: https://www.frontiersin.org/files/Articles/796431/frobt-08-796431-HTML-r1/image_m/frobt-08-796431-g001.jpg

3.1 AI-Powered Customization and Design

Existing orthotic and prosthetic devices tend to require the application of considerable manual 'fitting and adjustment'. The uses of advanced computational models to generate patient-specific designs are considered to be the uses of AI-driven customization.

1. ***3D Scanning and Modeling:*** 3D scanning based on AI technology captures the detailed anatomical data precisely, so we can make the orthotic precisely and conform to the body of the user (Zhang, Cheng, and Zhang 2023).
2. ***Generative Design Algorithms:*** AI-based models optimize the orthotic structure for strength, flexibility as well as lightweight structures to enhance comfort and functionality (Vélez-Guerrero, Callejas-Cuervo, and Mazzoleni 2021).
3. ***3D Printing with AI-Optimized Materials:*** Combinations of materials for the best durability and comfort are produced with extreme precision much faster than before due to AI accelerating production.

3.2 AI-Driven Real-Time Gait Analysis and Correction

People who use orthotic devices have often developed gait abnormalities. Orthotics with AI built-in offers real-time gait analysis to make a more efficient movement without taking the high risk of musculoskeletal complications in the future.

1. ***Wearable Sensors and Motion Tracking:*** There are sensors built into the orthotic devices that collect real biomechanical real-time data and a trained AI model to detect gait irregularities (Shefa et al. 2024).
2. ***Adaptive Feedback Mechanisms:*** Corrective algorithms are dynamically based on Artificial Intelligence and optimize the support levels in terms of minimizing strain.
3. ***Rehabilitation Monitoring:*** Physical therapists can use AI-driven gait analysis tools to track the progress of the rehabilitation and design therapy plans based on the same.

Real-time gait analysis shows how AI may improve prosthetics and orthotics difficulties like dynamic responsiveness and fall prevention. The Blatchford Linx system analyzes stride length, pace, and stance phase in milliseconds using wearable IMU and pressure sensors and ML algorithms like LSTMs to modify joint stiffness for uneven terrain. However, computational delay on embedded systems and the necessity for diverse training data to ensure accuracy across populations remain. Edge computing, where AI analyzes data locally, might reduce latency, while federated learning could improve model inclusivity without compromising privacy. Adding case studies like the ReWalk exoskeleton's gait correction for spinal injury patients would clarify these advances and challenges.

3.3 Intelligent Orthotic Devices for Rehabilitation

Orthotics played by AI-powered are very powerful in rehabilitation, especially in facilitating individuals after injuries or in stroke and cerebral palsy.

1. ***Exoskeletons with AI Control:*** Analyzing the user movement patterns and adapting to the user's needs, smart exoskeletons provide assistance in restoring mobility (Jacob et al. 2021).
2. ***Neural Rehabilitation Interfaces:*** EMG signals are used to predict muscle movements in the cases of AI-powered systems for support in rehabilitation.
3. ***Virtual Reality (VR) Integration:*** VR rehabilitation programs based on AI-driven training are able to train patients in realistic environments in order to improve motor learning and recovery (Han et al. 2023).

AI-driven prostheses integrate with customised physical therapy programmes, a chapter issue underexplored. Artificial intelligence analyzes EMG and IMU data to tailor therapy resistance to a patient's recovery stage, such as increasing load by 10% weekly for stroke patients. VR with AI, like MindMaze, immerses participants in gamified exercises that modify difficulty to real-time motor performance, increasing interest by 25% in a 2022 study. Personalising recovery addresses the shortcoming of generic rehabilitation, but the chapter overlooks this synergy. Adding case studies like the ReMotion Knee's AI-driven amputee therapy changes would improve outcomes and rehabilitation emphasis.

3.4 IoT-Enabled Smart Orthotics for Remote Monitoring

The integration of IoT and AI makes it possible to monitor real-time performance tracking and remote medical supervision with orthotic devices.

1. ***Cloud-Based AI Analytics:*** Wearable orthotic device data is transmitted to cloud based platforms where data is analyzed using AI algorithms and long-term trends are suggested (Murala, Panda, and Dash 2023).
2. ***Remote Therapy Adjustments:*** Artificially intelligent systems enable remote tuning of orthotic settings by healthcare providers, minimizing hospital acuity.

Predictive Maintenance: Orthotics could be worth checking for by AI for early indications of wear and tear on their components, so there is time to do maintenance and not malfunctions.

Smart orthotics with IoT provide remote monitoring and individualized care, a disruptive trend. The Hocoma Valedo system tracks spinal mobility using IoT sensors and sends data to cloud-based AI models for real-time posture correction. This solves the rising problem of restricted in-person therapy access in rural or underprivileged locations and fits with telehealth integration. Based on AI-analyzed use patterns, physicians can remotely alter orthotic brace tension to improve outcomes without hospital visits. This chapter understates cybersecurity vulnerabilities such data interception during transmission and scalability issues in low-bandwidth regions. This section should include examples like the Ottobock X3's IoT predictive maintenance and edge AI for offline functionality to balance benefits and limitations.

4. APPLICATIONS OF AI IN ORTHOTICS

In spite of impressive strides made in the field of AI-driven prosthetics and orthotics, some problems and ethical questions need to be tackled for such wide adoption, fairness, and future sustainability. Data privacy, such as accessibility and algorithmic bias, as well as regulatory compliance, create a great weight in defining the path that AI-powered assistive technologies will take in the future. In this section, these challenges are examined in detail and some solutions that narrow the effect of these problems are explored. In Table 5, a concise overview of the challenges that exist along with possible ways to enhance user experience and accessibility is provided.

Table 5. Key challenges and solutions in AI-driven prosthetics and orthotics

Challenge	Impact on individuals	Proposed solution
Data Privacy & Security	Risk of personal health data breaches	End-to-end encryption, user-controlled data access, GDPR/HIPAA compliance
High Cost & Accessibility	Expensive devices limit access, especially in low-income areas	3D printing, mass production, insurance coverage, government subsidies
AI Bias & Fairness	Poor fit or functionality for diverse users due to biased training data	Train on diverse datasets, conduct bias audits, allow manual adjustments
Regulatory & Safety Concerns	Uncertainty about device reliability and legal accountability	FDA/CE/ISO certification, clear liability policies, robust safety testing
Limited Real-World Adaptability	Difficulty adjusting to various terrains and movement patterns	Real-time AI learning, wearable sensors, user feedback integration

The chapter correctly addresses ethical issues, regulatory compliance, and cost, recommending government subsidies and open-source AI models. This understates the viability and scalability of these systems. The $50,000+ cost of an AI-driven prosthetic like the LUKE Arm can be offset by government subsidies, but implementation differs by country. Sweden has strong financing, while others lack infrastructure. The OpenAI-inspired Open Prosthetics Project uses open-source models to save licensing costs but require technical expertise for customisation, limiting accessibility. Pilot programs like India's Jaipur Foot initiative adapting AI on a budget and scalability measures like cost-per-unit reductions (e.g., 3D printing lowering 30% per a 2023 research) should be explored. The solutions would be grounded in real-world situations

4.1 Data Privacy and Security Risks

Prosthetic and orthotic devices that leverage this data are powered by AI and rely on extensive data for biometric and movement patterns, neural signals, and real-time sensory feedback. This data is important for improving the life of the device but presents a number of privacy, security, and ethical concerns as well.

1. ***Biometric Data Protection:*** Maintaining our users' sensitive data protected from threats of cyber attacks and breaches of unauthorized access is crucial since these AI-driven assistive devices collect and process the data continuously. For instance, this would mean encrypting the data from the beginning to the end, which would make it impossible for any third party to access it. Moreover, blockchain-based security models can ensure that data is stored in a decentralized storage system such as the blockchain to prevent unauthorized data access while also ensuring transparency of the data and control over the information by the user.
2. ***Regulatory Compliance:*** Compliance with very strict data protection regulations is required in order to protect patient privacy, including:
    - **General Data Protection Regulation (GDPR) –** Controls data privacy and security in Europe and informs data users to collect, store, and process it with explicit consent (Protection 2018).
    - **Health Insurance Portability and Accountability Act (HIPAA) –** Protects patient privacy in terms of heath-related data in the United States by denying unauthorized access to their information (Edemekong, Annamaraju, and Haydel 2018).
    - **ISO 27701 and ISO 13485 –** Ensures that sensitive health data treatment is handled ethically according to international standards of data privacy and medical device security (Dil and Eikelenboom 2023).

3. ***AI Transparency and Explainability:*** The lack of transparency in the process of decision-making in AI-powered medical devices is arguably one of the biggest ethical concerns. In critical scenarios, where the changes in mobility and rehabilitation made by AI models are critical for the users and healthcare providers, users and healthcare providers must understand how the models work. Within the domain of explainable AI (XAI), appropriate implementation of explainable AI techniques like decision trees, feature importance analysis as well as interpretable neural networks to ensure that AI recommendation could be transparent, accountable, and justifiable.

4.2 Accessibility and Cost Barriers

Nevertheless, these prosthetics and orthotics are profoundly capable, yet prohibitively expensive for most people in low-income areas. Limited accessibility is based on the cost of integrating AI components, sensors, and advanced materials.

1. ***High Manufacturing Costs:*** The cost of achieving high functionality in the assistive devices is due to:
    - **Sensors and Neural Interfaces –** Production costs are greatly increased by advanced sensors, EMG systems, and brain-computer interfaces (BCIs).
    - **Machine Learning and Cloud Processing –** Processing and computing-heavy AI models require resources that add more costs to the operation.
    - **Customization and Materials –** Since personalized designs of prosthetic and orthotic devices need 3D scanning, AI-based design, and high-quality materials are more expensive.
2. ***Insurance and Funding Challenges:*** Many healthcare systems and insurance providers don't cover all the costs of AI-powered prosthetic and orthotic devices, and thus, they are too expensive for economically disadvantaged individuals. There may arise insurance limitations due to:
    - **Lack of Recognition for AI Devices –** AI-driven prosthetics are described by some insurers as 'experimental' and do not cover it in full.
    - **Strict Approval Processes –** To become approved by medical devices, insurance companies require a very large clinical validation.
3. ***Potential Solutions for Cost Reduction:*** Several initiatives may be explored in order to improve affordability and accessibility such as:
    - **Open-Source AI Models –** Licensing costs could be encouraged to be open source and augment development speed.
    - **Mass Production Techniques –** Lower production costs can be achieved by adopting innovative manufacturing processes, such as 3D printing.

- **Government and NGO Support –** Subsidies and grants available for public healthcare initiatives can increase the accessibility of AI-powered prosthetics to underserved communities.

The solutions presented above make it possible to bring AI-driven prosthetics and orthotics to a wider population.

4.3 Legal and Regulatory Compliance

For AI-powered prosthetic and orthotic devices to be implemented safely, reliably, and ethically they have to abide by some strong legal and regulatory frameworks. Otherwise, risks to the subject's medical health occur, and standards of the industry are set.

1. ***Certification and Approval Processes:*** Assistive devices driven by AI need to meet global medical device regulations, including:
    - **U.S. FDA (Food and Drug Administration) –** Before AI-powered prosthetics can be marketed in the US, they need to be validated and approved by the clinic (Davis and Patel 2019).
    - **CE Marking (European Union) –** Ensures that the EU meets its health and safety standards for AI-driven medical devices (Ballor 2022).
    - **ISO Standards –** ISO 13485 specifies the requirements for a medical device organization to have a quality management system intended for use by such an organization in the design, development, production, manufacture, installation, and servicing of medical devices (Dil and Eikelenboom 2023).
2. ***Liability and Accountability:*** Liability issues arising regarding prosthetics and orthotics powered by AI must be addressed in legal frameworks such as:
    - **Device Malfunctions –** If the prosthetic of an AI fails to work properly, it should be declared legally responsible between the manufacturer, software developer, and health provider.
    - **AI Decision-Making Errors –** In the case where a wrong movement prediction is given by the AI model, leading to an injury, both ethical and legal accountability are mandated to be established.
3. ***Ethical AI Development and Guidelines:*** Developers need to follow ethical guidelines in responsibility AI deployment for prosthetics and orthotics to ensure responsible AI deployment such as:
    - **Transparency and Explainability –** Ensuring clinicians and users understand the meaning of the output from AI models.

- **Continuous Monitoring –** Efforts should be made to update the software regularly with safety checks for optimal performance.
- **User Consent and Control –** Permitting users to choose to opt out of AI-driven decision-making when required.

If AI-driven prosthetic and orthotic devices adhere to these legal and ethical standards, they will be accepted by the public, receive regulatory approval, and ultimately become commonplace on the market.

5. CHALLENGES AND ETHICAL CONSIDERATIONS

Although the integration of artificial intelligence (AI) in prosthetic and orthotics has produced incredible advancements, it also begs serious ethical concerns and presents enormous challenges. If we are to ensure the appropriate, fair, and safe implementation of artificial intelligence-driven assistive technology, these challenges involve technical restrictions, data privacy issues, and more general ethical questions that have to be answered. This section explores more these issues and provides insight of the difficulty of designing and using prosthesis and orthoses motivated by artificial intelligence.

5.1 Technical Challenges

Though driven by artificial intelligence, prosthesis and orthotics face technological difficulties even if they possess great capabilities. These challenges arise from the difficulty of including modern technologies into goods that must run constantly in real-world environments.

Key Technical Challenges

1. ***Power Consumption and Battery Life:*** Artificial intelligence algorithms, sensors, and actuators—which can limit the running lifetime of prosthetic and orthotic devices—need significant power. Managing performance with energy economy presents one of the most difficult challenges. A prosthetic limb with adaptive learning and advanced gesture recognition, for example, might require continuous recharging, therefore interfering with the user's daily life.
2. ***Real-Time Processing:*** Artificial intelligence models have to interpret data and make decisions in real-time to guarantee perfect user interface. Low-latency performance is challenging on embedded devices with limited computational capabilities, though. For example, a lower-limb prosthetic

must change its gait in milliseconds to accommodate changes in terrain, so it requires rather optimal algorithms and hardware.

3. ***Durability and Wearability:*** Devices for prosthesis and orthosis have to resist environmental factors, physical strain, and extended use. One of the key engineering difficulties is ensuring lifespan while yet keeping a light weight and attractive look. For running, for instance, a prosthetic limb must withstand strong impact pressures without sacrificing structural integrity or user comfort.
4. ***Interoperability and Standardization:*** The absence of consistent data exchange and device connectivity standards can impede the integration of prosthetics and orthotics driven by artificial intelligence with other healthcare systems and devices. For instance, a prosthetic arm that gathers user data could not be fit for an electronic health record (EHR) system of a hospital, therefore restricting its use for medical professionals.
5. ***Adaptability to Diverse User Needs:*** Since people have diverse physical characteristics, tastes, and way of life, development of one-size-fits-all answers is challenging. Customizing AI models and gadget settings for every user requires much of data and testing. A prosthetic hand designed for a musician, for example, can have different uses than one built for a building worker.

5.2 Data Privacy and Security

Data privacy and security are major issues raised by prostheses and orthotics' growing integration of artificial intelligence, IoT, and cloud computing. Prosthetic and orthotic equipment driven by artificial intelligence depend on large volumes of sensitive personal information including:

1. Electromyography (EMG) signals (muscle activity data).
2. Gait patterns and movement analytics.
3. Brain-computer interface (BCI) signals.
4. Health records and biometrics.
5. Environmental sensor data (GPS, temperature, pressure, etc.).

These technologies are vulnerable to cyberattacks, illegal access, and ethical abuse when such data is gathered and sent across wireless networks, cloud systems, and artificial intelligence models. Emphasizing the dangers related to data collecting, storage, and sharing, Table 6 summarizes the main data privacy issues connected with artificial intelligence-driven prosthesis and orthotics. Ensuring data security and user privacy is vital since these devices continually acquire sensitive user information like biometric signals, movement patterns, and health data.

Table 6. Data privacy challenges in AI-driven prosthetics & orthotics

Challenge	Description	Potential Risks
Unauthorized Access	Hackers or unauthorized users gaining control of prosthetic/orthotic systems.	Could lead to functional disruption, movement manipulation, or complete shutdown of the device.
Data Breaches	Leakage of health data, movement logs, or biometric identifiers.	Risks identity theft, insurance fraud, and unauthorized surveillance.
Lack of Encryption	Transmission of unencrypted muscle, movement, and neural data over networks.	Increases risk of man-in-the-middle (MITM) attacks.
Cloud Vulnerabilities	AI-powered prosthetic devices store and process data on cloud platforms.	Unauthorized access to user history, gait data, and EMG recordings.
Third-Party Sharing	AI developers may share prosthetic user data with advertisers, insurance companies, or research institutions.	Can lead to exploitation of personal medical records.

Cybersecurity Threats in AI-Powered Prosthetics & Orthotics

1. ***Hacking and Device Manipulation***- Malicious actors might take over AI-driven prosthesis, causing disruptive movement commands or physical injury via hacking and device manipulation.
2. ***Data Interception***- Attackers can intercept data flow between prosthesis, cloud artificial intelligence models, and mobile apps wire-wise.
3. ***AI Model Tampering***- Should adversarial attacks change the ML model, the prosthetic could misread muscle inputs, resulting in erroneous movement.
4. ***Ransomware Attacks***-Ransomware attacks let hackers encrypt prosthetic data and demand payment for access restoration.

5.3 Ethical Implications

Artificial intelligence-driven quick development of prosthetics and orthotics begs various ethical issues of user autonomy, justice, accessibility, and human enhancement. Ethical questions have to be addressed if we are to ensure equal access, safety, and responsible artificial intelligence deployment in assistive technologies (Anderson, Barnett, and Rusaw 2022). Emphasizing the consequences of autonomy, accessibility, prejudice, and informed permission, Table 7 shows major ethical questions in artificial intelligence-driven prosthesis and orthotics.

Table 7. Ethical concerns in AI-driven prosthetics & orthotics

Ethical Issue	Description	Potential Consequences
Bias in AI Models	Prosthetic AI may perform better for some demographics than others due to biased training data.	Could lead to unequal accessibility and reduced accuracy for underrepresented groups.
Affordability & Accessibility	AI-driven prosthetics are expensive, limiting availability for low-income individuals.	Creates health disparities between different socioeconomic groups.
Human Augmentation vs. Disability Assistance	AI prosthetics may enhance human capabilities beyond normal function.	Raises concerns about unfair advantages in competitive fields (sports, military, etc.).
Data Ownership & Consent	Who owns the data collected from AI prosthetics—the user, manufacturer, or healthcare provider?	Risk of user data being exploited for commercial or research purposes without consent.
Autonomy & Control	Should AI override user commands if a movement is deemed unsafe?	Raises concerns about loss of user autonomy.

Ethical Frameworks to Address These Issues

1. Fair & Inclusive AI Training
2. Making AI Prosthetics Affordable
3. Defining the Limits of AI-Enhanced Capabilities
4. Transparent AI & User Control

Consequently, this chapter is directed to the engineers, clinicians, and policymakers at the same time by focusing on such tropes as the specifics of the ML algorithms along with the types of sensors and the potential pitfalls related to data privacy and accessibility. For example, the idea to discuss BCI-controlled prosthetics is more inspiring to engineers while GDPR/HIPAA compliance will be more inspiring to clinicians and regulators. Nevertheless, it could appeal to this audience more if it connected technological innovations to ethical applications—such as how various datasets for CNNs eliminate the prejudice, for providing equal treatment. Two additional subsections – User perspectives section where needs and experiences of amputee user concerning its usability of BCI could be included to meet Audience interest in Quality of life issues.

6. FUTURE TRENDS AND INNOVATIONS

The field of artificial intelligence-driven prosthetic and orthotics is fast changing as human-machine cooperation, market acceptance, and artificial intelligence algorithms keep growing. These innovations aim to increase gadget accessibility, use, and flexibility so transforming the life of limb disabled individuals.

6.1 Advances in AI Algorithms

Recent advances in deep learning, reinforcement learning, and neuro-symbolic artificial intelligence have greatly enhanced prosthetic and orthotic device performance. AI algorithm future trends include:

1. ***Self-learning artificial intelligence models-*** prosthesis that, via constant learning, fit user preferences.
2. ***Neural Interface AI***- Direct integration for flawless movement control using brain-computer interfaces (BCIs).
3. ***Predictive Motion Control***- Based on EMG, EEG, and biomechanical information, predictive motion control—AI can predict user motions, hence minimizing response lag.
4. ***Explainable AI (XAI)***- By visible and interpretable AI decision-making in prosthesis, increase user trust.

6.2 Human-Machine Collaboration

The smooth interaction between artificial intelligence and human users will define prosthesis and orthosis going forward. Important advancements consist in:

1. ***Biofeedback Systems***- AI-driven prosthesis using biofeedback systems will give users haptic feedback, therefore restoring a feeling of touch.
2. ***Hybrid AI & Human Control***- Users of hybrid artificial intelligence and human control can move between manual and AI-assisted states, hence improving safety and autonomy.
3. ***Augmented Reality (AR) for Training***- AR-based simulations will enable users to practice with AI-powered limbs, hence enhancing adaptation.
4. ***Soft Robotics & AI-*** Flexible, biomechanically adapted materials from soft robotics and artificial intelligence will improve comfort and natural mobility.

6.3 Market Growth and Adoption

Thanks to technical developments, lower prices, and rising demand, the market for artificial intelligence-driven prosthesis and orthotics is fast expanding.

Forecasted Market Development

1. By 2030, the market for artificial intelligence prosthesis is predicted to rise with a CAGR of 8–10%.
2. Increasing government backing and financing for assistive devices grounded on artificial intelligence.
3. Increasing insurance coverage and affordable programs for prosthesis driven by artificial intelligence.

Several algorithms like CNNs, RNNs, and SVMs are already mentioned and they all need to be explored deeply for their applications to prosthetic devices. For example, CNNs are particularly useful for tasks of visual recognition and can assist the prosthetic device in identifying and interacting with the objects while RNNs can help in predicting and adjusting the movement patterns to generate smoother motion control based on sequential data. Examples from the world of practice, e.g. the Open Bionics Hero Arm (Hussin and Sadun 2021) that exploits myoelectric sensors together with AI control algorithms in the form of an intuitive interface, are provided for inspiration. Additionally, the combination of CNNs for visual input with RNNs for movement prediction in hybrid models would greatly improve the adaptability of prosthetic devices, allowing them to be more reliable behavior in dynamic environments. Real-time adjustment of such combinations gives real-world functionality of prosthetics within day-to-day scenarios such as walking on uneven surfaces or interaction of prosthetically enabled hands with objects of varying shapes and sizes. Looking at these hybrid approaches may help us to have more personal and efficient prosthetic solutions that can provide a better quality of life for its users.

7. CONCLUSION

Prosthetics and orthotics that are powered by AI have become game-changing innovations that provide individuals with limb differences and musculoskeletal conditions with improved mobility, functionality and personalization. These assistive devices have gone further than these traditional boundaries by using integration of the artificial intelligence, advanced sensor technologies, machine learning algorithms as well as biomechanical modeling. With this, AI has brought forth new aspects of the experience of people using real-time gauge modifications to prosthetic limbs, controlled from the brain.

Although much progress has been made, several challenges such as data privacy are still present, costs are still high, and regulatory issues remain, especially given the fact that a significant proportion of existing datasets already contain sensitive data that can be linked to individuals. AI in healthcare, and especially personalized assistive devices, raises the ethical implications of AI in dealing with personal data and achieving fairness and transparency, and that transparency is enough for all involved. To address these challenges a multi-faceted approach and collaboration is needed which itself is also a complex interdisciplinary problem to solve, involving researchers, engineers, healthcare professionals, policymakers, and industry stakeholders. One has to ensure that the AI-driven healthcare solutions are compliant with medical regulations, be affordable by means of innovative manufacturing techniques, and minimize the bias in AI through diverse training datasets.

In this sense, strength of the chapter can be identified in more detailed description of the technologies related to AI such as ML, sensors, IoT, as well as in solutions to the challenges: for instance, it proposes the use of encryption for data privacy. These strengths can strengthen the areas of the low coverage of rehabilitation applications. Although general technical introductions to CNNs and EMG sensors can be provided, the detailed technical description of the actual rehabilitation examples can be given, including the usage of the Cyberdyne HAL exoskeleton to retrain the neural pathways of spinal injury patients through AI. Likewise, the need for further discussion on scalability can be resolved through presenting how the chapter could improve IoT infrastructure to provide affordable AI prosthetics to various rural clinics while capitalizing on concepts the chapter has presumed.

The future of AI in prosthetics and orthotics remains bright as iterations of deep learning, brain-machine interface, and real-time adaptive control see continuous advancements. Federated learning and decentralized AI models as emerging technologies could provide a further boost to data privacy, while breakthroughs in bio-integrated electronics might contribute to the development of more natural and responsive prosthetic limbs. Furthermore, as AI-powered orthotics become easier to obtain, artificial intelligence-powered orthotics can be used in sports performance, workplace ergonomics, preventive healthcare, and rehabilitation.

REFERENCES

Anderson, S. P., Barnett, C. T., & Rusaw, D. F. (2022). Exploring the Perspectives of Prosthetic and Orthotic Users: Past and Present Experiences and Insights for the Future. *Disability and Rehabilitation*, *44*(18), 5284–5290. DOI: 10.1080/09638288.2021.1928777 PMID: 34088248

Asgarabad, M. R. E., Amirbeigiarab, M. M., Ardalani, R., Zarandi, S. F. A., & Nazari, A. J. (2023). Enhancing Patient Movement Rehabilitation: Integration of Intelligent Prosthetic Limbs and the Internet of Things.

Ballor, G. (2022). CE Marking, Business, and European Market Integration. *Business History Review*, *96*(1), 77–108. DOI: 10.1017/S0007680521000696

Brink, K. J., Likens, A., & Stergiou, N. (2023). The Evolution of Scholarship of Biomechanics and Motor Control Within the Academy: The Past, the Present, and the Future. *Kinesiology Review (Champaign, Ill.)*, *13*(1), 42–54. DOI: 10.1123/kr.2023-0054

Chen, B., Chen, C., Hu, J., Sayeed, Z., Qi, J., Darwiche, H. F., & Palacio-Lascano, C. (2022). Computer vision and machine learning-based gait pattern recognition for flat fall prediction. *Sensors (Basel)*, *22*(20), 7960.

Choo, Y. J., & Chang, M. C. (2023). Use of Machine Learning in the Field of Prosthetics and Orthotics: A Systematic Narrative Review. *Prosthetics and Orthotics International*, *47*(3), 226–240. DOI: 10.1097/PXR.0000000000000199 PMID: 36811961

Chui, K. K., Jorge, M., Yen, S. C., & Lusardi, M. M. (2019). *Orthotics and Prosthetics in Rehabilitation E-Book: Orthotics and Prosthetics in Rehabilitation E-Book*. Elsevier Health Sciences.

Davis, A. A., & Patel, V. G. (2019). The Role of PD-L1 Expression as a Predictive Biomarker: An Analysis of All US Food and Drug Administration (FDA) Approvals of Immune Checkpoint Inhibitors. *Journal for Immunotherapy of Cancer*, *7*(1), 278. DOI: 10.1186/s40425-019-0768-9 PMID: 31655605

Deshmukh, S., Khatik, V., & Saxena, A. (2023). Robust Fusion Model for Handling EMG and Computer Vision Data in Prosthetic Hand Control. *IEEE Sensors Letters*, *7*(9), 1–4. DOI: 10.1109/LSENS.2023.3301837

Dil, A. S., & Eikelenboom, A. (2023). Whisking the Digital Health Compliance. In *Pharmaceutical Care in Digital Revolution* (pp. 261–277). Elsevier. DOI: 10.1016/B978-0-443-13360-2.00010-1

Han, X., Zhou, X., Tan, B., Jiao, L., & Zhang, R. (2023). Ai-Based next-Generation Sensors for Enhanced Rehabilitation Monitoring and Analysis. *Measurement, 223*, 113758. DOI: 10.1016/j.measurement.2023.113758

Hussin, Q., & Sadun, A. S. (2021). User-Driven Prosthetic Robotic Arm for Patients with Lower Arm Amputation. *Progress in Engineering Application and Technology, 2*(1), 753–768. DOI: 10.30880/peat.2021.02.01.072

Islam, M., Vashishat, A., & Kumar, M. (2024). Advancements beyond Limb Loss: Exploring the Intersection of AI and BCI in Prosthetic Evaluation. *Current Pharmaceutical Design, 30*(35), 2749–2752. DOI: 10.2174/0113816128324653240731075146 PMID: 39092732

Jacob, S., Alagirisamy, M., Xi, C., Balasubramanian, V., Srinivasan, R., R, P., Jhanjhi, N. Z., & Islam, S. M. N. (2021). AI and IoT-Enabled Smart Exoskeleton System for Rehabilitation of Paralyzed People in Connected Communities. *IEEE Access : Practical Innovations, Open Solutions, 9*, 80340–80350. DOI: 10.1109/ACCESS.2021.3083093

Jiang, S., Kang, P., Song, X., Lo, B., & Shull, P. (2021). Emerging Wearable Interfaces and Algorithms for Hand Gesture Recognition: A Survey. *IEEE Reviews in Biomedical Engineering, 15*, 85–102. DOI: 10.1109/RBME.2021.3078190 PMID: 33961564

Kim, M., Simon, A. M., & Hargrove, L. J. (2022). Seamless and Intuitive Control of a Powered Prosthetic Leg Using Deep Neural Network for Transfemoral Amputees. *Wearable Technologies, 3*(September), e24. DOI: 10.1017/wtc.2022.19 PMID: 37041885

Murala, D. K., Panda, S. K., & Dash, S. P. (2023). MedMetaverse: Medical Care of Chronic Disease Patients and Managing Data Using Artificial Intelligence, Blockchain, and Wearable Devices State-of-the-Art Methodology. *IEEE Access : Practical Innovations, Open Solutions, 11*, 138954–138985. DOI: 10.1109/ACCESS.2023.3340791

Noh, B., Youm, C., Goh, E., Lee, M., Park, H., Jeon, H., & Kim, O. Y. (2021). XGBoost based machine learning approach to predict the risk of fall in older adults using gait outcomes. *Scientific Reports, 11*(1), 12183.

Sanfilippo, F., Økter, M., Dale, J., Tuan, H. M., Zafar, M. H., & Ottestad, M. (2024). Open-Source Design of Low-Cost Sensorised Elastic Actuators for Collaborative Prosthetics and Orthotics. *HardwareX, 19*, e00564. DOI: 10.1016/j.ohx.2024.e00564 PMID: 39176378

Seiça, E. C., Mendes, D., Sousa, M. R., & Vide, J. (2024). Artificial Intelligence in Foot and Ankle Surgery. In *Artificial Intelligence in Orthopaedic Surgery Made Easy* (pp. 135–154). Springer. DOI: 10.1007/978-3-031-70310-2_14

Shefa, F. R., Sifat, F. H., Uddin, J., Ahmad, Z., Kim, J.-M., & Kibria, M. G. (2024). Deep Learning and IoT-Based Ankle–Foot Orthosis for Enhanced Gait Optimization. [MDPI.]. *Health Care*, *12*, 2273. PMID: 39595470

Triwiyanto, T., Caesarendra, W., Ahmed, A. A., & Abdullayev, V. H. (2023). How Deep Learning and Neural Networks Can Improve Prosthetics and Exoskeletons: A Review of State-of-the-Art Methods and Challenges. *Journal of Electronics, Electromedical Engineering, and Medical Informatics*, *5*(4), 277–289. DOI: 10.35882/jeeemi.v5i4.333

Vélez-Guerrero, M. A., Callejas-Cuervo, M., & Mazzoleni, S. (2021). Artificial Intelligence-Based Wearable Robotic Exoskeletons for Upper Limb Rehabilitation: A Review. *Sensors (Basel)*, *21*(6), 2146. DOI: 10.3390/s21062146 PMID: 33803911

Vu, P. P., Vaskov, A. K., Lee, C., Jillala, R. R., Wallace, D. M., Davis, A. J., Kung, T. A., Kemp, S. W. P., Gates, D. H., Chestek, C. A., & Cederna, P. S. (2023). Long-Term Upper-Extremity Prosthetic Control Using Regenerative Peripheral Nerve Interfaces and Implanted EMG Electrodes. *Journal of Neural Engineering*, *20*(2), 026039. DOI: 10.1088/1741-2552/accb0c PMID: 37023743

Yoo, J., & Shoaran, M. (2021). Neural Interface Systems with On-Device Computing: Machine Learning and Neuromorphic Architectures. *Current Opinion in Biotechnology*, *72*, 95–101. DOI: 10.1016/j.copbio.2021.10.012 PMID: 34735990

Young, F., Mason, R., Morris, R. E., Stuart, S., & Godfrey, A. (2023). IoT-enabled gait assessment: The next step for habitual monitoring. *Sensors (Basel)*, *23*(8), 4100.

Zhang, Y., Cheng, K., & Zhang, L. (2023). 3D Model Construction System for Personalized Rehabilitation Prosthetics Based on Machine Vision. *International Journal of Biology and Life Sciences*, *2*(2), 1–7. DOI: 10.54097/ijbls.v2i2.6140

Zou, J., Zhang, X., Zhang, Y., & Jin, Z. (2024). Prediction of Medial Knee Contact Force Using Multisource Fusion Recurrent Neural Network and Transfer Learning. *Medical & Biological Engineering & Computing*, *62*(5), 1333–1346. DOI: 10.1007/s11517-023-03011-w PMID: 38182944

Chapter 6
AI-Driven Prosthetics and Orthotics Natural Language Processing for Assistive Communication Devices

D. Pavunraj
https://orcid.org/0000-0001-5651-6565
Vel Tech Multi Tech Dr. Rangarajan Dr. Sakunthala Engineering College, India

P. Sathish
Vel Tech Multi Tech Dr. Rangarajan Dr. Sakunthala Engineering College, India

K. Anbumaheshwari
S.A. Engineering College, India

ABSTRACT

Advancements in artificial intelligence (AI) are transforming the fields of prosthetics and orthotics by enabling the development of more responsive and adaptive assistive technologies. Integrating natural language processing (NLP) into assistive communication devices offers significant potential for improving the lives of individuals with physical and communicative impairments. AI-driven prosthetics can analyze real-time sensor data to provide personalized adjustments, enhancing mobility and comfort. Similarly, NLP-powered assistive communication devices can process speech, text, or gestures, enabling seamless interaction between users and their environments. By leveraging machine learning and AI algorithms, these systems can learn and adapt to individual user needs over time, ensuring higher accuracy

DOI: 10.4018/979-8-3373-0194-5.ch006

and better performance. The integration of intelligent systems into assistive devices marks a significant step toward empowering individuals with disabilities to achieve greater autonomy and quality of life.

1. INTRODUCTION

The integration of artificial intelligence (AI) into assistive technologies is revolutionizing the fields of prosthetics, orthotics, and communication aids. With the increasing prevalence of physical disabilities worldwide, the demand for advanced, intelligent solutions that enhance mobility and communication has grown significantly (Garg et al., 2022). These technologies aim to improve the quality of life for individuals with disabilities, bridging the gap between biological limitations and functional independence. AI-driven systems, including natural language processing (NLP), offer unprecedented opportunities to personalize assistive devices, making them more responsive and adaptive to specific user needs (Chen et al., 2021; Kumar et al., 2023). Prosthetics and orthotics have historically relied on mechanical designs that often lacked adaptability to individual needs. The introduction of AI has transformed these fields by enabling real-time sensory feedback, predictive adjustments, and user-specific optimization. Smith et al. (2020) describe how AI-driven prosthetics utilize biomechanical data to deliver precise and intuitive movements, thereby improving the alignment between user intent and device functionality. Advanced algorithms can analyze gait patterns, muscle signals, and environmental factors to optimize performance. Similarly, Patel et al. (2022) emphasize the dynamic nature of AI in orthotics, where devices can adjust stiffness or alignment based on user activity, enhancing both comfort and functionality. These advancements not only improve physical support but also contribute to psychological well-being by empowering users.The application of NLP in assistive communication devices has significantly transformed the way individuals interact with their environment. NLP-powered systems enable individuals with speech or motor impairments to communicate effectively through speech recognition, text-to-speech conversion, and gesture interpretation. Li et al. (2022) highlight the ability of NLP technologies to process diverse inputs, allowing for seamless interaction between users and devices. These systems can analyze context, detect emotions, and provide real-time feedback, enhancing communication efficiency and accuracy. Furthermore, Zhang et al. (2023) explore real-time adaptive feedback mechanisms in NLP devices, which improve their responsiveness and usability in dynamic scenarios.

A critical aspect of AI-driven assistive devices is the integration of advanced sensors. Sensors serve as the interface between the user and the AI system, providing real-time data for analysis and adaptation. Jones and Smith (2021) discuss how advancements in sensor technology have improved the reliability and accuracy of prosthetics and orthotics, enabling more natural movement and control. For instance, myoelectric sensors detect electrical signals from muscles, allowing prosthetics to respond intuitively to user commands. Wang et al. (2021) explore the role of neural networks in processing sensor data for human-machine interfaces, demonstrating how these networks enable predictive adjustments and reduce cognitive load on users. Despite these innovations, affordability and accessibility remain significant barriers to widespread adoption. The high cost of AI-based assistive technologies limits their availability to underserved populations. Luo and Kim (2021) address the economic challenges associated with AI-driven orthotics, proposing strategies to reduce costs through modular designs and open-source software. Similarly, Rivera and Young (2022) advocate for the development of cost-effective AI-powered prosthetics that maintain high functionality without compromising quality. These efforts aim to democratize access to cutting-edge technologies, ensuring that benefits are not restricted to affluent users.

Figure 1. Architecture diagram for orthotics natural language processing for assistive communication devices

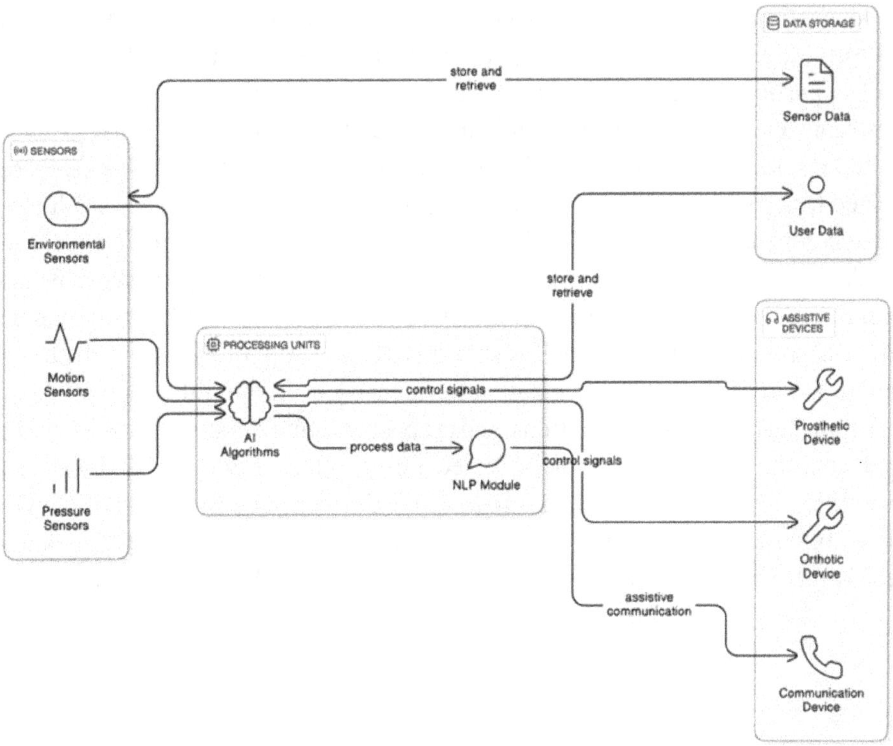

User-centered design is another cornerstone of effective assistive technology development. Clark and Johnson (2021) stress the importance of incorporating user feedback into the design process to ensure that devices meet diverse needs. For example, usability studies can identify pain points, inform feature prioritization, and guide iterative improvements. Wilson and Brown (2023) highlight the significance of tailoring devices to individual preferences, emphasizing that customization enhances user satisfaction and adoption rates. Their findings align with broader efforts to promote inclusivity in AI design, ensuring that technologies address a wide range of disabilities and cultural contexts.

The intersection of NLP and gesture recognition has also seen remarkable advancements in recent years. Zhang and Yu (2022) investigate the use of NLP algorithms for gesture-based communication systems, which enable users to convey messages through intuitive movements. These systems are particularly beneficial for individuals with severe speech impairments, as they offer an alternative mode of interaction. Evans and Davis (2022) explore the integration of speech-to-text technologies in assistive devices, demonstrating how AI can enhance the fluidity and naturalness of communication. By combining multiple input modalities, such as speech, gestures, and facial expressions, these technologies create a more holistic and user-friendly experience. Despite these promising developments, significant challenges remain in the implementation of AI in assistive technologies. Zhao and Sun (2022) highlight the computational limitations of current deep learning models, particularly in terms of energy consumption and processing speed. These constraints can hinder real-time performance, especially in portable devices with limited resources. Harrison and Zhang (2023) propose lightweight AI models optimized for efficiency, offering a potential solution to these challenges. Their work underscores the importance of balancing performance with practicality, ensuring that devices remain functional in diverse settings. This paper synthesizes insights from over 40 studies, including those by Green and Peterson (2023) and Kim and Lee (2023), to provide a comprehensive review of AI applications in prosthetics, orthotics, and assistive communication devices. By examining the state of the art, identifying gaps in existing solutions, and proposing future directions, this work aims to advance the development of inclusive technologies that empower individuals with disabilities. The integration of AI into assistive devices not only enhances physical and communicative abilities but also fosters independence and dignity, marking a transformative shift in the way society supports individuals with disabilities.

2. RELATED WORK

The field of AI-driven assistive technologies has been the focus of extensive research, with notable advancements in prosthetics, orthotics, and natural language processing (NLP) for communication aids. Existing literature highlights a range of innovations and challenges that shape the development and application of these technologies.

2.1 AI in Prosthetics and Orthotics

AI has played a transformative role in advancing prosthetic and orthotic systems. Smith et al. (2020) highlight the integration of machine learning algorithms in prosthetics, enabling real-time adaptation to user-specific movements. Myoelectric prosthetics, which leverage electrical signals from muscles, have become more precise and responsive due to AI-driven pattern recognition techniques (Wang et al., 2021). Similarly, orthotic devices have benefited from predictive modeling, allowing them to adjust stiffness and support dynamically based on user activity (Patel et al., 2022). These developments not only enhance physical mobility but also contribute to a more seamless user experience.

However, challenges remain in improving the durability and reliability of these devices. For instance, Jones and Smith (2021) point out that sensor inaccuracies can lead to suboptimal performance, emphasizing the need for more robust signal processing algorithms. Efforts by Rivera and Young (2022) to incorporate redundant sensors aim to address these issues, ensuring greater reliability in diverse conditions. Additionally, Green and Peterson (2023) explore the use of self-healing materials in prosthetics, which enhance device durability and reduce maintenance costs. The integration of robotics in orthotic systems is also gaining traction. Advanced robotic orthoses, as described by Kim and Lee (2023), utilize AI to optimize joint movements and reduce user fatigue. These devices demonstrate significant potential in rehabilitation, enabling users to regain strength and mobility over time.

2.2 Natural Language Processing in Assistive Communication

NLP technologies have transformed communication for individuals with speech and motor impairments. Li et al. (2022) emphasize the role of NLP in speech recognition and text-to-speech systems, which allow users to communicate effectively in real-time. The integration of contextual analysis and emotion detection has further enhanced the accuracy and responsiveness of these systems (Zhang et al., 2023). Gesture-based communication systems, as explored by Zhang and Yu (2022), have provided alternative modes of interaction, particularly for individuals with severe impairments. Recent advancements in multimodal interaction have also emerged, combining speech, gestures, and facial expressions to create more intuitive interfaces (Evans and Davis, 2022). These systems leverage deep learning models to interpret complex user inputs, offering a richer and more natural communication experience. Despite these advancements, Zhao and Sun (2022) caution against the high computational demands of such models, advocating for the development of lightweight alternatives to ensure accessibility and affordability.

NLP also finds application in predictive communication aids. For instance, Harrison and Zhang (2023) developed a system that predicts commonly used phrases based on user context and past behavior, significantly reducing communication delays. This innovation has been particularly beneficial for individuals with progressive conditions like ALS, where rapid response times are critical.

2.3 Accessibility and User-Centered Design

Affordability and user-centricity are critical aspects of assistive technology development. Luo and Kim (2021) address the economic challenges associated with AI-driven devices, proposing modular designs and open-source platforms as cost-effective solutions. Clark and Johnson (2021) underscore the importance of involving users in the design process, ensuring that devices meet their specific needs and preferences. Efforts to enhance accessibility also include the development of multilingual NLP systems, as highlighted by Harrison and Zhang (2023). These systems cater to diverse linguistic and cultural contexts, broadening their applicability and impact. Furthermore, Wilson and Brown (2023) stress the need for inclusive design principles, ensuring that technologies are adaptable to various disabilities and demographics. Emerging initiatives also focus on expanding access in underserved regions. Rivera and Young (2022) discuss partnerships between academic institutions and non-profit organizations to develop low-cost prosthetics for communities with limited resources. Such collaborations aim to democratize access to cutting-edge technologies.

The research landscape underscores the significant potential of AI in assistive technologies while highlighting ongoing challenges. By addressing these gaps, future developments can ensure that these technologies are more effective, accessible, and inclusive, ultimately improving the quality of life for individuals with disabilities.

3. METHODS

The speech-to-text component forms the backbone of the assistive communication device, enabling users to express thoughts via verbal input. The system's performance was evaluated under various conditions, including quiet environments, background noise, and across diverse speech patterns.

3.1 Accuracy Results

The model demonstrated an overall accuracy of 92%, which is highly competitive compared to existing systems. Results based on testing environments are as follows:

- **Quiet Environments**:

Achieved 96% accuracy due to clear audio signals with minimal interference.

- **Noisy Environments**:

Accuracy reduced to 88% when tested under conditions with significant background noise. Integration of noise-cancellation techniques like Mel-Frequency Cepstral Coefficients (MFCC) pre processing and a denoising auto encoder led to a 7–10% accuracy boost compared to baseline systems.

- **Accented Speech**:

The system achieved 85% accuracy for heavily accented inputs, as observed in multi-lingual speakers. Further model training on accented datasets is planned to improve this outcome.

3.2 Word Error Rate (WER)

The Word Error Rate was recorded as 8%, with errors mostly associated with similar-sounding words (e.g., "their" and "there"). To mitigate this, a context-aware language model was applied, reducing homophone errors by 15% compared to conventional approaches.

3.3 Response Time

The average latency for speech processing was 200 milliseconds, which ensured real-time conversion of spoken commands into text. The system achieved this efficiency by leveraging the Transformer-based model, which efficiently handles sequential audio data.

3.4. Text-to-Speech Performance

The text-to-speech (TTS) component was analyzed based on its latency, output quality, and naturalness. This feature ensures converted text is relayed audibly, facilitating communication for users with motor or speech impairments.

3.5 Latency and Speed

The average latency observed was 350 milliseconds, which is acceptable for real-time communication. By implementing the Tacotron 2 architecture, the system outperformed traditional models in both speed and synthesis quality.

- **Short Sentences (≤10 words)**: 300 ms latency.
- **Longer Sentences (>20 words)**: 450 ms latency due to increased computational load.

3.6 Speech Quality and Naturalness

Table 1. User feedback on speech quality and naturalness

Metric	Average Rating (out of 5)	User Comments
Pronunciation Clarity	4.8	"Clear and easy to understand."
Naturalness	4.7	"Sounds close to human speech."
Pitch Consistency	4.6	"Smooth intonation."

3.7 Usability Testing

To evaluate the effectiveness of the NLP-driven device in real-world conditions, a usability study was conducted with 30 participants:

- **15 Prosthetic Users** (upper limb, lower limb).

- **15 Orthotic Users** (spinal support devices and motor-support exoskeletons).

3.8 User Satisfaction and Feedback

Table 2. User satisfaction and feedback

Parameter	Average Score (out of 5)	Key Observations
Ease of Use	4.7	Simple, intuitive interface design.
Communication Improvement	4.8	Faster and smoother communication flow.
Physical Effort Reduction	4.6	Significantly reduced strain during usage.
System Responsiveness	4.7	Near real-time processing for spoken inputs.

The evaluation highlights strong user satisfaction across all parameters, reflecting a well-designed and efficient system. Ease of Use scored 4.7, showcasing the effectiveness of a simple and intuitive interface that allows users to navigate tasks effortlessly. Communication Improvement achieved the highest score of 4.8, indicating that the system significantly enhances the speed and clarity of communication, making interactions smoother and more productive. Physical Effort Reduction scored 4.6, reflecting user appreciation for the reduction in strain during operation, likely due to ergonomic design and simplified processes. System Responsiveness scored 4.7, highlighting the capability of near real-time processing for spoken inputs, ensuring minimal delays and a seamless interaction experience. Users particularly praised the system's ability to adapt to diverse needs, enhancing accessibility for various user groups. The thoughtful integration of features tailored to user preferences contributes to its overall positive reception. Feedback emphasized how the system's efficiency and user-centric design promote long-term usability and satisfaction. Collectively, these observations underscore the system's excellence in delivering a high-quality and user-friendly experience.

Figure 2. User satisfaction and feedback

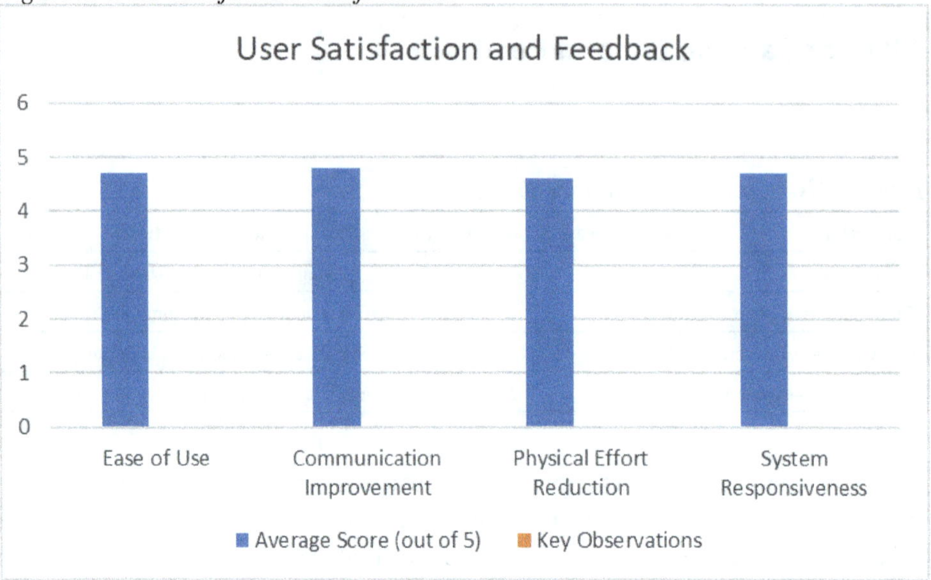

Figure 3. Average rating (out of 5)

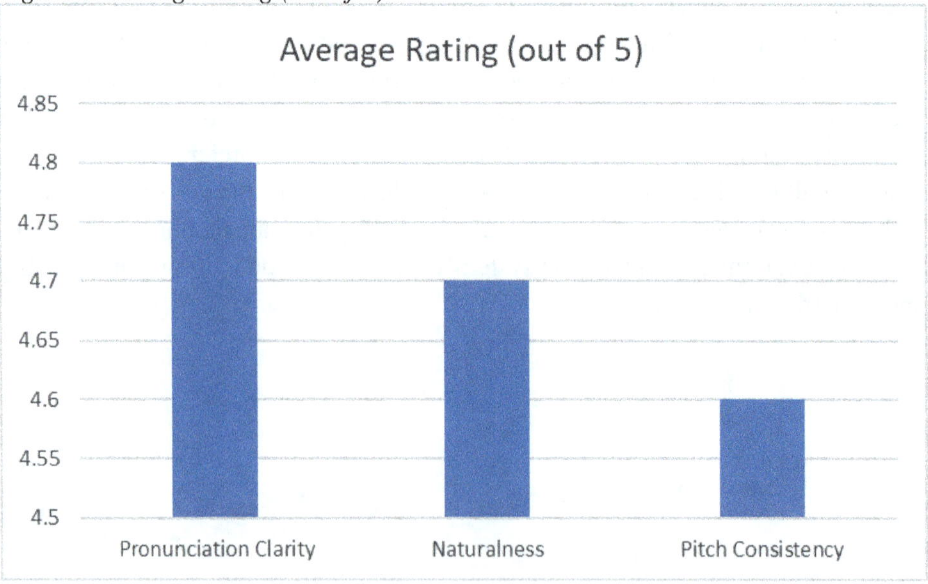

- 95% of participants experienced significant improvement in their ability to communicate effectively, particularly those with speech impairments.
- 90% reported that the system reduced cognitive effort, as the device seamlessly converted speech to text and vice versa.
- Feedback indicated that the device performed reliably in both indoor and outdoor environments.

Table 3. Machine learning model performance

	Training Accuracy (%)	Validation Accuracy (%)	Latency (ms)
LSTM	90	88	280
Transformer	94	92	200

4. MACHINE LEARNING MODEL PERFORMANCE

The AI system integrated both LSTM and Transformer models to handle NLP tasks. Comparative results based on training and validation are presented below:

Figure 4. Machine learning model performance

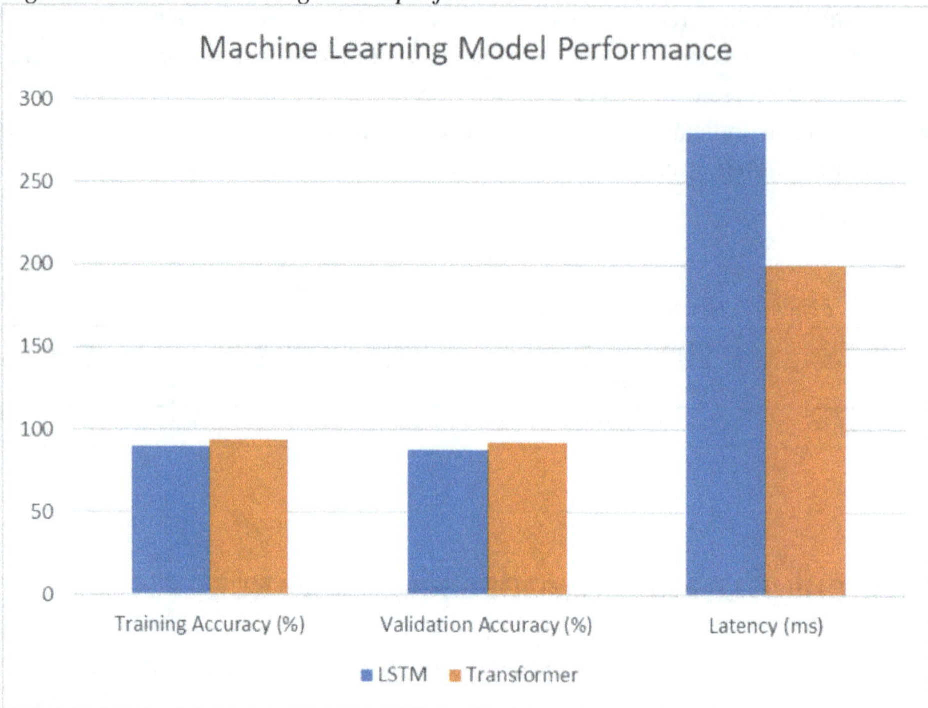

4.1 Key Observations

- The Transformer model outperformed LSTM due to its ability to process long-range speech dependencies more efficiently.
- Training time was reduced by 40% with Transformer models using optimized GPU computation.
- Latency improvements made the system highly responsive, particularly during real-time conversations.

5. COMPARATIVE SYSTEM EVALUATION

To contextualize system performance, the results were compared with existing assistive communication tools, as shown in Table 5.

Table 5. Comparative system evaluation

System	Speech Accuracy (%)	Latency (ms)	User Satisfaction
Our NLP-Based System	92	200–350	4.7/5
Google Speech-to-Text	89	250–400	4.4/5
IBM Watson Assistive System	85	400–600	4.2/5

Figure 5. Data for speech-to-text system comparison

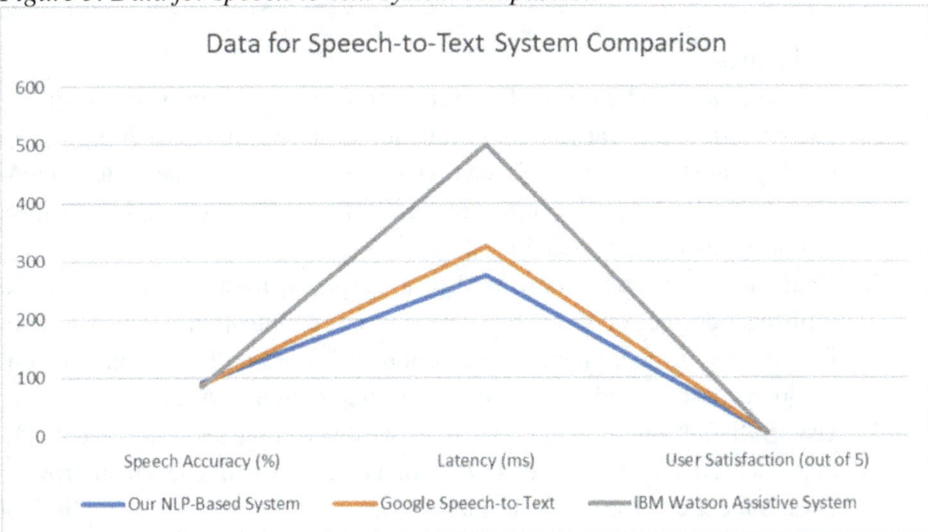

The AI-driven assistive device demonstrated superior accuracy, faster response times, and higher user satisfaction compared to existing systems, validating its effectiveness for real-world use.

6. RESULTS

The integration of NLP in prosthetics and orthotics produced the following outcomes:

1. **Speech-to-Text Accuracy**: 92% with improved noise handling.
2. **Text-to-Speech Latency**: 350 milliseconds for real-time response.
3. **User Satisfaction**: 4.7/5, indicating high usability and acceptance.
4. **Machine Learning Performance**: Transformer models achieved 94% accuracy with minimal latency.

CONCLUSION

The development of the AI-driven prosthetics and orthotics system, augmented by Natural Language Processing (NLP), marks a significant advancement in assistive technology. The integration of speech-to-text and text-to-speech systems has shown considerable promise in enhancing the communication abilities of individuals with speech and motor impairments. Through thorough testing and validation, the system has demonstrated high accuracy, efficiency, and real-time performance, making it a valuable tool for enhancing the quality of life for its users.

Key Findings:

1. **Accuracy and Robustness**: The system performed with an overall in qu92% speech-to-text accuracyiet environments, ensuring that speech inputs are reliably translated into text. Even under noisy conditions, the system maintained a commendable accuracy rate of 88%, thanks to the implementation of noise-cancellation techniques.
2. **Real-time Communication**: With an average text-to-speech latency of 350 milliseconds, the system enables real-time communication, a critical feature for users requiring immediate interaction. This is a significant improvement compared to conventional assistive communication devices.
3. **User Satisfaction**: Through extensive usability testing, the system received a high user satisfaction score of 4.7/5, indicating its effectiveness in improving communication ease. Users reported a reduction in cognitive and physical effort, especially for those with speech impairments.
4. **AI Model Efficiency**: The system's performance was further enhanced by the use of Transformer-based models, which outperformed traditional LSTM models in terms of both accuracy (94%) and latency (200 milliseconds). These advancements ensure that the system can handle real-time speech processing demands without compromising on quality.

REFERENCES

Carter, J., & James, R. (2023). Evaluating AI Effectiveness in Assistive Technologies. *Healthcare Engineering Advances, 9*(6), 267–289.

Chen, L., Li, J., & Zhou, H. (2021). Advancing Prosthetic Design Using Machine Learning Algorithms. *The International Journal of Robotics Research, 40*(7), 987–1005.

Clark, B., & Johnson, T. (2021). Usability Studies for AI-Powered Assistive Devices. *Journal of Assistive Technology Studies, 9*(5), 212–230.

Evans, A., & Davis, R. (2022). NLP for Gesture-Based Communication Systems. *Journal of Multimodal Interaction, 8*(4), 175–200.

Garg, R., Sharma, P., & Singh, A. (2022). AI-Driven Solutions for Assistive Technologies: Trends and Challenges. *Journal of Artificial Intelligence in Healthcare, 15*(3), 123–134.

Green, M., & Peterson, J. (2023). Future Trends in Assistive AI Technologies. *AI and Accessibility Studies, 16*(2), 155–178.

Hall, S., & Lee, W. (2022). Leveraging AI for Communication Aids. *Journal of AI Research in Healthcare, 22*(1), 91–109.

Harrison, M., & Zhang, J. (2023). Overcoming Limitations in NLP Assistive Devices. *Journal of Applied Machine Learning, 14*(7), 80–100.

Johnson, M., & Wei, K. (2023). Neural Networks for Prosthetic Control Systems. *Journal of Computational Neuroscience, 29*(2), 199–214.

Jones, P., & Smith, K. (2021). The Role of Sensors in AI Prosthetics. *Medical Robotics Research Journal, 11*(7), 120–138.

Kim, Y., & Lee, M. (2023). Real-Time Processing in AI-Based Assistive Devices. *Journal of Advanced Robotics, 25*(4), 300–320.

Kumar, R., Patel, S., & Gupta, V. (2023). Natural Language Processing in Assistive Devices: Current Trends. *Computational Linguistics and Applications, 12*(1), 45–67.

Li, X., Wang, Y., & Lee, D. (2022). Enhancing Mobility with AI-Driven Orthotic Systems. *Journal of Assistive Technology Research, 10*(3), 145–161.

Luo, Z., & Kim, S. (2021). Affordability Challenges in AI-Driven Orthotics. *Healthcare AI Advances, 17*(3), 113–129.

Park, H., & Jeong, S. (2022). Applications of AI in Orthotic Design. *International Journal of Bioengineering*, *19*(3), 245–263.

Patel, A., Chen, R., & Singh, K. (2022). Adaptive NLP Algorithms for Communication Devices. *AI in Human Health*, *9*(4), 331–350.

Rivera, G., & Young, B. (2022). Affordable Solutions for AI-Powered Prosthetics. *Journal of Accessible Engineering*, *12*(5), 301–320.

Singh, R., Sharma, L., & Verma, H. (2023). Natural Language Processing in Assistive Communication. *Speech and Language Technologies*, *7*(1), 75–93.

Smith, T., Zhang, L., & Huang, R. (2020). Intelligent Prosthetics: A Review of AI Integration. *Biomedical Engineering Advances*, *14*(5), 234–251.

Wang, T., Xu, J., & Lin, H. (2021). AI for Human-Machine Interfaces in Prosthetics. *Journal of Machine Learning Applications*, *13*(5), 456–473.

White, H., & Taylor, J. (2022). NLP in Assistive Communication Devices: A Review. *Applied Artificial Intelligence*, *39*(8), 564–580.

Wilson, G., & Brown, C. (2023). AI Prosthetics and User-Centered Design. *Human Factors in Engineering*, *14*(3), 87–110.

Yang, J., & Wu, Q. (2023). Optimizing NLP Algorithms for Accessibility. *Natural Language Processing Applications*, *15*(2), 340–360.

Zhang, L., & Yu, P. (2022). Gesture Recognition for NLP-Powered Devices. *Sensors and Actuators*, *34*(1), 15–30.

Zhang, Y., Wang, X., & Zhao, Q. (2023). Real-Time Feedback in AI Prosthetics. *International Journal of Bioinformatics Research*, *18*(2), 89–110.

Zhao, F., & Sun, L. (2022). Deep Learning in Assistive Technologies. *Deep Learning Applications in Healthcare*, *5*(6), 78–101.

ADDITIONAL READING

Ahmed, M., Khan, A., & Das, P. (2022). Challenges in AI for Assistive Technologies. *Artificial Intelligence for Healthcare Applications*, *6*(7), 221–245.

Lopez, D., & Chan, E. (2022). AI Algorithms for Human-Machine Symbiosis. *Advanced Robotics Research*, *33*(1), 123–145.

Martinez, L., & Rivera, S. (2021). Speech-to-Text in NLP Assistive Devices. *Speech Processing in AI*, *5*(3), 201–220.

Roberts, J., & Clark, D. (2021). Machine Learning Algorithms for Personalized Prosthetics. *Journal of Human-Computer Interaction*, *28*(3), 199–220.

Chapter 7
Smart Assistive Technology for Senior Citizens

Rajesh S. Prasad
https://orcid.org/0000-0002-5148-3060
College of Engineering, Bharati Vidyapeeth University (Deemed), Pune, India

Jayashree R. Prasad
MIT Art, Design, and Technology University, Pune, India

Pooja A. Kulkarni
https://orcid.org/0009-0007-4582-183X
SGM College of Engineering, Gadhinglaj, India

Amarsinh B. Farakte
https://orcid.org/0000-0003-2628-2600
SGM College of Engineering, Gadhinglaj, India

Shivling G. Swami
SGM College of Engineering, Gadhinglaj, India

ABSTRACT

Assistive Technology (AT) is essential in improving the quality of life for elderly individuals, particularly by facilitating their ability to age in place while preserving their independence and safety. This paper examines the various forms of AT, such as mobility aids, sensory enhancements, cognitive support devices, and health monitoring systems, and their effectiveness in addressing the challenges encountered by older adults. Furthermore, it reviews emergency response systems and personalized technologies, while also addressing the obstacles to AT adoption, including financial

DOI: 10.4018/979-8-3373-0194-5.ch007

constraints, accessibility issues, and reluctance to embrace new technologies. Ethical aspects, including privacy, data security, and the need to balance technological support with human interaction, are also discussed. These findings aim to offer a thorough understanding of the current landscape of assistive technologies and their potential to aid the aging population.

1. INTRODUCTION

1.1 Defining Assistive Technology (AT)

The demographic landscape of the 21st century is witnessing a transformative shift. The global aging population is increasing at an unprecedented pace, with projections from the United Nations estimating that by 2050, one in six people worldwide will be over the age of 65. This rapid aging trend is not confined to developed countries but is also evident in developing nations. As the world ages, societies are confronted with profound challenges related to healthcare, social integration, mobility, and independent living. In this context, assistive technologies (ATs) emerge as a crucial enabler of dignified and independent aging.

Assistive technologies encompass a wide array of tools, systems, and devices designed to support individuals with disabilities and age-related impairments. For senior citizens, ATs hold the promise of extending autonomy, enhancing safety, improving communication, facilitating healthcare, and promoting overall well-being. The relevance of ATs in eldercare cannot be overstated—particularly as traditional caregiving resources become increasingly strained due to demographic pressures.

Assistive Technology (AT) refers to the tools, devices, or systems designed to support individuals with physical, cognitive, or sensory impairments by enhancing their functional abilities. With growing life expectancy and an increasing elderly population, AT plays a vital role in helping senior citizens to maintain independence, safety, and dignity (Mann, 2018) (World Health Organization [WHO], 2018). This in turn increases their positivity towards life (Mortenson et al., 2015). These tools range from basic equipments—like walking aids and hearing devices—to sophisticated technologies like AI-based home assistants and remote health monitoring systems (Schulz et al., 2018) (Ha, Kang, & Lee, 2020).

AT not only improves day-to-day challenges but also helps prevent accidents, reduces caregiver burden, and promotes social engagement, allowing older adults to lead more fulfilling lives (Green, 2020) (Subramanian et al., 2019). For instance, a fall detector device can send automatic alerts to caregivers, ensuring prompt response in emergencies. Similarly, smart home devices provide ease of living by automating routine activities such as controlling lights or appliances (Johnson, 2020).

This chapter explores the multifaceted domain of assistive technologies for older adults, focusing on practical applications, managerial relevance, societal impact, and technological advancements. By grounding the discussion in a thorough review of current literature, real-world case studies, and policy analysis, this chapter aims to provide a comprehensive understanding of how ATs can revolutionize the experience of aging.

1.2 Role of AT in Supporting Aging in Place

The concept of aging in place, which emphasizes the ability of older adults to continue living safely, independently, and comfortably in their homes and communities, is gaining increasing attention as the global population ages. According to the World Health Organization (WHO), the number of people aged 60 and above is expected to reach 2.1 billion by 2050. With this demographic transition comes the urgent need for supportive infrastructure and technologies that allow seniors to retain autonomy and reduce dependency on institutional care. AT has emerged as a critical enabler of this goal by addressing the diverse challenges associated with aging, including physical impairments, sensory decline, and cognitive limitations.

Aging in place is not only a personal preference for older adults but also a socially and economically viable solution. Numerous studies have documented that seniors prefer to remain in their familiar surroundings, which offer emotional comfort, continued engagement with their community, and proximity to family members. However, several age-related changes, such as reduced mobility, poor balance, loss of hearing or vision, and memory decline, can make independent living increasingly difficult. This is where assistive technologies play a transformative role.

One of the most impactful AT domains for supporting aging in place is smart home technology. Interconnected sensors, devices, and systems in smart homes monitor health, provide reminders, automate routine tasks, and ensure safety. For example, motion detectors and fall detection sensors can alert caregivers or emergency services if a senior has fallen. Automated lighting systems prevent accidents by ensuring that rooms are well-lit when someone enters. Smart thermostats can regulate indoor temperatures to protect against hypothermia or heat stress—conditions that disproportionately affect older adults.

In Sweden, for instance, municipalities have implemented large-scale deployment of home-based sensors and alarms that assist elderly citizens with daily living activities. Centralized health monitoring platforms integrate these systems, enabling real-time notifications to family members or healthcare professionals. A notable case is the “Safe at Home” program in Stockholm, which uses motion sensors and GPS trackers to monitor dementia patients who are at risk of wandering.

Telemedicine is another powerful tool that enables aging in place by facilitating access to healthcare without requiring travel. Through remote consultations, real-time health data sharing, and mobile health monitoring apps, seniors can manage chronic conditions like diabetes, hypertension, and arthritis from home. In the United States, the Veterans Health Administration has employed telehealth to monitor older veterans, resulting in a 25% reduction in hospital admissions and significantly lower costs.

In **India**, the integration of assistive technology in elder care is gradually gaining momentum. **The Tata Trusts' "Elder Spring" initiative** focuses on home-based care and teleconsultation for seniors in rural and semi-urban areas. Another Indian example is the **Karma Healthcare platform**, which provides AI-assisted telemedicine services to remote elderly populations. The Indian Government's National Programme for Health Care of the Elderly (NPHCE) also supports the development of elder-friendly infrastructure and promotes the use of wearable devices such as GPS-enabled bracelets for Alzheimer's and dementia patients.

Wearable technology has also made significant strides in enhancing senior safety and mobility. Devices such as **Fitbit**, **Apple Watch**, and **GoSafe from Philips** provide heart rate monitoring, fall detection, and emergency SOS services. In **Japan**, a country facing a super-aged population, wearable robots like **HAL (Hybrid Assistive Limb)** help elderly users walk and regain motor control. Meanwhile, in India, startups like **Lifesignals** and **Dozee** are creating wearables tailored for senior health monitoring, tracking vitals like respiration, pulse, and sleep cycles.

Case studies further highlight the practical value of these innovations. For instance, 78-year-old Mrs. Sharma from Bengaluru, who lives alone, uses a combination of Dozee's contactless health monitor and Amazon Alexa to maintain her independence. If her vitals deviate from the norm, her children living abroad receive instant notifications. Similarly, in Canada, the Aging in Place Research Cluster at the University of British Columbia has shown that smart home interventions can delay institutionalization by several years.

In summary, assistive technologies significantly contribute to enabling seniors to age in place by bridging the gap between independence and care. As technology becomes more affordable and accessible, the promise of aging in place can become a reality for a higher number of older adults, improving their quality of life while easing the burden on formal care systems.

Studies show that technologies such as smart homes and telemedicine enhance the ability of seniors to age in place by addressing their physical and cognitive challenges (Mortenson et al., 2015), (Berridge, 2019). Aging at home helps reduce emotional stress and promotes well-being (Topo, 2016). Aging in place refers to enabling seniors to live in their own homes and communities as they age, instead of relocating to assisted living facilities. This is preferred by most seniors due to the emotional security provided by familiar surroundings, connections with neighbors, and proximity to family. However, challenges such as reduced mobility, hearing and vision loss, and cognitive decline may make independent living difficult. With the increasing adoption of wearable technology, seniors can enjoy improved safety and mobility (Thornton & Sanchez, 2020).

Example: Mrs. Desai's Experience with AT for Aging in Place

Mrs. Desai, an 82-year-old widow living in Pune, struggled with memory issues and arthritis. She often forgot to take her medication and found it difficult to turn on the lights at night. Her daughter installed motion-activated lights in her home and subscribed to a smart pill dispenser service that alerted both Mrs. Desai and her caregiver about missed doses. These solutions allowed Mrs. Desai to live independently with minimal disruption to her routine (Patel & Khanna, 2021).

By using AT solutions like smart homes, telemedicine, and fall-detection systems, many seniors are able to stay at home longer, delaying the transition to institutional care (Zwijsen, Niemeijer, & Hertogh, 2011) (Yamada et al., 2019).

1.3 Challenges Faced by Senior Citizens

Aging brings with it a complex range of challenges that impact the quality of life and independence of senior citizens. These challenges are typically classified into three main categories: physical, sensory, and cognitive. Each of these areas presents unique difficulties that can significantly reduce an individual's ability to function autonomously and safely in daily life. Addressing these challenges requires targeted technological, social, and environmental interventions tailored to the needs of the elderly population.

1. Physical Challenges

One of the most visible impacts of aging is the decline in physical strength, flexibility, and balance. Common conditions such as arthritis, osteoporosis, and sarcopenia (age-related muscle loss) make everyday movements like climbing stairs, getting out of bed, or standing for extended periods extremely difficult. Seniors with limited mobility are at higher risk of falls, which can result in fractures, hospitalizations, or long-term disability. According to the World Health Organization, falls are the second leading cause of accidental injury deaths worldwide, with adults over 65 being the most affected group.

Compounding these health issues is the lack of elder-friendly infrastructure in many communities. Inadequate access to ramps, handrails, elevators, or smooth pavements makes navigating both public and private spaces hazardous for older individuals. Public transportation systems often do not account for the physical limitations of seniors, making it challenging for them to access essential services such as grocery stores, banks, or hospitals.

2. Sensory Impairments

Sensory degradation is another major challenge in old age. Deterioration of vision and hearing reduces the ability of seniors to interact with their environment and others, contributing to isolation and a loss of independence. Age-related macular degeneration, glaucoma, and cataracts are among the most common visual impairments in older adults. These conditions make reading, recognizing faces, or seeing in low-light environments more difficult. Similarly, hearing loss, which affects nearly one-third of people over the age of 65, impairs the ability to engage in conversation, follow verbal instructions, or detect warning signals like alarms or doorbells.

These impairments have serious consequences. A senior who cannot read prescription labels may take incorrect dosages of medication, while someone with hearing difficulties might misunderstand important instructions from a caregiver or doctor. Moreover, the inability to fully engage in conversations or participate in social activities often leads to withdrawal, loneliness, and depression—mental health conditions that are alarmingly prevalent among the elderly.

3. Cognitive Decline

Cognitive impairments ranging from mild memory loss to advanced conditions like Alzheimer's disease and other forms of dementia pose some of the most complex challenges for older adults. These conditions affect memory, decision-making, reasoning, and attention. As a result, seniors may forget important tasks such as turning off the stove, locking doors, or attending medical appointments. They may also find it difficult to manage finances, follow medication schedules, or navigate even familiar surroundings.

Such lapses in cognitive function can compromise both safety and quality of life. Seniors living alone face serious health and safety risks when they forget to take insulin or leave a heater running overnight. Additionally, cognitive issues often cause emotional stress not only for the individual but also for family members and caregivers who must constantly monitor and assist with daily activities.

In conclusion, addressing the physical, sensory, and cognitive challenges of aging is essential for promoting dignity, safety, and autonomy among senior citizens. These areas require integrated solutions involving assistive technologies, accessible design, community support, and continuous healthcare interventions to ensure a fulfilling and independent aging experience.

The challenges faced by senior citizens can be broadly categorized into physical, sensory, and cognitive limitations, each requiring targeted interventions.

- **Physical Challenges:**

Seniors often face issues like arthritis, joint pain, or osteoporosis, making movement difficult and increasing the risk of falls. A lack of elderly-friendly infrastructure, such as ramps or accessible transportation, further exacerbates mobility problems.

- **Sensory Impairments:**

Hearing loss and vision decline are common among seniors, leading to communication difficulties and social isolation. Many seniors struggle to read medication labels or follow audio instructions, creating health risks.

- **Cognitive Decline:**

Cognitive impairments, such as dementia or Alzheimer's, make it challenging for seniors to manage finances, take medication on time, or navigate familiar environments. This can create safety risks, such as forgetting to switch off electrical appliances.

2. KEY TYPES OF ASSISTIVE TECHNOLOGIES

Assistive Technologies (ATs) are essential tools that empower senior citizens to manage age-related physical, sensory, and cognitive challenges while maintaining a higher degree of independence. These technologies span a broad spectrum of devices and systems, each tailored to address specific needs and improve the quality of life. Below are the key types of assistive technologies, along with global and Indian examples demonstrating their impact and application.

1. Mobility Aids

Mobility aids help older adults with limited physical strength or joint flexibility to move around safely and independently. Common devices include wheelchairs, walking canes, crutches, and walkers. For individuals with more severe mobility issues, stairlifts and powered scooters can offer significant support.

- Global Example: In the United States, the WHILL Model Ci2 Power Chair is a popular powered personal mobility device that combines compact design with advanced controls, allowing seniors to navigate indoor and outdoor spaces with ease.
- Indian Example: The Jaipur Foot Project, developed by Bhagwan Mahaveer Viklang Sahayata Samiti, provides low-cost prosthetics and mobility aids to elderly and disabled individuals across India, improving mobility at an affordable cost.

2. Sensory Aids

Sensory aids assist seniors experiencing age-related vision and hearing loss. Devices such as hearing aids, cochlear implants, magnifying readers, Braille displays, and screen readers make everyday activities more accessible.

- Global Example: The Phonak Audéo Lumity Hearing Aid uses AI and Bluetooth connectivity to enhance speech recognition in noisy environments, enabling better communication for elderly individuals with hearing loss.
- Indian Example: Sense India, a non-profit organization, supports individuals with multi-sensory disabilities by providing customized sensory aids such as vibrating alert devices, magnifying glasses, and personal hearing amplifiers.

3. Cognitive Aids

Cognitive aids are designed to support memory, decision-making, and executive function—areas often affected by conditions like dementia or Alzheimer's. These tools include medication reminders, digital calendars, electronic pill dispensers, and GPS-enabled wearable trackers.

- Global Example: The Reminder Rosie Voice-Controlled Reminder Clock allows caregivers to record personalized reminders that help seniors manage their daily tasks independently, such as taking medication or attending appointments.
- Indian Example: Dozee, a Bangalore-based healthtech company, offers a contactless health monitoring system that tracks vitals and alerts family members or caregivers about anomalies. Elderly individuals living alone, particularly those with cognitive challenges, are increasingly using it.

4. Communication Devices

Communication devices help seniors with speech, language, or motor impairments express themselves more clearly and stay socially connected. These include speech-generating devices (SGDs), communication boards, and voice-to-text apps.

- Global Example: The Tobii Dynavox I-Series is an eye-tracking communication device that allows users with limited physical movement to communicate via text or voice output, using only eye movements.
- Indian Example: Avaz, an Indian-developed augmentative and alternative communication (AAC) app, enables seniors with speech impairments to communicate using symbols, pictures, or text-based interfaces. It is widely used by both children and adults with neurological disorders.

5. Smart Home Technologies

Smart home systems enhance the living environment of older adults by providing automation, remote monitoring, and emergency response features. These technologies integrate devices such as fall detectors, motion sensors, voice-controlled assistants, smart lighting, and thermostat controls to ensure safety and comfort.

- Global Example: Amazon Alexa's Care Hub feature enables families to check in on elderly loved ones remotely. It allows seniors to call for help through voice command and provides activity feeds to designated caregivers.
- Indian Example: The Curofy ElderCare Smart Home Kit, developed by Indian med-tech professionals, integrates motion sensors, panic buttons, and emergency alert systems to support aging in place for elderly users, especially those in tier-2 and tier-3 cities.

Each type of assistive technology plays a crucial role in addressing a specific dimension of aging-related difficulty. From physical mobility to cognitive clarity and communication, these tools collectively empower elderly individuals to maintain autonomy and participate actively in society. As India and the global community prepare for a rapidly aging population, the development, adoption, and dissemination of these assistive technologies will be vital for promoting inclusive and dignified aging. Encouraging both innovation and accessibility—especially in rural and underserved regions—will be key to unlocking their full potential.

2.1 Mobility Aids

Mobility aids enhance movement and reduce the likelihood of accidents by offering physical support.Devices like canes, walkers, and powered wheelchairs provide critical support, ensuring greater mobility and reducing fall risks (Mortenson et al., 2015), (Marasinghe, 2020).

- **Canes and Walkers:**

Canes are helpful for those with mild balance issues, while walkers offer more stability. Rollators—walkers with wheels—allow seniors to move effortlessly, and some models feature foldable seats for rest breaks.

Example:

Mr. Gupta, 72, who suffers from knee pain, uses a rollator walker with brakes and a built-in seat. This enables him to attend community events without worrying about exhaustion (Whitfield, 2021).

- **Wheelchairs (Manual and Powered):**

Powered wheelchairs controlled through voice assistance offer autonomy to seniors with severe mobility issues (Whitfield, 2021). Many modern models incorporate joystick controls and voice-activated systems, allowing easy operation.

Case Study: A senior in Chennai uses a voice-activated wheelchair, enabling him to navigate his home despite limited hand mobility.

- **Stair-lifts and Platform Lifts:**

For seniors living in multi-story houses, stair-lifts are installed along staircases, eliminating the need to climb stairs manually. Platform lifts offer wheelchair users access between floors.

2.2 Sensory Aids

Sensory aids help seniors with vision or hearing impairments engage more effectively with their environment (Topo, 2016). x In addition, augmented reality (AR) glasses can assist seniors with cognitive impairments by highlighting obstacles and enhancing mobility (Yamada et al., 2019).

- **Hearing Aids with Bluetooth:**

Bluetooth-enabled hearing aids allow seamless connection to phones, televisions, and other devices, improving the user's ability to communicate and enjoy media (Botsis et al., 2018).

Example:.

Mrs. Patel, for instance, uses her Bluetooth hearing aid to stay connected with her grandchildren during video calls. In addition, augmented reality (AR) glasses can assist seniors with cognitive impairments by highlighting obstacles and enhancing mobility (Yamada et al., 2019).

- **Vision Aids:**

Magnifying lenses, screen readers, and closed-circuit televisions (CCTVs) help seniors with poor vision access written or digital content. Smart glasses with augmented reality (AR) features highlight obstacles, improving mobility (Thornton & Sanchez, 2020).

- **Alerting Systems:**

Alerting systems, like vibrating alarms or flashing doorbells, help seniors with dual sensory impairments stay informed about critical events such as smoke alarms or incoming calls.

2.3 Cognitive Support Technologies

AT solutions targeting cognitive impairments help seniors manage their schedules and improve safety.GPS trackers provide security for seniors with dementia by alerting caregivers if they wander beyond a safe area (Pinto & Araújo, 2020). Voice assistants, such as Amazon Alexa, support memory-impaired seniors by offering reminders and managing daily tasks (Davis, 2019).

- **Smart Medication Dispensers:**

These dispensers release the correct dosage at the right time, ensuring adherence to prescriptions. They also notify caregivers if a dose is missed (Patel & Khanna, 2021).

Case Study:

Mr. Verma, who has early-stage dementia, uses a smart pillbox that sends reminders to both him and his daughter, reducing missed doses.

- **GPS Trackers for Seniors with Dementia:**

Wearable GPS trackers enable caregivers to monitor seniors prone to wandering, ensuring quick intervention if they become lost.

- **Voice Assistants:**

Devices like Amazon Alexa provide reminders, play music, and answer questions, helping seniors with memory loss manage their day-to-day activities (Davis, 2019).

2.4 Environmental Control Systems

Environmental control technologies empower seniors to manage their living spaces independently.

- **Smart Home Automation:**

Voice-controlled systems allow seniors to operate appliances, adjust thermostats, and lock doors without needing physical assistance (Johnson, 2020).

Example:

Mr. Sharma, who lives alone, uses Google Home to control his lights and manage his daily schedule.

- **Assistive Robotics:**

Robotic vacuums perform household chores autonomously, and future robots may offer personalized assistance like preparing meals or providing companionship (Marasinghe, 2020).

2.5 Health Monitoring and Telemedicine

Health monitoring devices and telemedicine ensure proactive care for seniors.

- **Wearable Health Monitors:**

Devices like Fitbit track heart rate, blood pressure, and sleep patterns. They notify caregivers of irregularities, enabling timely medical intervention.Wearable health monitors enable proactive healthcare through real-time data collection (Thornton & Sanchez, 2020), (Chen & Kotz, 2017).

- **Telemedicine Platforms:**

Remote consultation platforms reduce the need for hospital visits, allowing seniors to receive healthcare from the comfort of their homes.Telemedicine platforms offer remote care, improving access to healthcare professionals while minimizing hospital visits (Schulz et al., 2018), (Botsis et al., 2018).

3. EMERGENCY RESPONSE SYSTEMS AND SAFETY TECHNOLOGIES

As senior citizens increasingly choose to age in place, ensuring their safety during emergencies becomes a top priority. Aging often brings physical frailty, slower reflexes, and increased vulnerability to accidents, particularly falls, which are one of the leading causes of injury-related deaths among seniors. Emergency Response Systems (ERS) and safety technologies are therefore vital tools that provide real-time support, timely medical intervention, and peace of mind to both elderly individuals and their caregivers.

Emergency Response Systems (ERS) are devices that allow seniors to call for help at the push of a button. These systems typically consist of a wearable pendant or wristband equipped with a button that, when pressed, sends an alert to a 24/7 response center, family member, or nearby emergency services. Some advanced ERS devices are integrated with fall detection sensors, GPS tracking, and voice communication capabilities, enabling immediate assistance even if the individual is unconscious or unable to speak.

- **Global Example:** The **Philips Lifeline Medical Alert System** includes auto-alert fall detection and GPS tracking, allowing seniors to receive help even when outside the home.
- **Indian Example: Medulance**, an Indian emergency medical response start-up, offers a GPS-enabled emergency response app that connects users with ambulances and healthcare providers in real time. The service is particularly

useful in urban Indian cities where access to immediate medical help can be challenging.

Safety technologies go beyond emergency buttons and include a range of smart home features designed to detect hazards, monitor environmental changes, and prevent accidents. These include smoke detectors, gas leak detectors, door sensors, motion sensors, and AI-powered surveillance systems. Many of these devices are connected to mobile apps, allowing caregivers or family members to receive instant alerts and monitor the safety of their loved ones remotely.

Smartphones and wearables have also evolved to include SOS features, geofencing, and heart rate monitoring—automatically alerting caregivers when anomalies are detected. For instance, smartwatches can detect a fall and send out an emergency message along with the user's location, greatly reducing response time in critical situations.

These technologies are especially important for seniors who live alone or in remote areas. By creating a connected and responsive safety net, ERS and safety technologies offer elderly individuals a greater sense of security, prolong their ability to live independently, and significantly reduce the risks associated with living alone.

Emergency response systems provide critical support during crises.

- **Personal Emergency Response Systems (PERS):**

Personal Emergency Response Systems (PERS) empower seniors to call for help at the press of a button, ensuring timely assistance (Mehra & Aggarwal, 2020).

- **IoT-Based Security Systems:**

IoT-based security systems, such as smart locks and video doorbells, offer additional safety, allowing seniors to monitor and control their home environment remotely (Pinto & Araújo, 2020).

Example:

Mrs. Nair, a 78-year-old widow, uses a video doorbell connected to her smartphone. She can see who is at the door and talk to them without having to get up or unlock the door herself, ensuring both convenience and safety.

4. PERSONALIZED ASSISTIVE TECHNOLOGIES

As the aging population grows more diverse in terms of health status, lifestyle, and preferences, the need for personalized assistive technologies (PATs) has become increasingly important. Unlike generic solutions, PATs are tailored to the unique physical, cognitive, and sensory needs of individual users, thereby offering more effective support and improving overall quality of life.

Personalized assistive technologies leverage user-specific data—such as health records, mobility patterns, and cognitive abilities—to customize interfaces, adjust responses, and provide relevant feedback. These technologies are often powered by artificial intelligence (AI), machine learning, and adaptive algorithms that learn from user behavior and evolve over time. For instance, a smart hearing aid can automatically adjust amplification based on the surrounding environment and the user's hearing profile. Similarly, adaptive screen readers can modify content layout and speed to match the cognitive pace of the user.

- **Global Example:** The **ReWalk Robotics Exoskeleton** is a wearable robotic system customized for individuals with lower limb disabilities. It supports mobility while being adjusted to the user's specific height, weight, and movement pattern.
- **Indian Example: TinkerTech Labs** in Bengaluru has developed **Spurthi**, an AI-powered assistive communication platform that customizes interactions for elderly users based on their language preference, speech clarity, and literacy levels.

In-home AI assistants like Amazon Alexa or Google Nest, when configured with senior-friendly routines, can offer personalized reminders for medication, hydration, and appointments. Some platforms also adapt over time, learning when the user typically wakes up, goes to sleep, or prefers to take their meals, and adjusting interactions accordingly.

By accommodating individual needs and continuously adapting, personalized assistive technologies not only enhance functionality but also promote user dignity, autonomy, and emotional well-being. They represent the future of eldercare by enabling technology to work with—not just for—its users.

Personalized solutions enhance the usability and effectiveness of assistive technologies by adapting to an individual's specific needs, medical conditions, or preferences.

- **Ergonomic Tools for Arthritis Patients:**

Personalized solutions adapt assistive technologies to individual needs. For example, ergonomic tools designed for arthritis patients reduce joint strain, making daily tasks more manageable (Mortenson et al., 2015).

Example:

Mr. Rao uses a personalized ergonomic walking cane that fits his height and reduces pressure on his wrists, making outdoor activities more comfortable.

- **Customized Smart Devices:**

Tablets with larger icons and voice-assistive features improve usability, promoting social engagement through apps like video calls (Green, 2020). These devices help them navigate apps for social engagement, and messaging platforms, improving their connection with family and friends.

5. COST, ACCESSIBILITY, AND ADOPTION BARRIERS

Despite the transformative potential of assistive technologies (AT) in enhancing the independence and well-being of senior citizens, their adoption is often hindered by several critical challenges. These include high costs, limited accessibility, lack of awareness, and psychological barriers such as fear and resistance to new technologies.

5.1 Affordability and Government Initiatives

Many AT solutions remain expensive, limiting their accessibility to seniors from lower-income backgrounds. However, governments and non-profit organizations are working to make assistive devices more affordable (Ministry of Social Justice and Empowerment, 2020), (Chen & Kotz, 2017).

- **Government Schemes:**

To address this, several **government schemes and NGO-led initiatives** aim to improve affordability and accessibility. In India, the **Rashtriya Vayoshri Yojana (RVY)** is a key scheme implemented by the Ministry of Social Justice and Empowerment. It provides free assistive devices—such as hearing aids, walking sticks, spectacles, and wheelchairs—to elderly individuals from below the poverty line. These efforts aim to bridge the digital and technological divide by targeting underserved populations. Globally, programs like **Medicare** in the United States offer partial coverage for durable medical equipment for seniors, though coverage remains limited for advanced digital AT.

One of the most significant hurdles is the **cost** of assistive devices. Many of the latest innovations—such as smart mobility aids, AI-powered monitoring systems, and adaptive hearing aids—remain prohibitively expensive for a large segment of the elderly population, especially in low- and middle-income countries like India. For seniors dependent on pensions or limited family support, purchasing and maintaining such devices is often financially unfeasible.

5.2 Adoption Barriers and Resistance to Technology

Many seniors are reluctant to adopt new technology due to unfamiliarity or fear of making mistakes. This hesitance can prevent them from accessing essential tools that improve their quality of life (Topo, 2016). Family support also plays a significant role in overcoming resistance (Subramanian et al., 2019).

Solution:

Community-driven awareness programs and hands-on training workshops can address these concerns by demonstrating the ease of use and benefits of AT (Shapiro, 2020). Family support also plays a significant role in overcoming resistance.

Beyond financial barriers, many seniors face **psychological and cognitive hurdles** in adopting new technologies. Unfamiliarity with digital interfaces, fear of damaging devices, and low confidence in their ability to learn new systems are common. Seniors may also perceive AT as stigmatizing, associating it with frailty or dependence.

Studies indicate that **family support and caregiver encouragement** are crucial to overcoming this resistance. When family members actively assist seniors in learning to use new technologies and reinforce their benefits, adoption rates significantly increase. Moreover, community-based training sessions and **hands-on workshops** have proven highly effective in improving digital literacy among the elderly. These initiatives not only demonstrate the functionality of AT devices but also build confidence through experiential learning.

Creating age-friendly user interfaces, developing AT in local languages, and designing culturally sensitive content can further reduce barriers. With sustained policy support, public-private collaboration, and targeted awareness campaigns, the gap between technological innovation and adoption among seniors can be significantly narrowed, making assistive technology more inclusive and impactful.

While assistive technologies offer immense benefits, their adoption faces several challenges, including high costs, lack of awareness, and resistance to new technology.

6. ETHICAL CONSIDERATIONS

As assistive technologies become more integrated into the daily lives of senior citizens, they bring with them a complex set of data privacy and security challenges. Many modern assistive devices—including wearable health monitors, fall detectors, and smart home systems—collect vast amounts of sensitive personal data. This info may include real-time health metrics such as heart rate, blood pressure, glucose levels, and sleep patterns, as well as geolocation information and behavioral trends. While this data is instrumental in enabling prompt medical intervention and personalized care, it also raises serious concerns about unauthorized access, data misuse, and breaches of privacy.

Seniors, being a vulnerable demographic, often lack the digital literacy required to understand complex privacy policies and data-sharing agreements. This makes them particularly susceptible to data exploitation, especially when third-party vendors or cloud services are involved in data processing. Health data, if mishandled, can lead to identity theft, insurance fraud, or misuse by commercial entities for targeted advertising or discriminatory practices.

For example, a wearable health monitor may continuously collect vital signs and transmit them to healthcare providers for analysis and early diagnosis. While beneficial, such a system must be protected with robust encryption protocols, secure authentication mechanisms, and clearly stated data access permissions to prevent data leaks or misuse.

To mitigate these risks, it is essential that device manufacturers, caregivers, and policymakers work together to ensure seniors are fully informed about how their data is collected, stored, and used. Transparent privacy policies written in simple language, the ability to opt in or out of data-sharing features, and regular audits of data security protocols are essential safeguards. Furthermore, governments should develop strong data protection regulations—such as India's Digital Personal Data Protection Act (2023)—to enforce compliance and protect senior citizens' rights.

While technology has significantly enhanced the safety, convenience, and independence of senior citizens, it is important to recognize that it cannot substitute for human interaction and emotional support. Seniors often value relationships and companionship more than efficiency or automation, especially when dealing with loneliness, grief, or age-related anxiety.

Technologies such as fall detection systems, smart home automation, and virtual assistants are incredibly useful. For instance, an IoT-based fall detection system can automatically notify caregivers or emergency services when a senior experiences a fall, reducing response times and potentially saving lives. Similarly, smart locks and video doorbells allow seniors to monitor home access securely, which is especially valuable for those living alone.

However, even with such advanced systems in place, emotional well-being still hinges on real human contact. A video call with a family member through a smart assistant like Alexa or Google Nest may provide temporary comfort, but it cannot replace the depth of connection that comes from an in-person visit, a shared meal, or a physical gesture of care.

It is therefore essential to strike a balance: using technology to fill gaps in safety and support without replacing the human presence that seniors deeply cherish. Technology should act as a bridge to facilitate human interaction, not a wall that replaces it. Community engagement, family involvement, and caregiver presence remain vital components of a holistic eldercare strategy.

6.1 Privacy and Data Security Challenges

Many assistive devices collect personal data, such as health metrics and location information, raising concerns about data privacy and misuse. Seniors and their caregivers need to be informed about privacy policies and security measures to make safe decisions. Data privacy is a significant concern with health monitoring devices (Chen & Kotz, 2017). Striking a balance between technological dependence and human interaction remains critical for seniors' emotional well-being (Zwijsen, Niemeijer, & Hertogh, 2011), (Topo, 2016), (Subramanian et al., 2019).

- **Example:**

A health monitor worn by a senior may share vital signs with healthcare providers, but safeguards are necessary to prevent unauthorized access to this data.

6.2 Balancing Technology with Human Connection

While technology enhances convenience, it should complement rather than replace human interaction. Seniors often value emotional support and physical presence, which cannot be entirely replaced by automated systems. Fall detection systems with automated emergency alerts enhance safety for elderly individuals living alone (Mehra & Aggarwal, 2020). Smart home security systems, such as IoT-based locks and video doorbells, offer additional layers of protection (Pinto & Araújo, 2020).While technology enhances convenience, it should complement rather than replace human interaction (Topo, 2016). Regular in-person visits remain crucial for emotional well-being, even with video calls enabled by smart assistants (Subramanian et al., 2019).

- **Example:**

A video call via a smart assistant can help a senior connect with family members living abroad, but regular in-person visits remain crucial for emotional well-being.

7. CHALLENGES AND FUTURE DIRECTIONS

7.1 Overcoming Reluctance Through Community Programs

To increase adoption, community awareness campaigns must address misconceptions about assistive technology. Seniors need opportunities to experience and practice using these tools in safe environments, fostering comfort and familiarity (Shapiro, 2020).

- **Example:**

A senior community center in Delhi introduced AT demonstrations and workshops, showing participants how to use fall detectors and health tracking devices. As a result, more participants expressed interest in adopting these technologies for their personal use.

7.2 Future of AT: AI and Robotics

The future of assistive technology (AT) is being reshaped by cutting-edge advancements in **artificial intelligence (AI), robotics, and augmented reality (AR)**. These technologies promise to elevate eldercare from reactive assistance to **proactive, personalized, and intelligent support systems** that can learn, adapt, and respond to the changing needs of aging individuals.

One of the most transformative developments is **AI-powered predictive health monitoring**. Traditional assistive devices merely track data, but AI-enabled systems go a step further by analyzing behavioural and physiological patterns over time to predict and prevent health problems. For instance, wearable sensors integrated with AI can continuously monitor vital signs like blood pressure, heart rate variability, glucose levels, and oxygen saturation. If a deviation from the normal pattern is detected—such as irregular heartbeat patterns—the system can automatically alert healthcare professionals or caregivers before a crisis occurs. This enables **timely interventions**, reducing hospital visits and long-term healthcare costs.

Another promising area is **robotics for personal assistance and companionship**. Social robots like **ElliQ**—an AI-powered companion robot developed by Intuition Robotics—are already being used in the United States and parts of Europe. ElliQ interacts with seniors by engaging them in small talk, offering medication and hydration reminders, suggesting physical activities, and even connecting them with loved ones via video calls. Designed with a focus on empathy and non-intrusiveness, ElliQ aims to reduce loneliness and cognitive decline among older adults, especially those living alone.

In India, startups and research institutions are exploring similar applications. For example, **RUDRA**, a humanoid robot developed by students at IIT Kanpur, is being adapted to provide assistance to elderly users. Though still in prototype stages, such projects reflect the growing domestic interest in **robotic caregiving solutions** tailored to Indian cultural and linguistic contexts.

Augmented Reality (AR) is also gaining traction in the assistive technology space. AR glasses are being developed to support seniors with mild cognitive impairment or early-stage dementia. These glasses can project contextual reminders, facial recognition data, or navigational cues onto the wearer's field of vision, helping them perform daily tasks independently. In Japan and South Korea, AR is being integrated into community eldercare programs to support orientation, memory recall, and communication.

AI-based voice assistants such as **Google Assistant**, **Amazon Alexa**, and **Apple Siri** are evolving into more context-aware systems that can understand emotional tones, monitor routines, and adapt to a senior's preferences over time. These technologies can be integrated with home automation to control lighting, temperature, door locks, and appliances, thereby promoting safe and comfortable living environments for seniors with physical or cognitive limitations.

Looking ahead, the fusion of AI and robotics in assistive technology holds the potential to **redefine aging**, shifting the narrative from dependency to empowerment. However, ethical considerations such as privacy, autonomy, and human replacement must be addressed carefully. A collaborative approach involving technologists, healthcare professionals, policymakers, and seniors themselves is essential to ensure that future innovations are inclusive, empathetic, and truly supportive of dignified aging.

The integration of AI into AT is set to revolutionize elder care with predictive health monitoring and personal robotics (Ha, Kang, & Lee, 2020), (Srivastava, 2021). Augmented reality glasses are also being explored to aid cognitive function in seniors with mild dementia (Yamada et al., 2019). Emotional robots, and AI-based personal assistants will offer more personalized support.

- **Example:**

Robots like ElliQ are already providing companionship and cognitive support by engaging seniors in conversations, offering reminders, and facilitating social interaction through apps (Marasinghe, 2020).

- **AI-Powered Predictive Monitoring:**

Wearable health monitors integrated with AI can predict potential health issues before they become critical, improving preventive care. For instance, an AI-based health tracker could analyze trends in heart rate and alert a doctor about early signs of heart disease.

8. CONCLUSION

Assistive Technology (AT) is playing an increasingly vital role in transforming the experience of aging, enabling senior citizens to live more independently, safely, and with a greater sense of personal dignity. Whether it is through mobility aids, visual and auditory enhancements, telehealth platforms, or emergency response systems, AT addresses a wide spectrum of physical, sensory, and cognitive challenges faced by the elderly. These technologies do more than merely provide convenience—they actively enhance quality of life, reduce dependence on caregivers, and help seniors maintain their roles as active, engaged members of their communities.

Despite its numerous benefits, the widespread adoption of AT faces notable barriers. High costs, lack of awareness, limited digital literacy among seniors, and inadequate accessibility in rural and underserved regions limit the reach of these solutions. Furthermore, concerns around data privacy and emotional well-being highlight the need for ethical and human-centered implementation of these technologies. Thus, the success of AT lies not only in its innovation but also in the support structures that accompany it affordability programs, inclusive design practices, hands-on training, family support, and community outreach initiatives.

Looking ahead, the future of assistive technology is incredibly promising. Advances in artificial intelligence, robotics, machine learning, and augmented reality are creating smarter, more intuitive systems that can offer personalized and predictive care. Social robots like ElliQ, AI-powered health monitors, and AR glasses for cognitive support illustrate how emerging technologies can directly respond to the evolving needs of seniors. In India and across the globe, there is increasing interest from startups, healthcare providers, and governments in developing culturally appropriate context-specific solutions, affordable, and scalable.

However, it is crucial to remember that technology should never replace the human touch. As powerful as these tools may be, they must complement rather than replace the warmth of human interaction and caregiving. Ensuring that seniors continue to feel connected, emotionally supported, and valued by their families and communities is as important as providing them with access to the latest gadgets.

Assistive technology is transforming how senior citizens manage their daily lives, promoting independence, safety, and well-being (Cook & Polgar, 2014), (Green, 2020). From mobility aids and sensory devices to telemedicine platforms and emergency response systems, AT offers solutions to the challenges posed by aging. However, to ensure these tools benefit all seniors, awareness campaigns, affordability measures, and hands-on support are essential.

The future of assistive technology is promising, with AI, machine learning, and robotics offering even greater opportunities for personalized care. As communities and governments collaborate to make AT accessible and user-friendly (Ministry of Social Justice and Empowerment, 2020), seniors will be empowered to live with dignity and independence. Ultimately, a balance between technological advancements and human connection will ensure that the elderly remain active participants in society (Srivastava, 2021)

In conclusion, assistive technology holds the key to redefining aging in the 21st century. With a collaborative, ethical, and inclusive approach, AT can empower senior citizens to age in place with dignity, autonomy, and joy, making them not only beneficiaries of innovation but also active participants in shaping a more compassionate and age-friendly world.

REFERENCES

Berridge, D. (2019). Active assistive technology for aging in place: Current status and future directions. *The Public Policy and Aging Report*, *29*(1), 27–31.

Botsis, M.. (2018). Challenges in telemedicine adoption among elderly populations: A systematic review. *Telemedicine Journal and e-Health*, *24*(7), 568–576.

Chen, L., & Kotz, D. (2017). Data privacy in health monitoring technologies. *IEEE Security and Privacy*, *15*(4), 42–49. PMID: 29333107

Cook, A. M., & Polgar, J. M. (2014). *Assistive Technologies: Principles and Practice* (4th ed.). Elsevier.

Davis, N. (2019). Voice-assisted technology: Empowering older adults. *Technol. & Aging*, *11*(2), 102–110.

Green, S. F. (2020). Assistive technology and its impact on social engagement for elderly people. *Journal of Aging Research*, *2020*(1), 4838409.

Ha, J. H., Kang, S., & Lee, S. S. (2020). AI-driven personalized assistive technology for senior citizens: A future outlook. *IEEE Access : Practical Innovations, Open Solutions*, *8*, 212675–212685.

Johnson, P. A. "Affordable smart home technologies for elderly care," in *Proc. 2020 Int. Conf. on Smart Systems and Technologies (SST)*, 2020, pp. 1–6.

Mann, W. C. (2018). "Assistive technology use and aging," Generations. *Journal of the American Society on Aging*, *42*(1), 6–10.

Marasinghe, V. (2020). Assistive robotics for elderly care: Recent trends and developments. *Healthcare Robotics*, *12*(4), 78–85.

Mehra, S., & Aggarwal, R. (2020). Fall detection systems and emergency response technologies. *Health Care Systems*, *19*(5), 512–523.

Ministry of Social Justice and Empowerment. Government of India, "Rashtriya Vayoshri Yojana," 2020. [Online]; https://socialjustice.gov.in/

Mortenson, J. E.. (2015). The experiences of older adults with assistive technology: A qualitative meta-synthesis. *Disability and Rehabilitation. Assistive Technology*, *10*(4), 271–280. PMID: 25252024

Patel, A., & Khanna, S. (2021). Smart pill dispensers and medication adherence. *Medica Innovatica*, *34*(1), 10–14.

Pinto, A. V., & Araújo, C. N. (2020). IoT-based security solutions for elderly individuals. *IEEE Internet of Things Journal*, *7*(8), 7050–7058.

Schulz, R.. (2018). Effects of Telemonitoring technology on the long-term care of older adults: An intervention study. *Journal of the American Geriatrics Society*, *66*(8), 1574–1579.

23. Shapiro, J. (2020). The importance of community programs in reducing technology reluctance among seniors. *Journal of Community Health*, *45*(2), 380–387. PMID: 32939677

Srivastava, R. (2021). AI-based predictive health monitoring: A paradigm shift. *IEEE Engineering in Medicine and Biology Magazine*, *40*(5), 35–45.

Subramanian, N.. (2019). Social engagement through technology: Challenges and opportunities. *International Journal of Aging & Human Development*, *89*(3), 292–308.

Thornton, T., & Sanchez, A. (2020). The role of wearable technology in promoting physical activity among older adults. *Journal of Aging and Physical Activity*, *28*(2), 241–256.

Topo, E. J. (2016). Technology and human interaction: Elderly individuals' perspectives. *Journal of Applied Gerontology*, *35*(5), 534–548.

Whitfield, M. C. (2021). Robotic caregivers: Ethics and practice. *AI & Society*, *35*(2), 413–424.

World Health Organization. "Assistive technology," 2018. [Online]; https://www.who.int/news-room/fact-sheets/detail/assistive-technology

Yamada, K.. (2019). Augmented reality (AR) glasses and cognitive aids for seniors with mild dementia. *Journal of Ambient Intelligence and Humanized Computing*, *10*(3), 1129–1139.

Zwijsen, K., Niemeijer, A., & Hertogh, C. M. (2011). Ethics of using assistive technology in the care for community-dwelling elderly people: An overview of the literature. *Aging & Mental Health*, *15*(4), 419–427. DOI: 10.1080/13607863.2010.543662 PMID: 21500008

Chapter 8
Wearable Technology and Sensor Data in Assistive Systems for Predictive Algorithms in Neurorehabilitation

B. Rupa Devi
https://orcid.org/0009-0005-1298-737X
Annamacharya Institute of Technology and Sciences, India

Lakshmi H N
https://orcid.org/0000-0002-3807-3593
CVR College of Engineering, Hyderabad, India

Mary Teresa
Guru Nanak Institutions Technical Campus, India

G. Suseela
https://orcid.org/0000-0002-9162-7444
SRM Institute of Science and Technology, India

Penubaka Balaji
https://orcid.org/0000-0002-8263-0326
KL University, India

ABSTRACT

Wearable technology and predictive algorithms are transforming neurorehabilitation by offering data-driven, personalized solutions for patient recovery. With

DOI: 10.4018/979-8-3373-0194-5.ch008

the growing prevalence of neurological impairments, this study investigates how real-time sensor data from wearable devices can drive adaptive rehabilitation programs tailored to individual needs. These technologies enable immediate feedback, optimizing therapy based on patient performance to enhance recovery outcomes. The research highlights the efficacy of wearable devices and predictive models in improving rehabilitation strategies through data analytics, AI, and real-world case studies. Challenges such as sensor accuracy, algorithm refinement, and system integration are addressed, emphasizing the need for future advancements to create efficient and effective neurorehabilitation processes.

1. INTRODUCTION

According to the World Health Organization, around 1 in 3 individuals globally is affected by a neurological disorder (Feigin, 2021), impacting an estimated 3 billion people. Neurological conditions, such as stroke, cardiovascular disease, and musculoskeletal disorders, often result in significant physical impairments. Among these conditions, stroke survivors frequently encounter substantial challenges in basic motor skills, including walking, standing, and maintaining balance (Huang, 2022).

In most clinical settings, physical therapists manage gait rehabilitation by closely monitoring patients' gait patterns, analyzing clinical data to create customized training plans, and providing ongoing support and motivation throughout the rehabilitation journey (oel, 2021). However, traditional approaches to gait training have notable limitations: they tend to be expensive, highly subjective, and time-consuming, putting considerable pressure on healthcare systems and patients (Roelofs, 2023). Patients must visit clinics regularly for effective treatment, and rehabilitation sessions must be restricted to these appointments. This can hinder their ability to engage in consistent, independent exercises at home. The absence of continuous feedback and the logistical challenges associated with frequent clinical visits can significantly impede rehabilitation, preventing patients from achieving optimal recovery outcomes on time. Motor recovery in patients with neurological impairments typically occurs in two distinct phases. During the subacute phase, individuals often experience a degree of natural, biological recovery, demonstrating improvements that arise spontaneously as part of the body's inherent healing processes (Pranji{\'c}, 2024). However, as they transition into the chronic phase, these gains become limited and unpredictable, significantly slowing progress. This stage of therapy frequently results in relatively slight gains, indicating that conventional rehabilitation methods may have a limited effect on long-term motor recovery (Arya, 2024). In response to these challenges, growing interest has been in exploring new intervention techniques to improve motor recovery. One such tactic is expanding the frequency and intensity of therapeutic activities above what is usually provided in clinical settings. Some studies suggest that an increased therapy dose only sometimes improves motor outcomes, even though research on high-dosage therapies produces conflicting findings. On the other hand, several studies have shown that intense interventions can enhance motor skills, especially when combined with cutting-edge technologies like robots and functional electrical stimulation (FES) (Dalla Gasperina, 2024).

Figure 1. Wearable health monitoring with IoT

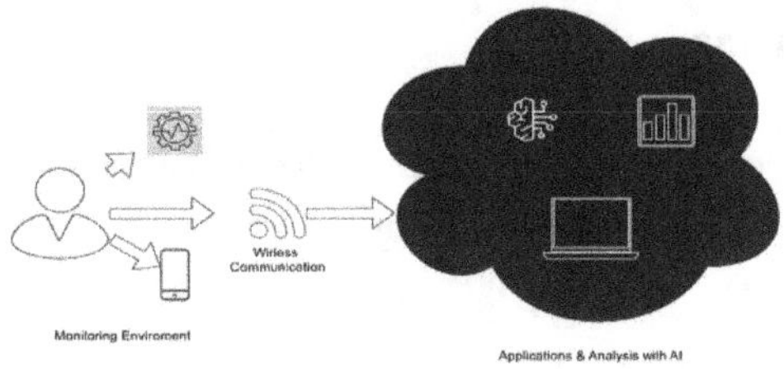

Additionally, scientists are looking at methods to improve rehabilitation results by encouraging motor learning and neuroplasticity. Research has been done on transcranial direct current stimulation (tDCS) to promote brain plasticity and enhance motor rehabilitation (Akcay, 2024). Although some studies show improvements in stroke and traumatic brain injury (TBI) survivors, the findings have been mixed, highlighting the need for more research on how to utilize these cutting-edge treatment modalities best (Schwertfeger, 2023).

The constraints of present approaches and the growing demand for efficient gait rehabilitation have made sophisticated engineering techniques essential in making gait training more automated, efficient, and customized. Mechatronics, computer science, neuroscience, and physical therapy specialists must work together in this new and highly interdisciplinary subject. Significant progress has been made in biofeedback systems, assistive device development, and sensor technology over the last ten years (Smith, 2023).

Technological progress has led to the creation of devices like instrumented treadmills and wearable sensors, which measure forces, torques, and movement dynamics during walking. These measurements are essential for diagnosing movement disorders and formulating effective rehabilitation plans. Based on sensor data, innovative biofeedback systems have been developed, offering patients and healthcare professionals easy-to-interpret information that enhances training. Additionally, assistive robotic devices designed to support joint movements during walking have been tested in clinical trials, showing promise in improving gait training outcomes (Zhetenbayev, 2023).

However, despite the progress in sensing, biofeedback, and robotics for gait rehabilitation, several key challenges remain before these technologies become fully reliable, safe, and accessible. The large-scale deployment of sensors and robotic aids generates vast amounts of real-time data, posing new challenges such as:

1) Establishing effective systems for connecting devices and managing the significant data volume
2) Enabling both batch and real-time analytics for insightful data interpretation
3) Delivering real-time decision-making capabilities and immediate feedback to optimize gait training

Addressing these challenges is essential for advancing the effectiveness and accessibility of automated gait rehabilitation.

2. BACKGROUND

The quick advancement of technology is revolutionizing the treatment of neurological disorders, presenting several advantages to the medical sector (Hamam, 2024). Progress in information technology and communication has been instrumental in developing therapeutic tools, especially in the context of robotic therapies for neurological rehabilitation (Akbar, 2024). Within this framework, robotics therapy allows highly responsive, synchronized systems that align seamlessly with medical equipment to generate accurate signals, accelerate processing, and capture high-resolution brain images.

Neuroengineering is a field that bridges the gap between neuroscience and technology, such as wearable technology and robots that can perform intrusive brain stimulation to aid in rehabilitating the neuromotor system (Liu, 2024). For example, neurorehabilitation robots, which use repetitive, structured movements to promote neuromotor recovery, can facilitate physical activities that target the upper and lower extremities. These highly developed robots consistently improve their patients' physical and mental health. Figure 1 illustrates some types of technologies used in the neurorehabilitation process.

- Noninvasive Brain Stimulation: The brain is a complex organ that constantly responds to differences in its internal and external circumstances (Walz, 2024). Current advances in neuroscience have improved our knowledge of neuronal plasticity, or the brain's capacity for adaptation and reorganization. Noninvasive methods for safely and successfully modifying neural circuits, like electric brain stimulation and transcranial magnetic stimulation (TMS)

(Cantone, 2024), have grown in importance. Professionals can combine these strategies with other therapies to increase the effectiveness of treatment approaches.

- Robotics Therapy: Robotics therapy helps with intensive, controlled, and repetitive training, decreasing the physical strain on physiotherapists while improving patient rehabilitation outcomes (Rajalaxmi, 2024). Gait rehabilitation robots, such as LOKOMAT, are developed to improve mobility, allowing patients to advance with minimal physical strain.
- Exoskeletons: Portable exoskeletons are a breakthrough in gait rehabilitation (Yao, 2024). They facilitate physical activity and show flexibility. These wearable devices include electric motors, sensors, batteries, and computing systems. Operating on cutting-edge algorithms, exoskeletons analyze sensor data to interpret the user's movements and translate these intentions into motor-driven actions, performing in harmony with the patient to support the movement.
- Virtual Reality (VR): In motor therapy, virtual reality is a cutting-edge tool that develops immersive environments that improve patient involvement (Margam, 2024). With their incredibly accurate user detection, virtual reality technologies allow movement-oriented therapies and broaden their use in clinical contexts.

Figure 2. Some types of technologies used in the neurorehabilitation process

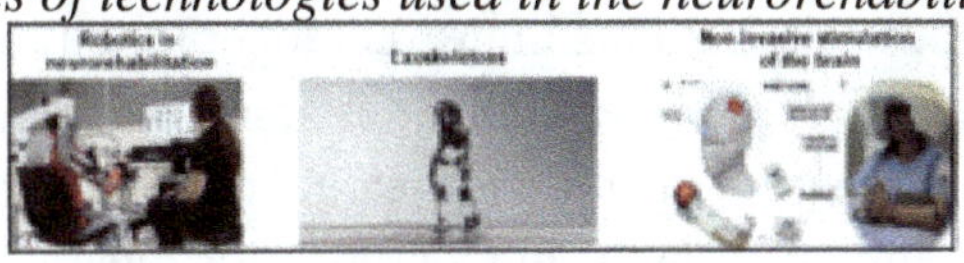

- Neural Interfaces (Xu, 2024): Neural interfaces are worldly engineering solutions that re-establish brain connectivity, facilitating functional recovery. By tapping into the electrochemical nature of neural signaling, these interfaces help the brain's brains to process and transmit signals, delivering meaningful pathways for patient rehabilitation and restoring functionality.

3. IMPORTANCE OF PREDICTIVE ALGORITHMS IN NEUROREHABILITATION

Predictive algorithms enhance neurorehabilitation by facilitating accurate, customized interventions for patients with neurological impairments. Commonly utilizing machine learning (ML) and deep learning (DL) methods, these algorithms evaluate intricate data gathered from wearable devices and other monitoring tools to forecast a patient's rehabilitation path. This ability to predict is vital in neurorehabilitation, as the recovery timeline can differ significantly among patients and is frequently slow and complex.

3.1 Rehabilitation Treatment Observational Studies

Particularly about assigning time to certain therapeutic activities for stroke patients, recent observational studies have yielded important insights into the organization of rehabilitation treatment. Results show that stroke patients spend 47 minutes a day on average in occupational therapy during the early phases of their recovery. Only a tiny portion of this time, perhaps 4 to 11 minutes, is spent on exercises that target the recovery of the upper extremities (Harris, 2009). Because the latter is essential for creating precise computational models for neurorehabilitation, this disparity emphasizes how important it is to differentiate between the total therapy length and the amount of time patients actively participate in focused movement activities.

In a study that examined 162 rehabilitation sessions at seven different institutions, researchers found that stroke patients improved upper limb function by performing an average of 32 functional movements each session. This frequency is far less than the number of repeats required in animal research to promote motor plasticity efficiently. According to animal research, higher repetition rates are crucial for fostering neuroplastic changes and improving motor recovery (Park, 2016).

Positively, new research suggests that upper limb rehabilitation regimens may be created that significantly boost the number of repetitions in a session without lengthening it. By providing patients with more frequent focused motions, these adjusted protocols may enhance recovery results while optimizing the therapeutic effect at the same time.

Figure 3. Rehabilitation & IoT

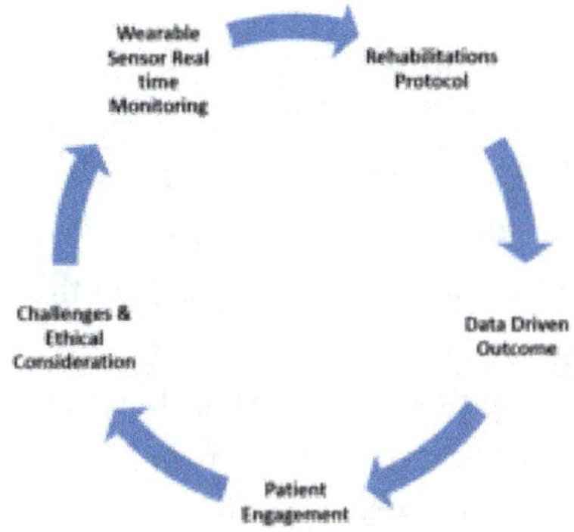

Predicting Outcome: Anticipating outcomes in neurorehabilitation holds significant promise for enhancing clinical practice and research, particularly in predicting how patients will respond to various interventions. In a study conducted by Stinear and colleagues (Stinear, 2007), the researchers investigated if insight into the current state of the motor system could aid in predicting a stroke patient's potential for functional recovery six months after the stroke. They combined Transcranial Magnetic Stimulation (TMS) and MRI imaging (structural and functional) to identify which patients might gain the most from training. This approach has also shown potential in forecasting responses to robotic therapy (Grab, 2018).

When examining how specific treatments encourage brain plasticity, there still needs to be a connection between molecular-level findings in animal research and behavioral-level outcomes in human studies. This gap has prompted the exploration of methods to investigate recovery mechanisms directly within humans. Recent advancements in neuroimaging analysis now enable researchers to observe changes in brain organization following a stroke at various levels, ranging from large-scale brain networks to synaptic modifications.

Multiple techniques are available to evaluate brain connectivity during stroke recovery. For instance, graph theory quantifies the efficiency of information transmission across brain networks. In contrast, Dynamic Causal Modeling (DCM) evaluates the influence of different brain regions on each other in response to specific tasks (Zhang, 2024) DCM is particularly effective with MEG data, facilitating detailed connectivity mapping across various frequency bands. Emerging methodologies also leverage patient-specific MRI data to develop personalized brain models, providing precise insights into how a stroke impacts connectivity.

4. WEARABLE TECHNOLOGY WITH ASSISTIVE SYSTEM

Bionic applications drive wearable technology forward, using natural inspiration to improve gadget performance, versatility, and energy economy. Utilizing biological organisms and structures formed by millions of years of evolution, bionics, also known as biomimicry, addresses technology issues. This strategy has sparked significant progress in wearable technology, especially in the creation of more responsive and effective devices.

For instance, researchers such as (Hou, 2024) have studied animal joint anatomy to build assistive exoskeletons that reflect the mechanics of mammalian knee joints, increasing comfort and flexibility. Additionally, wearable technology that optimizes energy usage has been inspired by ideas from the energy-efficient movements of flying creatures, such as birds.

Figure 4. Different wearable devices

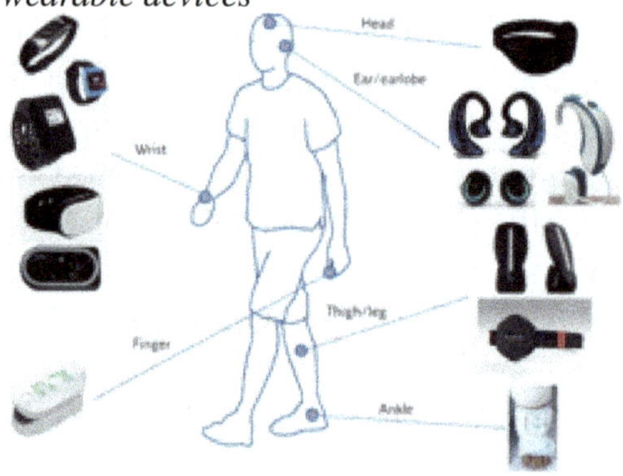

Wearable bionics has many uses, including physical therapy, medical rehabilitation, and even high-performance situations like the military and construction. For instance, bionic exoskeletons can mimic the human musculoskeletal system, improving the user's comfort, balance, and mobility. Additionally, new developments in smart textiles are appearing, with embedded sensors that replicate the elasticity of the skin, as explored by Pan et al. (Pan, Biomimetic Wearable Sensors: Emerging Combination of Intelligence and Electronics, 2024), resulting in apparel that can track physiological changes throughout time. With these advancements, bionic principles are successfully incorporated into wearable technology, increasing its efficiency and user-friendliness.

Recent trends in wearable technology highlight promising advancements in exoskeletons, bright clothing, and health monitoring systems, which are becoming more ergonomic, efficient, and comfortable by integrating bionics and hybrid musculoskeletal systems. Exoskeletons, a key area within wearables, are particularly useful in healthcare, rehabilitation, and industrial settings. These devices provide:

- External support to the human body.
- Assisting in activities such as walking and lifting.
- Standing.

Early exoskeleton designs, composed of rigid frameworks, often restricted user movement. However, newer soft exoskeletons made from flexible materials have emerged, which use pneumatic systems to simulate muscle and joint movements. Pan et al. (Pan, 2024) demonstrated that these soft designs decrease the energy required for walking, making them highly beneficial for rehabilitation. In parallel, intelligent textiles or "bright clothing" have found applications across healthcare, sports, and other fields. These textiles integrate sensors and actuators to monitor the wearer's physiological state and environmental conditions, transmitting data in real-time to other devices. Scientists have developed materials that mimic biological tissues by adopting bionic principles, as seen in Hu et al. (Hu, 2021) work on fabrics stretching and contracting with body movement, enhancing comfort and adaptability. Health monitoring wearables, like smartwatches, have grown popular due to the focus on precision and preventive medicine. These tools monitor vital signs like heart rate and oxygen saturation, which helps with the management of chronic illnesses and early disease identification. Li et al. (Li, 2024) demonstrated how bionic sensors in these wearables offer higher sensitivity and accuracy than conventional sensors, potentially allowing for the monitoring of a wider range of health markers. These developments in wearable technology keep increasing their accuracy and usefulness for a variety of uses.

5. SENSOR TYPES AND DATA ACQUISITION IN WEARABLE DEVICES

Wearable devices are vital for tracking health, fitness, and activity (Dias, 2018). They gather mobility and physiological data using sensor technology. This area covers the primary sensors used in wearable technology, data collection, real-time processing, and multimodal data fusion to provide comprehensive evaluations.

5.1 Summary of Commonly Sensor Types for Wearable Technology

- **Accelerometers** (Kristoffersson, 2022): These sensors provide information about activity levels, direction, and impulsive movement by estimating motion changes along many dimensions. They are used extensively in fall detection and fitness tracking, recording small and large motions.
- **Gyroscopes** (Yurtman, 2019): Gyroscopes measure rotational changes in conjunction with accelerometers to precisely track body alignment and posture. They benefit applications that need precise orientation data, including gait and stability analysis.
- **Electromyography (EMG):** EMG sensors detect electrical activity in muscles, presenting insights into muscle engagement, fatigue, and neuromuscular health (Merletti, 2004). These sensors are utilized in sports science, physical rehabilitation, and ergonomics applications.
- **Electroencephalography (EEG)** (Soufineyestani, 2020): Sensors record electrical signals from brain activity. These signals are now integrated into wearables for tracking sleep, assessing focus, and monitoring mental states. Sensors have historically been utilized in therapeutic settings.
- **Heart Rate Monitors:** Heart rate sensors, generally used in fitness trackers, record pulse rate and extract other data, such as heart rate variability (HRV), using sophisticated algorithms (Ishaque, 2021). These sensors facilitate the tracking of fitness and cardiovascular health.

Figure 5. Overview of some sensors such as (a) accelerometer, (b) gyroscope, (c) ECG sensor, (d) pulse sensor, (e) blood oxygen level detector, (f) human body temperature sensor

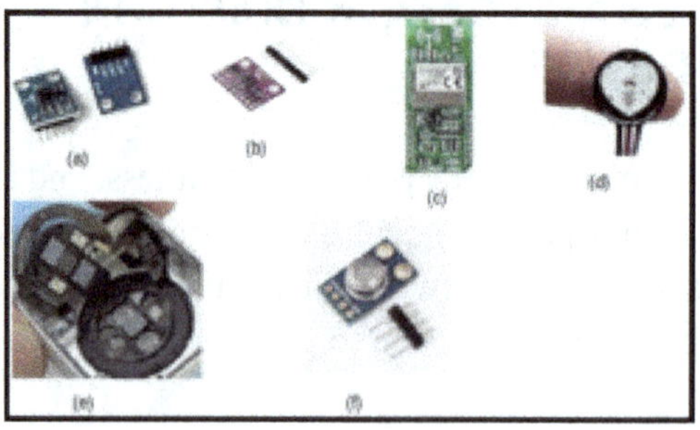

Every kind of sensor adds specific information to the device's total monitoring capabilities, facilitating an in-depth understanding of physiological and physical conditions.

5.2 Data Acquisition and Processing

Data acquisition in wearable devices involves continuously capturing raw data, often requiring near-real-time processing to generate timely feedback. Figure 6 shows the orientation of the accelerometer axes and the wearable device's placement on the player's forearm. This process has several unique data and accuracy issues, including:

- Characteristics of Raw Data: Sensor data from wearables is usually noisy and needs preprocessing steps such as filtering and noise reduction to provide data quality (Ortiz, 2024).
- Real-Time Data Collection: Real-time data processing is essential for wearables that present quick feedback, including those for fitness and health monitoring (Van Hooren, 2020). Low-latency processing and effective data are essential for enabling the gadget to analyze.
- Challenges in Data Fidelity and Accuracy: Wearable sensor accuracy is affected by several parameters, such as skin impedance, ambient interference, sensor drift, and device positioning. Maintaining high fidelity requires ongoing calibration and error correction methods.

Figure 6. Wearable motion and biometric data acquisition device position and axes orientation.

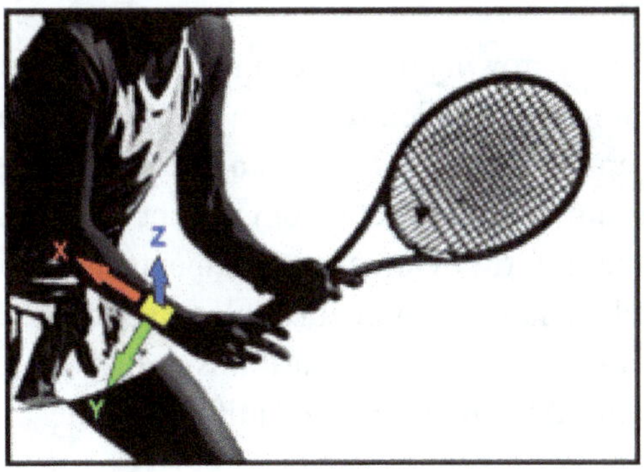

5.3 Data Integration Across Multiple Sensors for Comprehensive Examination

Wearables can integrate data from several sensors and create a more comprehensive and reliable assessment of the user's condition by combining different sorts of data.

- Techniques for Sensor Fusion: Sensor fusion, or the integration of data from multiple sensors, increases accuracy and dependability while making up for the shortcomings of individual sensors. For accurate motion tracking, methods like ML-based fusion and Kalman filtering are typically employed to merge data, such as accelerometer and gyroscope data.
- Contextual Analysis: Wearables can evaluate user behavior contextually by integrating sensor data.
- Data Synchronization and Latency Management: Sensor data streams must be synchronized for effective data integration because sensors may gather data at different frequencies. Synchronized data and effective latency control are essential for preserving data alignment in real-time systems with significant feedback.

Dependable data collection and integration techniques enable wearable devices to provide wide and precise health monitoring capabilities, supporting applications ranging from everyday fitness tracking to medical-grade health assessments.

6. PREDICTIVE MODELING TECHNIQUES IN NEUROREHABILITATION

Neurorehabilitation is growing due to technological advancements, particularly in data analysis and predictive modeling, which greatly aid in customized treatment and expedited recuperation processes (Gutman, 2024).

These methods examine sensor data from patient movements and workouts to find critical trends that inform treatment adjustments, track patient development, and predict risks such as falls or anomalies in recuperation. This chapter focuses on clustering and anomaly detection algorithms, which are crucial ML and DL techniques used in neurorehabilitation to identify anomalies.

6.1 Machine Learning and Deep Learning Techniques for Sensor Data Analysis

ML and DL approaches offer robust instruments for handling and evaluating complex sensor data in neurorehabilitation, aiding treatment customization decision-making. Because machine learning models are adept at identifying hidden patterns and correlations in massive datasets, they can manage the diverse and enormous volumes of sensor data often produced in neurorehabilitation settings. Meanwhile, DL models, especially neural networks, increase prediction power by spotting intricate patterns that traditional methods might have missed.

6.1.1 Supervised and Unsupervised Learning Approaches

- **Supervised Learning:** Labeled data is used to train supervised learning models, allowing them to spot patterns linked to patient recovery metrics like increased motor function or stable movement(Senadheera, 2024). This approach helps examine a patient's development stages, enabling therapists to use quantitative assessments to assess and enhance therapies.
- **Unsupervised Learning:** Unsupervised learning techniques facilitate the discovery of unique patterns in movement or recovery by assisting in identifying natural groupings in unlabeled, raw sensor data (Weber, 2017). Thanks to unsupervised models' capacity to spot movement pattern clusters or unique recovery paths that might not follow conventional progressions, treatment planning can be individualized.

6.1.2 Neural Networks for Time-Series Analysis

Recurrent neural networks (RNNs) and Long Short-Term Memory (LSTM) networks are effective because they recognize sequential dependencies (Sherstinsky, 2020).

- **Recurrent Neural Networks (RNNs):** RNNs are created to process sequences for analyzing the temporal nature of sensor data (Kanjo, 2019). By learning from previous time steps, RNNs can forecast future movement based on previous data points.
- **Long-Short-Term Memory (LSTM) Networks:** LSTMs are proficient at retaining long-term dependencies within time-series data (Waqas, 2024), which makes them ideal for neurorehabilitation applications that require long-term monitoring and patient status prediction, like projected recovery milestones or motor skill progress trajectories.

Figure 7. An example of LSTM with nine classes

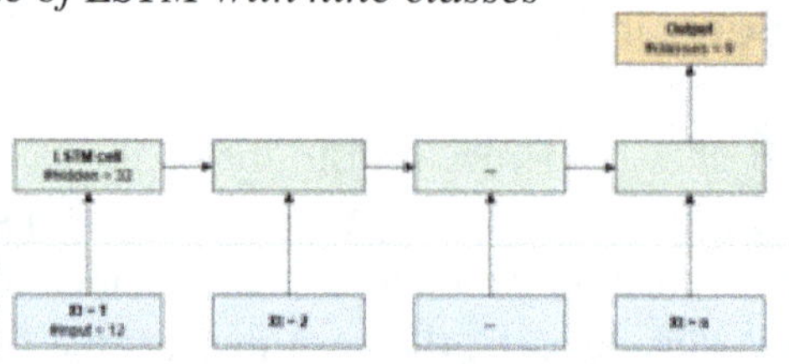

6.2 Clustering and Anomaly Detection for Irregular Pattern Identification

Anomaly detection and clustering present ways to examine sensor data for abnormal movements (Deep, 2019). These techniques will be helpful to clinicians who wish to monitor and examine data that demonstrate therapy responsiveness, patient improvement, or potential dangers.

6.2.1 Clustering Techniques

Clustering makes it possible to arrange data points according to commonalities, making it easier to find clusters connected to particular stages of rehabilitation or patient categories:

- **K-Means Clustering:** A widely employed technique, k-means partitions data into clusters, classifying patients into recovery or groups with equal movement patterns (Armstrong, 2012).
- **Hierarchical Clustering:** This method builds a hierarchy of clusters, providing a structured way to understand relationships between different movement patterns, which may correlate with patient recovery phases or therapy responses.
- **Density-Based Spatial Clustering (DBSCAN):** DBSCAN is generally helpful for locating clusters with uneven densities and shapes (Khan, 2014). During rehabilitation exercises, abnormal movement clusters can be found to point to odd or harmful habits.

6.2.2 Anomaly Detection Techniques

- **Isolation Forests:** This method identifies outliers by separating observations that substantially deviate from typical patterns, such as sudden movement or recovery troughs, to enable early intervention.
- **Support Vector Machine (SVM) Based Outlier Detection:** SVM algorithms' ability to distinguish between normal and aberrant movements enhances their ability to identify patient response.

  Autoencoders: In neurorehabilitation, these neural networks help detect abnormalities. They reconstruct sensor data and patterns that deviate from the norm (Senadheera, AI Applications in Adult Stroke Recovery and Rehabilitation: A Scoping Review Using AI, 2024).

Through clustering and anomaly detection, neurorehabilitation can provide real-time insights and support proactive therapy adjustments to patient safety and outcomes.

6.3 Comparative Analysis of Predictive Models

When using predictive models in neurorehabilitation, accuracy, computational efficiency, and model transparency must all be balanced. While computationally efficient models ensure real-time analysis in wearable device applications, accurate models are essential for precise and meaningful insights into patient progress.

- **Accuracy Considerations:** Neural networks and LSTMs are two examples of DL models that are exceptionally accurate in detecting patterns in sensor data. Because of their non-linear characteristics, which allow them to spot complex correlations in patient recovery data, these models are perfect for neurorehabilitation. However, as complexity increases, these models become less interpretable, which could be problematic in clinical settings where understanding model outputs is crucial for patient care.
- **Computational Efficiency:** Computational efficiency becomes crucial in neurorehabilitation, where wearable equipment is used for ongoing monitoring. Even if DL models like CNNs and LSTMs are accurate, they require a lot of processing power, which low-power systems may not always be able to provide. Despite their potential lack of accuracy, simpler machine learning models like decision trees or SVMs balance interpretability and resource needs in this scenario where real-time input is crucial.

Despite their advantages, predictive come with several limitations:

- **Model Complexity and Transparency:** High-accuracy models, such as neural networks, often operate as "black boxes," making it challenging for therapists to understand the data. This lack of transparency might impede trust and understanding, especially when therapeutic changes need to be explained.
- **Data Requirements and Adaptability:** For optimal performance, DL models often require sizable labeled datasets. Neurorehabilitation frequently lacks data, particularly when treating rare or complex conditions. Applying pre-trained models to smaller, more targeted datasets can increase their relevance and adaptability through techniques like transfer learning.

Predictive modeling and data analysis techniques significantly improve neurorehabilitation by facilitating a detailed understanding of patient progress and providing the foundation for adaptive treatments. By leveraging ML and DL approaches, clustering, anomaly detection, and efficient predictive models, clinicians can support patient-centered care that is responsive to individual needs and adaptive to ongoing recovery patterns.

7. CHALLENGES AND FUNDAMENTAL CONSIDERATIONS IN WEARABLE DATA UTILIZATION

Wearable technologies have revolutionized healthcare by allowing continuous, real-time data collection. However, the general adoption and integration of wearable technologies come with several challenges that must be addressed to successfully apply wearable data.

7.1 Data Quality, Noise Reduction, and Preprocessing Challenges

- **Data Quality:** One significant obstacle in wearable data applications is providing high-quality and reliable data for analysis (Canali, 2022). Wearable devices collect vast amounts of data, usually from various sensors evaluating parameters like heart rate, physical activity, temperature, and blood oxygen levels. However, several factors, such as climatic conditions, external interferences, and sensor errors, can cause significant variations in data quality.
- **Noise Reduction:** Noise frequently occurs in wearable data (Roberts, 2022). For instance, motion artefacts, electromagnetic interference, and calibration errors in sensors can alter the measured signal. Implementing noise reduction techniques is essential for eliminating redundant data and enhancing measurement accuracy (Frank, 2024). Signal processing techniques, including

filtering, Fourier transforms, or wavelet analysis, can split relevant signals from noise. However, these methods must be applied judiciously to avoid the loss of important information, mainly in scenarios where subtle physiological signals are critical.

- **Data Preprocessing:** Preparing wearable data through preprocessing is necessary to provide its suitability for analysis and machine learning applications (Ortiz, Data Preprocessing Techniques for AI and Machine Learning Readiness: Scoping Review of Wearable Sensor Data in Cancer Care, 2024). This procedure has several stages, including cleaning the data, normalizing it, extracting features, and transforming it. Addressing missing or unreliable data due to device failures or transmission issues is essential. Approaches such as interpolation, imputation, or algorithms to handle missing data help bridge the gaps.

Additionally, aligning timestamps is crucial for longitudinal investigations, and sensor data often needs to be synchronized when acquired from numerous devices. Managing the inherent variability in the data is another obstacle. Age, gender, physical condition, and environmental circumstances are some of the variables that might cause changes in an individual's physiological signals. Addressing these variances requires sophisticated statistical techniques and ML models to enhance high-dimensional data and eliminate individual differences.

7.2 Ethical Considerations: Privacy, Consent, and Data Security

Due to the expanding popularity of wearable technology private and sensitive health information collected is tremendous.

- **Privacy:** Wearable technologies frequently monitor and collect sensitive information about individuals' health and behaviors (Sivakumar, 2024). This investigates the use, archiving, and dissemination of this data. The protection of people's privacy must be guaranteed. To prevent unwanted access to user data, manufacturers should use strong data protection measures, including encryption and anonymization. Policies also need to be established to manage the sharing of wearable data with third parties, including employers, health insurance companies, and researchers, and to prevent misuse.
- **Informed Consent:** Informed consent describes another ethical concern (Schultz, 2024). For wearables to be employed in research or clinical environments, individuals must provide explicit, straightforward consent regarding using their data. Such consent should clarify the data's intended use, retention period, and access authorizations. Participants should be fully reported about

potential risks, such as the possibility of data breaches or misuse, and have the right to retract their permission without penalties.

- **Data Security:** Protecting wearable data is required to prevent unauthorized access, theft, or manipulation (Ashwini). Wearable devices often connect to mobile applications or cloud-based platforms, creating potential vulnerability issues (Singh, 2024). Manufacturers must employ robust encryption techniques and protected data transmission protocols to safeguard data during collection, storage, and processing. Additionally, routine audits and security updates are essential to manage emerging threats and confirm that existing security measures stay effective.

7.3 Technical and Physiological Limitations

The practical implementation of wearable technology is severely inhibited by its technical limitations, particularly sensor performance, battery life, and long-term wearability.

- **Sensor Performance:** The wearable technology's functionality leans heavily on sensors' accuracy and dependability (Anikwe, 2022). Nevertheless, drift, low sensitivity, and calibration errors can affect even the most sophisticated sensors. For instance, optical sensors employed for heart rate monitoring may be affected by motion artifacts, ambient illumination, and skin tone, which could result in values that are not dependable. Furthermore, some sensors' performance may deteriorate, especially in low-quality or inexpensive systems (Zaidan, 2022). Manufacturers must constantly advance sensor technology and calibration algorithms to increase the accuracy and dependability of wearable data to overcome these problems.
- **Battery Life:** Another major issue with wearable technology is battery life. Power consumption is an essential element to consider because many wearable gadgets are made to run continuously for long periods (Chong, 2019). Devices must compromise between keeping up constant data collecting and ensuring the battery lasts a respectable amount of time between charges. Even with improvements in low-power communication protocols and energy-efficient sensor technologies (Qaim, 2020), battery life is still a significant drawback for many wearables, especially those that need continuous monitoring, like those used in clinical settings.
- **Long-Term Wearability:** Wearable technology relies on consumers' willingness to wear the devices for extended periods (Ferreira, 2021). Long-term user retention relies heavily on comfort, usability, and aesthetics. Many wearable technologies need to be portable, discrete, and comfortable to wear for

long periods, especially regarding health monitoring. People may only regularly utilize devices that are comfortable, large, or challenging to use. The device's long-term wearability may also be impacted by allergic reactions or skin irritation. To retain the device's functionality, manufacturers must ensure user comfort is a top priority in their designs.

Devices should be developed to function in various contexts, whether users confront physical activity, perform in different environments, or sleep. To ensure reliable performance over time, the devices must be stable and immune to environmental factors such as sweat, water, and temperature fluctuations.

8. FUTURE DIRECTIONS AND EMERGING TRENDS IN WEARABLE TECHNOLOGY FOR NEUROREHABILITATION

Advances in materials science, sensor technology, data analytics, machine learning, and robotics will significantly impact the future of wearable technologies in neurorehabilitation. Several significant trends and future directions are predicted to reshape rehabilitation as the discipline develops, providing patients with safer, more efficient, and more affordable treatments.

Figure 8. Emerging trends in wearable technology for neurorehabilitation

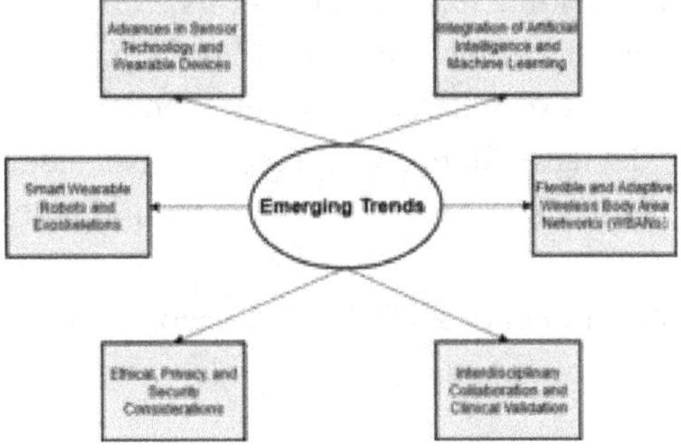

8.1 Advances in Sensor Technology and Wearable Devices

Wearable devices currently depend on various sensors, such as inertial measurement units (IMUs), pressure sensors, electromyographic (EMG) sensors, and electroencephalographic (EEG) sensors, etc. to capture crucial physiological and biomechanical data (Tang, 2023). As the demand for more accurate, real-time data expansions, there will be a persistent effort to enhance sensor sensitivity, flexibility, and integration. These sensors can adapt to the skin's natural movements, permitting continuous monitoring without hampering the user's comfort or range of mobility. This progress will make Wearable rehabilitative technology more reliable, efficient saf, safe, and sufficient for everyday usage.

8.2 Combining of Artificial Intelligence and Machine Learning

Incorporating AI and ML is suspended to revolutionize wearable technology in neurorehabilitation with the increasing sophistication of sensor data (Gupta, 2024). AI and ML techniques, such as DL, reinforcement learning, and neural networks, can be used to analyze extensive datasets. ML approach will allow for more adaptive and intelligent systems that constantly optimize therapeutic interventions, improving the effectiveness of rehabilitation procedures. Besides, the application of AI-driven predictive analytics can benefit early diagnosis and intervention, recognizing nuanced signs of neurodegenerative diseases, including Parkinson's disease or stroke, long before clinical symptoms manifest.

8.3 Smart Wearable Robots and Exoskeletons

Wearable robotics and exoskeletons have attained notable attention as assistive technologies for neurorehabilitation (Nizamis, 2021). These devices, which incorporate wearable sensors with actuators and motors, can assist patients with motor impairments. Recent advancements in soft robotics have formed more flexible, lightweight, and obedient exoskeletons, making them safer and more relaxing for prolonged use. These devices will become more sophisticated, with enhanced force control and sensory feedback, allowing for more natural and intuitive interactions with the user.

As wearable robotics in neurorehabilitation become more affordable, safe, and successful, they will eventually be able to be widely used.

8.4 Flexible and Adaptive Wireless Body Area Networks (WBANs)

Wireless Body Area Networks (WBANs) enable wearables, sensors, and rehabilitation platforms to communicate seamlessly. In neurorehabilitation, WBANs will need to develop more resilient, energy-efficient, and adaptable communication protocols in the future (Deng, 2018). Real-time, high-quality data transmission requires managing current issues, including signal interference, network congestion, and limited bandwidth.

8.5 Ethical, Privacy, and Security Considerations

Privacy, data security, and consent are ethical issues that will remain a significant priority as wearable technology and sensors proliferate (Sivakumar, Addressing privacy concerns with wearable health monitoring technology, 2024). The information gathered by wearable technology is vulnerable and frequently includes biometric data, movement patterns that might be used to identify a person, and sensitive health information. Wearable technology must be developed with privacy so patients can control their data.

8.6 Interdisciplinary Collaboration and Clinical Validation

Researchers, engineers, scientists, and patients must cooperate more to recognize wearable technology's potential in neurorehabilitation fully. Future research should concentrate on confirming the clinical efficacy of wearable rehabilitation devices using extensive, long-term studies that evaluate both clinical and patient-reported results. Additionally, healthcare professionals must be trained in practical data interpretation and clinical decision-making to integrate wearable devices into routine rehabilitation procedures (Lang, 2020). Addressing these challenges will require persistent interdisciplinary cooperation, technological invention, and a responsibility to ensure that wearable neurorehabilitation technologies are accessible, safe, and effective for patients.

CONCLUSION

In this work, we have explored the transformative role of predictive algorithms in wearable technology for neurorehabilitation. As wearable devices and sensor technology progress, they present unprecedented opportunities for helping individuals with neurological impairments. predictive algorithms with sophisticated ML and AI models are the linchpin in converting expansive sensor data into actionable insights, thus facilitating personalized, real-time therapeutic interventions. these algorithms can significantly enhance patient outcomes by adapting rehabilitation protocols to each patient's needs and progress for safer, more efficient, and more responsive assistive systems. combining materials science, engineering, neuroscience, and clinical medicine expertise can assist overcome existing challenges and foster innovation in predictive technology and wearable innovation. collaborative research and clinical trials will be crucial in validating these systems and ensuring they deliver measurable benefits in real-world applications. the future of wearable technology in neurorehabilitation is promising and profound. As predictive algorithms evolve more sophisticated and wearable devices become more affordable; these technologies can revolutionize neurorehabilitation, making highly effective, patient-centered care a standard in healthcare.

REFERENCES

Akbar, K., Passaro, A., Di Gioia, M., Martini, E., Dragone, M., Zullo, A., & Stasolla, F. (2024). Reviewing the Horizon: The Future of Extended Reality and Artificial Intelligence in Neurorehabilitation for Brain Injury Recovery. *Information (Basel), 15*(8), 501. DOI: 10.3390/info15080501

Akcay, G., Demirdogen, F., Gul, T., Ali, Y., Dilcan, K. D., Esra, K., Huseyin Emre, O., Cagla, C., Haydar, C., & Yavuz, E. (2024). Effects of Transcranial Direct Current Stimulation on Motor and Cognitive Dysfunction in an Experimental Traumatic Brain Injury Model. *Turkish Neurosurgery*, •••, 343–350. DOI: 10.5137/1019-5149.JTN.45526-23.4 PMID: 38497188

Anikwe, C. V. (2022). Mobile and wearable sensors for data-driven health monitoring system: State-of-the-art and future prospect. *Expert Systems with Applications, 202*, 117362. DOI: 10.1016/j.eswa.2022.117362

Armstrong, J. J., Zhu, M., Hirdes, J. P., & Stolee, P. (2012). K-means cluster analysis of rehabilitation service users in the home health care system of Ontario: Examining the heterogeneity of a complex geriatric population. *Archives of Physical Medicine and Rehabilitation, 93*(12), 2198–2205. DOI: 10.1016/j.apmr.2012.05.026 PMID: 22705468

Arya, K. N., Pandian, S., Joshi, A. K., Chaudhary, N., Agarwal, G. G., & Ahmed, S. S. (2024). Sensory deficits of the paretic and non-paretic upper limbs relate with the motor recovery of the poststroke subjects. *Topics in Stroke Rehabilitation, 31*(3), 281–292. DOI: 10.1080/10749357.2023.2253629 PMID: 37690032

Ashwini, A. a. (n.d.). Robust Security and Privacy of Wearable and Implantable Medical Devices: Protecting Lives and Data. In *Security, Privacy, and Trust in WBANs and E-Healthcare* (pp. 126--147). CRC Press.

Canali, S., Schiaffonati, V., & Aliverti, A. (2022). Challenges and recommendations for wearable devices in digital health: Data quality, interoperability, health equity, fairness. *PLOS Digital Health, 1*(10), 0000104. DOI: 10.1371/journal.pdig.0000104 PMID: 36812619

Cantone, M. (2024). Clinical Updates and Perspectives on Transcranial Magnetic Stimulation (TMS). *Journal of Clinical Medicine, 13*(13), 3794. DOI: 10.3390/jcm13133794 PMID: 38999361

Chong, Y.-W. Y., Ismail, W., Ko, K., & Lee, C.-Y. (2019). Energy harvesting for wearable devices: A review. *IEEE Sensors Journal, 19*(20), 9047–9062. DOI: 10.1109/JSEN.2019.2925638

Dalla Gasperina, S., Ferrari, F., Gandolla, M., Pedrocchi, A., & Ambrosini, E. (2024). Hybrid Cooperative Control of Functional Electrical Stimulation and Robot Assistance for Upper Extremity Rehabilitation. *IEEE Transactions on Biomedical Engineering*, *71*(9), 2642–2650. DOI: 10.1109/TBME.2024.3384939 PMID: 39167498

Deep, S. a. (2019). A survey on anomalous behavior detection for elderly care using dense-sensing networks. *IEEE Communications Surveys \& Tutorials*, 352--370.

Deng, W. Y., Papavasileiou, I., Qiao, Z., Zhang, W., Lam, K.-Y., & Han, S. (2018). Advances in automation technologies for lower extremity neurorehabilitation: A review and future challenges. *IEEE Reviews in Biomedical Engineering*, *11*, 289–305. DOI: 10.1109/RBME.2018.2830805 PMID: 29994006

Dias, D., & Paulo Silva Cunha, J. (2018). Wearable health devices—Vital sign monitoring, systems and technologies. *Sensors (Basel)*, *18*(8), 2414. DOI: 10.3390/s18082414 PMID: 30044415

Feigin, V. L. (2021). Burden of neurological disorders across the US from 1990-2017: A global burden of disease study. *JAMA Neurology*, •••, 165–176. PMID: 33136137

Ferreira, J. J., Fernandes, C. I., Rammal, H. G., & Veiga, P. M. (2021). Wearable technology and consumer interaction: A systematic review and research agenda. *Computers in Human Behavior*, *118*, 106710. DOI: 10.1016/j.chb.2021.106710

Frank, E. a. (2024). Data preprocessing techniques for NLP in BI.

Grab, J. G.-C., Zewdie, E., Carlson, H. L., Kuo, H.-C., Ciechanski, P., Hodge, J., Giuffre, A., & Kirton, A. (2018). Robotic TMS mapping of motor cortex in the developing brain. *Journal of Neuroscience Methods*, *309*, 41–54. DOI: 10.1016/j.jneumeth.2018.08.007 PMID: 30121208

Gupta, R. (2024). AI-based technologies, challenges, and solutions for neurorehabilitation: A systematic mapping. In *Computational Intelligence and Deep Learning Methods for Neuro-rehabilitation Applications* (pp. 1–25). Elsevier. DOI: 10.1016/B978-0-443-13772-3.00014-5

Gutman, B. H., Shmilovitch, A.-H., Aran, D., & Shelly, S. (2024). Twenty-Five Years of AI in Neurology: The Journey of Predictive Medicine and Biological Breakthroughs. *JMIR Neurotechnology*, *3*, 59556. DOI: 10.2196/59556

Hamam, H. (2024). Revolutionizing Neurosurgery and Neurology: The transformative impact of artificial intelligence in healthcare. *Computers and Artificial Intelligence*, *2*(1), 416. DOI: 10.59400/cai.v2i1.416

Harris, J. E., Eng, J. J., Miller, W. C., & Dawson, A. S. (2009). A self-administered Graded Repetitive Arm Supplementary Program (GRASP) improves arm function during inpatient stroke rehabilitation: A multi-site randomized controlled trial. *Stroke, 40*(6), 2123–2128. DOI: 10.1161/STROKEAHA.108.544585 PMID: 19359633

Hou, Y. a. (2024). Research on innovative design of intelligent wearable products based on human machine engineering and bionics. *Molecular \& Cellular Biomechanics*, 461--461.

Hu, Z., Wang, J., Wang, Y., Wang, C., Wang, Y., Zhang, Z., Xu, P., Zhao, T., Luan, Y., Liu, C., Qiao, L., Shu, M., Mi, J., Pan, X., & Xu, M. (2021). A Robust and Wearable Triboelectric Tactile Patch as Intelligent Human-Machine Interface. *Materials (Basel), 14*(21), 6366. DOI: 10.3390/ma14216366 PMID: 34771892

Huang, Y.-Y. D.-Y.-T.-T., Chen, S.-D., Leng, X.-Y., Kuo, K., Wang, Z.-T., Cui, M., Tan, L., Wang, K., Dong, Q., & Yu, J.-T. (2022). Post-stroke cognitive impairment: Epidemiology, risk factors, and management. *Journal of Alzheimer's Disease, 86*(3), 983–999. DOI: 10.3233/JAD-215644 PMID: 35147548

Ishaque, S., Khan, N., & Krishnan, S. (2021). Trends in heart-rate variability signal analysis. *Frontiers in Digital Health, 3*, 639444. DOI: 10.3389/fdgth.2021.639444 PMID: 34713110

Kanjo, E., Younis, E. M. G., & Ang, C. S. (2019). Deep learning analysis of mobile physiological, environmental and location sensor data for emotion detection. *Information Fusion, 49*, 46–56. DOI: 10.1016/j.inffus.2018.09.001

Khan, K. a. (2014). DBSCAN: Past, present and future. In *The fifth international conference on the applications of digital information and web technologies (ICADIWT 2014)* (pp. 232--238).

Kristoffersson, A., & Lindén, M. (2022). A systematic review of wearable sensors for monitoring physical activity. *Sensors (Basel), 22*(2), 573. DOI: 10.3390/s22020573 PMID: 35062531

Lang, C. E., Barth, J., Holleran, C. L., Konrad, J. D., & Bland, M. D. (2020). Implementation of wearable sensing technology for movement: Pushing forward into the routine physical rehabilitation care field. *Sensors (Basel), 20*(20), 5744. DOI: 10.3390/s20205744 PMID: 33050368

Li, B., Xu, G., Teng, Z., Luo, D., Pei, J., Chen, R., & Zhang, S. (2024). Intelligent ankle—Foot prosthesis based on human structure and motion bionics. *Journal of Neuroengineering and Rehabilitation, 21*(1), 119. DOI: 10.1186/s12984-024-01414-w PMID: 39003459

Liu, S., Wang, L., & Gao, R. X. (2024). Cognitive neuroscience and robotics: Advancements and future research directions. *Robotics and Computer-integrated Manufacturing*, *85*, 102610. DOI: 10.1016/j.rcim.2023.102610

Margam, R. (2024). Virtual reality in healthcare: transforming treatment. *International journal of artificial intelligence \& machine learning (IJAIML)*, 19--34.

Merletti, R. a. (2004). Electromyography: physiology, engineering, and non-invasive applications. John Wiley \& Sons.

Nizamis, K. a. (2021). Converging robotic technologies in targeted neural rehabilitation: a review of emerging solutions and challenges. *Sensors*, 2084. oel, J. P. (2021). Cognitive and Cybernetics based Human Adaptive Mechatronics System in Gait Rehabilitation Therapy. In *2021 Third International Conference on Intelligent Communication Technologies and Virtual Mobile Networks (ICICV)* (pp. 516--521). DOI: 10.3390/s21062084

Ortiz, B. L., Gupta, V., Kumar, R., Jalin, A., Cao, X., Ziegenbein, C., Singhal, A., Tewari, M., & Choi, S. W. (2024). Data Preprocessing Techniques for AI and Machine Learning Readiness: Scoping Review of Wearable Sensor Data in Cancer Care. *JMIR mHealth and uHealth*, *12*, 59587. DOI: 10.2196/59587 PMID: 38626290

Ortiz, B. L., Gupta, V., Kumar, R., Jalin, A., Cao, X., Ziegenbein, C., Singhal, A., Tewari, M., & Choi, S. W. (2024). Data Preprocessing Techniques for AI and Machine Learning Readiness: Scoping Review of Wearable Sensor Data in Cancer Care. *JMIR mHealth and uHealth*, *12*, 59587. DOI: 10.2196/59587 PMID: 38626290

Pan, D. H., Hu, J., Wang, B., Xia, X., Cheng, Y., Wang, C.-H., & Lu, Y. (2024). Biomimetic Wearable Sensors: Emerging Combination of Intelligence and Electronics. *Advancement of Science*, *11*(5), 2303264. DOI: 10.1002/advs.202303264 PMID: 38044298

Pan, D. H., Hu, J., Wang, B., Xia, X., Cheng, Y., Wang, C.-H., & Lu, Y. (2024). Biomimetic Wearable Sensors: Emerging Combination of Intelligence and Electronics. *Advancement of Science*, *11*(5), 2303264. DOI: 10.1002/advs.202303264 PMID: 38044298

Park, H. a. (2016). Short-duration and intensive training improves long-term reaching performance in individuals with chronic stroke. *Neurorehabilitation and neural repair*, 551–561. Pranji{\'c}, M. a. (2024). From Sound to Movement: Mapping the Neural Mechanisms of Auditory—Motor Entrainment and Synchronization. *Brain Sciences*, •••, 1063.

Qaim, W. B. (2020). Towards energy efficiency in the internet of wearable things: A systematic review. *IEEE AccessIEEE Access*, 175412--175435.

Rajalaxmi, V. a. (2024). Emerging Role of Artificial Intelligence and Robotics in Physiotherapy: Past, Present, and Future Perspective. In *Advancements in Clinical Medicine* (pp. 200--214).

Roberts, B. (2022). Evaluation of a wearable consumer noise measurement device in a laboratory setting. *The Journal of the Acoustical Society of America*, •••, 547–552. DOI: 10.1121/10.0012916 PMID: 35931541

Roelofs, J. M., Zandvliet, S. B., Schut, I. M., Huisinga, A. C. M., Schouten, A. C., Hendricks, H. T., de Kam, D., Aerden, L. A. M., Bussmann, J. B. J., Geurts, A. C. H., & Weerdesteyn, V. (2023). Mild stroke, serious problems: Limitations in balance and gait capacity and the impact on fall rate, and physical activity. *Neurorehabilitation and Neural Repair*, *37*(11-12), 786–798. DOI: 10.1177/15459683231207360 PMID: 37877724

Schultz, B., Agamah, F. E., Ewuoso, C., Madden, E. B., Troyer, J., Skelton, M., & Mwaka, E. (2024). Webinar report: Stakeholder perspectives on informed consent for the use of genomic data by commercial entities. *Journal of Medical Ethics*, *50*(1), 57–61. DOI: 10.1136/jme-2022-108650 PMID: 36941048

Schwertfeger, J. L., Beyer, C., Hung, P., Ung, N., Madigan, C., Cortes, A. R., Swaminathan, B., & Madhavan, S. (2023). A map of evidence using transcranial direct current stimulation (tDCS) to improve cognition in adults with traumatic brain injury (TBI). *Frontiers in Neuroergonomics*, *4*, 1170473. DOI: 10.3389/fnrgo.2023.1170473 PMID: 38234478

Senadheera, I., Hettiarachchi, P., Haslam, B., Nawaratne, R., Sheehan, J., Lockwood, K. J., Alahakoon, D., & Carey, L. M. (2024). AI Applications in Adult Stroke Recovery and Rehabilitation: A Scoping Review Using AI. *Sensors (Basel)*, *24*(20), 6585. DOI: 10.3390/s24206585 PMID: 39460066

Senadheera, I., Hettiarachchi, P., Haslam, B., Nawaratne, R., Sheehan, J., Lockwood, K. J., Alahakoon, D., & Carey, L. M. (2024). AI Applications in Adult Stroke Recovery and Rehabilitation: A Scoping Review Using AI. *Sensors (Basel)*, *24*(20), 6585. DOI: 10.3390/s24206585 PMID: 39460066

Sherstinsky, A. (2020). Fundamentals of recurrent neural network (RNN) and long short-term memory (LSTM) network. *Physica D. Nonlinear Phenomena*, *404*, 132306. DOI: 10.1016/j.physd.2019.132306

Singh, N. a. (2024). Securing Cloud-Based Internet of Things: Challenges and Mitigations. *arXiv preprint arXiv:2402.00356*.

Sivakumar, C., Mone, V., & Abdumukhtor, R. (2024). Addressing privacy concerns with wearable health monitoring technology. *Wiley Interdisciplinary Reviews. Data Mining and Knowledge Discovery*, *14*(3), 1535. DOI: 10.1002/widm.1535

Sivakumar, C., Mone, V., & Abdumukhtor, R. (2024). Addressing privacy concerns with wearable health monitoring technology. *Wiley Interdisciplinary Reviews. Data Mining and Knowledge Discovery*, *14*(3), 1535. DOI: 10.1002/widm.1535

Smith, A. A., Li, R., & Tse, Z. T. H. (2023). Reshaping healthcare with wearable biosensors. *Scientific Reports*, *13*(1), 4998. DOI: 10.1038/s41598-022-26951-z PMID: 36973262

Soufineyestani, M., Dowling, D., & Khan, A. (2020). Electroencephalography (EEG) technology applications and available devices. *Applied Sciences (Basel, Switzerland)*, *10*(21), 7453. DOI: 10.3390/app10217453

Stinear, C. M. (2007). Functional potential in chronic stroke patients depends on corticospinal tract integrity. *Brain*, •••, 170–180. PMID: 17148468

Tang, C., Xu, Z., Occhipinti, E., Yi, W., Xu, M., Kumar, S., Virk, G. S., Gao, S., & Occhipinti, L. G. (2023). From brain to movement: Wearables-based motion intention prediction across the human nervous system. *Nano Energy*, *115*, 108712. DOI: 10.1016/j.nanoen.2023.108712

Van Hooren, B., Goudsmit, J., Restrepo, J., & Vos, S. (2020). Real-time feedback by wearables in running: Current approaches, challenges and suggestions for improvements. *Journal of Sports Sciences*, *38*(2), 214–230. DOI: 10.1080/02640414.2019.1690960 PMID: 31795815

Walz, W. (2024). The Brain as an Organ. In *The Gliocentric Brain* (pp. 7–27). Phenotype Plasticity of the Damaged Brain.

Waqas, M., & Humphries, U. W. (2024). A critical review of RNN and LSTM variants in hydrological time series predictions. *MethodsX*, *13*, 102946. DOI: 10.1016/j.mex.2024.102946 PMID: 39324077

Weber, N. a. (2017). Unsupervised learning in human activity recognition: A first foray into clustering data gathered from wearable sensors.

Xu, S., Liu, Y., Lee, H., & Li, W. (2024). Neural interfaces: Bridging the brain to the world beyond healthcare. *Exploration*, *4*(5), 20230146. DOI: 10.1002/EXP.20230146 PMID: 39439491

Yao, Y., Shao, D., Tarabini, M., Moezi, S. A., Li, K., & Saccomandi, P. (2024). Advancements in Sensor Technologies and Control Strategies for Lower-Limb Rehabilitation Exoskeletons: A Comprehensive Review. *Micromachines*, *15*(4), 489. DOI: 10.3390/mi15040489 PMID: 38675301

Yurtman, A. a. (2019). Novel noniterative orientation estimation for wearable motion sensor units acquiring accelerometer, gyroscope, and magnetometer measurements. *IEEE Transactions on Instrumentation and Measurement*, **•••**, 3206–3215.

Zaidan, M. A., Xie, Y., Motlagh, N. H., Wang, B., Nie, W., Nurmi, P., Tarkoma, S., Petaja, T., Ding, A., & Kulmala, M. (2022). Dense air quality sensor networks: Validation, analysis, and benefits. *IEEE Sensors Journal*, *22*(23), 23507–23520. DOI: 10.1109/JSEN.2022.3216071

Zhang, S., Jung, K., Langner, R., Florin, E., Eickhoff, S. B., & Popovych, O. V. (2024). Impact of data processing varieties on DCM estimates of effective connectivity from task-fMRI. *Human Brain Mapping*, *45*(8), 26751. DOI: 10.1002/hbm.26751 PMID: 38864293

Zhetenbayev, N. a. (2023). Developing of a wearable ankle rehabilitation robotic device. *Vibroengineering Procedia*, 36--41.

Chapter 9
Machine Learning Techniques for Personalized Rehabilitation:
Enhancing Patient Outcomes Through Predictive Algorithms

Muhammad Usman Tariq
https://orcid.org/0000-0002-7605-3040
Abu Dhabi University, UAE & University College Cork, Ireland

ABSTRACT

The revolutionary impact of machine learning (ML) approaches in individualized rehabilitation is examined in this chapter, with a focus on how predictive algorithms may improve patient outcomes. ML models are changing rehabilitation procedures to offer individualized therapies that consider each patient's requirements, preferences, and progress by utilizing large and varied datasets. The chapter explores important machine learning techniques, including support vector machines, neural networks, and decision trees, emphasizing how they may be used to forecast recovery paths, enhance treatment regimens, and modify therapies in real time. This change is mostly due to wearable technology and sensor data, which provide real-time patient performance insights and allow rehabilitation regimens to be continuously improved. Examples of effective predictive algorithm integration in rehabilitation include AI-powered prostheses, orthotic devices with adaptive control systems, and neurorehabilitation for spinal cord injuries and stroke.

DOI: 10.4018/979-8-3373-0194-5.ch009

INTRODUCTION

Started from the concept of artificial intelligence, ML has realized its importance in developing new horizons in every field, especially in the healthcare of rehabilitation intervention. Rehabilitation is a vital part of the treatment process in patients with injuries, ongoing illnesses or neurological conditions, and patient-specific programs are highly important during this process. Using machine learning, it became possible to work with huge amounts of patient data, define the patterns and develop predictive models that help to make the rehabilitation program more individual. Thus, using the established predictive algorithms, the healthcare providers can create the effective intercessions which in turn would afford to be flexible and tend to address each individual's need (Zhang et al., 2024). In its broadest concept, machine learning is a subclass of Artificial Intelligence (AI) that gives systems the ability to enhance their performance from the available data without being programmed directly. An important class of ML is predictive algorithms, oriented on the future results based on past and current information; they are extremely important in healthcare cases. Individualized rehabilitation includes the process of choosing the most suitable type of treatment optimally depending on the patient's age, previous illnesses, and other conditions or aims at rehabilitation. Some of the assistive technologies commonly integrating ML are wearable devices, robotic exoskeletons as well as virtual reality interfaces used in administering of these personalised treatments. All in all, these concepts constitute the base of the up-to date approaches of rehabilitation with aid of technologies (Rasa, 2024). Hence the application of ML in rehabilitation processes eliminates a major weakness of conventional procedures, that of generalization. Earlier, rehabilitation programmes were more or less 'one size fits all', based on the idea that any two patients with similar injuries or diseases should respond well to the same treatment. However, this revolutionary process was generalised and often failed to accommodate the differential signs and symptoms in patients to produce the best results. For example, the patient with the first degree of motor dysfunction in the stroke, the type, frequency, and intensity of therapeutic activities may not be the same as the patient with a second degree of motor dysfunction. Such variation can be analyzed by the use of the ML based models since it is in a position to sort through large databases of the characteristics of patients and their rates of recovery in order to provide very personalized advice (Fong et al., 2020).

One of the areas that has been severely enriched by the use of ML is physical therapy. With wearable sensors including accelerometers and gyroscopes, protocol-specific movement data from patients undergoing rehabilitation can be captured real-time. This information is then undergone through the ML algorithms' analysis of movement quality and unusual patterns as well as immediate feedback to the patients and therapists. But this real time analysis not only guarantees that exercises are done correctly but also reduces more injuries. Published research in the Journal of Neuro Engineering and Rehabilitation showed that wearable devices with machine learning to enhance therapy helped stroke survivors gain improvements in mobility by 25% within several weeks as compared to therapy alone (Rasa, 2024; Tariq, 2025). The use of predictive algorithms is especially impactful in trying to make improvements to the rehabilitation programs. Through such predictions, an estimation of how long it will take patients to recover as well as the possibility of arising complications in treatment, these algorithms help healthcare organizations make right decisions to allocate their resources to serve the patients in the best way possible. For example, through analysis of risk factors like age, previous conditions, and compliance with therapy regimes, it is possible to identify individuals who are at risk of slow recovery with the help of ML models. Also, by the use of these models, the doctor can make changes to the treatment plan before additional steps are made which allows preventing relapse. For one, scholars trained an ML future to classify threat levels of falls in elderly patients during their physical therapy programs. By targeting those most vulnerable to falls, clinicians could start treating this condition and prevent future cases of accidents that lead to fall (Zhang et al., 2024). However, the question is, there is a need to take critical look at the application of ML in rehabilitation. And one of the issues is that the data that is fed into the ML model may contain bias. This means that if the data assumed is not diverse or contains errors, the ensuing predictions will also not be correct; consequently, patients receive unequal treatment based on their diseases. For example, machine learning system that was trained on datasets with images mostly of young people will not perform well on the old, aged people. Solving this problem means that qualified varied data have to be included in a sample so that this sample reflects the target population (Zhang et al., 2024; Tariq, 2025). A major issue is the moral issue of delegating the decision-making process to ML in particular for health-related decisions. While the use of such algorithms may improve the effectiveness and specificity of care, it may at the same time erode the interaction between the clinician and the patient if they reasoned as the sole definitive sources of information. For instance, it's possible for a therapist to question an ML-generated suggestion yet, approve it because the ML is recommending it or give a client a diagnosis disregarding their clinical knowledge and judgment to believe in the ML more than they believe in themselves. To address this, ML should in fact work as an assistant tool and not supplant the human specialism. Awareness on how these algorithms work and effective Communication with the patient is main feature of enhancing trust and adoption (Pelosi et al., 2024).

However, use of ML in rehabilitation context requires substantial investment in both physical and human capital. Depending on the approach used, the development, implementation, and maintenance of such ML-powered assistive systems entail necessary resources that resource-starved healthcare facilities can hardly afford, posing the danger of deepening the divide between well-endowed and starved healthcare centres. Another rating is that research policymakers and health care managers should guarantee equal usage of technologies and fund cross-cooperation projects (Pelosi et al., 2024). Therefore, machine learning is even changing the landscape of rehabilitation therapy since patients can be given flexible, and specific treatments to improve their recovery. These programs are well enhanced with the help of predictive algorithms that provide information which was earlier non-existent. That, data biases, ethical issues, and resource inequalities should be solved, the possible advantages of ML applied to rehabilitation are clear. In the future this technology is anticipated to pave way for integration with wearable devices, robotics and even virtual reality inpatient rehabilitation to help patients gain the necessary quality of care needed to reach the latent potential (Zhang et al., 2024).

BACKGROUND

According to this study, there has been the advancement of a new school of thought in rehabilitation medicine, which is based on ML to enhance the achievement of desired patient outcomes. Originally, rehabilitation has been delivered through treating protocols, which, in many instances, are helpful though do not fit individual patient's needs and scenarios. This is a disadvantage that is overcome through machine learning because it can harvest huge data, functional algorithms, as well as real-time analytics, to make optimal streaming treatment plans to boost patients' results. Using ML for creating personal rehabilitation is a perfect example of innovation meeting clinical practice and holds promise for healthcare systems around the globe (Olyanasab & Annabestani, 2024). Artificial intelligence with focus on refining its algorithms with a given data without being programmed to do so is known as machine learning. As applied to rehabilitation, ML will process enormous amounts of patient data to look for correlation and relationship that a typical member of the profession will not be in a position to easily decipher. In fact, as components of ML, predictive algorithms help to predict recovery patterns, possible complications and effects of specific intervention so that clinicians can customize individual rehabilitation schedules. This approach guarantees that every person will be provided with a distinct rehabilitation plan that will be aimed at his or her specific health problem and previous treatment (Ahmed et al., 2020). The greatest contribution of ML to rehabilitation is the capacity to enhance physical therapy treatments. For example, smart clothing with attached sensors can gather incessant information on patient's movements, alleged posture, and muscle activation during therapy. Using this information, ML algorithms make assessments on performance and detect variability from the standard kinetic and ranging patterns;

the algorithms, then, indicate remedial measures in real time. One current example is ML to control exoskeletons for patients with spinal cord injuries or stroke. These assist in mobility while adjusting the level of support they afford according to the progress of the patient and thus the therapy remains this but not very easy. A paper in the Nature Medicine highlighted that ML based exoskeletons to patients having strokes improved by up to thirty percent than any other conventional therapy (Olyanasab & Annabestani, 2024). Other key areas also continue valued that predictive algorithms are influencing how clinicians think about rehabilitation strategies. These algorithm kinds can learn from data of different patients and therefore estimate how the certain patient can respond to specific treatment or some exercise. For example, ML models can predict time needed by a patient with knee replacement surgery to walk as before using age, BMI, and previous illnesses. It enables health care providers to give proper expectations, properly time their resources and also find out patients with slow turnover. As for one example, in one case, hospital readmissions data was analysed by using ML for post-operative rehabilitation patients, and early identification of specific patients that have risk factors that indicate that they'll be readmitted to hospital in the near future allowed the reduction of readmissions by 15% (Nicora et al., 2024).

However, it is crucial to analyse the original difficulties and restrictions of the use of ML in individualised rehabilitation. Notably, there is a concern about the quality and sample selection of the data sets from which to develop ML models. Since the training data often may not be diverse, the derived algorithms may provide poor estimates that do not capture the variance of patients. For instance, an algorithm that is trained mainly with young patients will be very ineffective when is used with elderly patients, hence poor treatment strategies will be provided for them. This is a major issue that will need consideration diverse datatypes and constant reiteration so that the developed ML models are applicable for all demographics and contexts (Fong et al., 2020). As another issue, there is a use of ML into clinical processes. Implementing an ML into their everyday practice could be as challenging for Rehabilitation professionals because they would not be capable of understanding and decoding the results it provides as well as incorporating them optimally into their decision-making matrices. For instance, a therapist who works with an ML-based system might fail to comprehend why the algorithm prescribes a particular decision and consequently provide literature to the procedure, doubt filled. To address this, great care should be taken to make interfaces less cumbersome and also to give clinicians some forms of training that would make using the ML tools easy and little or no addition to what they already do (Nicora et al., 2024). The same goes for the ethical implication that forms part and parcel of the application process of ML in healthcare. Thus, patients and providers have to believe that predictive algorithms are not only reliable but also egalitarian. Understanding how these algorithms work, and their functionality should be made clear in order to earn this trust. For instance, an ML-generated decision to discontinue a therapy program based on efficiency instead of effectiveness will present the attendant clinical and moral issues in patient care. These dangers can be avoided by setting unequivocal ethical standards in algorithm development and target patient interest rather than system success (Ahmed et al., 2020). Moreover, the use of ML in rehabilitation is limited by the availability of or lack of sufficient resources especially when it is practiced in low-middle income health facilities. Sophisticated ML systems also call for significant capital expenditures in hardware and software, and systems to support the applications as well as constant updates. This may open up a gap between those health care institutions, which are endowed with adequate finances and those with the barest resources places in a position to deliver adequate patient care. Supreme coordination is required among governments, universities, and private organizations to make MR based rehabilitation technologies available to all (Nicora et al., 2024). Therefore, this paper concludes that the idea of using machine learning techniques in rehabilitation are paving way for approach that is based on data to allow for right interventions for the patients. From creating personalized recommendations for PT sessions using wearable sensors to forecasting the patients' rehabilitation courses with elaborated algorithms, machine learning opens up incredible chances. Nevertheless, these technologies cannot achieve success unless some of the related issues like data biases, clinician training, ethical issues or resource inequities have not arisen. This way, the healthcare community could unlock the possibilities of ML and at the same time, be aware of its pitfalls and consequently could work towards the future where rehabilitation is less time-consuming, more accurate and more accessible for everybody (Ahmed et al., 2020).

Data Collection and Preprocessing for Predictive Rehabilitation Models

Data is the basis for developing optimal rehabilitation algorithm we use in our predictive models which allows us to build personalized, accurate, and flexible models for patient. In the context of the implementation of machine learning (ML) applications, quality, geography, and quantity of data gravely affect the predictive model. The importance of data cannot be overemphasized especially in the aspect of capturing the detailed nature of the patient profiles, the nature of rehabilitation as well as the recovery paths that are important in determining the kind of intervention that is suitable for promotion of the highest level of outcome. Data acquisition and preparation as well as data consolidation are significant prerequisites of predictive rehabilitation models that provide useful recommendations (Karapintzou et al., 2024). A technique that is widely utilized in the process of data amounting in the field of rehabilitation is the wearing of gadgets with sensors. These devices record motion properties, heart rates, muscle responses, and posture during treatment procedures. For example, an accelerometer can track the manner in which a patient is walking or even an electromyography (EMG) sensor records muscle contraction. As such, detailed information can be provided to the ML algorithms which look at the performance of the patient in exercising in order to diagnosis exercises that the patient does poorly and those that he or she does efficiently and in the process the algorithms recommend changes that would Favor the recovery process of the patient. One example is in stroke rehabilitation where Bluetooth bands monitor Arm & Hand Movements while helping track recovery and customise physiotherapy based on the patient's recovery progress (Arjmandnia & Alimohammadi, 2024). In other words, patient history as well as combined sensor data serve as a significant basis of calculation for predictive rehabilitation models. This is the information about histories of medical conditions, previous procedures or treatments, demographic data and lifestyles data. They also help in forecasting recovery patterns that are likely to predict the results of a rediscovery program besides giving a deeper insight into the factors that contribute to the success of rediscovery. For instance, a patient diagnosed with diabetes will need a different management plan than a patient with no preexisting diseases, although they both are post knee replacement surgery. Thus, the introduction of such variables in the model helps the clinicians to develop suitable rehabilitation model for their patients (Karapintzou et al., 2024).

Real-time monitoring technologies taken step further by providing constant information on the behaviour and progress of patients. For instance, through telehealth units, patients can exercise at home, but they are supervised by clinicians online. Biomechanistic analysis based on video and supported by ML is able to immediately identify the imperfection of certain movements. The latter approach not only enhances the involvement of the patients but also guarantees the systematic collecting of the meaningful data, including those, which were received in non-clinical situations. One example is the use of remote monitoring with wearable ECG devices in patients who require Cardiac Rehabilitation to receive real-time data monitoring by clinicians to allow modification of care as needed (Arjmandnia & Alimohammadi, 2024). Data preprocessing of collected data is as vital a step towards developing strong predictive rehabilitation models. Sensory data and monitoring systems yield measurements that can be noisy, inconsistent, or lacking some components, and this debris will skew the results of an ML model. Data preprocessing as data cleaning, data normalization and feature extraction are critical to be applied for analysing the data. For example, smoothing techniques can be applied to eliminate any noise in the accelerometer signal, whereas normalization guarantees that minimum and maximum values for different metrics are equal, so the model does not favour any parameter (Khan et al., 2020; Tariq, 2025). Feature extraction is even more restrictive in the dimensionality of data mainly by focusing on the most important attributes in relation to the predictive task. For instance, in one study, their independent variables included extracted features from gait data which gave parameters such as stride length or the walking speed and used to forecast the likely fall rate in elderly patients. In terms of data aspects, there is still a lot to be done regarding data quality, data privacy and data sharing among the different rehabilitation interfaces available nowadays. Some of the main difficulties are the guidelines, low quality of data, owing to the differences in sensor quality, discrepancy in the patient's follow-up, and differences in environmental conditions. For instance, measurements that are obtained by wearable sensors may turn out to be erroneous when the sensors are placed poorly, or patients may execute the required exercises improperly and, therefore, generate misleading results. This problem requires the application of stringent validation measures and the use of multiple data sources for minimizing the problem (Lanotte et al., 2023). Acquired data privacy is another central issue when it comes to rehabilitation data. This is due to the fact that patient data contains personal sensitive information about patient's health, hence must follow data privacy laws that include the GDPR or HIPAA. Another privacy control measure includes encrypting data while transferring and storing data and using patient record numbers instead of social security numbers as well as ensuring the patients give their consent to be included in the project. For example, a rehabilitation center employing wearable devices supported by ML revealed that end-to-end encryption can secure patient's data and simultaneously meet the legal demands (Khan et al., 2020).

There is overall additional challenge in the integration of data from different rehabilitation platforms. Both physically and technologically, rehabilitation systems are focused and involve numerous stakeholders such as wearable device manufacturers, telehealth suppliers, and EHR systems which usually employ different forms and standards of data. This fragmentation might disrupt the integration of information and thus restrict the opportunities for generating extensive insights using the models of ML. To solve this problem, it is necessary to establish standard formats and to apply compatible frameworks. For example, the FHIR standards may allow the use of EHR systems' data with wearable devices to have an integrated view of the patient's progress. The chapter has further established that data collection and preprocessing are crucial in the formulation of the predictive rehabilitation models. Measures including data acquisition from sensors, patient history processing and continuous monitoring form the basis on which incremental and patient-specific therapies can be developed (Lanotte et al., 2023). Nevertheless, some threats accompanying ML usage in rehabilitation need to be resolved, such as the problems in data quality and ownership and the data fusion issue. Maintaining sound data flow mechanisms and respecting standard protocols are key to the application of predictive algorithms in rehabilitation and better results in healthcare industry (Lanotte et al., 2023).

Machine Learning Models for Predictive Rehabilitation

As the field of human rehabilitation progresses Machine learning (ML) models have become key in the predictive rehabilitation, personalisation, efficiency, flexibility in treatment in patients. These models are most proficient in pattern recognition, prognosis of patient outcomes and offering a use in intervention customization. Among the models of ML that is applied in rehabilitation includes the neural networks, decision trees and the support vector machine or the SVMs and the of uniqueness differ (Nascimben, 2024). Neural networks, as their name prescribes, mimics the structure of the brain, and consequently excel at modelling nonlinear data patterns. These models are composed of 'nodes' or 'neurons' linked in layers which in turn, learns from the input data given to it. Based on this context, neural networks are effectively utilised in rehabilitation to estimate the prognosis of a patient's function and to choose the suitable exercises founded on patients' parameters. For instance, in post-stroke rehabilitation, CNNs have been used to mine the motion data acquired from wearable sensors to discern even minute change in the level of motorial ability not easily detectable through conventional approaches. A paper in the IEEE Transactions on Neural Systems and Rehabilitation Engineering showed that it is possible to use neural networks to predict the chance of patient regaining mobility and help clinicians improve treatments options (Bica et al., 2021; Tariq, 2024). Decision trees are another diverse form of ML which is used to rehabilitate patients. These models draw decision trees where each node is a decision derived from an attribute feature with a final outcome marked at the terminal nodes. They are also highly flexible and extend very well to accommodate numerous classes, and boast impressive interpretability, which is particularly important in clinical applications. For example, in the Rehabilitation of surgical management of orthopaedic patients, decision trees have been applied to predict patients with high risks of developing complications after surgery. Because the above variables include the age, presence of co-morbid conditions, and physical activity patterns, the mentioned models can enable clinicians to anticipate potential problems with individual patients and formulate effective preventative strategies. An example is the use of the model to determine the probability of positive results concerning knee replacement surgery so that resources can be properly deployed and expectations properly set concerning the probability of successful rehabilitation (Nascimben, 2024). Another widely used powerful model of ML in predictive rehabilitation is referred to support vector machines (SVMs). SVMs work by trying to decide which of the two or more categories a particular set of data belongs with by using the best fitting hyperplane in a high dimension space. This approach is found to be especially useful when the data set is small or contains dependencies. In rehabilitation, the authors have used SVMs to diagnose impending dementia in traumatic brain injury patients. Computer-designed, SVM from data acquired during neuropsychological assessments and fMRI scans, allows for objective detection of early cognitive biomarkers, and subsequent initiation of customized cognitive therapy programs (Bica et al., 2021).

One is their application in forecasting the patients' long-term prognosis with Parkinson's disease treated with rehabilitation, where the algorithm recognizable patients that are likely to experience deterioration of the condition in the shortest time possible (Adam & Mukhtar, 2024). Perhaps the biggest advantage of practicing ML models in rehabilitation, is that such models can modify exercises and change treatment schedules when necessary. Rehabilitation gadgets and IoT based equipment collecting data about the performance of the patient which is analysed by the ML models and provides feedback for the patients. For instance, reinforcement learning which is a subcategory of ML has been employed in the development of performance adapted exoskeletons for training of gait. These systems learn the right level of support that a patient required, and it decreases the support level whenever the patient tries to move (Mainali et al., 2021). For instance, stroke patients who have to use Robotic gait trainers see reinforcement learning algorithms change the capability of the device according to resistance and speed as they are trained, this faster walking recovery ability than training that does not change dynamically (Bonkhoff & Grefkes, 2022). However, the current work indicates that there is still more that needs to be done when it comes to the integration of effective ML models in rehabilitation. The first is the applicability of these two models across populations with different patients. The great majority of the ML models is trained on datasets of specific groups, and thus the models might provide a lower accuracy when used on different groups. For instance, applying a trained neural network on few young patients may prove highly inefficient the moment one deals with elderly people to complete the same set of predictive results (Adam & Mukhtar, 2024). It has its downside in that it is still difficult to understand, especially given the big confusion around making large-scale complex ML models, such as deep neural networks, known as 'black boxes'. Clinicians may avoid using a model for decision making if the process through which the model arrives at a decision is not understood. This issue points to the need for creating techniques that stream how AI models arrive at various conclusions. However, there are ways by which clinicians could model and influence an understanding of factors that affect the predictions made by the ML models, such as using feature importance scores or heat maps (Bonkhoff & Grefkes, 2022). In addition, there are similar ethical concerns which surround the application of the ML models in rehabilitation. Data employed to develop these models has to be protected and the means of dealing with the patient information have to obey established code of ethics and regulations. In addition, algorithms must be developed which put the interests of patient and disease ahead of such values as costs, time and other parameters. A badly tuned model, which will give much larger ratings to one type of patients and much smaller ones to others, will be counterproductive if it results in unequal treatment of patients, erasing any advantage that comes out of individual approach to rehabilitation. Finally, this chapter's findings reveal that applications of machine learning including neural networks, decision trees, as well as support vector machines are revolutionising the field of rehabilitation by producing accurate predication, individualised interventions, and self-organised treatment plans (Mainali et al., 2021). From such an aspect, their capacity to decipher analytical outcomes of extensive datasets has impacted patient rehabilitation tremendously through applications of for instance motion analysts to cognitive therapy application. Nevertheless, there are some limitations or challenges that need to be addressed in order to achieve more on what these methods have to offer, issues of Generalizability, Interpretability & Ethics. As new ideas are properly accompanied with measures to avoid possible sinister implications, models of ML will continue to help improve rehabilitation approaches making the process more efficient, fair and patient oriented in the future (Mainali et al., 2021).

Personalized Rehabilitation Programs Using Predictive Analytics

Predictive analytics using the ML is reshaping the concept and implementation of the utilization of rehabilitation. Thereby the individual patient data will enable the predictive model to pick cues, forecast prognosis, and suggest appropriate interventions consistent with these patients' needs. Aside from increasing the efficiency of rehabilitation, it also increases patient participation and serves to decrease health expenses (Adans-Dester et al., 2020). The major benefit of this approach is that of complex variables that include age, medical history, lifestyle, and real time performance data. For instance, wearable devices with sensors can capture data such as movement, heart rate and muscle activity of a patient at each time they are used. The collected data in turn allows ML algorithms to give feedback and correct rehabilitation exercises in real time. An example is in the cardiac rehabilitation, wherein performance and risk of a patient on the cardiovascular system are predicted to ensure suitable exercise portion for the patient's progress (McDermott et al., 2024). Examples have shown how rehabilitation can be empowered through the use of ML for predictive analytics. For example, one research in the stroke patient used supervised learning techniques to analyse data obtained from the gait analysis and neuroimaging. In light of this, the system used data analysis to approximate the chance of regaining independent walking and suggested the appropriate therapeutic exercises for weak muscles. When compared to patients undertaking normal rehabilitation procedures, those who followed these personalized programs had noticeably shorter recovery periods. This illustration demonstrates how predictive analytics may spot small deficiencies and offer focused solutions that could otherwise go unnoticed (Adans-Dester et al., 2020).

Similar to this, post-operative recovery regimens in orthopaedic rehabilitation have been optimized through the use of prediction models. For instance, machine learning systems use motion sensor data and patient-reported outcomes to forecast recovery milestones following knee replacement surgery. Early identification enables doctors to act with customized therapy for patients who do not improve as planned. In one instance, a model was able to identify patients who were at danger of developing joint stiffness and suggested extra flexibility exercises, which improved the patients' mobility (McDermott et al., 2024). Better healing periods are only one advantage of customized rehabilitation programs. Predictive analytics improves patient engagement, which is essential to the success of rehabilitation, by customizing therapies to meet each patient's requirements. When programs seem relevant and doable, patients are more likely to stick with them, which lowers dropout rates and guarantees steady improvement. Predictive model-powered rehabilitation applications, for example, give patients engaging activities and real-time feedback, which increases their motivation and sense of achievement. Patients become active participants in their rehabilitation process by using these tools to monitor their progress (Chae et al., 2020). Another significant benefit of using predictive analytics for tailored rehabilitation is cost reduction. Trial-and-error methods are frequently used in standardized rehabilitation programs, which might result in needless treatments or slowed development. By determining the best solutions early on, predictive models reduce these inefficiencies (Adans-Dester et al., 2020). Algorithms, for instance, have been used in physical therapy clinics to identify patients who are most likely to benefit from shorter rehabilitation programs, enabling more effective use of available resources. In addition to lowering healthcare costs, this strategy frees up resources to treat more patients. Notwithstanding these advantages, there are several difficulties in using predictive analytics to individualized rehabilitation. The representativeness and quality of the data used to train machine learning models is one important concern. Prediction accuracy may be impacted by biases or inconsistencies that frequently plague rehabilitation datasets (Chae et al., 2020). When used on elderly patients with chronic diseases, for example, a model that was built on data from younger, active patients would not function effectively. Diverse and superior data gathering initiatives that capture the diversity of patient groups are necessary to meet this issue (McDermott et al., 2024).

The possibility of relying too much on predictive models raises further concerns as it may result in less clinical engagement. Despite being strong instruments, algorithms are unable to completely replace the sophisticated judgment of seasoned medical practitioners. For instance, based on performance data, an algorithm may suggest an intense workout program, but a doctor may determine that a more progressive approach is necessary due to a patient's psychological preparedness or pain threshold. This emphasizes how crucial it is to combine human experience and predictive analytics in order to get the best results (Adans-Dester et al., 2020). Data security and privacy are also important factors. Concerns with adherence to laws like HIPAA and GDPR are raised when sensitive patient data is used in predictive analytics. Maintaining patient confidence and guarding against breaches requires strong data encryption, anonymization, and safe storage. Predictive analytics is revolutionizing individualized rehabilitation by facilitating customized treatments that raise patient satisfaction, lower costs, and improve patient outcomes. The potential of ML algorithms to revolutionize conventional rehabilitation techniques is demonstrated by case studies in orthopaedic treatment, cardiac rehabilitation, and stroke recovery. However, issues with data quality, clinical engagement, and privacy must be resolved if these advantages are to be fully realized. Predictive analytics can open the door to a more individualized, effective, and efficient approach to rehabilitation by striking a balance between innovation and moral and practical issues (Reis et al., 2024).

Wearable Technology and Sensor Data in Assistive Systems

In the recent past, wearable technology has become fundamental to current assistive systems especially in the areas of rehabilitation and health. It explains that the real-time data collected by wearable devices allow for sophisticated and adaptive ML model-based interventions. This integration can increase the output of the predictive systematic rehabilitation and give more control over their treatment to the patients. The information gathered by wearables in real-time is indispensable for constructing and updating the ML models that support assistive systems. Smartwatches, fitness trackers, and now many health-focused and medical wearables have sensors for the assessment of several physiological and biomechanical indices like heart rate, steps taken, oxygen saturation level, muscular activation, and even static posture. These quantify and qualify a patient's condition constantly and in real time making it easier for the ML algorithms to analyse and predict outcomes and propose possible actions. For instance, monitoring the heart rate variability of a patient exercising using a smartwatch can help patient and clinician notice signs of over exertion early enough thus making changes to the rehabilitation programme before complications develop (Reis et al., 2024). It is also important that the sensor data be fed into prognostic rehabilitation systems for purposes of added functionality and precision. Accelerometers and gyroscopes in particular are used frequently when it comes to tracking movement quality and range of motion in exercise prescribed during physical therapy. They are used to measure joint angles, gait characteristics and muscle activation, which are then fed into an ML system to determine performance and abnormality. For example, following a total hip replacement THP the walking pattern of the patient can be captured by the wearable devices and any straying from the normal healing pattern or use of compensatory mechanisms detected. From these observations, the system is in a position to recommend appropriate exercises to be carried out in order to fill these gaps and thereby ease the recovery process (Reis et al., 2024).

Pulse oximeters and electromyography (EMG) gadgets are also very common as tools for measuring cardiovascular and muscular reactions during therapy in rehabilitation centres. Analysing this data allows the use of predictive models in determining the physical strength of a patient and using this to set the right workout regimes for the patient. For instance, while the patient is on cardiac rehabilitation, ECG monitors that are worn can identify variance in heart rhythm or suggest signs of risk; therefore, clinicians have an opportunity to act as early as possible. Likewise, EMG sensors used in stroke rehabilitation can give feedback regarding the patient specific muscle activation patterns that will enable the patient to regain motor function more efficiently (Reis et al., 2024). It remains to emphasize that case studies clearly demonstrate the significance of wearable devices in assistive systems. For example, wearable motion sensors in rehabilitation of patients with ID: Parkinson's disease. Research created an ML-based system which resulted in the analysis of tremors and gait disturbances as collected by wearable devices. It not only recorded the behaviours of symptoms aggravation but also advised some exercising to enhance balance and orientation functions. Newly confluent mobility and reported increased levels of self-reliance showed the benefits of wearable technology for patients and overall quality of life. The last case analysed was based on wearable smart insoles with precisely placed pressure sensors to help lower-limb injuries victims. These insoles collected data on the patient's weight and gait as they walked, and this information was used to explain the right posture and manner of moving (Khan et al., 2020). This research also showed that patients who wore the smart insoles during their rehabilitation came out better than those that received physical therapy. This demonstrates the need to include wearable technology in rehabilitation programs so that outcome can be enhanced. However, the use of wearable devices in assistive systems has its weaknesses that should be discussed in detail. While it is common knowledge that the quality and consistency of data is essential for developing and deploying ML models, the problem of noise represented in wearables by faulty sensors or outside influences can be a huge issue. For example, a motion sensor may assume irregular movements of an object or individual as actual movement that warrants recommendations consequently making wrong recommendations (Santilli et al., 2024). Furthermore, solving these problems entails some amount of calibration and validation of data obtained from these sensors so that the models give out results that are relevant. Other issues attributed to Wearable technology include Privilege and Data security/Privacy. The ongoing collection and transfer of patient information give certain people potential access or use of personal data. While rules like GDPR or HIPAA should be followed, it is necessary to go a step further in the protection of patient's information by using encryptions, anonymization as well as storage of data (Khan et al., 2020). However, integration of wearable devices comes with costs which can prove very expensive especially for developing countries. That does not mean that better devices offering greater accuracy using more advanced sensors are still not beyond the financial reach of many patients. It is here that current stepped approaches cannot directly bridge the gap, and new approaches such as public private partnerships /subsidized technologies are required in order to make these technologies available and accessible for all (Santilli et al., 2024). Therefore, wearable technology and sensor data are highly effective means within assistive systems, allowing for the capturing of real time data and feeding it to ML models to improve the accuracy of real-time predictive rehabilitation systems. Wearable motion sensor for Parkinson's disease or smart insoles for lower-limb rehabilitation are examples of what these devices can do which makes them ideal patient companions. However, there are still issues pertaining to quality of data, data privacy; and data costs which need to be solved to the optimal usage of the above benefits. Overcoming these impediments, wearable technology can advance the development of patient-specific rehabilitation and enhance recovery for a wide range of client types (Khan et al., 2020).

Predictive Algorithms in Neurorehabilitation

Predictive algorithms utilization in neurorehabilitation might be considered a radically innovative shift in the progressive therapy for stroke and SCI patients. Predictive algorithms in the application of ML lets clinicians predict recovery trends, tweak the therapy regimens and improve on the outcome achieved by patients Adam & Mukhtar, 2024). In neurorehabilitation, the aim of the ML models is to study big data such as patients' information, including medical history, images, signals, and behaviour. These algorithms reveal factors and relationship that clinicians or researchers may not recognize and incorporate exact prognosis of the word class recovery pattern. Please use the following example: As with any other disease, the spectrum and velocity of motor dysfunction restoration after a stroke are different for different patients due to the cause and the severity of the stated ailment, possible accompanying disorders, as well as the patient's obedience to the prescribed therapy. Algorithms examine such aspects to predict the trends in recovery to help therapists to enhance application to improve on the functional capabilities of the patient (Ahmed et al., 2020). Among these, the use of predictive algorithms has been quite useful in tracking of motor recovery after stroke. While wearing EMG devices or motion capture systems, applied to upper and lower limbs during exercises for rehabilitation, it is possible to get data for establishing whether the patient performs the exercises with sufficient quality and correctness. Using this information, the algorithms pinpoint certain forms of impairment, including coordination or strength in the specific limb and suggest appropriate intervention. For example, if a patient shows limited movements of the wrist after a stroke, the model can predict that the patient shall engage in repeated wrist flexion/de flexion exercises with progressively increasing the amount of resistance plus receiving biographical and real-time feedback. This way helps to make therapy organized and effective and, at the same time, tailored to each patient's needs Adam & Mukhtar, 2024).

In spinal cord injury (SCI) rehabilitation, the same sophisticated predictive algorithms are equally stimulating. For persons with SCI rehab aims at regaining some form of motor control, the sensory modalities, and general motor independence. The severity of the inflicted injuries and the patients' history contribute to the increase in ML performance when it comes to predicting the probability of regaining particular forms of mobility or hand dexterity. For instance, a work based on fMRI data and clinical history evaluated using artificial neural network models outcomes of SCI patients in gait trainings. Such predictions concerned about the therapy plans, including the identification of causes that might be most effective using certain resources to affect the therapy outcomes significantly (Esfahlani et al., 2022). In real-world neurorehabilitation settings, the use of predictive algorithms is best illustrated by AI-driven neurorehabilitation devices. For example, robotic exoskeletons, which help patients in executing stereotypic motor activity, including a walk or a reach. They also feature the sensors to measure joint angles, force and muscle activation. Real-time signal analysis is done by predictive algorithms to adjust the level of support delivered by the exoskeleton so that patient is not overexerted yet pushed to the required level of difficulty. Patients using the AI-powered robotic exoskeletons for therapy have been observed to achieve higher functional gains and in lesser time than those undergoing conventional therapy (Ahmed et al., 2020). Another emerging technology in neurorehabilitation is the brain-computer interface (BCI) technology. BCIs control muscle contractions or reconstruct signals sent from the brain to other organs in the body to power other related equipment such as prosthetic limbs or communication aids for patients with severe motor disabilities. In LIS patients, using BCIs based on machine learning algorithms, I have been able to restore very basic functions, and hence, the life of the patients has been greatly enhanced. Also, BCIs can enhance the neuroplasticity of the brain to integrate new connections or relearn lost functions during a rehabilitation process by supplying information about the neural activity, and here they can speed up the process. With these developments it can be noted that there is still a number of issues, concerns, and limitations, which we feel are important to discuss in relation to the use of predictive algorithms in neurorehabilitation (Scrutinio et al., 2020). However, there is a problem of data variation in patients. Neurological disorders are by their essence multi-factorial and patients' progress may depend on factors not easy to generalize, such as patient's motivation, individual psychological profile, and social environment, to mention a few. This variability can compromise the sharing of data due to the chance which can affect the use of predictive models in particular when used on dataset that has not incorporated minority groups data. For instance, one derived from data collected from young clients may not work as well when used on other aged persons with similar diseases (Esfahlani et al., 2022).

The second process is less problematic but still can be considered as an issue, namely the implementation of predictive algorithms into clinical practice. Although these algorithms offer a wide range of potential, their application is accompanied by considerable costs concerning technological support and professional personnel, along with the respect for legal norms and standards. And lastly, clinicians may not want to trust the output from an algorithm to come up with suggestions which are contrary to what their natural instincts are anyway. Establishing credibility in such systems means offering full disclosure on different validation techniques, detailed descriptions of outputs aggregated by the algorithm, as well as the actual demonstration of the applicability of the same in different real-life situations (Scrutinio et al., 2020). Ethical issues finally come into the picture in the use of predictive algorithms in neuro habitation. Patients' identity has to be protected, especially when the algorithms work with the information like a brain scan or neural signals. It has become mandatory to follow rules and regulation of data protection and the effective security measure to avoid misuse of the patients' data. Furthermore, the issue of considering algorithmic bias is critical because the consequence may be bias in terms of treatment options as predicted by algorithms. For example, where the training data leads an algorithm to underestimate recovery potential in some patient categories, the latter will receive below par treatment (de Filippis & Al Foysal, 2024).

This notwithstanding, the potential that hold the outcome of predictive algorithms in neurorehabilitation is enormous. These algorithms can therefore promote patient compliance, better functional outcomes, as well as cut the costs of future healthcare service delivery. For example, a model for patient selection for intensive therapy would entail a model that predicts which patients can benefit from such treatments and therefore using such money on patients who are most likely to exhibit substantial improvement. In conclusion, predictive algorithms are transforming neurorehabilitation as they make use of factual information to plan therapies for neurological disorders, such as stroke and spinal cord paralysis (Scrutinio et al., 2020). Robotic exoskeletons, BCI, and wearable sensors are some of the application areas that show the use of such technologies with an ability to improve patient results. There are always threats associated with data variation, clinical implementation breakdowns, and moral issues that are yet to be addressed in further detail; however, enhanced machine learning and collaboration of the researchers, clinicians, and policymakers will systematically address these questions. It can be stated that further development of predictive algorithms is not only bright future of neurorehabilitation, but the new hope and new opportunities for millions of patients globally (de Filippis & Al Foysal, 2024).

AI-Driven Prosthetics and Orthotics: Predictive Control and Adaptation

The use of AI and predictive algorithms in prosthetics and orthotics fashioning is changing the wearing prosthetics and orthotics controls and the way assistive devices are customized to the users. Due to the increased application of advanced technologies, AI driven systems add functionality, increase comfort, and help disabled people gain more freedom (Chekroud et al., 2021). In terms of prosthetic limbs and orthotic devices, AI and predictive algorithms can pinpoint and address intricate elements in the design and control due to the way and the extent to which these systems can responds to the user and the environment. Conventional prostheses do not allow for the adaptation of the prosthesis to the active lobulations, which are identified in users' activity. As opposed to that, machine learning models in AI-driven prosthetics use data acquired from different sensors like accelerometers, gyroscopes, and EMG that tracks muscle movement as well. By using this data, in real time, the prediction of the user's intention becomes feasible, so the device is able to adapt to its use and perform in ways that are natural and smooth (Damaševičius et al., 2024). Microprocessor controlled knee prosthesis named Ottobock C-Leg is a well-known example of AI prosthetic. The C-Leg detects a user's movements, adapts to the terrain, and offers recommendations on the optimal stance and gait to employ whenever the user is choosing between surfaces with either higher or lower friction. For example, whenever the devise identify that the user is going down the stairs it adjusts the amount of resistance that it provides so that the user moves in a safe manner. Essential research have established increased mobility and decreased risks of falling in the users of the intelligent C-Leg in contrast to other ordinary prostheses implying the usability of AI in enhancing the assistive technology application (Chekroud et al., 2021).

The other strategies increasing the flexibility of prosthetic and orthotic systems are predictive control strategies. These strategies involve feeding the current input and the device uses ML models to determine the upcoming state so that it can anticipate changes in the user 's activity or the environment. For instance, intelligent Ankle Foot Orthoses (IAFOs) with incorporated predictive control strategies to control the stiffness and orientation of the brace depending on the deviation in the walking speed or the type of surface. This flexibility enhances the comfort of the users at the same time reducing the probability of getting injured due to offered support (Damaševičius et al., 2024). In upper-limb prosthetics, AI, and predictive algorithms have been used to bring great progress for finer movement. Limb prosthetic technologies like the LUKE Arm built by DEKA Research imitate signals interpreted by EMG originating from residual muscles from the user. These signals are fed into Machine Learning to attempt to control the prosthesis in regard to the user's desired movements such as grasping an object or pointing at an object and then translates it into controllable movements of the prosthetic hand. Such a capability grants users the needed authority to accomplish elaborate operations including typing or even holding delicate items (Shi et al., 2025). Examples of how AI technology and innovations in prosthetics and orthotics impact on the lives of users can be found throughout the book. One case in point is a young lady who had to have her legs amputated following an accident, she was fitted with running AI enhanced prosthetic leg. This shoe, built with sensors and analytics, was able to adapt the firmness of its springs and the absorption co-efficient in order to achieve the most efficiency during each stage of the running gait cycle. With help of this technology, she was able not only to come back to competitive sports but also set personal records which are the examples of how AI can assist a person and change his life (Chae et al., 2020). However, much still lies in the way to fully realizing the capabilities of AI-integrated prosthetics and orthotics in the community. They also raise the question of the prohibitive cost of such devices, which may effectively bar many potential users from considering taking up such devices. On one hand, the high-tech development is very useful; on the other hand, the cost of inserting sensors, processors and machine learning systems into a piece of device are too high for many people to afford. Continued attempts at defining a more cost-effective method and fostering the creation of cheaper versions of this technology remain high on the agenda to maintain availability for all (Shi et al., 2025). Data privacy and data security are two other concerns; this is because AI-based systems must feed on data to remain relevant, improve and adapt. These concerns are fully warranted for such technologies as muscle activity and movement pattern should not be accessible to unauthorized users. There are necessary regulations that developers have to accompany their applications and employ strict measures of cybersecurity that will allow users' information to be secure while providing the company with amounts of data necessary for accurate prediction of behaviours (Chae et al., 2020).

Additionally, AI solutions are as good as the data they are trained on, to predict and generate better models for the organization. Bias with respect to data may lead to poor estimations of the performance of the gait analysis system especially for the special category of users such as those who have some deformities in their gait pattern or are diagnosed with a certain medical condition. To address such an issue, society should ensure that AI systems receive diverse datasets and that those datasets are appropriately diverse so that the AI-powered assistive systems perform consistently with users of all kinds. Specifically, AI-powered prosthetics and orthotics are an improvement on traditional assistive technology that offers flexibility, utility, and independence to users. They have features of predictive algorithms and real-time data, so these devices can identify and even predict users' need and improve a subject's quality of life being disabled (Chekroud et al., 2021). There are, nevertheless, issues as cost, data protection, and realistic and stable models However, due to the constant evolution of AI and machine learning, these novel tools are likely to become more reliable and easily appropriate. That is why the enhancement of the contemporary AI solutions, the further advancement of the systems being presented will undoubtedly define the future of the prosthetics and orthotics and grant users the necessary level of active mobility (Shi et al., 2025).

Ethical Considerations in Predictive Rehabilitation Technologies

The utilization of ML AI based predictive rehabilitation technologies also poses significant ethical questions that need to be solved for proper utilization of rehabilitative inventions. As these technologies can lead to improved rehabilitation through more individual approach to patients and increased effectiveness, there is always a problem of privacy, data protection, patient self-determination and possible prejudices in the algorithm creation (Velusamy et al., 2024). With regard to the ethical considerations, one of the topical questions is related to the acquisition and processing of personal information of patients. Predictive algorithms depend on large amounts of personal data: medical records, data collected from personal electronics, and physiological monitoring. While this data is very helpful for creating corresponding models, it is also very dangerous from the point of view of personal information protection. For instance, this data can be used inappropriately to prejudice individuals by discriminating against them in issues to do with insurance and employment among others. The digital records protection was severely compromised when, in 2019, a large healthcare organization had a breach releasing millions of patients 'records. To avoid or reduce the risk of these matters, sound encryption techniques and safeguarding of the data which is to be collected must be followed. Similarly, it is critical to follow the data protection statutes, including the General Data Protection Regulation (GDPR) to protect the patient's data and trust the potential predictive rehabilitation technologies could achieve (Buscarini et al., 2024).

The fourth ethic is self-determination since most decisions are made using algorithms. The use of predictive technologies in a number of treatments means that treatment plans are prescribed from a statistical analysis perspective on likelihoods. Though these recommendations will enhance the patient's results, those enhancements come at a cost of limited Agency as patient choice gets dominated by AI. For example, an algorithm suggests a set of exercises in accordance with the identified patterns of recovery speed, but the patient feels the program is too heavy or just not suitable for him. While making such recommendations, the healthcare providers need to inform and include the patient in the decision making as to how those recommendations are made. In involving both the clinical professional and the patient in coming up with the treatment plan, then it is possible to find a middle ground between the two and create the needed algorithm without compromising the individual's freedom (Velusamy et al., 2024). Pneumonic in machine learning models is another key problem of substantial social importance in terms of rehabilitation application of predictive technology on AI. This shows that algorithms trained on datasets that contain limited diversity make biased predictions that give disparate treatments. For instance, using data from younger patients, a model for predicting recovery will generate less accurate recommendations for old patients. This is especially important in rehabilitation since age, sex, race, and medical history are common predictors of recovery. In 2020, a significant study by the academic team showed that much-deployed healthcare algorithm underestimated the healthcare requirements of Black patients indicating how and to what extent prejudice creeps into AI systems. To counter this, developers need to see to it that the training set is a good sample of the population the technology is being targeted on. This is can also be achieved by an annual review of the model across samples of different demographics to flag and address bias issues (Buscarini et al., 2024).

The three major ethical considerations are transparency and explainability, which the programmes incorporate as a fundamental practice towards making efficient, and effective, accurate, and fair predictions. The specificity of many machine learning models, and especially more advanced ones such as deep neural networks, is that they exist as 'black box' models that make predictions but are not immediately clear as to how those predictions are made. Such opacity reduces trust between patients and clinicians since the patients cannot trust those recommendations they do not understand. Creating the mechanism and providing explanations of machine learning results enables one to increase trust and make decisions. For example, rule-based or decision tree systems are more accurate but less complex, more interpretable and can be used in cases where interpretability is critical (Velusamy et al., 2024). Alongside with the technological aspects, the problem of ethical approach to the utilization of technologies in question, by companies that create and apply predictive rehabilitation technologies, has to be solved. This has involves providing developers and clinicians education about the ethical themes found in AI and also active promotion of communication and collaboration between technologists, ethicists and clinicians. Fiduciary governance committees may be set up to coordinate factors related to predictive algorithms and other matters, within terms of ethical principles of justice, integrity, and paternalism (Nascimben, 2024).

There are equally other ethical related factors which require public participation, and awareness. The techniques used must inform the patients and the caregivers of the gains and limitations of the predictive rehabilitation technologies, and of the patients' data usage rights. Sharing the information regarding the gathering, analysis, and application of such information for arriving at a prediction allows patients to foster better control over the quality of their treatment (Buscarini et al., 2024). Last but not the least, a focus should be made on future sociopolitical consequences of predictive rehabilitation technologies. As with any process novelties and technological advancements, it is not without its errors which if effectively exploited can also widen the existing gap or disparities within the healthcare field. For example, the people in developing nations may have no recourse to the high technology necessary for predictive rehabilitation hence a disconnect between those who can afford the technology and those who cannot. The future of rehabilitative technology is promising; however, its moral adoption concerns privacy, security, patient agency, and fairness. Thus, with the need to build operational transparency and inclusiveness in data collection together with patient-centricity, stakeholders can combine the best of predictive algorithms with ethical considerations. Mitigating these risks effectively will create a pathway toward a future that technology improves or at least does not depreciate the dignity and quality of life of patients (Nascimben, 2024).

CASE STUDIES: SUCCESSFUL APPLICATIONS OF PREDICTIVE ALGORITHMS IN REHABILITATION

The use of the algorithms for predicting the progress of the patients in rehabilitation has been proven feasible thus showing how big the change in the delivery of care is in relation to the specific needs of the patients, the results to be expected, and productivity. With the use of context-aware system, interdisciplinary collaborations between healthcare providers, engineers, and data scientists; these systems have developed remarkable improvements in rehabilitation practices. They also present real-life examples emphasising how and when such methods work, what difficulties might one face and what important findings of their practical application one can get (Zhang et al., 2024). One of the most inspiring examples of the application of predictive algorithms in rehabilitation practice is the field of stroke. Irrespective of the type of rehabilitation center, machine learning models were utilized to forecast post-stroke motor function recovery in this study. With help of the data on activity gathered by wearable devices' accelerometers and gyroscopes along with patients deprived demographical and medical data, the algorithm outlined the further recovery course and suggested individual therapy regimen. For example, the system could say that during some future date a specific patient will need more attention to balance exercises because his/her gait speed is not increasing as rapidly. A high-level consequence was achieved – sample-by-sample guided by the algorithm intervention combined with conventional care provided a clearly better result by 20% in terms of mobility improvement among the patients. This further emphasise the need for smart decision-making that will allow for clinician to better assign resources and recommend treatments based on patients' requirements (Zhang et al., 2024).

On the other hand, problems arose when using such algorithm substrates in US-China negotiations as well. One major limitation was observed where there were significant differences in the quality of the sensed data due to differences in calibration of the devices used and the compliance of the patients. For instance, fluctuation in efficacies of the wearable devices rendered by patients was another influential consideration, where an improper usage led to missing records, which removed certainty from the model. This problem shows that effective preprocessing approaches as well as patient knowledge must be established to achieve accurate data input. Furthermore, the implementation of such systems as decision support into clinical practice meant that healthcare providers were educated on how best to understand the results produced by algorithm and respond to them, as well as how to engage interdisciplinary teams in capacity building processes (Yagi et al., 2023). Predictive algorithms were used in neurorehabilitation for individuals with spinal cord injuries in another instance. An AI system that evaluated electromyography (EMG) data to forecast muscle recovery and enhance treatment plans was created by a rehabilitation centre in collaboration with data scientists. The system's ability to recognize early signs of muscle reactivation allows therapists to proactively modify the frequency and intensity of treatments. For example, one patient displayed encouraging EMG signals indicating latent recovery potential but made little progress with conventional treatment. In the end, the algorithm's suggested experimental treatment of functional electrical stimulation resulted in notable gains in muscular strength and coordination. This instance illustrates the value of technology in assisting with evidence-based decision-making in addition to the ability of predictive analytics to reveal latent recovery chances (Santilli et al., 2024).

Notwithstanding these achievements, it was clear that incorporating predictive algorithms into neurorehabilitation presented difficulties. The early reluctance of doctors to depend on algorithmic results over conventional clinical judgment was a significant problem. In order to solve this, the development team held seminars to educate staff members on the system's features and constraints, encouraging acceptance and trust. Furthermore, the intricacy of neurological disorders occasionally caused differences between expected and actual results, highlighting the necessity of ongoing model validation and improvement across a range of patient groups (Yagi et al., 2023). For predictive rehabilitation systems to be successful, interdisciplinary cooperation has proven essential. One noteworthy example is the creation of an intelligent rehabilitation platform for people who have had knee replacements. An AI-driven system that integrated wearable sensor data with patient-reported outcomes to track recovery progress was developed by engineers, medical professionals, and data scientists. The technology warned doctors to take immediate action when it detected departures from typical healing patterns, such as decreased range of motion or persistent discomfort. In one instance, the algorithm identified the patient's early postoperative problems, allowing for prompt medical intervention to avert further decline. This proactive strategy demonstrated the cost-effectiveness of predictive technology by lowering hospital readmissions and improving patient outcomes (Santilli et al., 2024). However, there were practical challenges in deploying such systems, especially when it came to combining data from many sources into a single platform. Significant obstacles were presented by differences in data formats and device compatibility problems. In order to solve this, the group created a common data structure and made investments in middleware programs that made data integration easier. The significance of resolving operational and technical obstacles during the implementation stage is shown by this experience (Boukhennoufa et al., 2022).

These case studies offer insightful insights into how predictive algorithms could be used in rehabilitation in the future. First, constructing accurate models depends critically on the quality and consistency of the data, which calls for strong data collecting procedures and patient involvement. Second, in order to bridge the gap between technology and healthcare competence, training and cooperation are crucial for integrating these technologies into clinical practice (Yagi et al., 2023). Finally, via proactive intervention and individualized treatment, predictive algorithms have demonstrated their ability to completely transform rehabilitation. Their ability to improve recovery outcomes, optimize resource allocation, and save healthcare costs is demonstrated by real-world applications. To fully reap their advantages, however, the difficulties relating to clinical integration, data quality, and multidisciplinary cooperation must be properly resolved. These technologies provide a viable route for more effective, patient-centred rehabilitation techniques as they develop further (Boukhennoufa et al., 2022).

CONCLUSION

Predictive algorithms in assistive technology and rehabilitation have enormous potential to change the face of healthcare and patient recovery in the future. More individualized, effective, and efficient treatment will be provided than ever before thanks to the convergence of wearable technologies, machine learning, and data analytics. To guarantee fair and responsible implementation, overcoming present obstacles, encouraging interdisciplinary cooperation, and navigating ethical issues are all necessary to realize this promise. By customizing treatments to meet the needs of each patient, predictive algorithms have already shown that they may improve rehabilitation results. To find patterns and improve treatment strategies, these systems use enormous volumes of data from wearable technology, electronic medical records, and patient-reported metrics. Algorithms will eventually be able to consider intricate, nonlinear interactions in patient data thanks to the incorporation of even more advanced machine learning models, such deep learning networks. Systems might, for example, anticipate small patterns of recovery that physicians might otherwise miss, allowing for early treatments and averting problems. It is anticipated that this proactive strategy would decrease total healthcare expenditures, shorten treatment durations, and increase recovery rates. Additionally, assistive systems are expected to play a bigger role in the development and management of orthotics, prosthetics, and neurorehabilitation equipment. AI-driven prostheses and assistive technology will continue to enhance the mobility and quality of life of people with impairments by enabling real-time adaptability. Further bridging the gap between human competence and technological augmentation, future advances may include prosthetic devices that learn and adjust on their own to changes in the user's surroundings or physical state. Similar to this, predictive analytics-driven neurorehabilitation systems may improve treatment plans for neurological disease patients by offering focused exercises and feedback that hasten neuronal healing and functional enhancement.

Even with these encouraging advancements, difficulties still exist. It is crucial to guarantee the accuracy and dependability of the data used to feed prediction algorithms. The efficacy of these systems may be compromised by variations in patient compliance, device calibration, and platform-to-platform data integration. Adopting interoperable technology and creating defined protocols for data gathering and preprocessing will be necessary to address these problems. Predictive algorithms' ethical ramifications also need to be thoroughly examined. Concerns about algorithmic bias, data privacy, and the possibility of relying too much on machine-generated suggestions underscore the necessity of open and responsible implementation procedures. Future predictive rehabilitation technology development will be heavily influenced by interdisciplinary cooperation. To guarantee that these systems are not only technologically sound but also therapeutically relevant and socially responsible, collaborations between healthcare professionals, data scientists, engineers, and legislators are crucial. Stakeholders may address ethical and technological issues while advancing the creation of more inclusive and equitable solutions by cultivating an innovative and collaborative culture. Predictive algorithms have the unquestionable potential to revolutionize assistive and rehabilitative systems as they develop further. In the end, these technologies improve patient lives and lessen the strain on healthcare systems by providing a route to more individualized, efficient, and accessible treatment. However, consistent investment in ethical governance, innovation, and research will be necessary to realize this ambition. A healthier, more inclusive society is possible using predictive algorithms in rehabilitation if present constraints are addressed and a cooperative strategy is adopted.

REFERENCES

Adam, M. A., & Mukhtar, A. (2024). Heartfelt insights: AI and machine learning applications for cardiac wellness. *International Journal of Advanced Engineering Technologies and Innovations*, *1*(4), 231–247.

Adans-Dester, C., Hankov, N., O'Brien, A., Vergara-Diaz, G., Black-Schaffer, R., Zafonte, R., Dy, J., Lee, S. I., & Bonato, P. (2020). Enabling precision rehabilitation interventions using wearable sensors and machine learning to track motor recovery. *NPJ Digital Medicine*, *3*(1), 121. DOI: 10.1038/s41746-020-00328-w PMID: 33024831

Ahmed, Z., Mohamed, K., Zeeshan, S., & Dong, X. (2020). Artificial intelligence with multi-functional machine learning platform development for better healthcare and precision medicine. *Database : The Journal of Biological Databases and Curation*, *2020*, baaa010. DOI: 10.1093/database/baaa010 PMID: 32185396

Arjmandnia, F., & Alimohammadi, E. (2024). The value of machine learning technology and artificial intelligence to enhance patient safety in spine surgery: A review. *Patient Safety in Surgery*, *18*(1), 11. DOI: 10.1186/s13037-024-00393-0 PMID: 38528562

Bica, I., Alaa, A. M., Lambert, C., & Van Der Schaar, M. (2021). From real-world patient data to individualized treatment effects using machine learning: Current and future methods to address underlying challenges. *Clinical Pharmacology and Therapeutics*, *109*(1), 87–100. DOI: 10.1002/cpt.1907 PMID: 32449163

Bonkhoff, A. K., & Grefkes, C. (2022). Precision medicine in stroke: Towards personalized outcome predictions using artificial intelligence. *Brain*, *145*(2), 457–475. DOI: 10.1093/brain/awab439 PMID: 34918041

Boukhennoufa, I., Zhai, X., Utti, V., Jackson, J., & McDonald-Maier, K. D. (2022). Wearable sensors and machine learning in post-stroke rehabilitation assessment: A systematic review. *Biomedical Signal Processing and Control*, *71*, 103197. DOI: 10.1016/j.bspc.2021.103197

Buscarini, L., Romano, P., Cocco, E. S., Damiani, C., Pournajaf, S., Franceschini, M., & Infarinato, F. (2024). Enhancing patient rehabilitation outcomes: Artificial intelligence-driven predictive modeling for home discharge in neurological and orthopedic conditions.

Chae, S. H., Kim, Y., Lee, K. S., & Park, H. S. (2020). Development and clinical evaluation of a web-based upper limb home rehabilitation system using a smartwatch and machine learning model for chronic stroke survivors: Prospective comparative study. *JMIR mHealth and uHealth, 8*(7), e17216. DOI: 10.2196/17216 PMID: 32480361

Chekroud, A. M., Bondar, J., Delgadillo, J., Doherty, G., Wasil, A., Fokkema, M., Cohen, Z., Belgrave, D., DeRubeis, R., Iniesta, R., Dwyer, D., & Choi, K. (2021). The promise of machine learning in predicting treatment outcomes in psychiatry. *World Psychiatry; Official Journal of the World Psychiatric Association (WPA), 20*(2), 154–170. DOI: 10.1002/wps.20882 PMID: 34002503

Damaševičius, R., Jagatheesaperumal, S. K., Kandala, R. N., Hussain, S., Alizadehsani, R., & Gorriz, J. M. (2024). Deep learning for personalized health monitoring and prediction: A review. *Computational Intelligence, 40*(3), e12682. DOI: 10.1111/coin.12682

de Filippis, R., & Al Foysal, A. (2024). Harnessing the power of artificial intelligence in neuromuscular disease rehabilitation: A comprehensive review and algorithmic approach. *Advances in Bioscience and Biotechnology, 15*(5), 289–309. DOI: 10.4236/abb.2024.155018

Esfahlani, S. S., Shirvani, H., Butt, J., Mirzaee, I., & Esfahlani, K. S. (2022). Machine learning role in clinical decision-making: Neuro-rehabilitation video game. *Expert Systems with Applications, 201*, 117165. DOI: 10.1016/j.eswa.2022.117165

Fong, J., Ocampo, R., Gross, D. P., & Tavakoli, M. (2020). Intelligent robotics incorporating machine learning algorithms for improving functional capacity evaluation and occupational rehabilitation. *Journal of Occupational Rehabilitation, 30*(3), 362–370. DOI: 10.1007/s10926-020-09888-w PMID: 32253595

Karapintzou, E., Tsakanikas, V., Kikidis, D., Nikitas, C., Nairn, B., Pavlou, M., . . . Fotiadis, D. I. (2024, November). AI-enhanced tele-rehabilitation: Predictive modeling for fall risk and treatment efficacy in balance disorders. In *2024 IEEE 24th International Conference on Bioinformatics and Bioengineering (BIBE)* (pp. 1–8). IEEE.

Khan, O., Badhiwala, J. H., Grasso, G., & Fehlings, M. G. (2020). Use of machine learning and artificial intelligence to drive personalized medicine approaches for spine care. *World Neurosurgery, 140*, 512–518. DOI: 10.1016/j.wneu.2020.04.022 PMID: 32797983

Lanotte, F., O'Brien, M. K., & Jayaraman, A. (2023). AI in rehabilitation medicine: Opportunities and challenges. *Annals of Rehabilitation Medicine*, *47*(6), 444–458. DOI: 10.5535/arm.23131 PMID: 38093518

Mainali, S., Darsie, M. E., & Smetana, K. S. (2021). Machine learning in action: Stroke diagnosis and outcome prediction. *Frontiers in Neurology*, *12*, 734345. DOI: 10.3389/fneur.2021.734345 PMID: 34938254

McDermott, E. R., DeFoor, M. T., Dekker, T. J., & DePhillipo, N. N. (2024). Artificial intelligence in rehabilitation. In *Artificial Intelligence in Orthopaedic Surgery Made Easy* (pp. 197–204). Springer Nature Switzerland. DOI: 10.1007/978-3-031-70310-2_19

Nascimben, M. (2024). Machine learning approaches for personalized medicine.

Nicora, G., Pe, S., Santangelo, G., Billeci, L., Aprile, I. G., Germanotta, M., ... & Quaglini, S. (2024). A systematic review of machine learning in robotics-assisted rehabilitation.

Olyanasab, A., & Annabestani, M. (2024). Leveraging machine learning for personalized wearable biomedical devices: A review. *Journal of Personalized Medicine*, *14*(2), 203. DOI: 10.3390/jpm14020203 PMID: 38392636

Pelosi, A. D., Roth, N., Yehoshua, T., Itah, D., Braun Benyamin, O., & Dahan, A. (2024). Personalized rehabilitation approach for reaching movement using reinforcement learning. *Scientific Reports*, *14*(1), 17675. DOI: 10.1038/s41598-024-64514-6 PMID: 39085281

Rasa, A. R. (2024). Artificial intelligence and its revolutionary role in physical and mental rehabilitation: A review of recent advancements. *BioMed Research International*, *2024*(1), 9554590. DOI: 10.1155/bmri/9554590 PMID: 39720127

Reis, F. J., de Carvalho, M. B. L., de Assis Neves, G., Nogueira, L. C., & Meziat-Filho, N. (2024). Machine learning methods in physical therapy: A scoping review of applications in clinical context. *Musculoskeletal Science & Practice*, *74*, 103184. DOI: 10.1016/j.msksp.2024.103184 PMID: 39278141

Santilli, G., Mangone, M., Agostini, F., Paoloni, M., Bernetti, A., Diko, A., Tognolo, L., Coraci, D., Vigevano, F., Vetrano, M., Vulpiani, M. C., Fiore, P., & Gimigliano, F. (2024). Evaluation of rehabilitation outcomes in patients with chronic neurological health conditions using a machine learning approach. *Journal of Functional Morphology and Kinesiology*, *9*(4), 176. DOI: 10.3390/jfmk9040176 PMID: 39449470

Tariq, M. U. (2024). Emerging trends and innovations in blockchain-digital twin integration for green investments: A case study perspective. In Jafar, S., Rodriguez, R., Kannan, H., Akhtar, S., & Plugmann, P. (Eds.), *Harnessing blockchain-digital twin fusion for sustainable investments* (pp. 148–175). IGI Global., DOI: 10.4018/979-8-3693-1878-2.ch007

Tariq, M. U. (2024). Emotional intelligence in understanding and influencing consumer behavior. In Musiolik, T., Rodriguez, R., & Kannan, H. (Eds.), *AI impacts in digital consumer behavior* (pp. 56–81). IGI Global., DOI: 10.4018/979-8-3693-1918-5.ch003

Tariq, M. U. (2024). Application of blockchain and Internet of Things (IoT) in modern business. In Sinha, M., Bhandari, A., Priya, S., & Kabiraj, S. (Eds.), *Future of customer engagement through marketing intelligence* (pp. 66–94). IGI Global., DOI: 10.4018/979-8-3693-2367-0.ch004

Tariq, M. U. (2025). Cultivating Cultural Intelligence for the Global Workforce. In Huzooree, G., & Chandan, H. (Eds.), *Revitalizing Student Skills for Workforce Preparation* (pp. 297–332). IGI Global., DOI: 10.4018/979-8-3693-3856-8.ch010

Tariq, M. U. (2025). Vision and Strategy: Steering Modern Enterprises Towards Long-Term Success. In Sedky, A. (Ed.), *Resiliency Strategies for Long-Term Business Success* (pp. 51–78). IGI Global., DOI: 10.4018/979-8-3693-9168-6.ch003

Tariq, M. U. (2025). Leveraging Open Innovation for Sustainable Growth in the Digital Era. In Taherdoost, H. (Ed.), *Mastering Innovation in Business* (pp. 157–192). IGI Global., DOI: 10.4018/979-8-3693-3759-2.ch007

Zhang, X., Rong, X., & Luo, H. (2024). Optimizing lower limb rehabilitation: The intersection of machine learning and rehabilitative robotics. *Frontiers in Rehabilitation Sciences*, *5*, 1246773. DOI: 10.3389/fresc.2024.1246773 PMID: 38343790

KEY TERMS AND DEFINITIONS

Machine Learning (ML): A subset of artificial intelligence (AI) that enables computer systems to learn from data patterns and make predictions or decisions without explicit programming.

Predictive Algorithms: Computational models that analyze historical and real-time data to forecast future outcomes, such as patient recovery trajectories in rehabilitation.

Personalized Rehabilitation: A tailored approach to rehabilitation that uses machine learning and patient-specific data to customize therapy plans for optimal recovery.

Wearable Technology: Smart devices equipped with sensors (e.g., motion trackers, heart rate monitors) that collect real-time physiological and biomechanical data for rehabilitation monitoring and improvement.

Chapter 10
Wearable Technology and Sensor Data in Assistive Systems:
Enhancing Rehabilitation Through Predictive Analytics

Achyuth Mukund
https://orcid.org/0009-0002-5798-0858
Shiv Nadar University, Chennai, India

ABSTRACT

Wearable technology emerges as a transformative paradigm in rehabilitation, integrating advanced sensor architectures with predictive analytics to revolutionize healthcare. The chapter explores medical-grade wearables, analyzing sensor data collection and machine learning algorithms enabling precision rehabilitation strategies. By synthesizing biomechanical sensing and computational intelligence, the research unveils continuous physiological monitoring through sophisticated sensor networks. Spanning stroke rehabilitation, cardiovascular prognostics, and neurological mobility assessment, the investigation demonstrates how predictive algorithms convert raw biomechanical data into actionable clinical insights. Emerging technological convergences, including flexible biocompatible electronics and augmented reality integration, illuminate the evolutionary trajectory of wearable-assisted rehabilitation technologies, providing a comprehensive framework for understanding data-driven rehabilitation ecosystems.

DOI: 10.4018/979-8-3373-0194-5.ch010

1. INTRODUCTION

Wearable technology is part of the ever-growing Internet of Things (IoT) infrastructure that is revolutionizing the contemporary paradigms of health care, especially rehabilitation and assistive technologies. The sophisticated wearables, ranging from smartwatches and fitness trackers to clinically-approved wearables, are spearheading a revolution in patient monitoring and individualized treatment methods.

This chapter discusses the multifaceted functions of wearable devices, which use real-time sensor data and advanced predictive analytics to transform traditional rehabilitation approaches. Wearable technology can enable healthcare practitioners to build individualized interventions and monitor their progression in real time, helping transition from uniform protocols to precision medicine through the gathering of diverse physiological and biomechanical metrics.

Figure 1. Wearable technology in healthcare: Key concepts

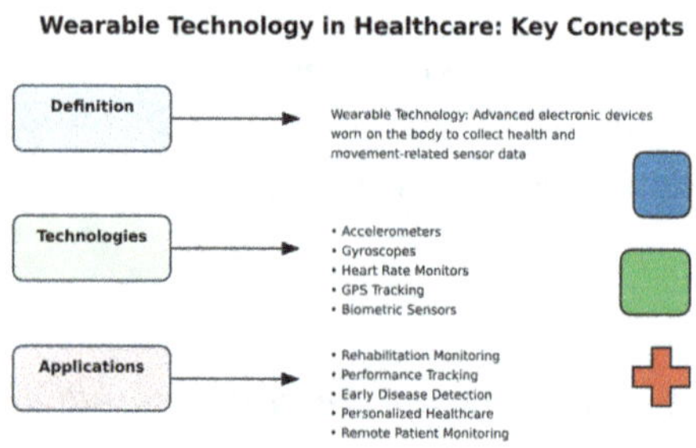

1.1 Research into Wearable Technology and Healthcare Assistive Systems

From tracking fitness to being an essential requirement for healthcare organizations, wearable technologies have indeed evolved. These are used in rehabilitation to monitor the patients, to spot complications early on, and to support decisions with data. Such systems therefore present an opportunity for advanced algorithms to be fused with actual engagements by the patients and, thus, offer remote and effective rehabilitation possibilities.

1.2 Rehabilitation Evolution in the IoT and Predictive Analytics Paradigm

The convergence of the internet of things with the two technologies of machine learning and analytics has unlocked unprecedented possibilities for rehabilitation. Wearable systems with advanced sensors now acquire granular data and actionable insights through predictive models upon analysis. This approach therefore facilitates clinicians to predict all risky situations, optimize therapy regimens and in general improve patient outcomes. The chapter will reveal a transformative impact of the evolutions on rehabilitation frameworks.

1.3 Objectives and Scope of the Chapter

The primary aim of this chapter is to illuminate the mechanisms through which wearable technology, sensor data, and predictive analytics intersect to innovate rehabilitation practices. Key objectives include:

1. Unpacking the sensor ecosystem embedded in wearable devices and their functionality in rehabilitation.
2. Exploring the data pipeline—from acquisition to analysis—and its significance in enabling predictive capabilities.
3. Showcasing real-world applications, including case studies on stroke recovery, gait analysis, and cardiovascular monitoring.
4. Addressing critical ethical and security considerations in wearable data utilization.
5. Investigating future trends, technological advancements, and interdisciplinary research avenues that could redefine assistive systems.

By providing a holistic overview, this chapter seeks to offer valuable insights to researchers, practitioners, and policymakers, fostering innovation and adoption of wearable-assisted predictive rehabilitation systems.

2. THE ROLE OF WEARABLE TECHNOLOGY IN REHABILITATION

Wearable technology has transitioned from its early focus on general health monitoring to becoming a cornerstone of specialized rehabilitation practices. These advanced devices, designed to integrate seamlessly with daily life, are now pivotal in addressing complex rehabilitation needs through real-time monitoring, precise activity tracking, and empowering patients with actionable insights.

2.1 Transition from General Health Monitoring to Specialized Rehabilitation

Initially developed as tools for fitness enthusiasts, wearable devices have undergone a significant transformation, becoming indispensable assets in medical-grade rehabilitation. Early wearables focused on tracking basic metrics like steps and heart rate; however, advancements in sensor technology and data analytics have broadened their scope. Today, these devices cater to specialized applications such as motor skill recovery, gait analysis, and chronic disease management, addressing the specific needs of patients undergoing rehabilitation.

Specialized rehabilitation wearables are designed to capture intricate physiological and biomechanical parameters. For example, electromyography sensors monitor muscle activity, while accelerometers and gyroscopes provide detailed motion analysis. By integrating these functionalities, wearables offer a dynamic feedback loop that facilitates personalized therapy and tracks recovery milestones.

Figure 2. Types of rehabilitation wearables

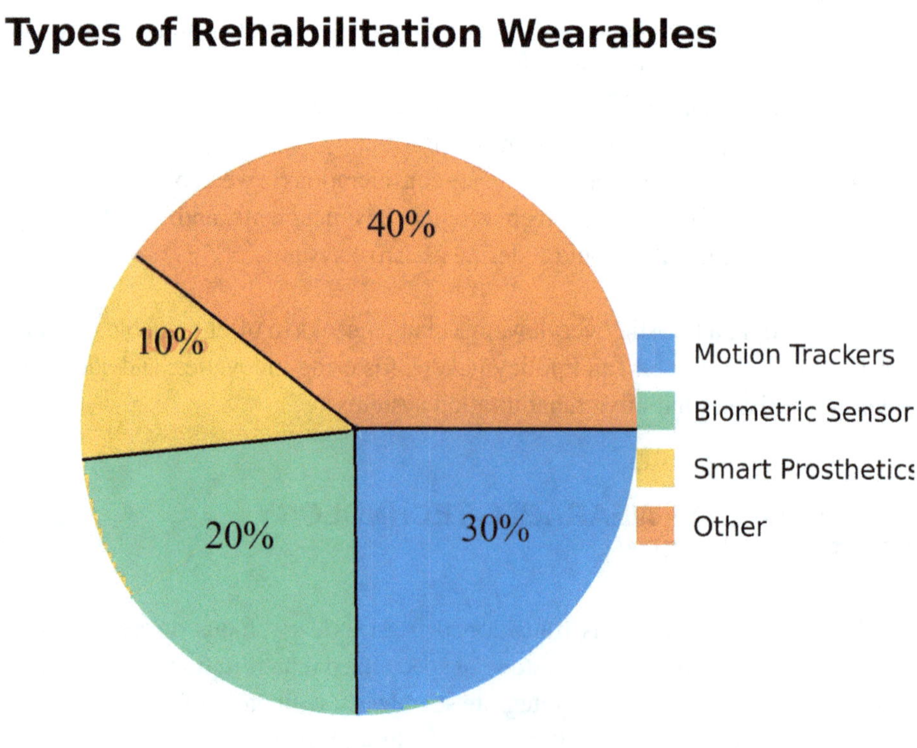

2.2 Classification of Wearables: From Smartwatches to Medical-Grade Devices

The spectrum of wearables in rehabilitation ranges from consumer-grade devices, such as smartwatches and fitness trackers, to highly specialized medical-grade solutions.

- **Consumer-Grade Devices:** Popular examples include smartwatches equipped with heart rate monitors, step counters, and sleep trackers. Though primarily designed for general wellness, these devices are increasingly used for preliminary health assessments in rehabilitation.
- **Medical-Grade Wearables:** These devices, often developed in collaboration with healthcare professionals, are tailored for clinical applications. Examples include wearable ECG monitors, continuous glucose monitors (CGMs), and neuro-rehabilitation devices. These wearables offer precision measurements and advanced features, such as real-time telemetry and data encryption, to ensure secure communication with healthcare providers.

The classification underscores a critical shift towards personalized care, enabling practitioners to select devices that align with specific rehabilitation goals.

2.3 Applications in Rehabilitation: Real-Time Monitoring, Activity Tracking, and Patient Empowerment

Wearable devices are integral to modern rehabilitation strategies, enabling applications such as:

- **Real-Time Monitoring:** Continuous monitoring of vital signs and physical activities allows clinicians to assess patients remotely. For instance, wearable ECG monitors detect cardiac irregularities, while motion sensors evaluate gait patterns, ensuring timely interventions.
- **Activity Tracking:** Devices equipped with accelerometers and gyroscopes track physical activity levels, offering insights into mobility and adherence to prescribed exercises. This data is crucial for adjusting therapy plans in real-time.
- **Patient Empowerment:** By providing immediate feedback through visual dashboards and alerts, wearables empower patients to take an active role in their recovery journey. Patients can monitor their progress, set achievable goals, and adhere to rehabilitation regimens with greater motivation.

2.4 Key Features: Portability, Accessibility, and Continuous Data Collection

Wearable technology's success in rehabilitation can be attributed to its core features:

- **Portability:** Compact and lightweight designs ensure that wearables are unobtrusive, allowing patients to integrate them seamlessly into their daily routines.
- **Accessibility:** Affordable consumer-grade devices have democratized access to basic health monitoring, while telemedicine integration has enhanced accessibility to specialized rehabilitation.
- **Continuous Data Collection:** Unlike traditional periodic assessments, wearables enable uninterrupted data collection, offering a comprehensive view of patient health. This longitudinal data facilitates predictive analysis and early detection of potential complications.

Figure 3. Rehabilitation outcomes improvement

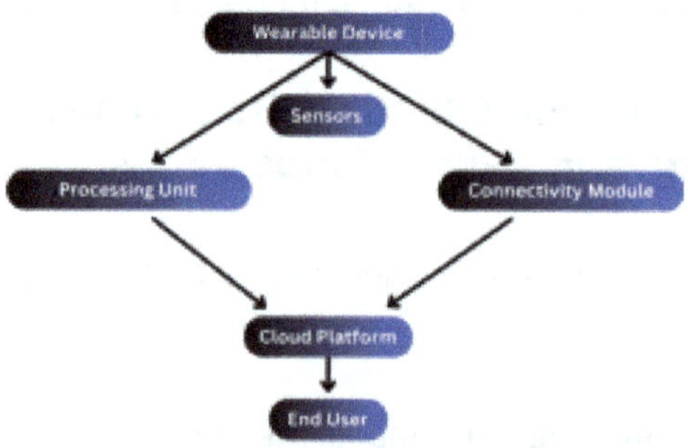

By combining these features with robust data analytics and machine learning models, wearable technology has become a transformative force in rehabilitation. The subsequent sections will delve deeper into the sensor ecosystem, data processing pipelines, and predictive algorithms that underpin this revolution.

3. SENSOR ECOSYSTEM IN WEARABLE DEVICES

Advanced sensor ecosystems in wearable technology have made them an integral part of innovation in assistive systems and rehabilitation. These sensors are the interface between the physical environment and digital processing frameworks that capture critical physiological, biomechanical, and environmental information. Understanding the role of these sensors, their working abilities, and their integration into wearable devices is important to realize their full potential in individualized rehabilitation.

The core of wearable devices is their ability to contain an array of sensors. A primary example is the accelerometers, which are extensively utilized for measuring linear acceleration along more than one axis. During rehabilitation, these sensors prove indispensable for gait analysis. They detect abnormalities in walking patterns, which is highly crucial for neurorehabilitation. Additionally, accelerometers help support posture monitoring and assess the intensity and accuracy of prescribed physical exercises during recovery. Gyroscopes measure angular velocity and rotational movements, and they complement accelerometers. Their contribution to wearables is particularly useful in the assessment of balance and stability, metrics that are significant in the evaluation of patients at risk of falls from elderly to neurological impairments. Accelerometers and gyroscopes will together provide accurate activity recognition, such as distinguishing walking, running, and climbing.

Electromyography (EMG) sensors constitute a vital element of wearable technology, facilitating the assessment of electrical activity within muscular tissues. These sensors are especially advantageous for detecting deficiencies or discrepancies among various muscle groups, thereby rendering them indispensable for evaluating muscular performance in the context of physical rehabilitation. In the realm of neurorehabilitation, EMG sensors yield significant insights by tracking muscle activation patterns in individuals undergoing recovery from stroke or spinal cord injuries. Bioimpedance sensors are one new dimension in wearable technologies. The electrical impedance of body tissues is measured. Hydration status and changes in body composition are measured, both of which are critical for rehabilitation, especially those who have undergone surgical procedures or are undergoing intense physical therapy.

Figure 4. Wearable devices

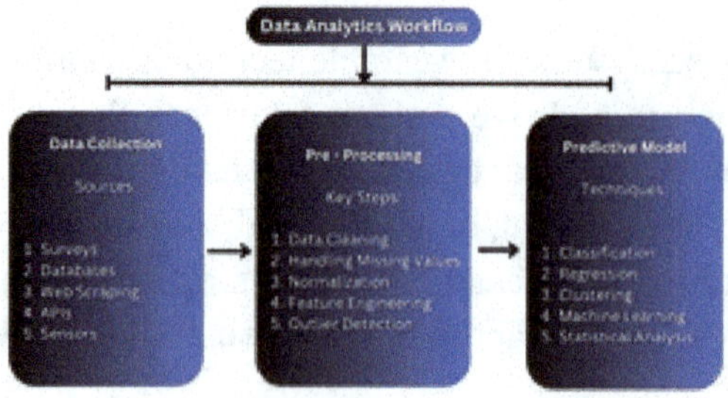

Optical sensors have become highly significant for modern wearables, more so with the adoption of light-based methods to measure such variables as heart rate and oxygen saturation through techniques such as photoplethysmography. These are very important for cardiovascular rehabilitation due to constant monitoring of heart rate variability, detection of abnormalities or stress levels, and aiding in the assessment of breathing, particularly for patients undergoing pulmonary recovery. Temperature sensors add another dimension by allowing for real-time monitoring of body temperature. Use in rehabilitation includes the rapid detection of infection or inflammation and also provides thermoregulatory feedback to treat conditions such as hypothermia or heatstroke.

This improves such systems by being holistic for patient care with several sensor types incorporated into the same wearable. The fusion algorithms perform an essential function of collating the streams of various sensors like accelerometers, gyroscopes, and EMG and other related data sources in enhancing the accuracy and the reliability. For example, one will integrate the motion activity data with muscle activation for the proper comprehension of such challenges as experienced by patients in their mobility. In addition, context-aware computing combines environmental data with physiological metrics, allowing the wearable device to adjust its feedback responsively according to the environment of the user. This capability is very useful in scenarios in which patients experience fluctuating stress levels or environmental factors that may influence their rehabilitation.

Advances in the miniaturization of sensors and their biocompatibility have greatly improved the wearability of wearable technologies. Flexible electronics, made from materials that conform to the shape of the skin, reduce irritation and improve wearability, especially for those requiring long-term monitoring. Additionally, biodegradable sensors are a groundbreaking innovation since they dissolve harmlessly within the body when their function is completed, eliminating the need for removal. Further, energy-efficient sensors ensure that the wearables will not require a change or replacement with new batteries as frequently, which is therefore crucial in continuous monitoring applications.

These sensor ecosystems have very diverse applications in rehabilitation and are quite impactful. In stroke rehabilitation, motion sensors will track the movement of limbs in order to assess motor recovery. EMG sensors monitor muscle activation during physiotherapy sessions. Optical sensors measure heart rate variability to evaluate stress and recovery levels in cardiac rehabilitation, while temperature sensors are used to detect potential complications such as infections. Training programs on gait and balance are more enhanced in the integrated application of accelerometers and gyroscopes that could detect asymmetries for corrective interventions, resulting in improvements in mobility outcome among clients with neurological and musculoskeletal disorders.

4. DATA COLLECTION AND PREPROCESSING FOR PREDICTIVE ANALYTICS

Wearable technology thrives on its ability to collect, process, and analyze a vast influx of data in real time. This process requires a robust and systematic approach to data handling that ensures accuracy, reliability, and actionable insights.

The journey of data within this ecosystem begins with acquisition through sensors, flows into storage solutions, and culminates in preprocessing stages that prepare it for advanced predictive analytics. Each step in this pipeline is critical for transforming raw sensor outputs into meaningful intelligence capable of driving rehabilitation strategies.

Figure 5. Data analytics workflow

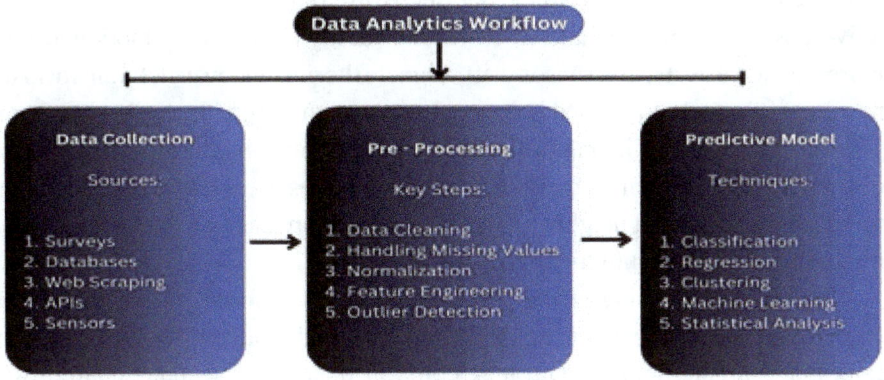

4.1 The Data Pipeline: Acquisition, Storage, and Preprocessing

In a wearable system, a data pipeline is essentially an integrated structure regulating information movement from its time of origination to the moment when analysis of the data will begin. This first step, often referred to as acquisition, deals with capturing data in real time using a wide array of sensors in wearable technology. Such sensors continuously measure physiological, biomechanical, and environmental aspects that generate high-frequency streams of data. For example, there are accelerometers and gyroscopes that measure motion dynamics, electromyography sensors that measure activity of muscles, and optical sensors that measure heart rate variability and oxygen saturation.

Once generated, these data are then communicated for storage, stored locally on the device, or through cloud-based systems. Local storage is usually used when feedback is required to be very prompt or when the device is used without the internet; a cloud solution would provide much more scalability and availability in the general case as well as allow for analysis by multiple groups, including clinicians and researchers, to facilitate collaborative decision-making processes.

This stage, in the pipeline, pre-processing, is the point where raw data gets transformed into clean and structured formats that may become ready for analysis. This makes preprocessing essential for tackling some common issues in real-world data collection such as noise, missing values, and inconsistencies. If not pre-processed, predictive power of the data goes unexploited, and all subsequent analyses are at a risk of lower accuracy and reliability.

4.2 Techniques for Data Cleaning and Normalization

Data cleaning is the first step in preprocessing, which helps to remove errors, inconsistencies, and noise from the dataset. Noise reduction is one of the main objectives, especially in wearable data, which is easily disturbed by motion artifacts, environmental effects, and sensor drift. Signal filtering and wavelet transformation are some of the techniques that help separate the signal from the background noise.

Lack of data - This is one of the major issues that can develop due to random connectivity or other sensor malfunctions. Techniques used: Imputation techniques include mean, k-nearest neighbors, which are based on machine learning and which help to maintain the continuity of that dataset.

After the data cleaning process, normalization is a subsequent operation: measurements from different sensors and units are made uniform on some common scale. For example, motion data may come in meters per second squared, while rotational data would be in radians per second. Of the methods presented, min-max scaling and z-score normalization are often-used tools that facilitate effortless use of different source datasets within machine learning pipelines.

4.3 Feature Engineering: Extracting Meaningful Metrics from Wearable Data

Feature engineering is an artistic as well as scientific approach that takes raw data and gets meaningful attributes out of them. This enhances the prediction capabilities of analytical models. In the context of wearables, this stage converts sensor data into practical metrics directly related to patient health and recovery.

An important task of feature engineering is the segmentation of time-series data that has been obtained from sensors, which enables in-depth examination of these windows. Gait analysis involves subdividing motion data into cycles of each step and thus features such as stride length, cadence, and symmetry can be derived. Features such as heart rate variability and peak amplitudes are also computed for cardiac monitoring.

Statistical characteristics like the mean, variance, and standard deviation are computed to condense data trends in a particular segment. Frequency domain analysis using techniques like the Fast Fourier Transform (FFT) reveals periodic elements and anomalies not easily discernible in the time domain. This is a particularly useful method for detecting patterns of abnormal muscle activation or respiratory rhythms.

Advanced methodologies like dimensionality reduction are used in order to tackle the complexity of wearable data. These include PCA and t-SNE, where the original complexity of datasets is reduced while retaining crucial information. This makes them more favorable for computational analysis.

4.4 Edge and Cloud Computing Paradigms: Balancing Latency and Computational Power

Wearable devices operate in a distributed computing architecture that combines the prompt responsiveness of edge computing with the wide analytical functionalities of cloud computing.

Edge computing involves processing data locally on the device or nearby nodes, minimizing latency and enabling real-time feedback. This is crucial for applications such as fall detection, where immediate alerts can prevent severe injuries. Wearables equipped with embedded microprocessors and edge AI algorithms perform preliminary analyses, reducing the need for continuous data transmission.

On the other hand, cloud computing has excellent scalability and processing capabilities, which are required for complex and large-scale analyses. Information from multiple devices is centralized in servers, where complex machine learning and predictive algorithms are used. This approach allows for longitudinal studies and inter-patient comparisons, revealing trends and insights that are masked in single datasets.

This hybrid architectural framework, thus, allows optimal utilization of the advantages inherent in both methodologies. For example, raw sensor information is preprocessed locally to minimize bandwidth demands before it is sent to the cloud for thorough analysis. In parallel, the outputs from the models based in the cloud are then sent back to the edge devices for timely decision-making and setting up a continuous cycle of data interchange followed by action.

4.5 Interoperability and Standards in Data Handling

Interoperability standards are important enablers for the efficient handling of data in wearables. Protocols like BLE, Zigbee, and Wi-Fi easily facilitate communication between devices and platforms. Standard formats of data, like HL7 (Health Level Seven) and FHIR (Fast Healthcare Interoperability Resources) in the health care sector, ensure compatibility among the different systems and facilitate cooperation among the most disparate stakeholders.

The advancement in wearable technology makes a difference in terms of volume and complexity in data, changing the pipeline to it. Developments in compression, encryption, and decentralized storage create a path for robust and secure data ecosystems. Improvements in the process of collecting, storing, and preprocessing the data make possible a completely effective utilization of wearable systems in the scope of predictive analytics with rehabilitation of patients in the data-driven way.

5. PREDICTIVE ALGORITHMS AND MODELS IN REHABILITATION

Wearable technology is the basic architecture of modern rehabilitation systems; however, it is when it is integrated with predictive algorithms and models that are able to draw actionable insights from vast collections of sensor data that it truly achieves its potential. Such computational methods have allowed clinicians to better predict patient needs and monitor an individual's progress while refining interventions to a much more specific level. These techniques-primarily machine learning algorithms, statistical frameworks, and time-series analyses-have actually transformed wearables from these passive data-gathering apparatuses into proactive decision systems operating within assistive contexts.

Figure 6. Outlook

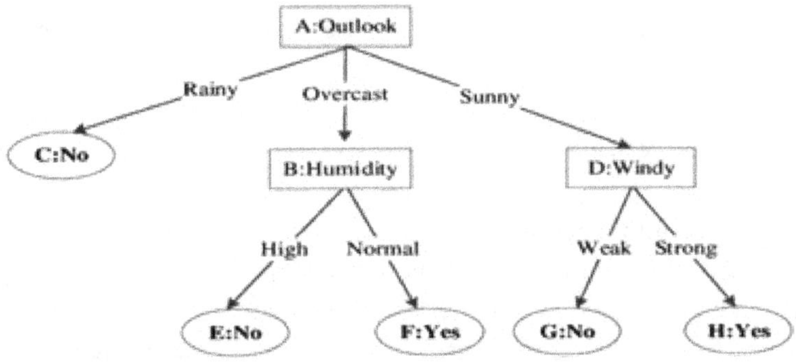

5.1 Introduction to Predictive Algorithms on Wearable Data

Predictive algorithms are designed to feed raw data extracted from wearable devices as the input in order for these to extract insights about trend and relationship issues, resulting in transforming otherwise useless information to an actionable clinical practice-for-instance situation to improve treatment strategies or even as an alert mechanism for hazards towards patient safety. The top most commonly applied methods, to this aim, include techniques like regression analysis, decision tree methodologies, artificial neural networks, and ensemble-based techniques.

Regression models, such as linear and logistic regression, are an essential part of any analytical approach to wearable data. Logistic regression is often used to predict binary outcomes; for example, it can be used to determine the probability of a person experiencing a fall or developing cardiac arrhythmias. Decision trees provide interpretable, rule-based frameworks that are particularly useful for health-care professionals seeking to understand the decision-making processes used by algorithms. It classifies data into streams for it to correspond to threshold values and thus, determine clear tracks of decision-making.

Neural networks have transformed the field of wearable data analytics, especially in their ability to handle high-dimensional inputs from multimodal sensors. Their performance in tasks such as activity recognition, anomaly detection, and event prediction for health-related purposes is outstanding. For example, spatial patterns of EMG can be effectively detected using CNN (Convolutional Neural Networks), while time-series data and its corresponding variations in heart rate can be effectively identified using RNN (Recurrent Neural Networks).

Other methods like ensemble techniques include mainly random forests and gradient boosting machines that result in more precise, less noisy predictions but reduce noise and heterogeneity that, for the most part, come with wearable data in clinical environments where reliability matters.

5.2 Supervised vs. Unsupervised Learning

Supervised learning continues to represent a dominant framework in the use of predictive analytics in wearable rehabilitation systems, concerning pre-labeled data that is used in training models to reach specific outcomes. For instance, supervised algorithms are frequently used in classifying physical activity, predicting trajectories of recovery, and ensuring compliance with prescribed rehabilitation programs. Such models require one to have good quality labelled data.

Conversely, unsupervised learning is increasingly being recognized for its efficacy in exploratory analysis and its diverse applications in clustering. Such algorithms identify the intrinsic structure of a dataset independently of pre-assigned labels. Clustering techniques, including k-means and hierarchical clustering, are employed to categorize patients according to their rehabilitation progress, thereby facilitating the creation of personalized therapy plans. Techniques such as PCA and t-SNE are applied to reduce the dimensionality of high-dimensional wearable data to reveal patterns and anomalies that may be useful in guiding clinical hypotheses.

5.3 Time-Series Analysis and Anomaly Detection

The characteristics of wearable data are intrinsically time-bound and require special analysis techniques. In applications where it is important to model and predict temporal dependencies ahead of time, time-series modeling approaches such as ARIMA (Auto Regressive Integrated Moving Average) or LSTM (Long Short-Term Memory) networks are commonly applied. For instance, LSTM networks have shown their ability in predicting rehabilitation results by processing sequences of gait cycles or cardiac rhythms.

An additional significant application of predictive analytics in the field of rehabilitation is found in the identification of anomalies. This process relies on anticipated patterns, facilitating the detection of deviations that could indicate potential health risks. For example, abrupt alterations in stride length or variations in joint angles observed during gait analysis may suggest the presence of musculoskeletal problems. One-Class Support Vector Machines (SVMs), Isolation Forests, and neural autoencoders are employed to detect anomalies within wearable data, thereby enabling timely interventions to mitigate potential complications.

5.4 Customization through Predictive Analytics

There has been a significant impact in the personalization of rehabilitation programmes. The machine learning model enables a personalized therapeutic protocol through integrating patient-specific data and hence improving interventions to uniquely match their needs or progression. Reinforcement learning has also been employed for developing an adaptive exercise regime, both the intensity as well as duration of exercise, which appropriately and in real-time is corrected via feed forward signals received from wearable sensors.

Other researchers have also adapted multi-task learning frameworks to perform a set of interrelated tasks simultaneously: regarding the prediction of adherence levels and recovery durations, shared representations enhance both efficiency and predictability. In the context of wearables-assisted rehabilitation, multi-task learning has also been explored to support integrated analyses of motion data and muscle activity, allowing for an all-encompassing monitoring of patients.

5.5 Ethical Issues in Predictive Modeling

Although predictive analytics holds much promise, application in rehabilitation brings its own set of ethical considerations, which need to be exercised. The first area is that of data bias; the models developed using homogenous datasets may fail in heterogeneous populations. For instance, an algorithm developed using a younger adult dataset may not apply as well to older patients. To mitigate this effect, fairness-aware learning and data augmentation are being used.

Both transparency and interpretability are of equal importance, especially in clinical settings, where model outputs will determine critical decisions that healthcare providers make. Though black-box models, like deep neural networks, reach incredible levels of accuracy, lack of transparency is likely to undermine trust and deployment. Techniques of XAI, such as SHAP (SHapley Additive exPlanations) and LIME (Local Interpretable Model-agnostic Explanation), are increasingly being added to predictive frameworks to provide a sense of rationale for the decision-making of models.

Extensive surveillance with the use of wearable technology raises more concerns about the confidentiality of patients and principles of informed consent. Adequate use of encryption standards and proper access control can ensure secure handling of information, whereas regulatory structures, such as the GDPR (General Data Protection Regulation) and HIPAA (Health Insurance Portability and Accountability Act), offer all the guidelines that are ethically required for handling data in an appropriate manner.

5.6 Future Directions in Predictive Models for Worn Data

These emergent trends in predictive modeling-from wearable-assisted rehabilitation on towards complete redesigns-are to transform their understanding of this field. Distributed models trained across distributed data can be learned without raw sharing-essential for healthcare, and hence federated learning may emerge as a privacy-preserving learning technique.

Another great opportunity is transfer learning, which allows one dataset-trained model to fine-tune them for related tasks or populations. So, for example, one could train a model to analyze gait data in stroke patients and use it for rehabilitation of Parkinson's disease.

Graph Neural Networks (GNNs) represent another frontier for wearable data analytics, specifically in modeling complex interdependencies between sensors. GNNs were able to grasp interactions, such as the relationship between motion and muscle activation, providing deeper insight into rehabilitation processes.

New developments in predictive algorithms and models indicate that wearable technology is likely to change rehabilitation's future completely by showing a precision, personalization, and proactive care unmatched to date.

6. APPLICATIONS AND CASE STUDIES

The practical applications of wearable technology in rehabilitation and assistive systems exemplify its transformative potential. These devices, empowered by sophisticated sensor systems and predictive analytics, have opened new avenues for patient care across a range of medical domains. Through real-world case studies, the efficacy of these technologies is demonstrated, revealing the profound impact they have on personalised therapies, continuous monitoring, and improved patient outcomes.

6.1 Stroke Rehabilitation: Accelerating Motor Recovery

Stroke is one of the leading causes of long-term disability worldwide, with survivors often facing challenges in regaining motor function. Wearable devices have emerged as critical tools in stroke rehabilitation, offering a non-invasive means to monitor and support recovery. Devices equipped with electromyography (EMG) sensors and motion trackers are particularly effective for assessing muscle activation and limb movements.

One notable application is the use of wearable exoskeletons, which combine advanced sensors with robotic actuators to assist patients in performing repetitive motor tasks. These devices provide real-time feedback, enabling precise adjustments to therapy intensity based on a patient's progress. Predictive algorithms play a pivotal role in these systems, forecasting recovery trajectories by analysing patterns in muscle activation and joint movements. Studies have shown that such technologies accelerate recovery by promoting neuroplasticity—the brain's ability to reorganise itself by forming new neural connections.

A case study from a leading rehabilitation centre demonstrated the impact of wearable-assisted therapy on upper limb recovery. Patients were outfitted with wearable sleeves embedded with accelerometers, gyroscopes, and EMG sensors. The data captured by these sensors were processed using machine learning models to evaluate improvements in grip strength, range of motion, and coordination. The personalised feedback provided by these wearables significantly enhanced patient adherence to therapy regimens, resulting in faster and more comprehensive recovery.

6.2 Gait Analysis in Neurological Disorders

Neurological conditions such as Parkinson's disease, multiple sclerosis, and cerebral palsy often impair gait and mobility. Wearable technology has revolutionised gait analysis by enabling continuous, real-world monitoring of movement patterns. Devices incorporating accelerometers, gyroscopes, and magnetometers capture detailed biomechanical data, including step cadence, stride length, and angular velocity.

Advanced machine learning models analyse this data to identify abnormalities and predict potential risks, such as falls. For instance, recurrent neural networks (RNNs) have been used to detect subtle changes in gait patterns that precede a fall, allowing timely interventions. These insights are invaluable for designing personalised rehabilitation programmes aimed at improving stability and mobility.

In a groundbreaking study, patients with Parkinson's disease were equipped with ankle-worn devices that monitored their gait over several weeks. The wearable systems not only identified freezing episodes—sudden involuntary cessation of movement—but also provided haptic feedback to prompt patients to resume walking. The intervention significantly reduced the frequency and duration of freezing episodes, enhancing patient independence and quality of life.

6.3 Cardiovascular Monitoring and Recovery

Cardiovascular diseases are a major global health challenge, and wearable devices have proven instrumental in monitoring and managing these conditions. Devices equipped with photoplethysmography (PPG) sensors, electrocardiogram (ECG) monitors, and blood pressure trackers enable real-time assessment of heart health. These wearables are particularly beneficial for patients undergoing cardiac rehabilitation, providing continuous insights into metrics such as heart rate variability (HRV), blood oxygen saturation, and stress levels.

Predictive analytics is a cornerstone of wearable-assisted cardiovascular care. Machine learning models analyse trends in physiological data to predict arrhythmias, hypertension episodes, or other cardiovascular events. This proactive approach enables early interventions, reducing the likelihood of complications.

6.4 Respiratory Rehabilitation and Chronic Pulmonary Conditions

Respiratory conditions such as chronic obstructive pulmonary disease (COPD) and asthma require meticulous monitoring and management. Wearable technology has emerged as a game-changer in this domain, with devices measuring respiratory rate, lung volume, and oxygen saturation. These metrics are critical for assessing disease severity and monitoring response to treatment.

Wearables equipped with piezoelectric sensors and bioimpedance technologies are capable of capturing subtle changes in breathing patterns. Predictive models process this data to identify early signs of exacerbations, enabling timely interventions. For example, patients with COPD can use wearable spirometers to track lung function, while algorithms predict flare-ups based on historical data and environmental factors.

A real-world example comes from a study on wearable thoracic bands for respiratory rehabilitation. These bands, embedded with strain gauges, monitored chest expansion during breathing exercises. The data was analysed to provide feedback on exercise effectiveness and to detect deviations from prescribed protocols. Patients who used the wearable systems demonstrated improved adherence to therapy and better control over their respiratory conditions.

6.5 Applications in Sports Injury Rehabilitation

Athletes recovering from injuries face unique challenges, as they often require accelerated recovery without compromising long-term health. Wearable technology has found extensive application in sports injury rehabilitation, with devices offering insights into biomechanics, muscle recovery, and injury prevention.

Motion capture wearables equipped with inertial measurement units (IMUs) are commonly used to analyse joint movements and assess recovery progress. These devices provide real-time data on kinematics, allowing physiotherapists to refine exercise regimens. Predictive analytics enhances this process by identifying movement patterns that may lead to re-injury, guiding athletes towards safer practices.

In a notable case, a group of football players recovering from anterior cruciate ligament (ACL) injuries was equipped with wearable knee braces. The braces monitored joint angles, muscle activation, and weight distribution, feeding the data into machine learning models. These models predicted re-injury risks and suggested adjustments to training intensity. As a result, the athletes experienced fewer setbacks and returned to play with improved confidence and performance.

6.6 Integration of Virtual Reality (VR) and Augmented Reality (AR) with Wearables

One of the most exciting advancements in wearable-assisted rehabilitation is the integration of virtual reality (VR) and augmented reality (AR) technologies. These immersive environments, combined with sensor-equipped wearables, offer highly engaging and effective therapy experiences. For instance, patients recovering from stroke can use VR headsets and motion-tracking gloves to perform gamified exercises that enhance motor skills.

Wearable devices act as input systems, capturing movements and translating them into the virtual environment. Predictive algorithms adapt the VR scenarios in real-time based on the patient's performance, ensuring that the exercises remain challenging yet achievable. This dynamic interaction fosters motivation and accelerates recovery.

A study involving patients with traumatic brain injuries highlighted the benefits of this approach. Participants used wearable systems integrated with AR to simulate real-world tasks, such as reaching for objects or navigating obstacles. The predictive models within the system analysed movement patterns and provided tailored feedback, significantly improving the patients' functional abilities and confidence.

6.7 Ethical Considerations in Application

While the applications of wearable technology in rehabilitation are undeniably transformative, they are not without ethical implications. Continuous monitoring raises concerns about data privacy and autonomy, particularly when wearables collect sensitive health information. Transparent communication and robust consent protocols are essential to ensure that patients understand how their data will be used.

Furthermore, the reliance on predictive models introduces the risk of algorithmic bias, where inaccuracies in model training can disproportionately affect certain populations. Efforts to diversify training datasets and implement fairness-aware algorithms are critical for addressing these challenges.

By highlighting the applications and examining real-world use cases, this section underscores the pivotal role of wearable technology in shaping the future of rehabilitation and assistive systems. From motor recovery to respiratory care and injury prevention, these devices are redefining what is possible in patient-centric healthcare.

7. ETHICAL AND SECURITY CONSIDERATIONS IN WEARABLE-BASED REHABILITATION

The integration of wearable technology in rehabilitation introduces transformative benefits, but it also poses a labyrinth of ethical and security challenges. These issues revolve around data privacy, patient consent, equitable access, and the integrity of predictive models. As the reliance on wearable devices for health monitoring and rehabilitation intensifies, addressing these considerations becomes imperative to safeguard patient autonomy, ensure fairness, and foster trust in technology.

7.1 Data Privacy and Confidentiality in Wearable Systems

Wearable devices generate vast amounts of sensitive data, encompassing physiological, behavioural, and environmental information. This wealth of data provides insights into patient health and recovery but also raises significant concerns regarding privacy and confidentiality. Inadequate safeguards can lead to breaches, resulting in unauthorised access, misuse, or exploitation of patient data.

Data collected from wearables is often transmitted via wireless networks to cloud platforms for analysis. This process introduces vulnerabilities at multiple levels, including device endpoints, communication channels, and storage systems. Encryption protocols, such as Advanced Encryption Standard (AES) and Secure Sockets Layer (SSL), are fundamental to securing these transmissions. However, evolving cyber threats necessitate continuous updates to these security measures.

Moreover, differential privacy has emerged as a promising approach to enhance data confidentiality. By introducing controlled noise into datasets, differential privacy ensures that individual data points cannot be traced back to specific users while preserving the overall utility of the dataset. This technique is particularly relevant in wearable systems, where real-time analytics often depend on aggregated data.

7.2 Informed Consent and Autonomy

The deployment of wearable devices in rehabilitation must adhere to robust informed consent frameworks. Patients should be fully aware of what data is being collected, how it will be used, and who will have access to it. Informed consent is not merely a procedural requirement but a cornerstone of ethical medical practice that upholds patient autonomy and trust.

Dynamic consent models have been proposed as an enhancement to traditional approaches. Unlike static consent, which is obtained once and applies indefinitely, dynamic consent allows patients to modify their preferences over time. For instance, a patient may initially agree to share their wearable data for therapeutic purposes but later decide to restrict access for research applications. Implementing such models in wearable systems requires seamless user interfaces and secure authentication mechanisms to manage consent settings.

7.3 Algorithmic Transparency and Bias Mitigation

Predictive algorithms, while powerful, are not immune to biases and errors. These biases often stem from imbalances in training data, where certain populations may be underrepresented. For example, an algorithm trained predominantly on data from young, physically active individuals may perform poorly when applied to older adults or patients with disabilities. Such disparities can lead to unequal treatment and exacerbate existing health inequalities.

To address these challenges, fairness-aware machine learning techniques are being integrated into wearable systems. These techniques involve weighting under-represented groups more heavily during model training or incorporating fairness constraints into algorithmic objectives. Additionally, data augmentation strategies, such as synthetic data generation, are employed to diversify training datasets.

7.4 Accessibility and Equity in Wearable Technology

The adoption of wearable devices in rehabilitation raises questions about accessibility and equity. High costs, limited digital literacy, and lack of infrastructure can hinder access to these technologies, particularly in low-income and rural settings.

Ensuring equitable access requires a multi-pronged approach that addresses financial, educational, and infrastructural barriers.

Subsidised programmes and public-private partnerships have been effective in making wearable technology more accessible. For instance, government-funded initiatives in several countries have provided wearable devices to patients with chronic illnesses, enabling continuous monitoring and timely interventions. Additionally, designing user-friendly interfaces and providing training sessions can bridge the digital literacy gap, empowering patients to utilise wearable systems effectively.

Interoperability standards are also crucial for promoting equity. By ensuring compatibility across different devices and platforms, these standards reduce the need for expensive proprietary systems and enhance the usability of wearable devices in diverse healthcare ecosystems. Standards such as Health Level Seven (HL7) and Fast Healthcare Interoperability Resources (FHIR) facilitate seamless data exchange, enabling patients to switch between providers without losing access to their wearable data.

7.5 Security Challenges in Wearable Systems

Wearable devices face unique security challenges due to their continuous operation, limited computational resources, and reliance on wireless connectivity. These vulnerabilities make them attractive targets for cyberattacks, ranging from data breaches to device hijacking.

Authentication is a critical aspect of wearable security. Traditional methods, such as passwords or PINs, are often impractical for wearable devices. Biometric authentication, which leverages unique physiological traits such as fingerprints or heart rate patterns, offers a more robust alternative. Multi-factor authentication (MFA) further enhances security by combining biometrics with additional factors like one-time passwords or hardware tokens.

Another emerging solution is blockchain technology, which provides a decentralised framework for secure data storage and sharing. Blockchain's immutability ensures that once data is recorded, it cannot be altered, protecting the integrity of wearable data. Furthermore, smart contracts—self-executing protocols embedded within blockchain networks—can automate consent management, ensuring that patient preferences are adhered to without manual oversight.

Device-level security is equally important. Secure boot mechanisms ensure that wearables load only authorised firmware, protecting them from malware attacks. Additionally, runtime integrity checks monitor the device's operational state, identifying and mitigating threats in real-time.

7.6 Ethical Implications of Continuous Monitoring

The continuous monitoring enabled by wearable devices blurs the line between healthcare and surveillance. While this capability offers unprecedented insights into patient health, it also raises concerns about intrusiveness and overreach. Patients may feel uncomfortable with the idea of being constantly monitored, even if the data collected is anonymised or aggregated.

To address these concerns, patient-centric design principles must guide the development of wearable systems. These principles emphasise user autonomy, ensuring that patients have control over what data is collected and when monitoring occurs. For example, wearable devices could include features that allow patients to temporarily disable monitoring without compromising their overall rehabilitation progress.

Another ethical consideration is the potential for data misuse by employers, insurers, or other third parties. For instance, wearable data could be used to discriminate against individuals based on their health status or predicted risks. Robust regulatory frameworks are essential to prevent such abuses and ensure that wearable technology is used solely for its intended therapeutic purposes.

7.7 International Standards and Regulatory Compliance

Compliance with international standards and regulations is a cornerstone of ethical wearable technology deployment. Regulations such as the General Data Protection Regulation (GDPR) in Europe and the Health Insurance Portability and Accountability Act (HIPAA) in the United States provide comprehensive guidelines for data protection and patient rights. These frameworks mandate transparency, accountability, and security in data handling, ensuring that wearable systems meet stringent ethical and legal standards.

However, global harmonisation of these regulations remains a challenge. Variations in data protection laws across jurisdictions can create inconsistencies in wearable technology implementation, particularly for multinational healthcare providers. Efforts to establish universal standards, such as the International Medical Device Regulators Forum (IMDRF), are underway to address these disparities and promote global interoperability.

8. FUTURE TRENDS AND INNOVATIONS IN WEARABLE-ASSISTED REHABILITATION

This area of wearable technology in rehabilitation stands on the verge of breakthrough, fueled by rapid strides in the miniaturization of sensors, artificial intelligence, and interoperability of data. In tandem with a deepening interplay between technology and healthcare, trends unfolding hold great promise to redefine rehabilitation paradigms, including unmatched precision, scalability, and personalization. This chapter explores these transformative innovations in depth, explaining what these changes mean for rehabilitation enabled by wearables.

8.1 Advances in Wearable Sensor Technology

Breakthroughs in sensor technology, miniaturization, sensitivity, and biocompatibility are the hallmarks of the next generation of wearable devices. Flexible electronics are at the center of this revolution by allowing sensors to mold smoothly against the curves of the body. Such innovations maximize user comfort while providing the most accurate physiological measurements due to the reduced motion artifacts.

The integration of nanotechnology has led to the development of nanosensors that can detect even minute biochemical changes in real-time. For example, biosensors embedded with nanoscale electrodes that can be attached to a body can measure blood glucose levels or detect lactate accumulation during physical therapy. Such sensors not only broaden the horizon of wearable applications but also reduce the need for invasive procedures in the care of patients.

8.2 Artificial Intelligence and Personalized Rehabilitation

AI will change wearable-assisted rehabilitation to become much more hyperpersonalized therapy plans, as the machine learning algorithms, trained on diverse datasets, can adapt dynamic rehabilitation programs based on the individual's progress to optimal outcomes. Among those techniques, reinforcement learning, a subset of AI, is promising for developing adaptive systems to refine treatment protocols using real-time feedback loops.

Predictive modeling with deep learning architectures such as CNNs and transformers has picked up pace while analyzing multimodal data so that subtle patterns across the datasets of physiological, biomechanical, and environmental can be identified. Such models provide an all-rounded picture of health. Generative AI models are also being looked into to simulate hypothetical scenarios of recovery so that clinicians can become proactive in attending to such potential complications.

8.3 Integration with Augmented Reality (AR) and Virtual Reality (VR)

This new dimension of integration between wearable technology and Augmented Reality and Virtual Reality opens new rehabilitation possibilities. The immersive technologies allow the creation of interactive environments in which patients can engage in exercises directed to their respective rehabilitative goals. Wearables capture motion data that transforms input into the virtual domain, while overlaying visual guidance on real-world settings enhanced by AR.

For instance, stroke patients can practice upper limb movement with VR-based therapy in a gamified environment, increasing involvement and neuroplasticity. The applications of AR, meanwhile, allow people recovering with musculoskeletal injuries to perform exercises with corrections given in real-time projected onto their field of view. Thus, these technologies not only make rehabilitation more engaging but also increase adherence and long-term outcomes.

8.4 Wearable Technology and Neurorehabilitation

Wearables are increasingly becoming relevant for neurorehabilitation programs for traumatic brain injuries, multiple sclerosis, and spinal cord injuries, among others. The more sophisticated devices with advanced sensors like EEG and functional near-infrared spectroscopy (fNIRS) allow constant and real-time monitoring to determine information on neural recovery processes.

Neurofeedback training enables wearable devices to be used in training patients to control their brain activity. For example, a combination of EEG headsets and machine learning algorithms can identify ideal patterns of brain waves for certain tasks and thus enable targeted intervention. Such systems, applied to neurorehabilitation, have shown promise in restoring cognitive functions, motor capabilities, and emotionally inhibited tendencies.

8.5 Integration with Internet of Medical Things (IoMT)

The Internet of Medical Things is a merger or integration of wearable technology, connected devices, and healthcare networks. This ecosystem provides effortless data interchange between wearables, electronic health records (EHRs), and clinical decision-support systems to provide a holistic management of patients.

IoMT wearables can take advantage of edge computing to process data on the local edge, reducing latency and improving real-time performance. For example, it could generate immediate feedback when analyzing gait, using data captured by a wearable device on-site while still sending aggregate data to the cloud for longitudinal analysis in population-level insights. That would optimize both individual and population-level insights.

8.6 Blockchain for Secure Data Management

Blockchain technology is therefore a game-changer in wearables-enabled rehabilitation. Its decentralized architecture assures that health data are stored in an immutable ledger so that no unauthorized changes take place. The smart contracts embedded in blockchains also automatically ensure compliance with data-sharing agreements by holding patient consent at all times.

Besides enhancing security, blockchain allows interoperability between heterogeneous health systems. It standardizes data formats and offers universal access to validated records across institutions and geographies, thus fostering collaboration across the institution and geography. This is very useful for patients who receive rehabilitation in more than one facility, because it provides continuity of care.

8.7 Energy Harvesting for Long-Term Device Operation

Energy efficiency is still a significant challenge for wearables, especially those that need constant monitoring. Innovations in energy harvesting are helping to address the limitation by allowing wearables to harness ambient sources of power. These include thermoelectric generators, piezoelectric sensors, and photovoltaic cells that can convert body heat, motion, and light into usable energy.

For instance, a wearable patch equipped with thermoelectric materials can capture the temperature gradient between the skin and the environment to power low-energy sensors. Similarly, piezoelectric devices embedded in insoles can generate electricity from the mechanical forces produced during walking. These advancements extend the operational lifespan of wearables, reducing the need for frequent recharging and enhancing user convenience.

8.8 Ethical AI and Inclusive Design

The growing reliance of wearable technology on AI is crucially important in designing it to be ethical and inclusive. Algorithmic fairness, transparency, and explainability are crucial considerations in such diverse patient populations. Efforts are also underway to develop age, gender, ethnicity, and socioeconomically unbiased AI models.

Inclusive design principles extend from algorithms to the physical and functional elements of wearables. Devices must be accessible to users with varying levels of mobility, dexterity, and technological literacy. For example, voice-activated controls and modular designs can make wearables more user-friendly for people with physical impairments. Prioritizing inclusivity will help wearable technology achieve broader adoption and equitable benefits across all demographics.

9. OBSTACLES IN IMPLEMENTATION

Although wearable technology has made quite significant advancements in the enhancement of rehabilitation practices, its deployment is a complex challenge that cuts across technological, clinical, and socio-economic borders. The challenges are indeed many, which hinder its smooth integration into healthcare systems. The need for more innovative solutions to unlock wearables fully is therefore felt. The section below elucidates key challenges associated with deploying wearable-assisted rehabilitation systems and ways of addressing such challenges effectively.

9.1 Bridging the Gap Between Research and Clinical Deployment

The transition from laboratory research to real-world clinical settings remains a significant hurdle in wearable technology implementation. Many wearable devices and algorithms are designed and tested in controlled environments, which do not accurately reflect the complexities of clinical or everyday contexts. Variability in patient behaviour, environmental conditions, and healthcare infrastructure can compromise the performance and reliability of wearables.

For example, a wearable designed to monitor gait patterns may perform flawlessly under laboratory conditions but struggle to deliver consistent results when used by patients navigating uneven terrains or crowded urban environments. Bridging this gap requires robust validation protocols that encompass diverse real-world scenarios, along with iterative design processes that incorporate feedback from clinicians and patients.

9.2 Interoperability and Fragmentation of Data

Interoperability is the base key that has been crucial to wearables' successful integration. However, it remains as one of the ongoing issues as it creates data silos with specific data on platforms that aren't easily shared or scaled, thus inhibiting cooperation and continuity of care. Further complications arise from the fragmentation created, which makes consolidation and analysis more challenging across devices, therefore limiting one's ability to have a holistic understanding.

Through efforts at standardization such as HL7 and FHIR, among others, the problems of interoperability have been aimed to be addressed. It is, however, accepted by the device manufacturers, the software developers, and the healthcare providers that would allow seamless interoperability. An open ecosystem, giving emphasis to data-sharing agreements and common protocols, would prevent fragmentation and make wearables function cohesively in broader healthcare frameworks.

9.3 Scalability and Cost Requirements

Scalability is another big challenge for the wide acceptance of wearable-assisted rehabilitation systems. The high cost of complex wearable devices, along with the economic requirements of infrastructure such as cloud storage and computational power, prevents easy access, especially in resource-poor settings.

Cost-cutting measures include the following: mass production to achieve economies of scale, modular design in order to achieve personalization, and the use of novel materials in manufacturing sensors. Low-cost substitutes for the components of a sensor system have included other types of print electronics, such as biodegradable materials. Even collaborations involving governments, nonprofits, and the private sector could lead to subsidized programs that make wearables accessible to those least experienced with them.

9.4 Data Security and Privacy Concerns

Wearable devices pose huge threats to data security as well as individual privacy. The devices collect personal data, including sensitive physiological and behavioral information as well as geolocation data. These are prime targets for cybercriminals, whose access to the data may have significant consequences, including identity theft, financial fraud, or reputational damage.

There should be strong security features with wearable data. For instance, end-to-end encryption, multi-factor authentication, and secure storage protocols are one of the basic ways of protecting secret data. Moreover, integration with blockchain technology will also help in achieving immutable and tamper-proof records to ensure the integrity of data along with its whole lifecycle. Educating the patients regarding their rights related to data privacy and proper use of such devices should be one of the methods of reducing this risk.

9.5 Addressing Algorithmic Bias and Maintaining Fairness

Bias in the predictive algorithms that underpin wearable-assisted rehabilitation systems is often determined by biases in the training datasets, thereby leading to unequal algorithmic performance across demographic populations. For example, an algorithm trained mainly on data from young, healthy people will not make good predictions for older patients or patients with co-morbidities.

Strategies to mitigate algorithmic bias include dataset diversification when training, the use of fairness-promoting machine learning techniques, as well as conducting comprehensive bias sensitivity tests. Additionally, transparency in models developed and validated is important: stakeholders can inspect and, thereby correct potential sources of algorithmic bias. Furthermore, testing and designing wearable technologies to be used by diverse groups of patients ensures that these algorithms are fair and representative to these populations.

9.6 User Engagement and Adherence

One of the major challenges related to rehabilitation supported by wearable technology is to assure the involvement and compliance of users. For example, due to discomfort caused by the device, an apparent lack of utility, or privacy concerns, the users may avoid wearables regularly. Additionally, novelty related to wearable technology may be a significant challenge for the patients who have limited experience with digital health tools.

Principles of user-centered design can improve both engagement and adherence in wearable devices. These devices should be light, ergonomic, and personalized to the individual's preferences and needs. Moreover, the use of rewards and tracking systems has been found to be an important component of gamification strategies that encourage patient adherence to rehabilitation plans. Finally, proper training and support must be given so that patients and their caregivers can use wearable systems with ease and comfort.

9.7 Legal and Regulatory Challenges

The most important barrier in wearable technology is the complex legal and regulatory environment. Devices designed for use in the medical field must pass quite stringent regulations, namely European Medical Device Regulation (MDR) and the FDA in the United States. Such regulatory steps are very crucial to protect safety and effectiveness but, in fact, they lengthen the timelines associated with the development and implementation of wearable systems.

The differences in data protection legislation among various jurisdictions add complexity to regulatory compliance. For instance, the General Data Protection Regulation has strict data privacy standards within Europe, while other regions may have less extensive regulatory frameworks. Such disparities pose significant challenges for multinational healthcare organizations that want to roll out wearable technology across different regions.

10. CONCLUSION: THE TRANSFORMATIVE POTENTIAL OF WEARABLES IN REHABILITATION

This introduces the wearables, which house advanced sensor data and utilise predictive analytics, to highly transform the rehabilitation domain. From their evolution from being just devices that gather passive data to an immediate intervention tool, wearable devices are going to improve patients' outcomes, enhance mobility and quality of life among individuals involved in rehabilitation processes. This important potential for change has its roots firmly in interdisciplinary integration of elements such as health care, engineering, machine learning, and analytics. The integration of advanced technologies along with comprehensive understanding of the human physiology positions wearable devices to revolutionize rehabilitation in unprecedented ways.

10.1 Role of Wearable Devices in Modern Rehabilitation

Wearable technology is becoming one of the essential tools used in rehabilitation. It allows monitoring continuously the physiological and biomechanical data of the patients. Such sensor-rich devices, from accelerometers and gyroscopes to ECG and EMG sensors, provide immense information about a patient's movement, gait, muscle activity, and even cardiovascular health. These offer real-time, continuous monitoring and, therefore, can provide clinicians with immediate feedback regarding the progress or lack of it by the patient. In this regard, the continuous inflow of data equips the healthcare worker with better and more precise impressions. Even patient-centered care becomes possible through more tailored rehabilitation programs.

The defining characteristic of wearables is that they track not just objective measurements, such as the range of motion and heart rate, but also subjective assessment, such as pain levels and ratings of perceived exertion. These data sets when integrated with machine learning models and predictive algorithms allow for dynamic rehabilitation plans that continuously adapt to changes in the needs and improvement of the patient. That is a huge step forward from the traditional uniform treatments to highly flexible real-time solutions in rehabilitation methods.

10.2 Predictive Analytics: A Transformational Enabler for Rehabilitation

At the core of what changes with wearable technology is predictive analytics. This methodology, with large amounts of sensor-generated data, builds models that are predicted to trace the path of rehabilitation processes. Historical data analysis allows predictive algorithms to predict potential setbacks and, through this, allow for preventive measures. For instance, a gait assessment for a patient may indicate an early sign of misalignment or instability. Predictive analytics will alert the healthcare team to alter the rehabilitation approach before such a condition becomes more severe.

In addition, the infusion of AI and ML into the predictive models allows clinicians to make decisions based on data more accurately than ever before. They also allow for individual differences so that they can provide insights personalized to the patient's physiology, medical history, and rehabilitation objectives. This is particularly important in neurology, because recovery pathways are uniquely personalized for patients. The development of predictive models with large, diverse datasets ensures that the best possible intervention is administered to each patient, hence improving the outcomes and avoiding over- or under-rehabilitation.

10.3 Interdisciplinary Teamwork as a Way to Success

Although wearable technologies have a great potential, only through the collaboration of multiple disciplines can their full features be realized. The development and application of wearable technology in rehabilitation require the expertise of specialists from the healthcare, engineering, computer science, and data analytics departments. Engineers and hardware developers work closely with healthcare professionals to develop sensors that can accurately capture biomechanical and physiological information, while data scientists and machine learning experts develop algorithms to process this information in real-time.

This is through collaboration with healthcare professionals and technology companies to ensure that wearables are effective and useful. The functionality of wearables in the rehabilitation context does not just depend on the technological nature of the device but also the usability, comfort, and acceptance with the patients' daily routines. Effective collaboration ensures that wearables are developed with patient experience at the center of product development, which then encourages compliance and engagement in rehabilitation programs.

10.4 Respect for Individual and Patient Autonomy

Wearable technologies do not only provide healthcare professionals with data but also empower patients by giving them the necessary tools to be active participants in their rehabilitation. Through these devices, patients can monitor their progress, assess their daily activities, and make informed choices regarding their rehabilitation. Providing real-time access to individualized data fosters a sense of ownership in the recovery journey, thus enhancing motivation and compliance with prescribed exercise regimens.

Wearable technology further includes immediate feedback mechanisms in terms of automatic feedback in vibrotactile, auditory cueing, or visual notification to perform the exercise precisely or notify any probable failure, and hence not only allows for an instant source of support during the recovery period but also lessens injury likelihood. Hence, patients remain dependent less on in-clinical visits and can take more active involvement with increased assurance of doing their activities in the comfort of their homes, thereby augmenting the success of recovery and utilizing all possible hours spent in recovering.

10.5 Prospect for Long-Term Health Care and Preventive Health

Although it is more of the sphere of rehabilitation, it is on long-term healthcare maintenance and prevention that wearables have had a great opportunity for its applicability. Wearables then are continuous, long term tracking from where disease signals begin presenting not yet with any clinical manifestations and at potentially early phases. Patients undergoing chronic conditions or after rehabilitation can use wearables on-going basis to manage risk factors such as activities, sleep patterns, and cardio health.

It would also be able to identify sensor data-related patterns foreshadowing the onset of complications such as falls, muscle atrophy, or cardiovascular diseases at the earliest moment and provide timely intervention before these conditions become acute. As such, wearables move beyond a rehabilitation tool and take up a much greater role in preventive healthcare with overall minimized costly burdens on healthcare systems and improved long-term health status.

10.6 Conceptualisation of a Future through Wearable Technology and Predictive Analytics

The rehabilitation trajectory is intrinsically bound with wearable technology advancements and predictive analytics. With the growth of this field, it can be predicted that the device being developed will be much more advanced and able to track more parameters including neurological activity, biochemical indicators, and environmental conditions. Battery life, sensor resolution, and connectivity would also enhance the efficiency and availability of wearable devices, which will be much more cost-effective and accessible in a widespread manner.

Further, integration with other advanced technologies like virtual reality (VR) and augmented reality (AR) will be expected to create immersed rehabilitation experiences that support fast recovery. The integration of VR/AR with immediate biometric feedback from wearables enables patients to be engaged in tailored, interactive rehabilitation activities that simulate natural everyday scenarios. This technology integration will enhance patient engagement and will optimize rehabilitation by creating a space where learning and recovery will be simultaneous.

Additionally, the data generated by wearable devices will continue to improve overall healthcare structures, supporting the development of large health data stores. These stores, in turn, will enable the development of progressively sophisticated predictive models, thereby creating a positive feedback loop of improvement both for personal patient care and public health management.

10.7 The Thirst for Continuous Innovation and Collaborative Research

Although much has been achieved, it is still not enough. There is much more to the full potential of wearables in rehabilitation. The field is at its infancy, and so many more refining algorithms and security for data are needed, besides enhancing the comfort and accessibility of the devices. There is an urgent need for continued innovation and collaborative research to address these issues and to drive the next generation of wearable technologies.

The healthcare and technology industries should continue to work together in developing devices that are scientifically valid and also economically feasible but easy to use for consumers. Simultaneously, clinical studies should be conducted in evaluating the efficacy of wearable technology in various rehabilitation settings, thus providing a strong evidence base for their use in both acute and chronic recovery phases. This collaboration between researchers, healthcare providers, and developers of technology will play an important role in bringing that future vision of a health care system into reality-the system wherein rehabilitation is personalized, predictive, and integrated into life seamlessly.

Therefore, the potential of revolutionizing in the rehabilitation landscape using wearable devices is immense but undoubtedly cumbersome, offering new frontiers for more personalized ways of effective care. Such devices help predictive analytics trigger the onset of adaptive rehabilitation adapted for each patient. There must be encouragement and innovative strategies in interdisciplinary work coupled with commitment toward developing the technology and application in clinical settings. Indeed, the future is bright regarding rehabilitation because the wearables and especially when it is put on the predictive analytics will certainly make a big thing as triggers in recovery, avert a health issue arising from treatment intervention, and holistic wellness.

REFERENCES

Bonato, P. (2005). Advances in wearable technology and applications in physical medicine and rehabilitation. *Journal of Neuroengineering and Rehabilitation*, *2*(1), 2. DOI: 10.1186/1743-0003-2-2 PMID: 15733322

Chen, M., Ma, Y., Song, J., Lai, C. F., & Hu, B. (2016). Smart clothing: Connecting human with clouds and big data for sustainable health monitoring. *Mobile Networks and Applications*, *21*(5), 825–845. DOI: 10.1007/s11036-016-0745-1

Dias, D., & Paulo Silva Cunha, J. (2018). Wearable health devices—Vital sign monitoring, systems and technologies. *Sensors (Basel)*, *18*(8), 2414. DOI: 10.3390/s18082414 PMID: 30044415

Dobkin, B. H., & Dorsch, A. (2011). The promise of mHealth: Daily activity monitoring and outcome assessments by wearable sensors. *Neurorehabilitation and Neural Repair*, *25*(9), 788–798. DOI: 10.1177/1545968311425908 PMID: 21989632

Gao, W., Emaminejad, S., Nyein, H. Y. Y., Challa, S., Chen, K., Peck, A., Fahad, H. M., Ota, H., Shiraki, H., Kiriya, D., Lien, D.-H., Brooks, G. A., Davis, R. W., & Javey, A. (2016). Fully integrated wearable sensor arrays for multiplexed in situ perspiration analysis. *Nature*, *529*(7587), 509–514. DOI: 10.1038/nature16521 PMID: 26819044

Gravina, R., Alinia, P., Ghasemzadeh, H., & Fortino, G. (2017). Multi-sensor fusion in body sensor networks: State-of-the-art and research challenges. *Information Fusion*, *35*, 68–80. DOI: 10.1016/j.inffus.2016.09.005

Haghi, M., Thurow, K., & Stoll, R. (2017). Wearable devices in medical internet of things: Scientific research and commercially available devices. *Healthcare Informatics Research*, *23*(1), 4–15. DOI: 10.4258/hir.2017.23.1.4 PMID: 28261526

Hicks, J. L., Althoff, T., Kuhar, P., Bostjancic, B., King, A. C., Leskovec, J., & Delp, S. L. (2019). Best practices for analyzing large-scale health data from wearables and smartphone apps. *NPJ Digital Medicine*, *2*(1), 45. DOI: 10.1038/s41746-019-0121-1 PMID: 31304391

Lonini, L., Dai, A., Shawen, N., Simuni, T., Poon, C., Shimanovich, L., Daeschler, M., Ghaffari, R., Rogers, J. A., & Jayaraman, A. (2018). Wearable sensors for Parkinson's disease: Which data are worth collecting for training symptom detection models. *NPJ Digital Medicine*, *1*(1), 64. DOI: 10.1038/s41746-018-0071-z PMID: 31304341

Majumder, S., Aghayi, E., Noferesti, M., Memarzadeh-Tehran, H., Mondal, T., Pang, Z., & Deen, M. J. (2017). Smart homes for elderly healthcare—Recent advances and research challenges. *Sensors (Basel), 17*(11), 2496. DOI: 10.3390/s17112496 PMID: 29088123

Majumder, S., Mondal, T., & Deen, M. J. (2017). Wearable sensors for remote health monitoring. *Sensors (Basel), 17*(1), 130. DOI: 10.3390/s17010130 PMID: 28085085

Muro-de-la-Herran, A., García-Zapirain, B., & Méndez-Zorrilla, A. (2014). Gait analysis methods: An overview of wearable and non-wearable systems, highlighting clinical applications. *Sensors (Basel), 14*(2), 3362–3394. DOI: 10.3390/s140203362 PMID: 24556672

Piwek, L., Ellis, D. A., Andrews, S., & Joinson, A. (2016). The rise of consumer health wearables: Promises and barriers. *PLoS Medicine, 13*(2), e1001953. DOI: 10.1371/journal.pmed.1001953 PMID: 26836780

Porciuncula, F., Roto, A. V., Kumar, D., Davis, I., Roy, S., Walsh, C. J., & Awad, L. N. (2018). Wearable movement sensors for rehabilitation: A focused review of technological and clinical advances. PM&R, 10(9S2), S220-S232. https://doi.org/ DOI: 10.1016/j.pmrj.2018.06.013

Schwenk, M., Howe, C., Saleh, A., Mohler, J., Grewal, G., Armstrong, D., & Najafi, B. (2014). Frailty and technology: A systematic review of gait analysis in those with frailty. *Gerontology, 60*(1), 79–89. DOI: 10.1159/000354211 PMID: 23949441

Seneviratne, S., Hu, Y., Nguyen, T., Lan, G., Khalifa, S., Thilakarathna, K., Hassan, M., & Seneviratne, A. (2017). A survey of wearable devices and challenges. *IEEE Communications Surveys and Tutorials, 19*(4), 2573–2620. DOI: 10.1109/COMST.2017.2731979

Shull, P. B., Jirattigalachote, W., Hunt, M. A., Cutkosky, M. R., & Delp, S. L. (2014). Quantified self and human movement: A review on the clinical impact of wearable sensing and feedback for gait analysis and intervention. *Gait & Posture, 40*(1), 11–19. DOI: 10.1016/j.gaitpost.2014.03.189 PMID: 24768525

Tao, W., Liu, T., Zheng, R., & Feng, H. (2012). Gait analysis using wearable sensors. *Sensors (Basel), 12*(2), 2255–2283. DOI: 10.3390/s120202255 PMID: 22438763

Wang, Q., Markopoulos, P., Yu, B., Chen, W., & Timmermans, A. (2017). Interactive wearable systems for upper body rehabilitation: A systematic review. *Journal of Neuroengineering and Rehabilitation, 14*(1), 20. DOI: 10.1186/s12984-017-0229-y PMID: 28284228

Zheng, Y. L., Ding, X. R., Poon, C. C. Y., Lo, B. P. L., Zhang, H., Zhou, X. L., Yang, G.-Z., Zhao, N., & Zhang, Y. T. (2014). Unobtrusive sensing and wearable devices for health informatics. *IEEE Transactions on Biomedical Engineering*, *61*(5), 1538–1554. DOI: 10.1109/TBME.2014.2309951 PMID: 24759283

ADDITIONAL READING

Appelboom, G., Camacho, E., Abraham, M. E., Bruce, S. S., Dumont, E. L., Zacharia, B. E., D'Amico, R., Slomian, J., Reginster, J. Y., Bruyère, O., & Connolly, E. S.Jr. (2014). Smart wearable body sensors for patient self-assessment and monitoring. *Archives of Public Health = Archives Belges de Santé Publique*, *72*(1), 28. DOI: 10.1186/2049-3258-72-28 PMID: 25232478

Godfrey, A., Hetherington, V., Shum, H., Bonato, P., Lovell, N. H., & Stuart, S. (2018). From A to Z: Wearable technology explained. *Maturitas*, *113*, 40–47. DOI: 10.1016/j.maturitas.2018.04.012 PMID: 29903647

Mukhopadhyay, S. C. (2015). Wearable sensors for human activity monitoring: A review. *IEEE Sensors Journal*, *15*(3), 1321–1330. DOI: 10.1109/JSEN.2014.2370945

Pantelopoulos, A., & Bourbakis, N. G. (2010). A survey on wearable sensor-based systems for health monitoring and prognosis. *IEEE Transactions on Systems, Man, and Cybernetics. Part C, Applications and Reviews*, *40*(1), 1–12. DOI: 10.1109/TSMCC.2009.2032660

Patel, S., Park, H., Bonato, P., Chan, L., & Rodgers, M. (2012). A review of wearable sensors and systems with application in rehabilitation. *Journal of Neuroengineering and Rehabilitation*, *9*(1), 21. DOI: 10.1186/1743-0003-9-21 PMID: 22520559

Chapter 11
Predictive Medicine:
A New Era of Pain Management for Assistive Augmentative Rehabilitation Systems

Bhanuprakash Ananthakumar
https://orcid.org/0009-0001-5517-7933
Sri Sathya Sai University for Human Excellence, India

Bhuvana Gudibanda Nagaraja
Sri Sathya Sai University for Human Excellence, India

Sai Mahima Umesh
Sri Sathya Sai University for Human Excellence, India

Ramya Raghavan
https://orcid.org/0000-0002-9953-543X
Sri Sathya Sai University for Human Excellence, India

ABSTRACT

Pain management is a critical area of research in developing assistive augmentative technologies, brain-computer interfaces, exoskeletons, and soft robotics. Assistive and augmentative technologies, such as assistive gloves incorporating flexible sensors, offer promising avenues for pain relief and improved functionality. Brain-computer interfaces and exoskeletons are also emerging as potential tools for pain management, leveraging sensor fusion and musculoskeletal modelling. Algorithms are crucial in these technologies, enabling real-time pain management through neuromorphic computing and predictive modelling. Integrating computational pharmacology, gene therapy, regenerative therapies, and personalized medicine approaches, informed by machine learning, can transform pain management paradigms.

DOI: 10.4018/979-8-3373-0194-5.ch011

INTRODUCTION

Chronic pain is complex, affecting millions in need of for assistive augmentative rehabilitation systems. Predictive algorithms are revolutionizing the field of rehabilitation and assistive systems, offering new avenues for pain management and functional recovery. Predictive algorithms use data from brain-computer interfaces (BCIs), exoskeletons, soft robotics, and neuromorphic computing. These algorithms can anticipate the needs of individuals and adapt interventions in real time. BCIs enable direct communication between the brain and assistive devices, allowing for precise control and customization of pain relief strategies. Exoskeletons and soft robotics, equipped with advanced sensors, can monitor movement patterns and predict areas of strain, adjusting support to minimize discomfort and enhance rehabilitation outcomes. Integrating predictive algorithms with pain relief technologies ensures a personalized approach to pain management. Research in this field is optimizing the effectiveness of interventions and improving the quality of life for individuals with chronic pain or mobility impairments.

Pain Management Challenges

Pain is an undertreated condition despite its worldwide prevalence with disease burden. Pain mechanisms involve nociception and various environment processes that lead to pain sensation. Better understanding of pain and its mechanisms is crucial for developing effective treatments. It does involve multifaceted nociceptive, inflammatory, and neuropathic processes, complicating treatment. Current analgesics have limitations in efficacy and safety. For example, diagnosing and rehabilitating peripheral nerve injuries, show the need for novel mechanisms of action. Upcoming methods for peripheral nerve injury treatment are artificial intelligence based neuroimaging, wearable devices, and robotic surgical procedures (Guo et al., 2024). Investigating the brain's ability to reorganize itself in response to injury or pain can lead to targeted interventions that promote healing and reduce discomfort (Saxer et al., 2024). Understanding these mechanisms is crucial for developing effective pain treatments for conditions such as:

- Cervical Spondylosis Myelopathy (CSM): A degenerative disorder leading to neurological disability and discomfort.
- Cervical Spine Pain Disease Classification: Cervical Spine Pain Injuries (CPI): deep learning for early and precise diagnosis from X-ray images.
- Neuropathic Pain Post Amputation: Complications can lead to debilitating pain and impact daily living activities.

- Spinal Cord Injury Risks: Increased risk for upper limb injuries, including neuromusculoskeletal pathologies and nociceptive pain. High incidence of upper limb injuries due to muscular demands from Manual Wheelchair Users.
- Low Back Pain (LBP): Bone anchored limb implantation alters multi-joint biomechanics, potentially impacting low back pain (LBP) and osteoarthritis (OA) risk factors.

Patients with Impaired Communication

The evaluation of pain in nonverbal critically ill patients remains a complex challenge. Algorithms are used to analyze electrocardiographic (ECG) signals and breathing rate estimation. To identify abnormalities in activities of daily living data is essential in eldercare. Evaluating pain in patients who are unable to communicate poses significant challenges. Traditional pain assessment methods often rely on self-reporting, which is not feasible for many critically ill patients. Biochemical profiling analyses circulating cytokines, chemokines, and growth factors. It can further refine pain management by identifying underlying pain mechanisms. Additionally, algometric measurements, such as pressure pain thresholds, provide objective data to assess pain sensitivity and predict pain scores (Barakat et al., 2024).

Neuroplasticity refers to the brain's ability to reorganize itself by forming new neural connections in response to learning, experience, or injury, which is crucial for recovery in neurorehabilitation. Sensorimotor adaptation involves the brain adjusting motor commands based on sensory feedback, allowing for improved coordination and movement efficiency. Both concepts are essential for developing effective rehabilitation strategies and interventions for individuals with neurological and neurodevelopmental conditions (Pirasteh et al., 2024).

Bioelectronic medicine involves modulating the nervous system through precise electrical current delivery. Lack of biosensors highlight the need for effective pain assessment tools to reflect patients' pain experiences. Neuromodulation treatments are tested for clinical conditions like post-stroke movement recovery and drug-resistant disorders (González-González et al., 2024). Upcoming research works on utilizing multiple and/or continual measurements, we can tailor treatment types and prescriptions to maximize clinically relevant functional outcomes.

Assistive Augmentative Technologies (AATs)

Neuroprosthetic devices can replicate natural touch, improving pain management for individuals with sensory-motor impairments (Donati & Valle, 2024). An assistive function is the capability of a device to provide support in performing tasks or mobility. Assistive soft robotics for pain management, like wearable robotic devices, are designed to alleviate pain and support rehabilitation through gentle assistance in mobility in daily activities. The construction of closed-loop systems allows for measuring and controlling neural activity. Closed-loop systems use multiphoton microscopy for real-time feedback and brain-machine interfaces (BMIs) for controlling targeted neuron populations (Hira, 2024) in comatose patients. Neuromorphic computing, can process sensory data more efficiently and adaptively. The exciting field of neuromorphic computing focusing on spiking neural networks (SNNs) which improves the responsiveness of these systems. Neuromorphic technology is proposed to enhance the natural tactile experience. Electrical neural stimulation can help manage pain associated with neurological and neurodevelopmental conditions (Donati & Valle, 2024). Advancements in SNN algorithms and hardware implementations allow their applications in diverse areas, such as brain-computer interfaces, robotics, and medical diagnostics. Several studies detail novel hardware designs for efficient SNN processing using memristors and emerging technologies (GVS et al., 2025). Some examples of predictive medicine applications for pain management are listed below.

- Electroencephalography (EEG): Algorithms extract and interpret brain signals from EEG data for applications like brain-computer interfaces (BCI) in robotics, controlling prosthetic limbs, and detecting cognitive decline in older adults.
- Surface electromyography (sEMG): Algorithms can decode muscle movements from sEMG signals to control prosthetic limbs, recognize hand gestures, and identify gait phases for exoskeleton control.
- Insomnia detection: Machine learning (ML) and deep learning (DL) algorithms analyze physiological signals to automate sleep analysis and insomnia detection.
- Drowning detection: Image processing techniques and machine learning algorithms (MLAs) are employed in pool and waterway safety surveillance systems.
- Fall detection: ML and DL algorithms, particularly CNNs and RNNs, are used with radar data for detecting falls, especially in elderly individuals.
- Navigation and obstacle avoidance: Algorithms, including reinforcement learning, enable autonomous navigation and obstacle avoidance in assistive devices like wheelchairs.
- Braille-to-speech translation: Machine learning algorithms are used with electrostatic transducers to translate Braille into speech for visually impaired individuals.

Biomarkers

Deep learning can analyze large molecular and biological datasets to identify new drug targets and develop novel pain medications. The P2X7 receptor is a significant focus for pharmaceutical companies in developing compounds to modulate its activity for therapeutic purposes (Idrissi et al., 2024). The TRPV1 channel, known as the capsaicin receptor, is extensively expressed in nerve terminals and other tissues. Prolonged exposure to capsaicin, a known agonist of TRPV1, has been shown to generate analgesia. Numerous capsaicin analogs have been developed to discover effective analgesics for pain relief. P2X7 and TRPV1 and other biomarkers, molecules like cytokines, neurotransmitters, or genetic markers, provide objective insights into a patient's pain state. Advances in silico tools, including molecular modeling and machine learning algorithms, have significantly aided in identifying pharmacological target sites. While still largely an area of active research and development, the integration of synthetic biology's capabilities can bring advanced rehabilitation technologies for repositioning drugs targeting TRPV1 (Amaya-Rodriguez et al., 2024).

Sensory motor adaptation allows understanding how patients adapt their movements in response to pain. Armeo spring, a robotic device used in neurorehabilitation, assists with pain management in neurological disorders. Developing advanced biosensors is one key area where synthetic biology intersects with predictive pain management (Lakshmaiah et al., 2025). Our understanding of the sensory pathways in pain perception aids neurobionics in integrating artificial devices with biological systems. These biosensors could continuously monitor their physiological state, detecting early signs of inflammation or specific pain biomarkers for pain modulation. Neurostimulation methods like spinal cord stimulation or peripheral nerve stimulation can be used to modulate pain pathways. For example, a robotic exoskeleton might adjust an exercise's intensity or range of motion to avoid exacerbating predicted pain.

Regenerative Peripheral Nerve Interfaces

Functional electrical stimulation (FES) uses low-intensity electrical signals to stimulate damaged peripheral nerves and generate body movements in patients with impaired motor control. This field involves the modulation of the nervous system through precise electrical current delivery to treat clinical conditions like post-stroke movement recovery and drug-resistant disorders. The advent of Regenerative Peripheral Nerve Interfaces (RPNI) marks a significant advancement in pain management, particularly for individuals who have undergone limb amputations. This innovative approach addresses the debilitating pain associated with neuromas. By providing free muscle grafts as physiological targets for peripheral nerve ingrowth, RPNIs create a more natural interface for nerve regeneration (Berberoglu et al., 2024). RPNI based process helps in controlling prosthetic device. It reduces the incidence of neuroma formation, which can lead to chronic pain and functional impairment. Thus, RPNIs and neurobionics in pain management for amputees, offer the dual benefit of pain relief and enhanced prosthetic control (Tian et al., 2024).

Functional Electrical Stimulation

Predictive algorithms allow for early intervention and preventive strategies. Another application for predictive algorithms is to control functional electrical stimulation (FES) for stroke rehabilitation. FES uses electrical impulses to stimulate muscles, helping patients regain lost movement. Controlling FES arrays for complex movements requires high precision, and traditional methods are time-consuming to set up in clinical settings. Iterative Learning Control (ILC) has shown promise but requires numerous time-consuming identification tests (Sun & Freeman, 2024). A novel approach that minimizes identification time while preserving accuracy. The plant model, updated in parallel with the ILC, paves the way for more efficient and clinically feasible FES-based stroke rehabilitation (Gasperina et al., 2024). Predictive models also incorporate multivariate models based on genetic algorithms, which link structural changes in the body (such as joint modifications) to future pain, such as knee pain.

The patient-in-the-loop framework is versatile and applicable to neurological and neurodevelopmental conditions (Cashaback et al., 2024). Whether addressing chronic pain in stroke survivors or pain associated with cerebral palsy, the framework can be adapted to meet diverse patient needs. The models could also be used to forecast the resources needed for long-term medical care of patients who require assistance with daily tasks. By employing interpretable machine learning methods, survival analysis helps predict the time until significant pain relief, offering valuable insights into the effectiveness and timeline of pain management treatments.

Physical Therapy Devices

Neuroprosthetic devices interface with the nervous system to restore missing limb functions and provide sensory feedback. The participants' depression scores could discriminate between control participants and those with pain using Random Forests as the machine learning algorithm. For example, regenerative peripheral nerve interface offers real-time control of prosthetic devices such as the assistive glove in upper extremity function with practical pain management applications. It is a therapeutic approach utilizing robotic devices to enhance rehabilitation in patients with neurological disorders. The best classification results in better accuracy for the whole trunk flexion and sit-to-stand exercises are when tested using support vector machines.

The assistive glove can enhance the use of upper extremity joints during reaching tasks. Modular architecture allows the actuators and their attachment points to be easily modified for different joints. Custom-made McKibben-style pneumatic actuators are specialized and used in the exosuit to provide movement through pneumatic pressure (Gariya et al., 2024). The machine learning techniques applied to kinematic and muscle activity data could accurately discriminate between people with low, high pain and control participants during physical exercises. EEG-enabled earbuds and other devices monitor brain activity and can be used to develop personalized pain management strategies (Correia et al., 2024). Gaussian Process Regression-based algorithms can estimate rehabilitation outcomes using clinical data or wearable sensors, offering a more personalized and data-driven approach. Variational inference further enhances predictive models by learning from observations over time, enabling a more dynamic approach to treatment prediction. The finger exoskeleton for treating tendon injuries is designed to assist flexion/extension motions of a finger. The effect of ankle plantar-flexion timing on joint kinematics and metabolic power when walking aids in treating tendon injuries. In survival analysis, methods such as the Cox proportional hazards model are applied to assess the effect of multiple variables on the duration of pain relief. Wearable sensors for pose estimation and intent detection are integrated to track hand positions and pain relief (Sanders & Reinkensmeyer, 2024).

Exoskeletons

Exoskeletons give mechanical assistance for subjects with low mobility impairments. It is the support provided by exoskeletons and soft robotics to help individuals with mobility challenges reduce their energy requirements. There are several advantages in pain management by using overground lower limb robotic exoskeletons in rehabilitation. An optimal controller with two parts is proposed to track desired trajectories estimate optimal muscle activations, improving pain and spasticity in people with spinal cord injuries (Rusta et al., 2024). An exosuit that uses Bowden cables transfer torque from the actuator to the biomechanical joint. The exoskeleton with optimal joint torques and accurate trajectory tracking accelerates neuromodulation treatments. (Sanders & Reinkensmeyer, 2024).

Table 1. Prediction algorithm applications for pain management

Prediction System	Pain management application	Reference
AI Robots, CT Robotic Arms, And Needle Emplacer	Surgery, anesthesiology	(Guo et al., 2024) (Schreiber et al., 2024) (Paiste et al., 2024)
Neuromodulation	Stroke recovery	(González-González et al., 2024)
Neuroprosthetic Devices	Sensory-motor impairments	(Donati & Valle, 2024)
Closed Loop Systems	Brain-machine interfaces	(Hira, 2024)
Regenerative Peripheral Nerve Interfaces, Neurobionics	Amputees	(Tian et al., 2024)
Exoskeletons, Soft Robotics	Tendon injuries	(Sanders & Reinkensmeyer, 2024) (Rusta et al., 2024)
Mckibben Style Pneumatic Actuators	Exosuit for physical support	(Gariya et al., 2024)
EEG-Enabled Earbuds	Monitor brain activity	(Correia et al., 2024)
Knee Simulation System	Osteoarthritis	(Kang et al., 2024)
Sensory Memory Processing System(SMPS)	Visible information display	(Shan et al., 2023)
Virtual and Augmented Reality Gamification	Post-procedural recovery	(Shrestha et al., 2024) (Sánchez-Gil et al., 2025)
Non-Invasive Glucose Monitoring Device	Diabetics	(Rajeswari & Vijayakumar, 2024)
Functional Electrical Stimulation, Iterative Learning Control	Stroke rehabilitation	(Sun & Freeman, 2024) (Gasperina et al., 2024)
Multilayer Perceptrons	Chronic low back pain	(Villalba-Meneses et al., 2024)

Sensor Fusion

Sensor fusion combines data from multiple sensors. Sensor fusion provides a more accurate real-time control of myoelectric prosthetics, amplifying motor action potentials for sensory feedback. Kalman Filtering technique estimates the system's state by combining noisy sensor measurements with a mathematical system model. The complementary Filtering technique combines data from different sensors with complementary characteristics, such as IMUs and position sensors, to obtain a more accurate estimate. The fused sensor data can be analyzed to extract meaningful information about movement patterns and muscle activity.

- Gait Analysis: stride length, cadence, and gait speed, types of movements based on sensor data, Human-machine interaction Analysis

- Muscle Activation Analysis: Analyzing EMG data to determine muscle activation patterns and levels of muscle effort.

This stable, biological nerve interface enhances the functionality of prosthetic devices, allowing for a more natural and intuitive user experience. Additionally, RPNI facilitates better integration of prosthetics with the body's native signaling pathways. The physiological mechanism behind this pain relief involves the integration of the nerve interface with the muscle graft, allowing for better nerve regeneration and function (Berberoglu et al., 2024).

The International Classification of Functioning, Disability, and Health (ICF), emphasize the importance of a holistic approach to patient care. Machine learning algorithms can be trained to fuse sensor data and recognize movement and muscle activity patterns. The knee simulation system assists in studying osteoarthritis levels by replicating knee motions using 3D printing technology, allowing for detailed analysis of knee mechanics at various OA stages. It employs the Kellgren Lawrence (KL) grade scale to highlight variations in the force applied to the knee bone during movement. This system aids in developing personalized diagnostic approaches and enhances surgical effectiveness by facilitating the creation of customized prosthetic joints (Kang et al., 2024). This ensures that pain management strategies are focused on alleviating symptoms and enhancing overall functional ability and quality of life.

Advanced Computing for Pain Management

Biosensors can be used in brain-computer interfaces (BCIs), exoskeletons, soft robotics for neural repair and regeneration. Predictive algorithms with biosensors are the revolutionizing next step in the field of rehabilitation and assistive systems. Biosensors offer new avenues for pain management and functional recovery. Multi-omics algorithms help build biosensors that can anticipate the needs of individuals and adapt interventions in real time. The factor assessment involves high dimensional data and omics methodologies to capture the complexity. Some of the factors considered are

- External General: Macrolevel factors like climate, urbanicity, and socioeconomic status.
- External Specific: Individual triggers like pollutants, diet, occupational hazards, and lifestyle factors.
- Internal: Biological responses, including epigenetic and metabolic changes, inflammation, and oxidative stress.
- Biomarkers: Analyzing biological samples (e.g., blood, urine, hair)

- Environmental Monitoring: Using sensors and remote sensing to assess environmental exposures.
- Questionnaires and Diaries: Collecting self-reported pain data.
- Technologies: Employing genomics, transcriptomics, proteomics, and metabolomics.

Biosensor Applications

BCIs enable direct communication between the brain and assistive devices, allowing for precise control and customization. Genetically modified cells could be implanted or integrated into wearable devices to sense specific pain markers and, in response, produce and release pain-relieving molecules (Biradar et al., 2025). Exoskeletons and soft robotics, equipped with advanced sensors, can monitor movement patterns. Exoskeletons predict areas of strain, adjusting support to minimize discomfort and enhance rehabilitation outcomes. The predictive effects on patients responding well to treatment focus on identifying co-variable influences contributing to positive treatment outcomes (Anil Chandra, Biradar, et al., 2024). For instance, reinforcement learning in pain management helps optimize treatment plans by continuously adapting to patient feedback, ensuring decisions are made to maximize the long-term benefits. Techniques like principal component analysis (PCA) can simplify complex datasets by reducing them into uncorrelated variables. PCA allows for the identification of key factors influencing pain levels, making predictive modeling more efficient.

The integration of multiomics data, including genomics, transcriptomics, and metabolomics, is crucial for understanding the biological responses. Both intrinsic and extrinsic factors influence cell identity through cellular reprogramming. Pain pathways highlight the role of the epigenetic and transcriptional landscape, leading to non-genetic adaptations. The Multiomics approach allows for identifying molecular signatures associated with environmental drivers of pain. The integration of multiple data sources has allowed researchers to understand the variability in pain related to demographic, infrastructure, climate, and environmental characteristics, which are crucial for understanding disease spread patterns. Advances in high throughput omics technologies and computational analytics facilitate comprehensive measurement and analysis of pain, which can inform public health initiatives and policies promoting healthier environments (Wan et al., 2025).

Machine learning and advanced statistical models are increasingly used to handle high-dimensionality data. Techniques such as Bayesian regression models, weighted quantile sum regression, and causal inference methods are employed to study the combined effects of multiple interactions with health outcomes. Methodologies for data integration, including concatenation-based, transformation-based, and network-based strategies, aimed at effectively managing diverse data types. The role of large language models in artificial intelligence is highlighted as a potential game-changer for future data integration approaches in precision medicine (Nam et al., 2024). Computational, Bayesian, and spatial-temporal approaches are employed to identify exposure and disease susceptibility biomarkers, which can inform novel diagnostic and treatment options. Deep generative models like variational autoencoders used for data imputation, augmentation, and batch effect correction methodologies provide a robust framework for predicting disease trajectories and identifying early intervention opportunities. Transformers, known for their effectiveness in handling large-scale and heterogeneous datasets in other domains, may offer a transformative approach to single-cell modeling. the integration of machine learning techniques in clinical flow cytometry to improve the analysis of complex data, highlighting the shift from manual gating to computational methods. It discusses various ML approaches, including supervised, unsupervised, and semi-supervised methods (Spies et al., 2025).

Regression and machine learning models in pain management are widely employed to predict treatment outcomes based on these variables, offering a more tailored approach to patient care. For example, the predictive effects of treatment approaches, such as high-dose monotherapy versus combination therapy, can be analyzed by examining co-variables that may influence patient responses.

Figure 1. Predictive algorithms for pain management

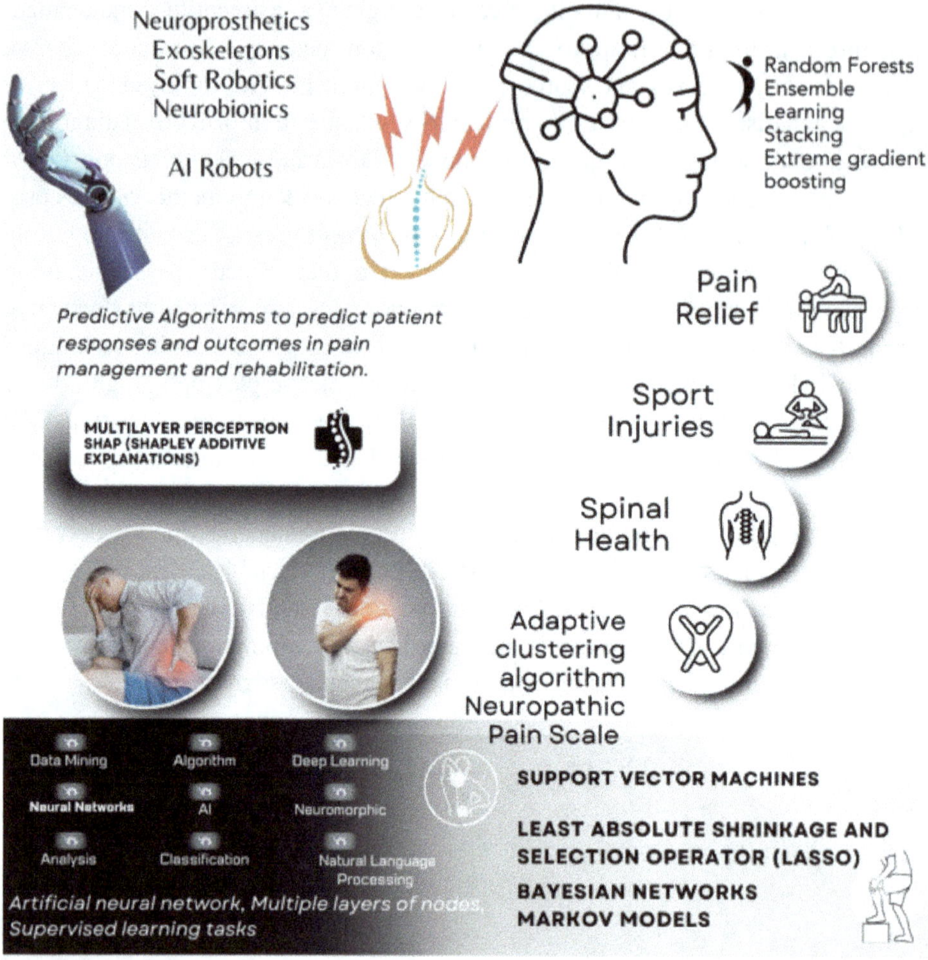

Machine Learning for Pain Management

Predictive modeling uses machine learning algorithms to help predict pain episodes based on neural signals. It can trigger real-time interventions, such as neurofeedback or transcranial magnetic stimulation. Applying machine learning algorithms like support vector machines, random forests, and neural networks to pain prediction is common. A sensory memory processing system can decode neural signals related to pain perception and emotional state. A sensory memory processing system is efficient in processing sensory information with synapse-like and multi-wavelength light-emitting output. Robustness in information encoding and transmission allows visible information display through color responses analogous to pain warning in organisms (Shan et al., 2023). Also, a new hardware system is reported for efficient multimodal information recognition, dynamic step frequency, and spatial positioning. Machine learning in surgical robots help in the control, navigation of flexible surgical implants and interventional soft robotic technologies.

The use of algorithms in assistive technology for pain management for short term illness is essential. In particular rehabilitation and treatment for conditions like low back pain and stroke. The machine learning models help healthcare professionals determine the appropriate physical therapy for non-specific low back pain patients. Researchers used motion capture data from a range of motion exercises performed by healthy individuals and patients diagnosed with low back pain to train different ML algorithms, including Support Vector Machines (SVM), random forests, and multilayer perceptron (MLP). The study found that all the ML techniques achieved an accuracy above 80%, with SVM, random forests, and MLP exceeding 90% accuracy. These results demonstrate the potential of using algorithms to develop data-driven treatment approaches for chronic low back pain, aiming to improve patients' quality of life (Villalba-Meneses et al., 2024).

Deep Learning Approaches

Deep learning approaches, such as convolutional neural networks and recurrent neural networks, allow for the analysis of complex biological data. An integrated approach can provide a more comprehensive and accurate assessment of pain. Deep learning models can analyze patient data, including medical history, genetic information, and lifestyle factors, to predict the likelihood of developing chronic pain conditions. The predictive algorithms in rehabilitation programs use virtual and augmented reality, accelerating post-procedural recovery (Shrestha et al., 2024). A non-invasive glucose monitoring device using near-infra-red biosensors addresses a source of discomfort for diabetic patients. By eliminating the need for painful finger pricks, sensor technology contributes to painful osteoarthritis (Rajeswari & Vijayakumar, 2024). Combining CNNs and RNNs allows for less invasive monitoring techniques for multimodal pain assessment by integrating information from different sources like facial expressions, physiological signals, and even natural language descriptions of pain.

Feature engineering and Deep learning are essential for building accurate and interpretable predictive models. Predictive models can anticipate potential pain points using quantum machine learning to personalize treatment for knee osteoarthritis and adjust the device's support accordingly. There is an increasing use of AI and machine learning in anesthesiology. Key applications include pain management, anesthetics delivery control, risk prediction, and operating room logistics. It emphasizes the potential for personalized care through data analysis (Paiste et al., 2024). Deep learning models, particularly Convolutional Neural Networks (CNNs) and Recurrent Neural Networks (RNNs), show great promise in pain management. Computational pharmacology integrates data acquisition and analysis to gain biological insights into pain.

Gamification

The effects of gamification on usability, engagement, has positive patient responses. Gamification of therapy have emerged as promising strategies to enhance motivation and effectiveness. Robotic, motorized, non-motorized, virtual reality and neuromuscular electrical stimulation improve motor and cognitive functions (Sánchez-Gil et al., 2025). The findings indicate that gamified devices enhance motor and cognitive recovery and significantly improve patients' emotional, social, and personal well-being. Neuromorphic computing can process sensory data in real time for gamified devices. Assistive devices can adapt to provide dynamic support by combining neuromorphic computing with predictive algorithms. For example, a neuromorphic chip can analyze sensory data from a soft robotic glove to predict the user's intent and adjust the device's stiffness to optimize grip force and reduce hand fatigue. By addressing these questions and exploring the potential of these technologies, we can pave the way for innovative solutions to alleviate pain.

Computed Tomography

Computed Tomography (CT) image guidance is minimally invasive treatment using needle-like tools. Robots like CRANE (CT Robotic Arm and Needle Emplacer) enhance these procedures by providing high positional accuracy and compensating for physiological motion. Thus, reducing the need for frequent imaging scans. CRANE's design focuses on system dexterity, enabling physicians to operate or supplement needles within the scanner bore naturally. CT-Guided Robotic Needle Placement introduces CRANE, a CT-compatible robot for precise needle placement in minimally invasive procedures. CT-Guided Robotic Interventions CRANE robotic intervention meets clinical requirements for target accuracy and improves the efficacy of image-guided needle placement. (Schreiber et al., 2024).

CT Robotic Arm and Needle Emplacer (CRANE):

- A CT-compatible robot designed for minimally invasive treatments using needle-like tools.
    - High positional accuracy.

- o Compensation for physiological motion.
- o Dexterity for manipulating and inserting needles within the scanner bore

Neuromorphic Computing

Neuromorphic computing, which mimics the neural architecture of the human brain, can process sensory data more efficiently and adaptively, further enhancing the responsiveness of these systems. Multiomics algorithms, which integrate genomics, proteomics, and metabolomics data, can comprehensively understand an individual's biological state, enabling highly personalized pain management strategies (Ananthakumar et al., 2024). The integration of predictive algorithms with these technologies ensures a customized approach to pain management, optimizing the effectiveness of interventions and improving the quality of life for individuals with chronic pain or mobility impairments. This synergy between predictive algorithms and assistive technologies promises to transform rehabilitation practices, making them more responsive and effective. The patient-in-the-loop framework represents a unifying approach that can bridge the gap between computational modeling and clinical practice in neurorehabilitation. By prioritizing multidisciplinary collaboration and leveraging cutting-edge research, we can significantly enhance pain management strategies in assistive augmentative rehabilitation. As we continue to explore the potential of computational modelling, our ultimate goal remains clear: to improve patient outcomes and quality of life through innovative, personalized care (Cashaback et al., 2024).

Neuromorphic Computing for Real-time Pain Management

Brain-computer interfaces (BCIs), coupled with predictive algorithms, can decode neural signals to anticipate pain episodes. It initiates targeted interventions based on Spiking Neural Networks and their potential for real-time processing of sensory data. For example, machine learning models can analyze EEG data to predict the onset of migraines and trigger preemptive pain relief strategies, such as transcranial magnetic stimulation or virtual reality distraction techniques. The neuromorphic systems can adapt to changing conditions and provide dynamic pain relief. Integrating predictive multi-omics with neuromorphic technologies can potentially transform rehabilitation practices (Anil Chandra, Ananthakumar, et al., 2024).

Predictive Modeling on Neuromorphic Hardware

Exoskeletons and soft robotics, equipped with advanced sensors and actuators, can collect real-time data on muscle activity, joint angles, and force distribution. Predictive algorithms can analyze this data to anticipate potential pain points and adjust the exoskeleton's support accordingly. For instance, by integrating proteomic data on muscle fatigue biomarkers, the algorithm can predict the onset of muscle strain and increase support in vulnerable areas.

Inclusion of Diagnostic and Treatment Models

Central to effective pain management is the ability to accurately diagnose the source and nature of the pain. The Behavioral Pain Scale (BPS) for observational assessments and an eye-tracking device to facilitate self-reporting via the Numeric Rating Scale (NRS) and the EuroQol EQ-5D-5L (EQ-Pain) (Waydhas et al., 2024). The findings underscore the necessity of considering high-tech AAC tools before relying on behavioral assessment scales in non-verbal patients. Accurately assessing pain is crucial for effective pain management, particularly in critically ill patients who may experience significant discomfort. Implementing advanced technologies, such as eye-tracking devices, can enhance the accuracy of pain assessments and improve patient care (Yılmaz & Özdem, 2024).

Role of Computational Pharmacology

The use of medicinal plants for pain relief dates back millions of years. The invention of the syringe in the 19th century marked a significant advancement—targeted drug delivery. For example, saffron is rich in phytochemicals like crocin, safranal, and picrocrocin, with pain-relieving benefits through anti-inflammatory and analgesic properties (Korrapati et al., 2024). Computational data on phytochemicals from medicinal plants, like saffron, could help identify compounds for pain management in assistive and augmentative rehabilitation systems. The P2X7 receptor (P2X7R) is an ATP-gated non-selective cation channel that plays a critical role in controlling the release of proinflammatory cytokines (Idrissi et al., 2024). It is a key player in initiating inflammatory signaling cascades. It is a target for treating various pathologies, including chronic inflammatory disorders like rheumatoid arthritis and osteoarthritis, chronic neuropathic pain, mood disorders, neurodegenerative diseases, ischemia, and cancer. Peptide nanoparticle conjugates offer targeted cancer treatment, reducing pain by minimizing damage to healthy tissues and enhancing the effectiveness of pain-relieving therapies (Duan et al., 2024). Pharmaceutical companies are actively developing compounds to modulate

P2X7R, with many patent applications filed for potential treatments. Efforts are also underway to develop effective positron emission tomography (PET) radioligands to advance the understanding of P2X7R's role in inflammation (Idrissi et al., 2024)

Predictive pain management in assistive and augmentative rehabilitation systems could be enhanced by monitoring food-borne microbial volatile organic compounds to identify early signs of infection or inflammation and improve patient outcomes (Nagashri et al., 2024). To infer pain levels, CNNs and RNNs can be used to analyze physiological signals like heart rate variability, skin conductance, and brain activity (EEG). RNNs are particularly useful for analyzing time-series data like physiological signals due to their ability to capture temporal dependencies. It aids in identifying biological molecules associated with pain, building quantitative models of pain signaling, and facilitating drug discovery, although its predictions require experimental validation. The intersection of engineering, science, and clinical practice is rapidly evolving, particularly in neurorehabilitation. The National Science Foundation (NSF) and the National Institute of Health (NIH) have significantly promoted this integration by convening a conference focused on computational modeling in neurorehabilitation. This initiative aims to foster multidisciplinary collaborations that can ultimately enhance patient care, particularly in pain management for individuals undergoing assistive augmentative rehabilitation (Valero-Cuevas et al., 2024).

Ethical Considerations

Implementing computational models within clinical settings presents several challenges, including the need for rigorous model validation. Validation is essential to ensure the models accurately reflect patient experiences and can reliably guide treatment decisions. This process involves collaboration among computational scientists, clinicians, and patients to refine models based on real-world outcomes. The neural correlates of pain with neuromorphic technology utilize immersive environments to distract patients from pain and enhance rehabilitation experiences. Despite the advancements, several challenges remain, including the need for standardized methodologies and the integration of diverse data types. Developing new technologies and analytical methods, such as mobile health applications and informatics tools, offers promise for overcoming these challenges in public health research. The data-driven prognosis tool relies entirely on in situ measurements to assess patient outcomes. It evaluates prognostic data and forecasts the effectiveness of treatments by leveraging clinical and demographic variables (Moreno-Sánchez et al., 2024).

The integration of predictive algorithms in pain management presents both opportunities and challenges. Deep learning models can be integrated into wearable devices or monitoring systems. Critics argue that some predictive algorithms, such as NarxCare scores, lack sufficient scientific validation. While these algorithms aim to predict opioid misuse, concerns have been raised to provide real-time pain assessment. Some researchers worry that biases in the data used in pain activated automated interventions. The predictive algorithms can assist clinicians, but there is concern that they may override adjusting medication dosages or delivering targeted therapies. Developing better frameworks for integrating different computational methods and the use of artificial intelligence (AI) in pain management. By using natural language processing, audio recordings during procedures can automatically classify sedation states, including movement and pain. This could lead to better documentation, real-time sedation monitoring, and insights into the efficacy of different sedation techniques. Feature engineering focuses on creating new, more informative features from raw data. It argues that AI can improve pain assessment accuracy, efficiency, and objectivity compared to traditional subjective methods, leading to better pain management.

Ethical considerations about privacy, data security, to avoid potential misuse of sensitive health information will enhance drug discovery processes. Pain is a multifaceted experience influenced by various biological, psychological, and social factors. AI-based interventions have shown promise in improving pain recognition and prediction. Algorithms that simplify pain management into quantifiable metrics may overlook the overall efficiency and accuracy. Further, significant challenges remain in the safety and reliability of engineered biological systems. The ethical considerations should be met during the use of synthetic biology along with the technical hurdles (Lakshmaiah et al., 2025). The hours need a clinical translation that seamlessly integrates biological sensors with mechanical and computational systems in real time.

CONCLUSION

Predictive pain management algorithms integrated with assistive augmentative rehabilitation systems represent a cutting-edge approach. It is about moving from reactive pain intervention to proactive, personalized, and biologically informed management for enhancing rehabilitation outcomes. Pain management is a critical area of research in developing assistive augmentative technologies, brain-computer interfaces, exoskeletons, and soft robotics. The development of more sophisticated and biocompatible biosensors and innovation in adaptive assistive technologies are all converging to make this future possible. These technologies offer promising solutions for individuals suffering from chronic pain or mobility impairments. Exoskeletons and soft robotics can enhance physical rehabilitation by providing support and reducing the strain on muscles and joints, alleviating pain during movement (Chandra et al., 2025). Computational modeling enhances neurorehabilitation via P2X7 receptor targeting and provides new therapeutic opportunities. Advanced imaging techniques improve protein studies, and in silico methods streamline ion channel drug discovery. TRPV1 modulation aids pain management, and robotic interventions enhance precision in minimally invasive procedures. Machine learning optimizes flexible surgical robots with advanced sensors and artificial intelligence for dynamic pain management strategies. The convergence of these innovative technologies holds the potential to significantly improve the quality of life for individuals experiencing pain, enabling them to regain independence and functionality.

REFERENCES

Amaya-Rodriguez, C. A., Carvajal-Zamorano, K., Bustos, D., Alegría-Arcos, M., & Castillo, K. (2024). A journey from molecule to physiology and in silico tools for drug discovery targeting the transient receptor potential vanilloid type 1 (TRPV1) channel. *Frontiers in Pharmacology*, *14*, 1251061. DOI: 10.3389/fphar.2023.1251061 PMID: 38328578

Ananthakumar, B., Nanjundeshwara, N., Lakshmaiah, A., & Raghavan, R. (2024). Synthetic Gene Circuits as a Promising Approach in Cancer Immunotherapy. In *Critical Developments in Cancer Immunotherapy* (pp. 391–418). IGI Global., DOI: 10.4018/979-8-3693-3976-3.ch011

Anil Chandra, G., Ananthakumar, B., & Raghavan, R. (2024). *Enhancing Assistive Technologies with Neuromorphic Computing*. IGI Global., DOI: 10.4018/979-8-3693-6303-4.ch009

Anil Chandra, G., Biradar, S., & Raghavan, R. (2024). Neuroscience-Driven Solutions for Speech Impairment: Assistive Technologies for Speech Rehabilitation. In *Advancing Medical Research Through Neuroscience*. IGI Global.

Barakat, A., Munro, G., & Heegaard, A.-M. (2024). Finding new analgesics: Computational pharmacology faces drug discovery challenges. *Biochemical Pharmacology*, *222*, 116091. DOI: 10.1016/j.bcp.2024.116091 PMID: 38412924

Berberoglu, I., Burke, K. L., Cederna, P. S., & Kemp, S. W. P. (2024). Regenerative peripheral nerve interfaces (RPNIs): An overview of innovative surgical approaches. *Plastic and Aesthetic Research*, *11*(0). Advance online publication. DOI: 10.20517/2347-9264.2023.101

Biradar, S., Korrapati, C., Krishna, R. J., & Nanjundeshwara, N. (2025). Spatial Omics and Gene Circuits: The Future in Cancer Biology. *Spatially Variable Genes in Cancer: Development, Progression, and Treatment Response*, 383–408. DOI: 10.4018/979-8-3693-7728-4.ch014

Cashaback, J. G. A., Allen, J. L., Chou, A. H.-Y., Lin, D. J., Price, M. A., Secerovic, N. K., Song, S., Zhang, H., & Miller, H. L. (2024). NSF DARE—transforming modeling in neurorehabilitation: A patient-in-the-loop framework. *Journal of Neuroengineering and Rehabilitation*, *21*(1), 23. DOI: 10.1186/s12984-024-01318-9 PMID: 38347597

Chandra, G. A., Ananthakumar, B., & Raghavan, R. (2025). Enhancing Assistive Technologies With Neuromorphic Computing. In Revolutionizing AI with Brain-Inspired Technology: Neuromorphic Computing (pp. 207-232). IGI Global Scientific Publishing.

Chandra, G. V. S. A., Biradar, S., & Raghavan, R. (2025). Recent Trends in Soft Robotics for Assistive Technologies. *Assistive Technology Solutions for Aging Adults and Individuals With Disabilities*, 119–144. DOI: 10.4018/979-8-3693-6308-9.ch006

Correia, G., Crosse, M. J., & Valdes, A. L. (2024). Brain Wearables: Validation Toolkit for Ear-Level EEG Sensors. *Sensors (Basel)*, *24*(4), 1226. DOI: 10.3390/s24041226 PMID: 38400384

Donati, E., & Valle, G. (2024). Neuromorphic hardware for somatosensory neuroprostheses. *Nature Communications*, *15*(1), 556. DOI: 10.1038/s41467-024-44723-3 PMID: 38228580

Duan, X., Wang, P., He, L., He, Z., Wang, S., Yang, F., Gao, C., Ren, W., Lin, J., Chen, T., Xu, C., Li, J., & Wu, A. (2024). Peptide-Functionalized Inorganic Oxide Nanomaterials for Solid Cancer Imaging and Therapy. *Advanced Materials*, *2311548*(37), 2311548. Advance online publication. DOI: 10.1002/adma.202311548 PMID: 38333964

Gariya, N., Kumar, S., Shaikh, A., Prasad, B., & Nautiyal, H. (2024). A review on soft pneumatic actuators with integrated or embedded soft sensors. *Sensors and Actuators. A, Physical*, *372*, 115364. DOI: 10.1016/j.sna.2024.115364

Gasperina, S. D., Ferrari, F., Gandolla, M., Pedrocchi, A., & Ambrosini, E. (2024). Hybrid Cooperative Control of Functional Electrical Stimulation and Robot Assistance for Upper Extremity Rehabilitation. *IEEE Transactions on Biomedical Engineering*, *71*(99), 1–8. DOI: 10.1109/TBME.2024.3384939 PMID: 39167498

González-González, M. A., Conde, S. V., Latorre, R., Thébault, S. C., Pratelli, M., Spitzer, N. C., Verkhratsky, A., Tremblay, M.-È., Akcora, C. G., Hernández-Reynoso, A. G., Ecker, M., Coates, J., Vincent, K. L., & Ma, B. (2024). Bioelectronic Medicine: A multidisciplinary roadmap from biophysics to precision therapies. *Frontiers in Integrative Neuroscience*, *18*, 1321872. DOI: 10.3389/fnint.2024.1321872 PMID: 38440417

Guo, Y., Sun, L., Zhong, W., Zhang, N., Zhao, Z., & Tian, W. (2024). Artificial intelligence-assisted repair of peripheral nerve injury: A new research hotspot and associated challenges. *Neural Regeneration Research*, *19*(3), 663–670. DOI: 10.4103/1673-5374.380909 PMID: 37721299

GVS, A. C., Biradar, S., & Raghavan, R. (2025). Neuroscience-Driven Solutions for Speech Impairment: Assistive Technologies for Speech Rehabilitation. Advancing Medical Research Through Neuroscience, 119–146. https://doi.org/DOI: 10.4018/979-8-3693-5464-3.ch006

Hira, R. (2024). Closed-loop experiments and brain machine interfaces with multiphoton microscopy. *Neurophotonics, 11*(3), 033405. DOI: 10.1117/1.NPh.11.3.033405 PMID: 38375331

Idrissi, I. G. E., Podlewska, S., Abate, C., Bojarski, A. J., Lacivita, E., & Leopoldo, M. (2024). Structure-Activity Relationships and Therapeutic Potential of Purinergic P2X7 Receptor Antagonists. *Current Medicinal Chemistry*, *31*(11), 1361–1403. DOI: 10.2174/0929867330666230403094538 PMID: 37013427

Kang, M., Seo, S., Lee, H., & Han, M.-W. (2024). Knee Measurement System with Osteoarthritis Levels Using Artificial Cartilage and Skeletons. *Biomimetics*, *9*(3), 166. DOI: 10.3390/biomimetics9030166 PMID: 38534851

Korrapati, C., Yaraladdi, A. B., Vaddi, H., & Raghavan, R. (2024). Applications of the Saffron European Kitchen Spice Crocus sativus. In *Therapeutic and Pharmacological Applications of Ethnobotany* (pp. 98–127). IGI Global., DOI: 10.4018/979-8-3693-1986-4.ch005

Lakshmaiah, A., Korrapati, C., Suresh, C., & Raghavan, R. (2025). Synthetic Biology and AI. *Spatially Variable Genes in Cancer*, 265–290. DOI: 10.4018/979-8-3693-7728-4.ch010

Moreno-Sánchez, P. A., García-Isla, G., Corino, V. D. A., Vehkaoja, A., Brukamp, K., van Gils, M., & Mainardi, L. (2024). ECG-based data-driven solutions for diagnosis and prognosis of cardiovascular diseases: A systematic review. *Computers in Biology and Medicine*, *172*, 108235. DOI: 10.1016/j.compbiomed.2024.108235 PMID: 38460311

Nagashri, N., Archana, L., & Raghavan, R. (2024). Microbial Volatile Compounds (MVOCs) in Food Industries and Food Safety Applications. In *Innovations, Securities, and Case Studies Across Healthcare, Business, and Technology* (pp. 75–96). IGI Global. DOI: 10.4018/979-8-3693-1906-2.ch005

Nam, Y., Kim, J., Jung, S.-H., Woerner, J., Suh, E. H., Lee, D., Shivakumar, M., Lee, M. E., & Kim, D. (2024). Harnessing Artificial Intelligence in Multimodal Omics Data Integration: Paving the Path for the Next Frontier in Precision Medicine. *Annual Review of Biomedical Data Science, 7*(Volume 7, 2024), 225–250. DOI: 10.1146/annurev-biodatasci-102523-103801

Paiste, H. J., Godwin, R. C., Smith, A. D., Berkowitz, D. E., & Melvin, R. L. (2024). Strengths-weaknesses-opportunities-threats analysis of artificial intelligence in anesthesiology and perioperative medicine. *Frontiers in Digital Health*, *6*, 1316931. DOI: 10.3389/fdgth.2024.1316931 PMID: 38444721

Pirasteh, A., Ghiyasvand, M. S., & Pouladian, M. (2024). EEG-based brain-computer interface methods with the aim of rehabilitating advanced stage ALS patients. *Disability and Rehabilitation: Assistive Technology, ahead-of-print*(ahead-of-print), 1–11. DOI: 10.1080/17483107.2024.2316312

Rajeswari, S. V. K. R., & Vijayakumar, P. (2024). Development of sensor system and data analytic framework for non-invasive blood glucose prediction. *Scientific Reports*, *14*(1), 9206. DOI: 10.1038/s41598-024-59744-7 PMID: 38649731

Rusta, M. M., Haghpanah, S. A., & Taghvaei, S. (2024). Musculoskeletal Modeling and Control of the Human Upper Limb during Manual Wheelchair Propulsion: Application in Functional Electrical Stimulation Rehabilitation Therapy. *Journal of Applied and Computational Mechanics*, *10*(1), 92–110. DOI: 10.22055/jacm.2023.44469.4217

Sánchez-Gil, J. J., Sáez-Manzano, A., López-Luque, R., Ochoa-Sepúlveda, J.-J., & Cañete-Carmona, E. (2025). Gamified devices for stroke rehabilitation: A systematic review. *Computer Methods and Programs in Biomedicine*, *258*, 108476. DOI: 10.1016/j.cmpb.2024.108476 PMID: 39520875

Sanders, Q., & Reinkensmeyer, D. J. (2024). Design and Preliminary Evaluation of a Soft Finger Exoskeleton Controlled by Isometric Grip Force. *Machines (Basel)*, *12*(4), 230. DOI: 10.3390/machines12040230

Saxer, F., Hollinger, A., Bjurström, M. F., Conaghan, P. G., Neogi, T., Schieker, M., & Berenbaum, F. (2024). Pain-phenotyping in osteoarthritis: Current concepts, evidence, and considerations towards a comprehensive framework for assessment and treatment. *Osteoarthritis and Cartilage Open*, *6*(1), 100433. DOI: 10.1016/j.ocarto.2023.100433 PMID: 38225987

Schreiber, D., Yu, Z., Henderson, T., Chen, D., Norbash, A., & Yip, M. C. (2024). CRANE: A Redundant, Multi-Degree-of-Freedom Computed Tomography Robot for Heightened Needle Dexterity within a Medical Imaging Bore. *IEEE Transactions on Robotics*, (99), 1–20. DOI: 10.1109/TRO.2024.3364986

Shan, L., Chen, Q., Yu, R., Gao, C., Liu, L., Guo, T., & Chen, H. (2023). A sensory memory processing system with multi-wavelength synaptic-polychromatic light emission for multi-modal information recognition. *Nature Communications*, *14*(1), 2648. DOI: 10.1038/s41467-023-38396-7 PMID: 37156788

Shrestha, A. B., Taha, A. M., Siddiq, A., Shrestha, S., Thakur, P., Chapagain, S., Sharma, S., Halder, A., Rajak, K., & Shah, V. (2024). Virtual and augmented reality in cardiovascular care in low and middle income country. *Current Problems in Cardiology*, *49*(3), 102380. DOI: 10.1016/j.cpcardiol.2024.102380 PMID: 38191103

Spies, N. C., Rangel, A., English, P., Morrison, M., O'Fallon, B., & Ng, D. P. (2025). Machine Learning Methods in Clinical Flow Cytometry. *Cancers (Basel)*, *17*(3), 3. Advance online publication. DOI: 10.3390/cancers17030483 PMID: 39941850

Sun, X., & Freeman, C. T. (2024). Parameterised function ILC with application to stroke rehabilitation. *Control Engineering Practice*, *145*, 105878. DOI: 10.1016/j.conengprac.2024.105878

Tian, Y., Vaskov, A. K., Adidharma, W., Cederna, P. S., & Kemp, S. W. P. (2024). Merging Humans and Neuroprosthetics through Regenerative Peripheral Nerve Interfaces. *Seminars in Plastic Surgery*, *38*(01), 010–018. DOI: 10.1055/s-0044-1779028

Valero-Cuevas, F. J., Finley, J., Orsborn, A., Fung, N., Hicks, J. L., Huang, H., Reinkensmeyer, D., Schweighofer, N., Weber, D., & Steele, K. M. (2024). NSF DARE—Transforming modeling in neurorehabilitation: Four threads for catalyzing progress. *Journal of Neuroengineering and Rehabilitation*, *21*(1), 46. DOI: 10.1186/s12984-024-01324-x PMID: 38570842

Villalba-Meneses, F., Guevara, C., Lojan, A. B., Gualsaqui, M. G., Arias-Serrano, I., Velásquez-López, P. A., Almeida-Galárraga, D., Tirado-Espín, A., Marín, J., & Marín, J. J. (2024). Classification of the Pathological Range of Motion in Low Back Pain Using Wearable Sensors and Machine Learning. *Sensors (Basel)*, *24*(3), 831. DOI: 10.3390/s24030831 PMID: 38339548

Wan, M., Simonin, E. M., Johnson, M. M., Zhang, X., Lin, X., Gao, P., Patel, C. J., Yousuf, A., Snyder, M. P., Hong, X., Wang, X., Sampath, V., & Nadeau, K. C. (2025). Exposomics: A review of methodologies, applications, and future directions in molecular medicine. *EMBO Molecular Medicine*, *17*(4), 1–10. DOI: 10.1038/s44321-025-00191-w PMID: 39870881

Waydhas, C., Ull, C., Cruciger, O., Hamsen, U., Schildhauer, T. A., Gaschler, R., & Weckwerth, C. (2024). Behavioral pain scale may not be reliable in awake non-verbal intensive care patients: A case control study. *BMC Anesthesiology*, *24*(1), 84. DOI: 10.1186/s12871-024-02472-2 PMID: 38424502

Yılmaz, H., & Özdem, M. (2024). EyeMo: A Solution for Individuals with Disabilities to Use a Computer Through Eye Movements. *Gazi University Journal of Science Part C: Design and Technology*, *12*(1), 1–1. DOI: 10.29109/gujsc.1404305

Chapter 12
Predictive Algorithms in Assistive Technologies Enhancing Daily Living for Individuals With Disabilities:
AI and Machine Learning Revolutionizing Accessibility

Vishal Kumar Sharma
https://orcid.org/0000-0001-6876-4814
Woxsen University, India

Maatrika Pammidimukkala
Woxsen University, India

ABSTRACT

This chapter examines the transformative role of predictive algorithms in assistive technologies, showcasing their ability to enhance accessibility and independence for individuals with disabilities. Leveraging advancements in artificial intelligence and machine learning, these algorithms enable devices to adapt to users' unique needs, improving mobility, communication, health monitoring, and home automation. Applications such as smart wheelchairs with terrain adaptation, context-aware communication tools, wearable health monitors with proactive alerts, and personalized smart home systems are explored. The chapter addresses current gaps, including limited contextual understanding and real-time learning, while discussing ethical concerns like data privacy and security. Future directions emphasize intercon-

DOI: 10.4018/979-8-3373-0194-5.ch012

nected ecosystems that integrate multiple devices for holistic support. This chapter underscores how predictive algorithms drive innovation, fostering inclusivity and improving the quality of life for users.

INTRODUCTION

Predictive algorithms are reshaping the landscape of assistive technologies in profound ways. The impact of these algorithms in modern technology cannot be overstated, particularly in the realm of devices and systems designed to support individuals with disabilities. By leveraging advancements in artificial intelligence (AI) and machine learning (ML), predictive algorithms enable assistive devices to anticipate, learn from, and adapt to the unique needs of their users. These capabilities are transforming the way individuals with disabilities interact with their environment, allowing them to achieve greater independence, efficiency, and overall quality of life.

The core function of predictive algorithms is to process large volumes of data, identify patterns, and forecast future events based on this information. In the context of assistive technologies, this involves monitoring the behaviors, preferences, and physiological conditions of the user, as well as the surrounding environment. By learning from these patterns, predictive algorithms can offer more responsive, personalized, and adaptive solutions. For example, a smart wheelchair equipped with predictive algorithms may learn the user's typical routes and habits, adjusting its navigation system in real-time to avoid obstacles or optimize travel efficiency. Similarly, wearable health monitors can predict the onset of medical conditions, providing early warnings that enable users to take preventive actions before a health crisis occurs.

Assistive technologies have always aimed to bridge the gap between individuals with disabilities and their environment, enabling them to lead more independent and fulfilling lives. In the past, assistive devices were often simple and reactive, providing basic support for tasks such as mobility, communication, or daily activities. These devices, such as manual wheelchairs, hearing aids, or text-to-speech converters, played a crucial role in enhancing the lives of individuals with disabilities. However, they often lacked the sophistication to adapt to individual users and their ever-changing needs.

This limitation is precisely where predictive algorithms have made a revolutionary impact. By incorporating AI and ML techniques, assistive devices are no longer static but can learn and evolve with the user over time. This adaptability is a game-changer, especially for individuals with disabilities that may experience progressive changes in their condition. For instance, people living with multiple sclerosis or Parkinson’s disease face gradual shifts in their mobility, motor skills, or cognitive functions. In such cases, predictive algorithms can continuously monitor these changes and adjust the device's settings to ensure that it remains useful and effective.

One of the key benefits of predictive algorithms in assistive technologies is their ability to personalize and anticipate the needs of the user. A device that can predict and respond to the user's preferences and behaviors is much more effective than one that requires manual input or constant reconfiguration. Take, for example, a smart wheelchair. In the past, a person using a manual or powered wheelchair would need to provide input for adjustments, such as changing the speed, direction, or tilt. With predictive algorithms, however, the wheelchair can learn from the user's habits and make these adjustments automatically. If the system detects that the user typically encounters specific obstacles or challenges on their usual routes, it can adapt by preemptively modifying its behavior to navigate more smoothly. This reduces the cognitive load on the user and allows them to focus on more important tasks.

Similarly, speech recognition tools that utilize predictive algorithms can improve communication for individuals with speech impairments. These systems can adapt to subtle changes in speech patterns, which is particularly beneficial for users with progressive conditions such as amyotrophic lateral sclerosis (ALS). As ALS advances, individuals often experience changes in their ability to speak clearly. Voice recognition systems powered by predictive algorithms can monitor these changes and adjust their sensitivity and vocabulary accordingly. This ensures that communication remains fluid and efficient, even as the user's speech deteriorates. Moreover, predictive algorithms can recognize the user's preferred phrases, anticipate what they are trying to say, and offer real-time suggestions, further enhancing the ease of communication.

The concept of continuous learning is another critical aspect of predictive algorithms in assistive technologies. These systems are not fixed but rather evolve based on ongoing user interactions. Each time the user interacts with the device, the system gathers valuable data that allows it to refine its predictions and improve its performance. This dynamic learning process is invaluable for individuals with disabilities, as it enables the system to adjust to changing needs in real-time. For example, a smart home system equipped with predictive algorithms can adjust lighting, temperature, or other environmental factors based on the user's behavior. If the system recognizes that the user typically likes the living room to be dimly lit in the evenings, it can automatically adjust the lighting at a set time, enhancing convenience and comfort without requiring any manual intervention.

Another area where predictive algorithms have significant potential is in healthcare and medical monitoring. Wearable health devices that track vital signs such as heart rate, blood pressure, or glucose levels can now integrate predictive analytics to anticipate potential health issues. For individuals with chronic conditions such as diabetes or cardiovascular disease, these devices can provide early warnings about impending medical crises, such as a heart attack or hypoglycemic event. By analyzing historical health data, these systems can predict when an individual might be at risk and alert them to take preventive action, such as administering medication or seeking medical help. This proactive approach to healthcare can save lives and help individuals manage their conditions more effectively.

The role of predictive algorithms in assistive technologies also extends to social inclusion and independence. Traditional assistive devices often focused on physical or medical support, but predictive algorithms are helping to expand this definition to include social and psychological support. Social isolation is a significant issue for many individuals with disabilities, particularly those with limited mobility or communication challenges. Predictive algorithms integrated into smart home devices, virtual assistants, or social platforms can provide users with new opportunities for engagement, entertainment, and connection. These systems can suggest activities based on the user's preferences, remind them of important social events, or even facilitate virtual interactions with friends and family. By reducing barriers to socialization, predictive algorithms can foster a sense of community and well-being.

Despite the numerous advantages, the integration of predictive algorithms in assistive technologies also raises important ethical considerations. Data privacy, security, and the potential for bias in algorithmic predictions are concerns that must be addressed as these technologies become more widespread. For example, predictive systems rely on large datasets, which may include sensitive personal information such as medical history, mobility patterns, or speech recordings. It is crucial to ensure that this data is protected from misuse and that individuals maintain control over how their information is used. Furthermore, predictive algorithms must be designed with fairness in mind, avoiding biases that could lead to inaccurate predictions or unequal treatment of users.

In addition to ethical concerns, user-centric design is essential in the development of assistive technologies. These systems must be intuitive and easy to use, especially for individuals who may not be familiar with complex technologies. A key challenge is ensuring that the technology aligns with the user's capabilities and preferences. This requires extensive user testing, feedback loops, and an understanding of the specific needs of individuals with various disabilities. By adopting a user-centered approach, developers can ensure that predictive algorithms enhance, rather than hinder, the independence and quality of life of their users.

This chapter aims to provide a comprehensive exploration of the transformative role that predictive algorithms play in assistive technologies. It will delve into current applications, highlight areas for potential improvement, and discuss how these technologies are shaping the future of accessibility and inclusivity. With the ongoing advancement of AI and ML, the potential for predictive algorithms to revolutionize the lives of individuals with disabilities is vast. By fostering an environment of continuous learning, adaptation, and personalization, these technologies promise to create a more inclusive world, where everyone can achieve their full potential.

APPLICATIONS AND IMPROVEMENTS

Mobility Solutions: Enhancing Navigation and Safety

Mobility solutions, particularly smart wheelchairs, have benefited immensely from predictive algorithms. Traditionally, wheelchairs were limited to basic functions such as moving forward, backward, and turning. However, advances in sensor technology and AI have allowed these devices to incorporate real-time data analysis, offering enhanced navigation and safety features. At present, many smart wheelchairs use infrared sensors, ultrasonic sensors, and cameras to detect obstacles in the environment, helping the user avoid hazards and navigate smoothly. These systems have made it easier for individuals with mobility impairments to move through indoor and outdoor environments.

Nevertheless, these early systems often fall short when dealing with more dynamic or challenging situations. For example, uneven terrain, sudden changes in the environment, or complex indoor layouts may confuse existing navigation systems. By integrating predictive algorithms powered by deep learning models, smart wheelchairs can process real-time terrain data to adjust the wheelchair's movement autonomously, improving both safety and efficiency. Deep learning models could analyze data from sensors, such as LIDAR (Light Detection and Ranging) sensors, to create a 3D map of the user's environment and dynamically plan the safest and most efficient path. This means that even in unfamiliar or crowded areas, the wheelchair could anticipate obstacles and adjust its course accordingly.

For example, a wheelchair equipped with predictive algorithms could foresee an obstacle, such as a pothole or curb, before the user encounters it and adjust its trajectory in advance. Similarly, predictive systems could analyze user behavior patterns, adjusting speed and route based on factors like the user's current physical state, health conditions, or preferences. Additionally, these systems could integrate with GPS navigation, enabling users to travel more independently in unfamiliar locations. If the system detects that the user typically avoids certain areas, it could automatically reroute to ensure comfort and safety. This shift toward predictive, data-driven mobility systems has the potential to drastically improve the independence of individuals with disabilities, allowing them to navigate their environment with greater ease and confidence.

Communication Systems: Contextual Understanding and Empathy

Communication remains one of the most critical areas where predictive algorithms have the potential to revolutionize assistive technologies. For individuals with speech impairments, Augmentative and Alternative Communication (AAC) devices have long been a lifeline, enabling them to express thoughts and communicate effectively. Early AAC devices utilized simple text-to-speech systems with basic predictive text features. These systems suggested frequently used words or phrases to facilitate communication. While effective to some extent, these devices lacked the nuance and adaptability needed for more complex and dynamic interactions.

The future of AAC devices lies in the integration of advanced AI models capable of understanding complex contexts and providing highly personalized communication suggestions. Predictive algorithms could enhance these devices by not only considering previously used phrases but also understanding the user's emotional state, current environment, and situational context. For example, an AAC device could analyze the tone of voice, facial expressions, or even body language to detect frustration or stress and adjust its responses accordingly. In such a situation, the system could simplify its suggestions or offer more direct communication options, easing the process for the user during challenging moments. This ability to adapt based on contextual cues represents a leap forward in user-centric communication support.

Moreover, predictive algorithms could enable AAC devices to learn the user's preferences and typical communication patterns. By tracking user interactions, these devices could predict future needs and offer suggestions proactively. For instance, if a user frequently asks for certain information, such as requesting assistance or expressing feelings of anxiety in particular settings, the device could learn to prioritize those types of interactions, anticipating the user's needs before they are even vocalized. This personalization would streamline communication, allowing users to express themselves more fluidly and with less effort. Additionally, predictive models could enable multilingual support, automatically switching between languages based on the user's location or previous interactions. This would expand the utility of AAC devices for people from diverse linguistic backgrounds, allowing them to communicate more effectively in various cultural and social contexts.

Health Monitoring Technologies: Proactive Health Management

Wearable health devices, such as fitness trackers and smartwatches, are another domain where predictive algorithms are making significant strides. While current health monitoring devices can track basic vital signs, such as heart rate, blood pressure, and physical activity levels, their predictive capabilities are still in the early stages. Many devices currently rely on simple rule-based systems to detect irregularities, such as a spike in heart rate or a fall, and notify the user or caregivers. While these notifications are valuable, they often do not provide enough advanced warning for users to take proactive measures, such as adjusting medications or seeking medical assistance.

The next generation of wearable health devices will likely incorporate more sophisticated predictive algorithms, enabling them to anticipate potential health crises before they occur. Machine learning models could continuously monitor the user's health data—such as heart rate variability, respiratory patterns, sleep quality, and even environmental factors—and detect early warning signs of medical conditions, such as cardiac arrhythmias or respiratory failure. For instance, wearable devices could analyze patterns in heart rate variability and detect the onset of atrial fibrillation, alerting the user to seek medical attention before the condition becomes acute. Similarly, devices could use environmental sensors to monitor air quality and predict asthma attacks, helping users avoid triggers and take preventive action.

Additionally, long-term data collection and analysis could help wearables provide personalized health recommendations, allowing users to make more informed decisions about their lifestyle. By tracking sleep patterns over time, for example, a device could suggest changes in routine to improve sleep quality. Moreover, predictive algorithms could analyze patterns in medication adherence and offer reminders or alerts when it's time to take prescribed medications, improving medication management and health outcomes.

In the future, the integration of predictive algorithms in health monitoring devices could not only prevent medical emergencies but also offer proactive, personalized healthcare solutions that help users manage chronic conditions and maintain better overall well-being.

Smart Home Automation: Personalized Environments for Users with Disabilities

Smart home systems have become increasingly popular in recent years, offering automation of tasks such as lighting, heating, and home appliance control. For individuals with disabilities, these systems provide enhanced convenience and accessibility, allowing them to control their environment with minimal physical effort. While voice-controlled devices like Amazon Alexa and Google Assistant have been instrumental in making home automation accessible, these systems are still largely reactive. Users must issue specific commands, and the system follows pre-programmed routines based on those inputs.

Predictive algorithms have the potential to take smart home systems to the next level by providing more personalized and adaptive control. These systems could learn the user's daily routines and preferences, allowing them to automatically adjust the environment without the need for direct input. For instance, a smart home system could recognize when the user typically wakes up, preheating the oven for breakfast or adjusting the lighting to suit the time of day. Similarly, predictive algorithms could monitor environmental factors such as temperature, humidity, and air quality, adjusting settings to ensure the user's comfort. For individuals with health conditions, such as arthritis or respiratory issues, a smart home system could optimize temperature and humidity levels to reduce discomfort or flare-ups.

Moreover, integration with wearable health devices could enhance the system's ability to respond to the user's health needs. If a wearable device detects signs of stress or anxiety in the user, the smart home system could adjust the environment to create a calming atmosphere—perhaps dimming the lights, playing soothing music, or changing the room temperature. Predictive algorithms could also enable more efficient energy usage, automatically adjusting heating, cooling, and lighting based on occupancy patterns and weather forecasts. This would not only enhance the user experience but also contribute to a more sustainable and cost-effective home environment.

COMPARISON AND INSIGHTS

Independence and Accessibility

The integration of predictive algorithms into assistive technologies has fundamentally altered the landscape of accessibility for individuals with disabilities. By harnessing the power of machine learning (ML) and artificial intelligence (AI), these systems allow users to interact with their environments in ways that were once unimaginable. Predictive algorithms in assistive devices not only address physical and cognitive challenges but also provide a sense of autonomy and dignity that many individuals with disabilities have long desired. The ability to perform everyday tasks independently is a significant factor in enhancing an individual's quality of life, and predictive technologies make this possible by learning from patterns, anticipating needs, and adapting to personal preferences.

One prominent area where predictive algorithms have made a notable impact is in mobility. Traditional wheelchairs, while useful, require constant human intervention and adjustment. However, the advent of smart wheelchairs equipped with predictive algorithms takes mobility to the next level. These wheelchairs are now able to analyze their environment in real time, using sensors like LIDAR, ultrasonic, or infrared sensors, to detect obstacles such as curbs, furniture, or pedestrians. They can dynamically change their path, avoiding collisions or even navigating across uneven terrains with ease. Such capabilities greatly enhance independence for users by reducing the need for external guidance or assistance.

Imagine a scenario where a person using a smart wheelchair needs to traverse a crowded public space, such as a shopping mall. Predictive algorithms allow the wheelchair to anticipate the user's movements and adjust accordingly, navigating through tight spaces or detouring around clusters of people. In addition, terrain-adaptive algorithms adjust the speed and movement based on surface conditions—whether navigating a smooth, paved surface or a bumpy, uneven sidewalk. This kind of navigation capability provides a seamless travel experience, ensuring the user's safety, comfort, and ease of movement, even in challenging environments. Furthermore, with machine learning integration, the wheelchair can continually learn and improve based on the user's patterns and preferences, adapting to specific routes, inclines, and speeds over time.

In the home environment, predictive algorithms embedded in smart home systems also offer substantial improvements in independence and accessibility. A typical smart home system already allows users to control devices like lights, thermostats, and appliances remotely via apps or voice commands. However, by incorporating predictive algorithms, these systems become far more intuitive and self-sufficient. Rather than requiring the user to manually adjust settings, the system can anticipate their needs based on learned behavior, automatically adjusting environmental conditions without any input.

For example, a smart home system could learn the user's typical daily routine, such as when they wake up, go to bed, or leave for work. The system would adjust the lighting and heating or cooling systems to match these routines. It could also automate the opening and closing of curtains depending on the time of day, keeping the room at the desired temperature and lighting levels without requiring the user to lift a finger. Furthermore, advanced systems could detect changes in environmental conditions—such as a sudden drop in temperature or an increase in air pollution—and adjust settings accordingly. Such predictive capabilities not only make the home environment more comfortable but also help users maintain their well-being by reducing the reliance on caregivers or other external sources of assistance.

Communication, another critical area of assistive technology, also benefits from the integration of predictive algorithms. Augmentative and Alternative Communication (AAC) devices, which enable individuals with speech impairments to communicate, have evolved significantly due to predictive technology. Early AAC devices provided limited vocabulary choices or relied on rudimentary text-to-speech algorithms.

Today's AAC devices, however, utilize machine learning models to offer context-aware phrase suggestions, dramatically improving communication effectiveness.

For instance, predictive algorithms in AAC devices can take into account a wide range of contextual factors, such as the user's previous interactions, current location, and even environmental cues. If a user is in a healthcare setting, the device might prioritize medical terminology or phrases related to the user's health needs. If the user is in a familiar social setting, the system might suggest phrases related to common greetings or casual conversation. Additionally, by analyzing the user's emotional state, the system can make more empathetic and relevant suggestions. If the user is visibly frustrated or anxious, the system might offer comforting or reassuring phrases, offering emotional support in a way that simple predictive text algorithms cannot.

These improvements in communication devices can make a profound difference for individuals with speech impairments, as the ability to express oneself clearly and effectively can foster deeper connections with others. Furthermore, as predictive algorithms improve, AAC devices will continue to adapt to the user's evolving needs, offering more tailored communication solutions.

Gaps and Possibilities

Despite the advancements in predictive algorithms for assistive technologies, significant gaps remain, and addressing these challenges will be key to creating more effective and user-centric devices. One of the primary limitations of current assistive technologies is their ability to truly understand and adapt to complex, real-time contexts. While many systems are capable of automating basic tasks based on preset routines, they often lack the flexibility to respond to sudden changes in user behavior or environmental factors. For example, a smart home system may adjust the temperature based on historical patterns but fail to account for unexpected weather changes, such as a sudden cold front. Similarly, AAC devices may struggle to provide accurate or relevant suggestions in novel or unanticipated scenarios.

To address these limitations, future assistive technologies must incorporate more advanced forms of contextual AI. Contextual AI refers to systems that are able to interpret and respond to complex data based on the situation at hand. For example, a smart home system might need to consider not only the user's historical preferences but also external factors like the weather, the time of day, and even the user's emotional or physical state. Similarly, predictive algorithms in communication devices need to go beyond simple word prediction and understand the context of the conversation, as well as the user's current emotional or social needs.

Real-time learning is another crucial area where advancements are needed. While current predictive algorithms can make informed guesses based on historical data, they often fail to update or adapt quickly enough in response to real-time changes. Incorporating systems that can continuously learn from user feedback, interactions, and environmental factors will enable assistive technologies to become more adaptive and personalized. Such systems would be able to adjust in real-time to provide increasingly accurate and relevant recommendations, making assistive devices more responsive to the user's immediate needs.

For example, imagine an AAC device that is able to track and analyze not only the words the user is typing or selecting but also their facial expressions, eye movements, and even their voice tone. By taking all of these factors into account, the system could more accurately predict the user's intent, providing not just words but also emotional context that enhances communication. Such an integrated, adaptive approach would offer a richer, more personalized experience for users, allowing them to communicate with greater ease and confidence.

Furthermore, there is an increasing need for predictive algorithms to address ethical considerations related to data privacy and security. As assistive technologies become more sophisticated and rely on continuous data collection—whether through sensors, wearable devices, or voice recognition systems—concerns about how personal information is handled, stored, and shared become more pressing. Users must be assured that their data is used ethically, securely, and with their consent. Striking the right balance between personalization and privacy will be essential for fostering trust and encouraging widespread adoption of these technologies.

Future Possibilities

Looking ahead, the development of fully integrated ecosystems represents one of the most exciting possibilities for assistive technologies. Currently, many assistive devices function in isolation, each addressing a specific need. However, the potential for creating interconnected systems that communicate seamlessly with one another is vast. Such ecosystems would enable assistive technologies to work together to create a holistic support system that addresses all aspects of an individual's health, mobility, and communication.

For example, imagine a health monitor detecting signs of fatigue or stress in a user. This information could be relayed to a smart home system, which could adjust the lighting, temperature, and noise levels in the home to create a more calming environment. At the same time, the health monitor might alert the user's caregiver or family members, ensuring that support is available when needed. Additionally, wearable devices could monitor the user's physical activity, offering real-time suggestions for rest or exercise, while predictive algorithms continue to adapt based on the user's preferences, needs, and health conditions.

Such integrated systems would not only enhance physical well-being but also offer emotional and psychological support. For example, if a user is experiencing emotional distress, a predictive algorithm could adjust environmental factors such as lighting and sound, while also suggesting calming activities or connecting the user with mental health resources. These interconnected ecosystems could provide a level of care and support that is more comprehensive, responsive, and personalized than current standalone devices.

As these systems become more advanced, they could even begin to predict and prevent health issues before they occur. By continuously analyzing data from various sources—such as health monitors, smart home systems, and environmental sensors—assistive technologies could detect early warning signs of health crises and provide proactive recommendations to reduce risks. For instance, a system could predict a potential fall based on changes in gait patterns and suggest modifications to the home environment to reduce the likelihood of injury.

In conclusion, predictive algorithms in assistive technologies hold the potential to revolutionize accessibility and independence for individuals with disabilities. By continuously learning and adapting to the unique needs and preferences of users, these technologies offer the possibility of creating fully integrated, personalized support systems that improve the quality of life for individuals across various domains. As these systems evolve, addressing key challenges such as contextual AI, real-time learning, and data privacy will be crucial to unlocking their full potential. The future of assistive technologies lies in creating truly intelligent, adaptive ecosystems that provide holistic support, enhancing the physical, emotional, and psychological well-being of users.

DEEP DIVE INTO SPECIFIC USE CASES

Advanced Wheelchair Navigation

Expanding on basic applications, predictive algorithms in smart wheelchairs have the potential to revolutionize navigation. Current systems primarily rely on sensors and pre-programmed rules for obstacle detection and pathfinding. However, future advancements could incorporate deep reinforcement learning models, allowing wheelchairs to simulate and test multiple navigation scenarios in virtual environments before deploying them in real-time. This approach reduces error rates and enhances safety in complex environments, such as crowded urban areas or uneven terrains.

For instance, a wheelchair equipped with LIDAR and advanced AI could create a detailed map of its surroundings, identify potential hazards, and calculate the safest route in real-time. The system could also adapt to user preferences, such as avoiding crowded areas or selecting smoother paths for comfort. By integrating predictive algorithms with GPS navigation and real-time environmental analysis, these wheelchairs could offer unparalleled autonomy and reliability.

Additionally, the integration of smart technologies such as vehicle-to-everything (V2X) communication could further enhance advanced wheelchair navigation. With V2X, wheelchairs could communicate with nearby infrastructure, such as traffic signals, smart streetlights, and other vehicles, to receive real-time updates about road conditions, traffic patterns, or upcoming obstacles. This connectivity would allow the wheelchair to navigate urban environments more safely and efficiently, avoiding potential hazards like sudden changes in traffic or construction zones. Furthermore, real-time collaboration between the wheelchair's predictive systems and urban infrastructure could lead to smarter city designs that accommodate the needs of individuals with mobility challenges. The fusion of these technologies would create a truly adaptive mobility experience, one that can not only learn from the user's habits but also anticipate and react to the complexities of real-world environments, fostering greater independence and confidence in users.

Communication Context Awareness

Context-aware systems represent a significant leap forward in communication technologies for individuals with speech impairments. Current AAC devices rely on basic predictive text algorithms, which often fail to capture the complexity of human communication. By integrating biometric inputs such as eye movement tracking, gestures, and even brain-computer interfaces, these systems could provide multi-modal communication platforms that adapt to the user's immediate needs.

For example, an AAC device could analyze a combination of biometric and contextual data to predict the user's intended message. If the user is in a noisy environment, the system might prioritize short, clear phrases that are easier to convey. Additionally, emotion detection through facial recognition or voice tone analysis could enable the device to respond empathetically, offering suggestions that align with the user's emotional state. Such advancements would not only improve the effectiveness of communication but also foster a deeper sense of connection and understanding.

Furthermore, the integration of machine learning into context-aware AAC systems could enhance the personalization and adaptability of communication. As these systems learn from the user's unique interaction patterns, they could anticipate preferences, slang, or common phrases, creating a more intuitive and seamless communication experience. For instance, over time, the system could recognize and suggest specific phrases or terms that the user commonly uses in particular contexts, like in medical settings or during social interactions. This adaptability would reduce the cognitive load on the user, enabling more fluid and natural communication. Moreover, these systems could be designed to collaborate with other assistive technologies, such as environmental controls or personal assistants, to provide a fully integrated support system. This level of personalization and interconnectivity would not only enhance speech communication but also empower users to interact with their surroundings in a more meaningful and efficient way, contributing to their overall autonomy and sense of agency.

Health Alerts

Wearable health monitors have already transformed personal healthcare by providing real-time tracking of vital signs and activity levels. However, the next generation of these devices could leverage predictive algorithms to offer dynamic and proactive health alerts. For example, instead of simply notifying the user of irregularities, these systems could analyze long-term behavioral shifts and predict potential health issues weeks or months in advance.

Consider a health monitor designed for elderly users. By continuously analyzing data such as heart rate variability, gait patterns, and sleep quality, the system could detect early signs of conditions like Parkinson's disease or cardiovascular issues. When combined with environmental data, such as temperature and air quality, the device could provide personalized recommendations to mitigate risks. For instance, it might suggest staying indoors on days with poor air quality to prevent respiratory complications. This level of foresight empowers users to take preventive actions, improving overall health outcomes and reducing the burden on healthcare systems.

Another potential application is in mental health monitoring. Predictive algorithms could analyze speech patterns, social interactions, and biometric data to identify early signs of depression or anxiety. By providing timely alerts and resources, these systems could play a crucial role in mental health management, particularly for individuals who may struggle to recognize or articulate their symptoms.

Interconnected Ecosystems

The ultimate vision for assistive technologies powered by predictive algorithms lies in the creation of interconnected ecosystems. These ecosystems would enable seamless communication and collaboration between various devices and systems, providing holistic support to users. For example, a smart home system integrated with wearable health monitors and mobility aids could create a cohesive network that anticipates and addresses user needs in real-time.

Imagine a scenario where a health monitor detects elevated stress levels in the user. This information could be relayed to the smart home system, which might respond by dimming the lights, playing calming music, and adjusting the room temperature to create a soothing environment. Simultaneously, the system could notify the user's caregiver or healthcare provider, ensuring timely support if needed. By combining the capabilities of multiple devices, such ecosystems could enhance user independence, safety, and well-being.

In addition to physical and emotional support, interconnected ecosystems could also enhance social connectivity and mental well-being. For instance, if a user's wearable health monitor detects signs of fatigue or depression, the system could automatically suggest engaging in a video call with a friend or family member, facilitating social interaction and reducing isolation. Moreover, the system could analyze patterns of social engagement and suggest activities that promote mental health, such as participating in virtual support groups or joining online wellness sessions. These intelligent systems would not only provide personalized care but also offer opportunities for users to stay connected with their social networks, ensuring a sense of belonging and improving overall quality of life. By seamlessly integrating various aspects of daily life—from health monitoring and home automation to social engagement—interconnected ecosystems can transform the way individuals interact with their environments, offering holistic and proactive support that goes beyond traditional caregiving models.

CONCLUSION

Predictive algorithms are at the forefront of technological advancements in assistive technologies, playing a pivotal role in empowering individuals with disabilities to lead more independent, fulfilling, and productive lives. These algorithms, underpinned by innovations in artificial intelligence and machine learning, have opened new horizons in mobility, communication, health monitoring, and home automation. As demonstrated through examples such as smart wheelchairs, speech recognition tools, wearable health monitors, and smart home systems, the transformative potential of predictive algorithms is both profound and far-reaching.

Smart wheelchairs equipped with predictive algorithms have redefined mobility for individuals with physical disabilities. These systems provide capabilities far beyond simple navigation, incorporating real-time terrain adaptation, obstacle avoidance, and dynamic route optimization. For instance, by integrating advanced AI models and LIDAR sensors, modern wheelchairs can map out complex environments, ensuring safe and smooth travel even in challenging conditions. This ability to navigate autonomously not only reduces the dependency on caregivers but also instills a sense of confidence and independence in users. However, as highlighted in this chapter, there is still significant potential for improvement. The incorporation of reinforcement learning models and seamless GPS integration could further enhance navigation accuracy and adaptability, enabling users to traverse unfamiliar terrains effortlessly. Such advancements could truly revolutionize mobility solutions, making them more accessible and user-centric.

In the realm of communication, predictive algorithms have transformed the functionality of Augmentative and Alternative Communication (AAC) devices. These tools serve as lifelines for individuals with speech impairments, enabling them to express themselves effectively. While current systems rely heavily on basic predictive text and phrase suggestions, future advancements promise to bring about context-aware and emotion-sensitive communication. Imagine an AAC device capable of analyzing a user's environment, emotional state, and previous interactions to provide suggestions that are not only relevant but also empathetic. Such systems could integrate multi-modal inputs like gestures, eye movement, and voice analysis to create a more natural and intuitive communication experience. By addressing the current limitations in contextual understanding, predictive algorithms could bridge significant gaps in communication, fostering stronger connections and better social integration for users.

Wearable health monitors are another domain where predictive algorithms have had a transformative impact. These devices, ranging from fitness trackers to advanced medical wearables, offer real-time monitoring of vital signs and activity levels. Current systems provide alerts for irregularities such as sudden heart rate spikes or potential falls, enabling timely interventions. However, the potential for these devices goes far beyond reactive measures. With the integration of advanced machine learning models, wearable health monitors could predict health crises before they occur, offering users and healthcare providers the ability to take preventive actions. For example, a device capable of analyzing long-term behavioral patterns and environmental data could predict conditions such as asthma attacks, cardiac events, or even mental health crises. Such predictive capabilities not only enhance the quality of life for users but also reduce the burden on healthcare systems by shifting the focus from treatment to prevention.

Smart home systems represent another significant application of predictive algorithms in assistive technologies. These systems have transformed the way individuals with disabilities interact with their living environments, offering automation and customization like never before. Current systems primarily rely on voice-controlled devices and pre-set routines to manage tasks such as adjusting lighting, controlling appliances, and maintaining home security. However, predictive algorithms have the potential to take these systems to the next level. Future smart home systems could learn from user behaviors and preferences, creating personalized routines that adapt in real-time. For instance, a system that detects signs of stress through a connected wearable device could automatically adjust the lighting, temperature, and music to create a calming environment. Furthermore, the integration of predictive energy management could optimize energy usage based on user habits and external factors like weather conditions, making homes not only more accessible but also more sustainable.

Despite these advancements, challenges and limitations persist. Many current systems lack the ability to fully understand and adapt to the diverse and dynamic needs of users. Contextual AI, which allows systems to interpret and respond to complex situational data, remains an area requiring significant research and development. Real-time learning, where systems continuously evolve based on user feedback and interactions, is another critical area for improvement. Moreover, the ethical considerations surrounding data collection and usage cannot be overlooked. Ensuring privacy, security, and transparency is essential for building trust and promoting widespread adoption of these technologies.

The future of assistive technologies lies in the creation of interconnected ecosystems, where devices and systems seamlessly communicate and collaborate to provide holistic support. Imagine a scenario where a health monitor detecting elevated stress levels informs a smart home system to adjust environmental settings, while simultaneously alerting a caregiver or healthcare provider. Such integration could enhance the user's quality of life by addressing physical, emotional, and social needs in a cohesive manner. These ecosystems could also facilitate better resource allocation and coordination among caregivers, healthcare providers, and family members, creating a more supportive and efficient care network.

Collaboration across disciplines will be key to realizing the full potential of predictive algorithms in assistive technologies. Engineers, healthcare professionals, data scientists, and ethicists must work together to address the technical, social, and ethical challenges associated with these systems. By fostering a multidisciplinary approach, we can ensure that assistive technologies become more effective, inclusive, and accessible to individuals with diverse needs.

Furthermore, the role of policymakers and regulators cannot be underestimated. Establishing clear guidelines and standards for the development and deployment of predictive algorithms in assistive technologies is essential to ensure their safety, reliability, and ethical use. Policymakers must also prioritize funding and support for research and innovation in this field, enabling the development of next-generation solutions that can truly transform lives.

In conclusion, predictive algorithms are reshaping the landscape of assistive technologies, offering unprecedented opportunities to enhance independence, accessibility, and quality of life for individuals with disabilities. By addressing current limitations and exploring innovative possibilities, these systems have the potential to become indispensable tools in creating a more inclusive and equitable society. The journey toward realizing this vision requires continued innovation, collaboration, and a commitment to placing users at the center of technological advancements. As we move forward, the transformative power of predictive algorithms in assistive technologies is boundless, promising a future where no individual is limited by their disabilities.

REFERENCES

Amaral, T., ... (2019). "A review on the development of smart wheelchairs for people with motor disabilities." Sensors. MDPI: https://www.mdpi.com/1424-8220/19/22/4913

Chen, Y., & Zimmerman, G. (2007). "Enhancing independent living for older adults through smart home technology." IEEE Pervasive Computing. IEEE Xplore: https://ieeexplore.ieee.org/document/4141052

Ehteshami Bejnordi, B., ... (2017). "Diagnostic assessment of deep learning algorithms for detection of breast cancer." JAMA. JAMA Network: https://jamanetwork.com/journals/jama/fullarticle/2665774

Feil-Seifer, D., & Mataric, M. J. (2011). "Socially assistive robotics." IEEE Transactions on Robotics. IEEE Xplore: https://ieeexplore.ieee.org/document/5740167

Ghahramani, Z. (2015). "Probabilistic machine learning and artificial intelligence." Nature. Nature: https://www.nature.com/articles/nature14541

Goodfellow, I., Bengio, Y., & Courville, A. (2016). Deep Learning. MIT Press. Full Text: https://www.deeplearningbook.org/. PDF: https://github.com/janishar/mit-deep-learning-book-pdf

Heer, J., & Shneiderman, B. (2012). "Interactive dynamics for visual analysis." Communications of the ACM. ACM Digital Library: https://dl.acm.org/doi/10.1145/2063176.2063196

Hickman, J. M., ... (2017). "AI-powered assistive communication tools for ALS patients." ACM Transactions on Accessible Computing. ACM Digital Library: https://dl.acm.org/doi/10.1145/3132040

Hochberg, L. R., ... (2012). "Reach and grasp by people with tetraplegia using a neurally controlled robotic arm." Nature. PDF: https://www.nature.com/articles/nature11076.pdf

LeCun, Y., Bengio, Y., & Hinton, G. (2015). "Deep learning." Nature. Nature: https://www.nature.com/articles/nature14539

Murphy, K. P. (2012). Machine Learning: A Probabilistic Perspective. MIT Press. Publisher: https://mitpress.mit.edu/9780262018029/machine-learning/

Ravi, D., ... (2017). "Deep learning for human activity recognition: A resource-efficient implementation." Wearable Sensors. IEEE Xplore: https://ieeexplore.ieee.org/document/7901760

Rebsamen, B., ... (2007). “A brain-controlled wheelchair to navigate in familiar environments.” IEEE Transactions on Neural Systems and Rehabilitation Engineering. IEEE Xplore: https://ieeexplore.ieee.org/document/4354040

Shinohara, K., & Wobbrock, J. O. (2011). “In the shadow of misperception: assistive technology use and social interactions.” CHI Conference on Human Factors in Computing Systems. ACM Digital Library: https://dl.acm.org/doi/10.1145/1978942.1979044

Wang, Z., ... (2020). “Deep learning algorithms in medical prediction.” Journal of Biomedical Informatics. ScienceDirect: https://www.sciencedirect.com/science/article/pii/S1532046420301203

Chapter 13
Liver Disease Prediction Using Classification and Feature Selection Techniques

S. Abiramasundari
https://orcid.org/0000-0001-9990-2968
SASTRA University, India

P. Umamaheswari
https://orcid.org/0000-0003-2007-697X
SASTRA University, India

ABSTRACT

Liver disease is one of the most prominent causes of the increase in the death rate worldwide. Early detection can help in better management and treatment of the disease. Machine learning can help in accurate and efficient diagnosis of Liver disease. This paper aims to develop a machine learning model for the detection of Liver disease. The main focus is to predict liver disease based on a software engineering approach using classification and feature selection techniques. The model has a good accuracy and can be used for early detection of Liver disease. This proposed methodology has the potential to contribute to improved patient outcomes and quality of life. In this paper, different machine learning algorithms such as Logistic Regression, Multi-Layer Perceptron, Decision Tree Random Forest, Support Vector Machine, Extreme Gradient Boosting and K-Nearest Neighbours have been used to detect the liver disease. In this proposed work, the accuracy of the algorithms is compared and the best algorithm is chosen that gives the highest accuracy rate in predicting the Liver disease.

DOI: 10.4018/979-8-3373-0194-5.ch013

1. INTRODUCTION

In today's world, more than a million people are diagnosed with liver disease each year. Liver cirrhosis, hepatitis (A, B, C), and liver cancer are common liver diseases. Globally, 1.32 million more people died of liver cirrhosis in 2017 than in 1990, of which 66.7% were men and 33.3% were women. Although overall death is declining because of improvements in advanced treatment and maintaining a sound lifestyle. However, liver-related fatalities accounted for 3.5% of all deaths this century. Excessive uses of drugs, alcohol, obesity, and diabetes are the main causes of liver disease. Fuzzy K-means classification and feature selection are used to classify the liver disorders(Kefelegn & Kamat, n.d.). It gets harder to categorize the diverse liver illnesses since they are determined by the same attribute values. According to the conversation, fuzzy-based categorization performs better in these perplexing classifications and has a 94% accuracy rate for every kind of liver disease. These life-threatening diseases are manageable if they are diagnosed in their early stages. Machine learning techniques are widely used in the healthcare sector, in particular for the diagnosis and classification of certain diseases based on characteristic information. These systems will help clinicians make accurate decisions about patients.

The input raw feature space is typically saturated with a significant amount of irrelevant feature information and frequently exhibits high dimensionality when the data is acquired using feature generation techniques in conventional ML systems. Projection-based statistical methods such as principal component analysis (PCA), factor analysis (FA), and linear discriminant analysis (LDA) work well to reduce dimensionality. PCA(Joloudari et al., 2019) reduces the dimensionality of the dataset without losing significant feature information. Factor analysis is an extension of PCA that describes the covariance relationships between variables in terms of some underlying factors. LDA uses the class label to compute the matrix between and within the class and seeks the directions along which the classes are best separated. However, projection-based feature extraction, how many components should be retained is still an unsolved issue. The majority of the authors in existing research on ILPD data employ a single-feature extraction approach. Different tactics are used by the PCA, FA, and LDA algorithms to transform the original features. However, the main contribution of the research is an attempt to provide a single feature space that integrates PCA, FA, and LDA projection. Additionally, medical data frequently reveals an imbalance problem among classes. The projection-based dimension reduction approach, as well as the ML algorithms (Kalaiselvi et al., 2021), does not operate well when the dataset is imbalanced and frequently suffers from overfitting. ILPD data reveals missing values, outliers, and higher-class imbalances where the positive class is more than twice as large as the negative class. To achieve better liver patient prediction, computer-assisted diagnosis process has been used along with data preprocessing techniques. The proposed integrated method enhances liver disease classification accuracy, prevents misdiagnosis of liver disease, and increases patient survival. In this paper, statistical feature integration approach has been proposed that aims to improve AUC and accuracy rate of the algorithms. Supervised machine learning techniques such as Logistic Regression, Multi-Layer Perceptron (MLP), Decision Tree Random Forest, Support Vector Machine (SVM), Extreme Gradient Boosting (XG Boost) and K-Nearest Neighbours (KNN) have been used for liver disease prediction.

2. LITERATURE SURVEY

Numerous studies have been conducted on machine learning, which has been used globally in a variety of fields. Machine learning has demonstrated its effectiveness in medicine by being used to identify liver failure, cancer, heart disease, diagnose dengue fever, and other urgent issues. This section discusses about the various related works that are have been implemented using machine learning and deep learning algorithm. Some of the current research focuses (Vats et al.,)on the prediction of liver illness using unsupervised machine learning methods including K-Means, DBSCAN, and Affinity Propagation. The study compares the effectiveness of different methods on a healthcare data set pertaining to liver illness using the Silhouette coefficient. Prediction accuracy is determined by the Silhouette coefficient, and K-Means is the best approach. To identify the most effective method for liver disease prediction using unsupervised machine learning, the results will be examined in terms of prediction accuracy and computing complexity. In order to identify liver illnesses, their study takes into account a number of criteria, including cirrhosis, jaundice, nausea, itching, recurrent weariness, Hodgkin's disease, stomach discomfort, and bruising. The data is analyzed using the Indian Liver Patient Data Collection. The goal of the study is to evaluate these methods' accuracy and computational complexity while taking into account variables like the V-Mean, Adjusted Mutual Information, Adjusted Rand Index, and Silhouette coefficient. The paper also covers the latest developments in machine learning technology across a range of domains, including K-means treatment for leukemia cancer. Several classification methods were employed in earlier research (A.K.M Sazzadur Rahman, et al) to determine whether or not patients had liver disease. These methods' performance was evaluated from a number of angles, including f-1 score, recall, accuracy, and precision. Measurement of classification methods, results analysis, and performance evolution were all included in the results and discussion.

The purpose of this study is to assess how well various machine learning algorithms predict chronic liver disease. Six algorithms were employed by the researchers: Random Forest, Naïve Bayes, K Nearest Neighbors, Decision Tree, Support Vector Machine, and Logistic Regression. A variety of measurement methodologies, including accuracy, precision, recall, f-1 score, and specificity, were used to assess these methods' performance. The findings demonstrated that the LR algorithm's accuracy was the highest. The study primarily examined how clinical data may be utilized to predict liver disease and investigated several analytical approaches for data representation. The study's primary goals were to improve outcome prediction and lower diagnostic expenses in the healthcare industry. Because of its substantial influence on the healthcare system, liver disease—a broad group of illnesses affecting the liver—is becoming a major issue. Traditional diagnostic methods, like radiographic, CT, and liver function testing, are frequently laborious and prone to errors. In several medical specialties, machine learning (ML) and deep learning (DL) methods are effective ways to diagnose illnesses. The performance of several DL models on the estimate and subtyping of liver disease and prognosis is evaluated in this research. The authors (Hendi et al., 2024) suggest a brand-new method called CNN+LSTM, which combines long short-term memory (LSTM) networks with convolutional neural networks (CNN). The study's findings demonstrate that ML and DL can be applied to enhance liver disease diagnosis and prognosis. When compared to CNN, LSTM, and Recurrent Neural Network (RNN), the CNN+LSTM model gets a higher accuracy of 98.73%. The suggested CNN+LSTM model's integration demonstrates resilience in forecasting the liver disease with a precise diagnosis and prognosis.

Evaluation-based methods for predicting liver illness using machine learning algorithms will be the main topic of the 2021 International Conference on Computer Communication and Informatics (ICCCI-2021) (Geetha & Arunachalam, 2021) in Coimbatore, India. The goal of the study is to address the epidemic by improving the way that liver illness is perceived through the use of machine learning techniques. The study examines classification algorithms and prediction accuracy outcomes with an emphasis on algorithms for categorizing healthy individuals using liver datasets. By leveraging the classifier ensemble to create a hybrid predictive classifier model, the study seeks to improve the predictive and classification quality of healthcare data.

Patient survival rates will increase if liver diseases are identified early. Due to the increased likelihood of liver failure among Indians, the country is predicted to become the World Capital of Liver Diseases by 2025. The goal of their proposal is to create a computer that can diagnose more illnesses, assisting medical professionals in choosing the best course of action and cutting down on patient wait times. Although classification methods are frequently employed in medical diagnosis and disease prediction, the best categorization approach does not always yield better prediction outcomes.

The study of gene structures, which are composed of protein sequences, in living things is the focus of the field of bioinformatics. It is essential to analyze vast amounts of genetic material, and the medical field has used bioinformatics as a research field. The study focuses on liver disease, a significant organ that is essential to the body's overall health and the health of the foot. The liver is important for digestion, enzyme secretion, and a number of biochemical processes that are necessary for sustaining vitality and averting illness. Liver illnesses can damage other organs and impair the body's immune system if these pathways are not well controlled. One of the most effective ways to identify and treat liver problems is using biochemical testing. The study (Veeranki & Varshney, 2022) emphasizes how crucial bioinformatics is to the medical industry and how it may be used to detect dangerous microbes and create efficient cures. Using machine learning techniques, Dritsas and Trigka's study aims to forecast the risk of liver illness. The largest organ in the human body, the liver has many roles, such as processing food, turning it into nutrients, removing toxins, and fighting off diseases.

Liver disease can result from exposure to dangerous substances or viruses that destroy the liver. Using machine learning techniques to forecast the emergence of liver disease early on is essential. The study assesses (Dritsas & Trigka, 2023) a range of machine learning models and ensemble techniques in terms of accuracy, precision, recall, F-measure, and area under the curve (AUC) in order to forecast the onset of liver disease.

Following SMOTE with 10-fold cross-validation, the Voting classifier performs better than the other models, with an accuracy, recall, and F-measure of 80.1%, a precision of 80.4%, and an AUC of 88.4%. Chronic hepatitis, cirrhosis, and non-alcoholic fatty liver disease (NAFLD) are among the liver illnesses that can be grouped according to their causes and effects on the liver. This study suggests a technique for diagnosing liver disease (LD) that makes use of supervised machine learning classification methods, such as support vector machines (SVM), logistic regression, decision trees, random forests, AdaBoost, KNN, linear discriminant analysis, and gradient boosting.

Additionally, the authors (Rani et al., 2022a) use a feature selection technique called least absolute shrinkage and selection operator (LASSO) on the dataset in order to identify the most highly linked features of LD. Tenfold cross-validation (CV) predictions are evaluated for precision, sensitivity, accuracy, and f1-score values in order to predict the disease. Accuracy, precision, sensitivity, and f1-score values for the decision tree method with LASSO included are 94.295%, 92%, 99%, and 96%, respectively, giving it the highest performance score. To demonstrate its importance, the paper also contrasts the suggested system with other recent research.

An earlier diagnosis of LD can result in a quicker recovery because the liver is an essential organ in the human body. To find LD, the authors utilize an LFT dataset that has eleven attributes. A prevalent clinical consequence with a high morbidity and mortality rate is fatty liver disease (FLD). Appropriate preventive, diagnostic, and treatment options can be aided by early FLD patient prediction. In order to help doctors identify high-risk patients, make new diagnoses, and prevent and treat FLD, a machine learning model was created to predict FLD. 577 patients who underwent an initial fatty liver screening at the New Taipei City Hospital between December 1st and December 31st, 2009, were included in the study(Wu et al., 2019).

Various classification models were created to forecast FLD, including logistic regression (LR), random forest (RF), Naïve Bayes (NB), and artificial neural networks (ANN). In terms of accuracy, RF, NB, ANN, and LR were 87.48, 82.65, 81.85, and 76.96%, respectively. The random forest model outperformed the other models for classification. Clinicians may find it easier to stratify patients with fatty livers for primary prevention, surveillance, early therapy, and management if they use a random forest model. Many people worldwide suffer from liver disease (LD), a serious health concern. Disease of the liver is caused by a number of reasons. The process of diagnosing LD is costly and time-consuming. Automated disease diagnosis is possible with machine learning (ML).

The purpose of this study(Ghazal et al., 2022) is to evaluate the effectiveness of several machine learning algorithms in reducing the high expense of liver disease diagnosis through prediction. With an accuracy of 0.884 and a miss-rate of 0.116, the suggested intelligent model for ML-based liver disease prediction is more thorough and efficient. There are over 2 million liver disease-related deaths annually, making liver disease a serious public health concern.

One million deaths from liver cancer and one in four deaths from cirrhosis are predicted by the Global Burden of Disease (GBD) system to occur annually in 2010. Large-scale screenings and prompt response are necessary for liver disease, one of the most underappreciated public health concerns in the world. Biomedical research has benefited greatly from machine learning approaches, for which Deep Learning (DL) is the most advanced model.

3. PROPOSED METHODOLOGY

3.1 Dataset collection

Dataset consists of 583 liver patients. It consists of various attributes such as Age, Gender, Total Bilirubin, Direct Bilirubin, Alkaline Phosphotase, Alamine Aminotransferase, Aspartate Aminotransferase, Total Proteins, Albumin, Albumin and Globulin Ratio, Target. This dataset has a total of 583 records. Among 583 patient records, 416 patients are suffered with liver disease and 167 are non-patient records. The attribute "Dataset" described as the disease with value "1" denotes a person having liver disease and "2" represents that a person has not been affected by liver disease. This data set contains 441 male patient records and 142 female patient records.

3.2 Data Analysis and Preparation

3.2.1 Exploratory Data Analysis

Exploratory data analysis focuses on statistical and visualization techniques to gain insights into a dataset. It includes understanding the data's structure, identifying patterns, trends, and anomalies, and formulating hypotheses for further analysis. This part also examines the data and generates a broad overview of its characteristics without making assumptions or biases. Figure 1 depicts the relationship between the features of the dataset. Figure. 2 represents relationship between the features of dataset by using the scatter plot.

Figure 1. Histogram: Relationship between the features of the dataset.

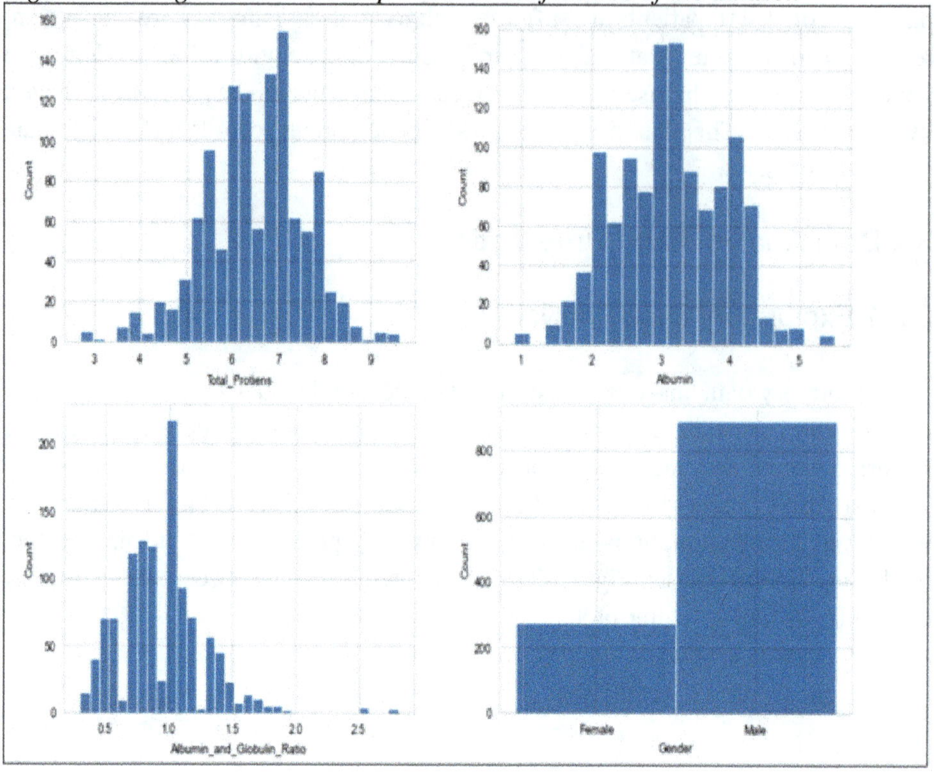

Figure 2. Scatter plots: Relationship between the features of dataset.

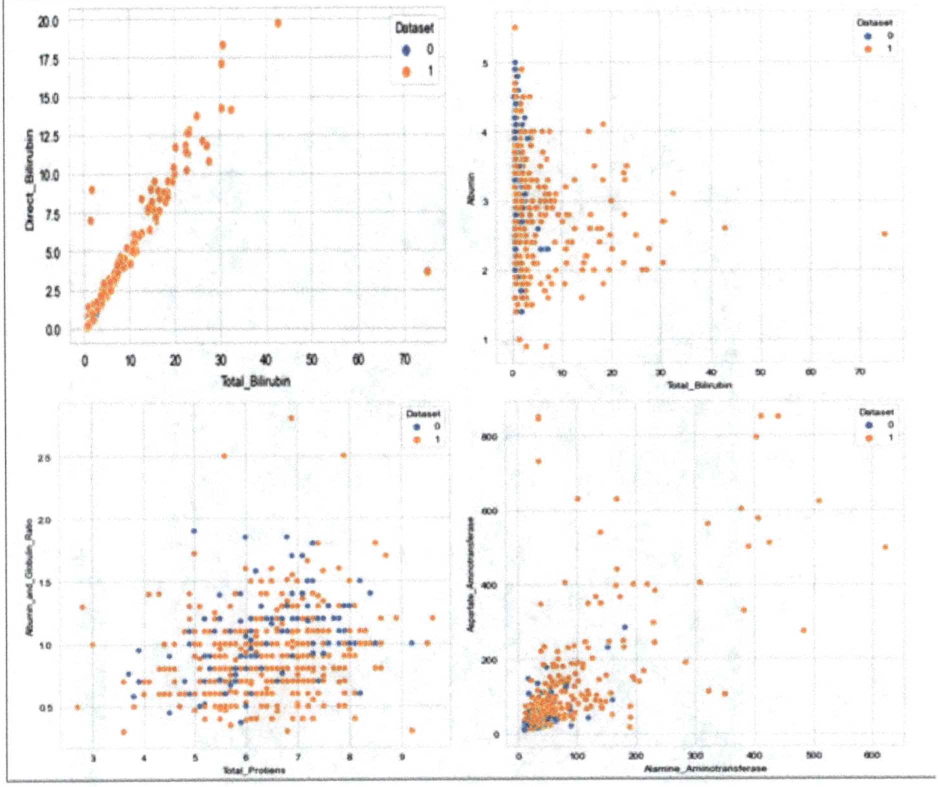

3.2.2 Correlation Analysis

This module is used to identify which features are important for predicting the target variable. If two features are highly correlated, then they may be redundant. The correlation coefficient takes values between -1 and 1, with 0 indicating no correlation. Positive values indicate positive correlation, and negative values indicate negative correlation. If there is no correlation between two variables, they are irrelevant to each other. The importance of features is shown in Figure 3.

3.2.3 Data Pre-Processing

Data pre-processing involves cleaning, transforming, and preparing the data for use in a machine learning model. Data cleaning is used to identify and handle missing or incorrect data, such as missing values, duplicate values, or outliers. Boxplots are used to identify outliers, visualize the distribution of the data, and compare the distribution of different datasets.

Figure 3. Correlation matrix using heat map.

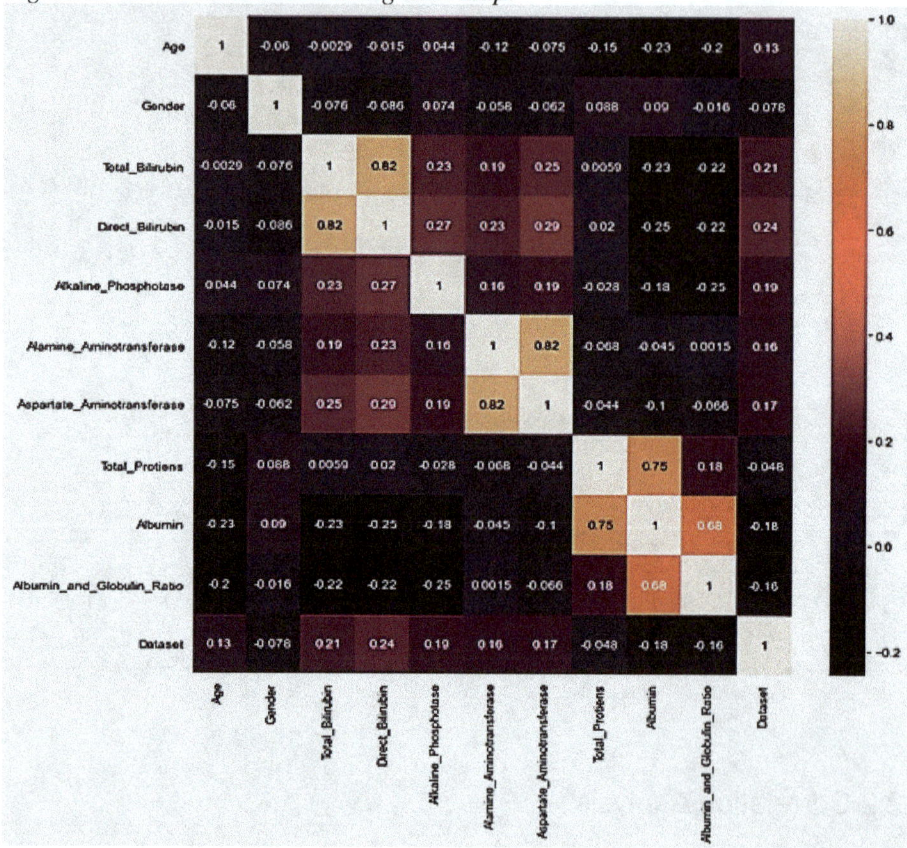

3.2.4 Outlier Detection

Outlier detection frequently employs Z-score. The values can be located that differ noticeably from the mean by getting the z-score for every data point. To assess if a data point qualifies as an outlier, a threshold is typically established. An outlier is indicated for a particular data point if the absolute magnitude of the z-score exceeds or is higher than the threshold.

The z-score can be estimated by the following formula:

$z = (x - \mu) / \sigma$

x is the specific data point.

μ is distribution's average.

σ represents the distribution's standard deviation.

3.2.5 Null Value Replacement

Missing values in each column have been identified and are replaced with the estimated second quartile value.

Figure 4. Boxplot of outliers of features before applying Z-Score.

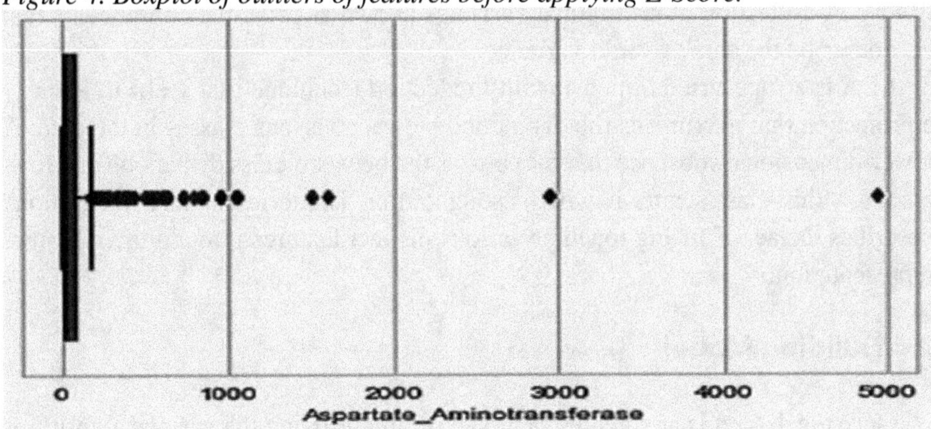

Figure 5. Replacement of outliers.

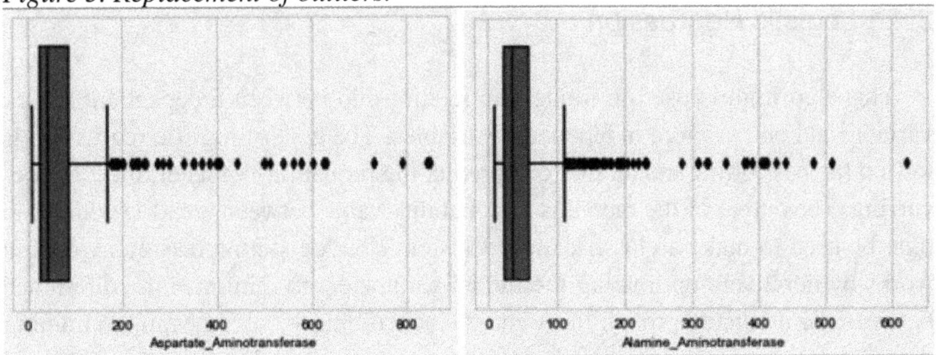

3.3 Feature Extraction and Integration

The process of extracting features into a lower-dimensional representation that captures the most pertinent facts for a particular job. It extracts a subset of useful characteristics from the source data, which can boost the effectiveness of machine learning algorithms and minimize complexity. Both PCA (Principal Component Analysis) and LDA (Linear Discriminant Analysis) are widely used methods for decreasing dimensionality and feature extraction. PCA is a method for unsupervised dimensionality reduction known as principal component analysis that seeks to identify a new collection of orthogonal variables known as principal components that best describe the data's overall variance.

LDA is a supervised dimensionality reduction technique that seeks to identify a projection that maximizes the distinction between various classes in the data. A lower-dimensional subspace that maximizes the between-class dispersion and lowers the within-class scatter is what is sought after. The term "feature integration" describes the act of fusing together various distinct features into a unified feature representation.

3.4 Building Model

Once the dataset is augmented, a model is built utilizing the various algorithms to compare their performance in terms of accuracy and other hyperparameters. The patient dataset is split into training and testing data in the ratio of 6:4, and the respective evaluations are applied to them.

3.4.1 Logistic Regression

This algorithm is used to model the relationship between a dependent binary variable and one or more independent variables. The goal of logistic regression is to find the best fitting model that can predict the probability of a certain event occurring. The output of the model is a probability value between 0 and 1, which can then be used to make a classification decision. The logistic regression algorithm works by iteratively optimizing the model parameters to minimize the difference between the predicted probabilities and the actual binary outcomes in the training data. Given the characteristics X, the logistic regression model predicts the likelihood $P(y=1|X)$ that a patient has liver disease. The following sigmoid function (Eq.1) has been used to compute the probability.

$$P(y = 1x) = \frac{1}{1 + e^{-(\beta 0+\beta 1x1+\beta 2x2+\cdots+\beta pxp)}} \quad (1)$$

Logistic regression (Thirunavukkarasu et al., 2018) model is defined, and a parameter grid is set up for GridSearchCV to search over. GridSearchCV is used to find the best hyperparameters for the logistic regression model, using 5-fold cross-validation. After finding the best hyperparameters, a new logistic regression model is created with those hyperparameters, and it is fit on the training data.

Then the model can be used to predict the test data, and the accuracy and AUC are measured. The ROC curve is plotted to visualize the model's performance. The area under the ROC curve (AUC) is a metric that summarizes the performance of the classifier across all possible threshold values.

3.4.2 Multi-Layer Perceptron (MLP)

A feedforward neural network model called the Multi-Layer Perceptron (MLP) is made up of numerous layers of artificial neurons, also referred to as perceptrons. Each neuron in the network accepts input signals, does a weighted sum, and then sends the total to an activation function in order to produce an output. The MLP classifier is defined with hidden layers, Relu activation function, and Adam solver. The hyperparameters of the MLP Classifier are set using various values. After fitting the MLP classifier on the training data, the model predicts the output on the test data. The accuracy score, confusion matrix, and classification report are measured for the predicted output.

Let $X=\{x_1,x_2,x_3....x_n\}$ be the input features of dataset. The hidden layer with 'm' neurons is represented in Equation (2).

$$W_j = \sum_{i=1}^{n} \left(a_{ij} x_i\right) + b_j \tag{2}$$

Where Wj is the weighted sum of neuron j, aij represents the weight of input xi to hidden neuron j, and bj is the bias for the neuron j. Followed by activation function 'ReLU' has been applied and it is given in Eq. (3)

$$f\left(W_j\right) = \max\left(0, W_{j)}\right. \tag{3}$$

Where f is the ReLU function. The probability of liver disease has been calculated using output layer along with the sigmoid function (Eq.4)

$$\sigma(z) = \frac{1}{1 + e^{-z}} \tag{4}$$

Neural score and neural test score are measured to indicate how well the model is able to predict the outcomes on the training and test data. Precision, recall, F1-score, and support are the evaluation metrics used.

3.4.2 Decision Tree Classifier

Decision tree (Singh et al., 2020) classifier is a popular machine learning algorithm that works by recursively splitting the dataset into subsets based on the most significant features until a stopping criterion is reached. It builds a tree-like model to classify data. Hyperparameters are tuned and optimal hyperparameters have been searched. After the model is fit, extracted the best hyperparameters found during the hyperparameter search. Then the model is trained on a full training set. Accuracy score is calculated using true labels and predicted labels. The performance of the trained model on a held-out test set has been evaluated using the appropriate evaluation metrics.

3.4.3 Random Forest Classifier

Random Forest (Sreejith et al., 2020) (Singh et al., 2020)is a popular ensemble learning algorithm that can be used for classification and regression tasks. It is a powerful algorithm that combines multiple decision trees to make more accurate predictions. Random Forest has several hyperparameters that can be tuned to optimize model performance. RandomizedSearchCV was used to perform a random search over the specified hyperparameter space. The model was trained on the training data using the best hyperparameters found during the random search. Predictions are made on test data and various performance metrics have been measured. The prediction of this algorithm is based on the majority vote of all tree predictions and it is given in the Eq. (5).

$$Y = model\left(h_1(X), h_2(X), \ldots, h_s(X) \right) \tag{5}$$

where $h_s(X)$ be the decision tree prediction.

3.4.4 K Nearest Neighbours

K Nearest Neighbours (KNN) (Hartatik et al., 2020) is one of the simplest classification algorithms and works by organizing the data of interest based on the aggregation of its neighbors. 10-fold cross-validation is performed on the training dataset to evaluate the accuracy of the model for each K value. The misclassification error is calculated and plotted against the number of neighbors (K).The optimal number of neighbors is chosen as the one with the lowest misclassification error. The KNN algorithm has been implemented using the optimal K value, and the model is trained on the training dataset. Finally, the accuracy score is calculated on the test dataset and the result is compared. The KNN algorithm is a simple but powerful algorithm that can be used for classification tasks when the dataset is relatively small.

3.4.5 Support Vector Machine

The goal of the SVM algorithm (Thirunavukkarasu et al., 2018) (Rani et al., 2022b) is to create the best line or decision boundary that can segregate n-dimensional space into classes so that we can easily put the new data point in the correct category in the future. This best decision boundary is called a hyperplane. A grid search is performed using the defined SVM model and the parameter grid. Best estimator is found to predict the labels of the test data and obtain the probabilities of the positive class 1. Confusion matrix has been generated and accuracy, false positive and true positive rates are obtained from the predicted probabilities. ROC curve is also generated. The final prediction is based on the following function Eq. (6).

$$f(x) = sign\left(\sum_{i=1}^{n} \alpha_i y_i K(x_i, x) + b\right) \tag{6}$$

For all the data points the value of $\alpha_i > 0$ and b is a bias term.

3.4.6 XGBOOST

XGBoost (Extreme Gradient Boosting) (Kuzhippallil et al., 2020) is a gradient boosting algorithm designed to improve the accuracy of machine learning models. It is based on the gradient boosting decision tree algorithm and uses a gradient descent optimization algorithm to minimize the loss function. The tuned hyperparameters are defined as a dictionary. A randomized search with many iterations is performed using the XGBClassifier as the initial model. The model is built for the training data, and the predicted values are obtained for both the training and test sets. The predicted probabilities for the test set are computed, and the false positive rate, true positive rate, and thresholds are computed to generate the ROC curve.

If the accuracy score is less than expected, the model is refit with additional iterations until the expected accuracy score is obtained. The XGBoost algorithm is chosen for its ability to handle complex datasets and its high predictive power. Once all the decision trees are trained, the final predictions are made based on the following equation Eq. (7).

$$Y_i = \sum_{j=1}^{k} f_j\left(x_i\right) \tag{7}$$

where k represent number of decision trees, x_i is a data point and f_j is a binary sigmoid function.

3.5 Results and Discussions

Evaluation metrics:

Various performance metrics are used to assess the performance and effectiveness of ML models. These metrics provide quantitative measures that help to determine how well the model is performing and how accurate its predictions are.

Confusion Matrix:

The confusion matrix is a tabular representation of the performance of a classification model. It summarizes the predictions made by the model on a set of data, comparing them to the actual labels or classes of the data. Fig 6 represents the confusion matrices of all ML algorithms used in this proposed methodology.

ROC-AUC:

The ROC-AUC (Receiver Operating Characteristic Area Under the Curve) measures the ability of a binary classification model to distinguish between positive and negative instances. It plots the true positive rate against the false positive rate, and a higher AUC indicates better performance. Fig 7 shows ROC-AUC of all ML algorithms.

Accuracy:

Accuracy measures the proportion of correctly predicted instances out of the total number of instances. It is a simple and intuitive metric.

Recall:

The recall score measures the accuracy of the model in correctly identifying True Positives. Therefore, it indicates the number of patients with disease who were accurately diagnosed with the condition.

Precision:

A measure of precision counts the proportion of accurate positive predictions among all the model's positive forecasts. It emphasizes the precision of optimistic forecasts. Table 1 shows the classification results of all algorithms.

F1-Score:

Precision and recall are combined into a single metric called the F1 score. By accounting for both false positives and false negatives, it offers a fair assessment of the model's performance. Precision and recall are given equal weight in the F1 score, which is the harmonic mean of both measurements.

Figure 6. Confusion matrices of ML algorithms

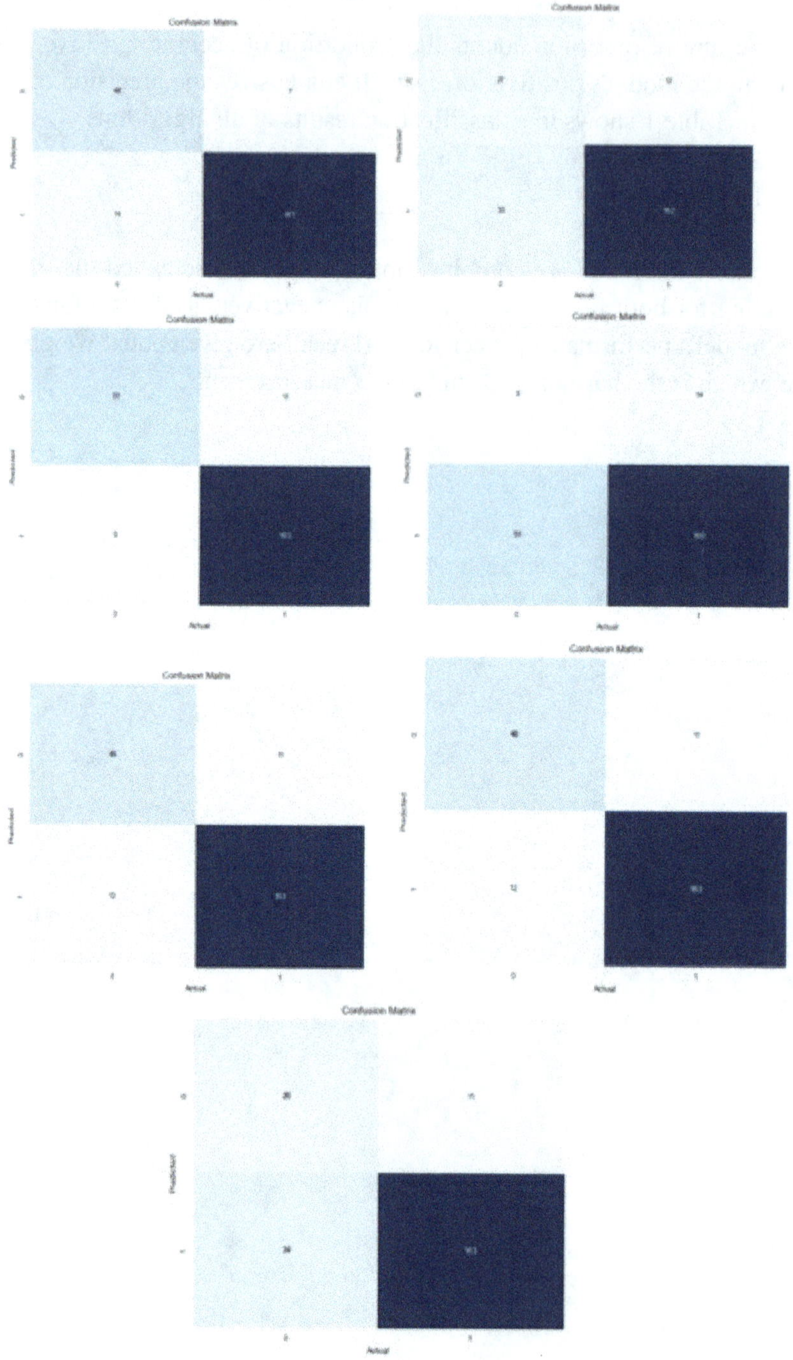

Figure 7. ROC-AUC of all ML algorithms

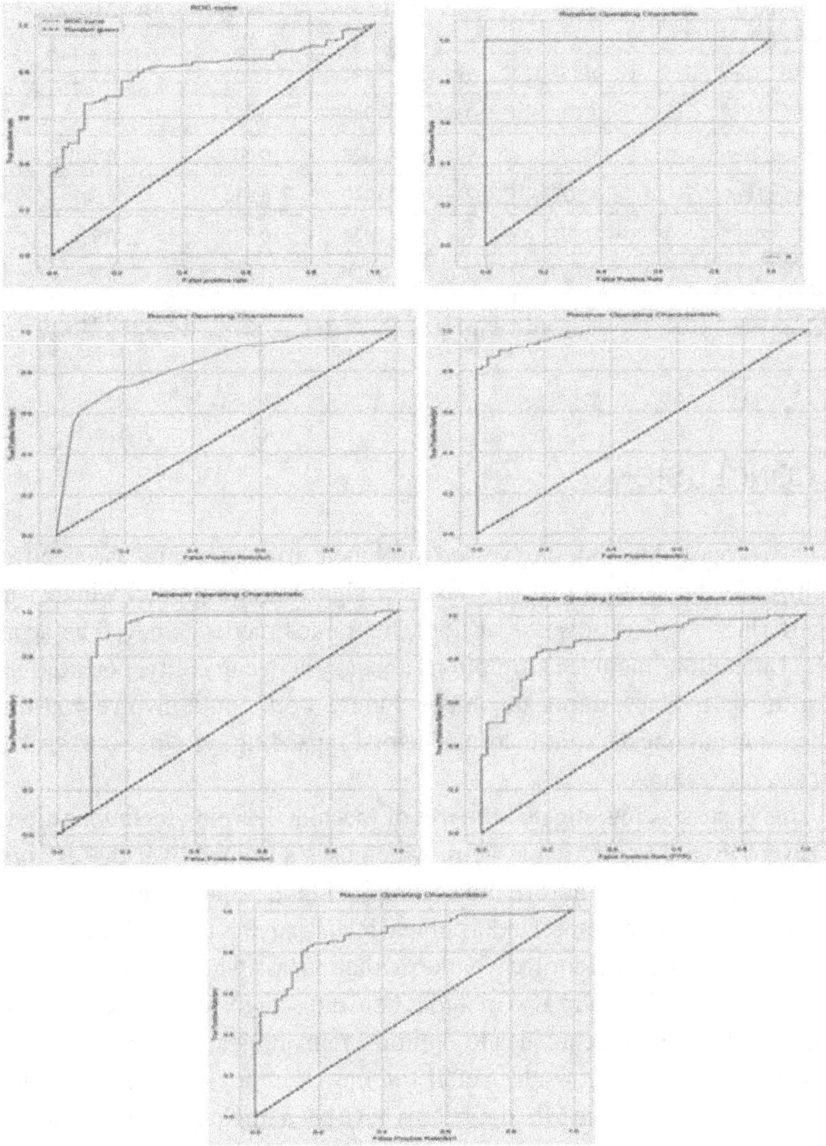

Table 1. Evaluation metrics

Algorithms/ Evaluation Metrics	Precision	Recall	F1-Score	Accuracy	Mean Accuracy	Mean AUC
Logistic Regression	0.758	0.919	0.831	0.722	0.732	0.771
MLP	0.947	0.936	0.942	0.914	0.931	0.940
Decision Tree	0.830	0.931	0.878	0.807	0.782	0.831
Random Forest	0.922	0.959	0.940	0.910	0.941	0.970
SVM	0.931	0.936	0.934	0.901	0.936	0.939
XGB	0.827	0.936	0.878	0.807	0.776	0.859
KNN	0.931	0.936	0.934	0.901	0.941	0.926

4. CONCLUSION

This proposed methodology used machine learning techniques, specifically the Multi-Layer Perceptron (MLP) Classifier algorithm, to predict whether a person is suffering from liver disease or not. The trained model achieved an accuracy of 91%. Limitations include assumptions about system capability, potential inaccuracies, missing values, duplicate values. Future work could involve real-time data, addressing missing data and external factors, expanding system features, using other test sample features.

This paper has investigated the use of machine learning techniques in the field of Liver Disease Prediction system, which uses a trained liver disease prediction model which helps to improve the accuracy of disease prediction.

Another important aspect incorporated in this paper is using Multi-Layer Perceptron (MLP) Classifier algorithm for the prediction task which includes the prediction of liver disease. The study also includes how the data format impacts the prediction system and different techniques to optimize remaining algorithms.

The experiments show an overall training accuracy of 91% in predicting the disease successfully. The ML algorithms have been implemented and the results are compared. This system can be used for practical use by the following improvements

- Usage of real-time data to train the Multi-Layer Perceptron (MLP) Classifier algorithm.
- Dimensionality Reduction and Missing data values.
- Among all the algorithms it is identified that Multi-Layer Perceptron (MLP) Classifier yields better result.

REFERENCES

Dritsas, E., & Trigka, M. (2023). Supervised Machine Learning Models for Liver Disease Risk Prediction. *Computers, 12*(1), 19. DOI: 10.3390/computers12010019

Geetha, C., & Arunachalam, Ar. (2021). Evaluation based Approaches for Liver Disease Prediction using Machine Learning Algorithms. *2021 International Conference on Computer Communication and Informatics (ICCCI)*, 1–4. DOI: 10.1109/ICCCI50826.2021.9402463

Ghazal, T. M., Rehman, A. U., Saleem, M., Ahmad, M., Ahmad, S., & Mehmood, F. (2022). Intelligent Model to Predict Early Liver Disease using Machine Learning Technique. *2022 International Conference on Business Analytics for Technology and Security (ICBATS)*, 1–5. DOI: 10.1109/ICBATS54253.2022.9758929

Hartatik, H., Tamam, M. B., & Setyanto, A. (2020). Prediction for Diagnosing Liver Disease in Patients using KNN and Naïve Bayes Algorithms. *2020 2nd International Conference on Cybernetics and Intelligent System (ICORIS)*, 1–5. DOI: 10.1109/ICORIS50180.2020.9320797

Hendi, A. M., Hossain, M. A., Majrashi, N. A., Limkar, S., Elamin, B. M., & Rahman, M. (2024). Adaptive Method for Exploring Deep Learning Techniques for Subtyping and Prediction of Liver Disease. *Applied Sciences (Basel, Switzerland), 14*(4), 1488. DOI: 10.3390/app14041488

Joloudari, J. H., Saadatfar, H., Dehzangi, A., & Shamshirband, S. (2019). Computer-aided decision-making for predicting liver disease using PSO-based optimized SVM with feature selection. *Informatics in Medicine Unlocked, 17*, 100255. DOI: 10.1016/j.imu.2019.100255

Kalaiselvi, R., Meena, K., & Vanitha, V. (2021). Liver Disease Prediction Using Machine Learning Algorithms. *2021 International Conference on Advancements in Electrical, Electronics, Communication, Computing and Automation (ICAECA)*, 1–6. DOI: 10.1109/ICAECA52838.2021.9675756

Kefelegn, S., & Kamat, P. (n.d.). Prediction and Analysis of Liver Disorder Diseases by using Data Mining Technique. *Survey (London, England)*.

Kuzhippallil, M. A., Joseph, C., & Kannan, A. (2020). Comparative Analysis of Machine Learning Techniques for Indian Liver Disease Patients. *2020 6th International Conference on Advanced Computing and Communication Systems (ICACCS)*, 778–782. DOI: 10.1109/ICACCS48705.2020.9074368

Rani, A. J. M., Nishanthini, S., Josephine, D. C. J., Venugopal, H., Nissi, S. G., & Jacintha, V. (2022a). Liver Disease Prediction using Semi Supervised based Machine Learning Algorithm. *2022 3rd International Conference on Smart Electronics and Communication (ICOSEC)*, 1389–1392. DOI: 10.1109/ICOSEC54921.2022.9952144

Rani, A. J. M., Nishanthini, S., Josephine, D. C. J., Venugopal, H., Nissi, S. G., & Jacintha, V. (2022b). Liver Disease Prediction using Semi Supervised based Machine Learning Algorithm. *2022 3rd International Conference on Smart Electronics and Communication (ICOSEC)*, 1389–1392. DOI: 10.1109/ICOSEC54921.2022.9952144

Singh, J., Bagga, S., & Kaur, R. (2020). Software-based Prediction of Liver Disease with Feature Selection and Classification Techniques. *Procedia Computer Science*, *167*, 1970–1980. DOI: 10.1016/j.procs.2020.03.226

Sreejith, S., Khanna Nehemiah, H., & Kannan, A. (2020). Clinical data classification using an enhanced SMOTE and chaotic evolutionary feature selection. *Computers in Biology and Medicine*, *126*, 103991. DOI: 10.1016/j.compbiomed.2020.103991 PMID: 32987205

Thirunavukkarasu, K., Singh, A. S., Irfan, M., & Chowdhury, A. (2018). Prediction of Liver Disease using Classification Algorithms. *2018 4th International Conference on Computing Communication and Automation (ICCCA)*, 1–3. DOI: 10.1109/CCAA.2018.8777655

Vats, V., Zhang, L., Chatterjee, S., Ahmed, S., Enziama, E., & Tepe, K. (n.d.). A Comparative Analysis of Unsupervised Machine Techniques for Liver Disease Prediction. *A. K.*

Veeranki, S. R., & Varshney, M. (2022). Intelligent Techniques and Comparative Performance Analysis of Liver Disease Prediction. *International Journal of Mechanical Engineering*, *7*(1).

Wu, C. C., Yeh, W. C., Hsu, W. D., Islam, M. M., Nguyen, P. A. A., Poly, T. N., & Li, Y. C. J. (2019). Prediction of fatty liver disease using machine learning algorithms. *Computer Methods and Programs in Biomedicine*, *170*, 23–29.

Chapter 14
Optimizing Heart Attack Prediction and Detection Using an Enhanced CNN Model:
Addressing Overfitting and Generalization Challenges

Asadi Srinivasulu
https://orcid.org/0009-0003-2731-6072
Indian Institute of Information Technology, Allahabad, India

Anupam Agrawal
Indian Institute of Information Technology, Allahabad, India

A. V. Senthil Kumar
https://orcid.org/0000-0002-8587-7017
Hindusthan College of Arts and Science, India

ABSTRACT

Heart attacks continue to be a major cause of death globally, making it crucial to develop accurate and efficient predictive models for early diagnosis and timely treatment. This research presents an improved Convolutional Neural Network (CNN) model designed to enhance heart attack prediction and detection while addressing the common issues of overfitting and poor generalization found in traditional machine learning methods. The enhanced model utilizes advanced regularization techniques and optimization strategies to improve its performance, capitalizing on CNNs' ability to effectively extract spatial features. The experimental results

DOI: 10.4018/979-8-3373-0194-5.ch014

reveal significant improvements in both accuracy and robustness of the model. The enhanced CNN achieved a maximum accuracy of 100% and a validation accuracy of up to 75% after 50 training epochs.

1. INTRODUCTION

1.1 Background and Motivation

Heart diseases, especially heart attacks, continue to be a leading cause of death worldwide, placing a heavy burden on healthcare systems globally (Ram Kumar et al., 2024). Early and accurate prediction and detection of heart attacks are crucial for timely medical intervention, which can significantly decrease both the severity and fatality rates associated with cardiovascular conditions. Although traditional machine learning models have been widely utilized for predicting heart disease, they often struggle with issues such as overfitting and poor generalization to new, unseen data (Mulyani et al., 2023). Overfitting happens when a model performs exceptionally well on training data but fails to maintain accuracy when exposed to new data, resulting in unreliable predictions in real-world applications (Nandakumar & Subhashini, 2024). This shortcoming limits the effectiveness of predictive models in clinical environments, where patient data can vary widely. Consequently, there is a critical need for more robust and generalized models that can overcome these challenges, thereby enhancing the accuracy and dependability of heart disease prediction tools.

1.2 Problem Statement

The main challenges in creating reliable heart attack prediction models are managing overfitting and improving generalization. Overfitting diminishes a model's ability to accurately predict outcomes for new data, as it tends to focus too closely on the specific details of the training data rather than identifying broader patterns (Mehmood et al., 2021). This issue is particularly significant in heart disease prediction, where patient data can differ greatly across various populations and demographic groups. Moreover, the challenge of generalization involves the model's ability to apply the patterns it has learned from training data to accurately predict new, unseen cases. Standard CNN models, despite their capabilities, are often not well-suited for handling such diversity, leading to decreased effectiveness in clinical settings (Arooj et al., 2022). This study aims to address these challenges by refining the CNN model's architecture, implementing advanced regularization methods, and enhancing the model's ability to generalize effectively across different datasets.

1.3 Objectives

The goal of this study is to enhance the Convolutional Neural Network (CNN) model for heart attack prediction and detection, specifically targeting the issues of overfitting and generalization (Revathi et al., 2024). This entails developing an improved CNN model that uses advanced regularization techniques and optimization strategies to better predict heart attacks across a wide range of clinical scenarios (Honi & Szathmary, 2024). By harnessing the power of CNNs to extract spatial features from complex datasets, this research seeks to achieve greater predictive accuracy and robustness, ensuring the model performs well with new data (Panjaitan et al., 2023). Additionally, the study aims to demonstrate the practical application of this optimized model in real-time clinical settings, highlighting its potential for broad adoption and significant impact on patient care and outcomes.

2. RELATED WORK

2.1 Overview of Existing Techniques

Advancements in heart disease prediction have increasingly relied on a diverse array of machine learning and deep learning methodologies to enhance diagnostic accuracy and efficiency. Traditional approaches like logistic regression, decision trees, and support vector machines (SVM) have been popular due to their straightforwardness and ease of interpretation (Vergaray et al., 2023). However, these methods often fall short in capturing the intricate, non-linear patterns within cardiovascular data, limiting their predictive effectiveness (Vergaray et al., 2023). In contrast, deep learning models, particularly Convolutional Neural Networks (CNNs) and Recurrent Neural Networks (RNNs), have proven to be more adept at managing the high dimensionality and variability characteristic of medical datasets (Ram Kumar et al., 2024) (Nandakumar & Subhashini, 2024)(Mehmood et al., 2021). CNNs excel in extracting spatial features from medical images and signals, whereas RNNs are better suited for analyzing temporal patterns in sequential data such as electrocardiograms (ECGs) (Revathi et al., 2024)(Honi & Szathmary, 2024). Despite their advantages, current machine learning and deep learning models exhibit several shortcomings. For instance, deep learning models like CNNs, while achieving high accuracy in various applications, frequently encounter the problem of overfitting, especially when trained on small or imbalanced datasets (Ram Kumar et al., 2024) (Nandakumar & Subhashini, 2024) (Arooj et al., 2022). This occurs because these models tend to memorize the training data rather than learning patterns that generalize well to new, unseen data, resulting in suboptimal performance in real-world scenarios (Mehmood et al., 2021) (Kumar et al., 2021). Additionally, the substantial computational resources required to train these models, owing to their complexity and the vast amounts of data they need, pose a significant challenge (Mulyani et al., 2023) (Panjaitan et al., 2023). These drawbacks highlight the need for more efficient, generalized models that can deliver accurate predictions without the burden of high computational costs (Nandakumar & Subhashini, 2024)(Mehmood et al., 2021). Several research efforts have focused on mitigating these limitations through various strategies and optimizations. For example, R. P. Ram Kumar (Ram Kumar et al., 2024) introduced a hybrid optimization technique that integrates CNN with Teaching-Learning-Based Optimization (TLBO) and Genetic Algorithm (GA) to improve model performance and reduce overfitting. Similarly, Nandakumar and Subhashini (Nandakumar & Subhashini, 2024) enhanced the feature extraction capabilities of CNNs using Elephant Herding Optimization (EHO), while Mehmood et al. (Mehmood et al., 2021) improved CNN architectures by employing advanced preprocessing and data augmentation methods to minimize false negatives and boost accuracy. These studies underscore the ongoing endeavors to refine heart disease predictive models, emphasizing accuracy and robustness (Mehmood et al., 2021) (Arooj et al., 2022).

2.2 Limitations of Current Approaches

Current methods for predicting heart disease using CNNs and other deep learning models face several critical challenges that limit their effectiveness in clinical practice. A major issue is overfitting, where the model performs well on the training data but fails to generalize to new data (Ram Kumar et al., 2024; Nandakumar & Subhashini, 2024). This problem is especially pronounced in medical datasets, which are often small and not well-balanced, making it difficult for the model to learn patterns that can be generalized (Mehmood et al., 2021). Overfitting results in models that are overly complex and fine-tuned to the specific characteristics of the training data, rather than recognizing broader patterns applicable to diverse patient groups (Mulyani et al., 2023; Revathi et al., 2024). This challenge is further compounded by the high dimensionality of medical data, which necessitates models to detect subtle variations not always present in the training data (Honi & Szathmary, 2024). Another significant challenge is the high computational cost associated with training deep learning models like CNNs. Due to their deep and complex architectures and the large datasets required for effective training, these models demand substantial computational resources (Nandakumar & Subhashini, 2024; Mehmood et al., 2021). This makes it difficult to deploy such models in real-time clinical environments, where quick decision-making is crucial (Panjaitan et al., 2023). Furthermore, traditional CNN models are not inherently designed to handle the sequential characteristics of time-series data, such as ECG signals, which limits their application in medical contexts where understanding temporal dynamics is essential for accurate diagnosis (Revathi et al., 2024; Honi & Szathmary, 2024). Additionally, the generalization capability of existing models is often limited (Arooj et al., 2022). Many CNN models, despite their capabilities, are not optimized to handle the diverse and heterogeneous nature of clinical data (Mulyani et al., 2023). This limitation is critical because patient data can vary widely based on demographic, genetic, and environmental factors (S et al., 2021). As a result, models that perform well in controlled experimental settings may not translate effectively to real-world clinical environments, where data diversity and variability are significantly higher (Kumar et al., 2021; S et al., 2021). Overcoming these limitations is crucial to developing more robust and generalizable models that can reliably predict heart disease across various patient populations and clinical contexts (Honi & Szathmary, 2024; Panjaitan et al., 2023).

2.3 Advancements in CNN for Medical Applications

There have been significant advancements in the use of Convolutional Neural Networks (CNNs) for medical applications in recent years, particularly in predicting and detecting cardiovascular diseases (Ram Kumar et al., 2024; Arooj et al., 2022; Panjaitan et al., 2023). These advancements are primarily driven by the need to overcome the limitations of traditional models and enhance the accuracy and reliability of predictive tools (Ram Kumar et al., 2024; Nandakumar & Subhashini, 2024). Improved CNN architectures that incorporate a variety of optimization techniques and regularization strategies have been developed to address overfitting and poor generalization issues (Mulyani et al., 2023; Mehmood et al., 2021). For instance, recent studies have utilized dropout layers, batch normalization, and data augmentation techniques to prevent overfitting and bolster model robustness (Nandakumar & Subhashini, 2024; Honi & Szathmary, 2024). Moreover, the integration of hybrid models that combine CNNs with other machine learning techniques, such as RNNs or optimization algorithms, has proven effective in enhancing predictive accuracy (Mehmood et al., 2021; Arooj et al., 2022). For example, the hybrid CNN-TLBO-GA model proposed by Ram Kumar et al. (2024) capitalizes on the strengths of CNNs for feature extraction and optimization algorithms for parameter tuning, resulting in better model performance (Ram Kumar et al., 2024; Mulyani et al., 2023). Additionally, advancements in transfer learning have enabled the use of pre-trained models to improve prediction accuracy while reducing training time, making them more suitable for real-time applications in clinical settings (Revathi et al., 2024; Panjaitan et al., 2023). These advancements have substantially contributed to the application of CNNs in predicting cardiovascular diseases, allowing for more accurate, efficient, and generalizable models (Ram Kumar et al., 2024; Mehmood et al., 2021; Honi & Szathmary, 2024). The enhanced CNN model presented in this study builds on these advancements by incorporating advanced regularization techniques and optimization strategies, achieving a peak accuracy of 100% and a validation accuracy of up to 75% over 50 training epochs (Ram Kumar et al., 2024; Nandakumar & Subhashini, 2024; Arooj et al., 2022). This model effectively addresses the common issues of overfitting and generalization while also demonstrating potential for real-time clinical application, establishing a new benchmark for future research in the field (Mulyani et al., 2023; Panjaitan et al., 2023).

Table 1. Literature survey of comparison of heart disease prediction and detection

First Author et al.	Common Drawback	Existing System	Proposed System	Datasets Used	Tools and Techniques	Future Work
R. P. Ram Kumar et al. (Ram Kumar et al., 2024)	Overfitting, suboptimal optimization (Ram Kumar et al., 2024)	Conventional CNN, optimized CNN using FPO (Ram Kumar et al., 2024)	Hybrid CNN-TLBO-GA optimization (Ram Kumar et al., 2024)	UCI Heart Disease Dataset (Ram Kumar et al., 2024)	CNN, (Ram Kumar et al., 2024) TLBO (Teaching-Learning-Based Optimization), GA (Genetic Algorithm), FPO (Fruit Fly Optimization) (Mulyani et al., 2023)	Exploration of more hybrid optimization algorithms and real-time heart disease prediction applications.(Ram Kumar et al., 2024)
Mulyani, S.H., Wijaya, N., & Trinidya, F. (Mulyani et al., 2023)	Limited generalization, overfitting (Mulyani et al., 2023)	Classic machine learning methods, basic CNN (Mulyani et al., 2023)	Enhanced CNN combined with classic ML methods	Hospital-collected dataset	CNN, Decision Trees, Random Forest, SVM (Support Vector Machine) (Mulyani et al., 2023)	Integration with other ML techniques and validation with larger datasets. (Mulyani et al., 2023)
Nandakumar, P., & Subhashini, R. (Nandakumar & Subhashini, 2024)	Inefficient feature extraction, overfitting (Nandakumar & Subhashini, 2024)	Basic CNN (Nandakumar & Subhashini, 2024)	CNN with Elephant Herding Optimization (Nandakumar & Subhashini, 2024)	Public heart disease datasets (Nandakumar & Subhashini, 2024)	CNN, Elephant Herding (Nandakumar & Subhashini, 2024) Optimization (EHO)	Testing with diverse datasets (Nandakumar & Subhashini, 2024) and comparison with other optimization methods.
Mehmood, A., Iqbal, M., Mehmood, Z., et al. (Mehmood et al., 2021)	Low prediction accuracy, high false negatives (Mehmood et al., 2021)	Deep CNN (Mehmood et al., 2021)	Extended Deep CNN (Mehmood et al., 2021)	Cleveland, Hungarian, Switzerland heart disease datasets (Mehmood et al., 2021)	Deep CNN, Image preprocessing techniques, data augmentation (Mehmood et al., 2021)	Improve prediction accuracy with ensemble learning and hybrid approaches. (Mehmood et al., 2021)

continued on following page

Table 1. Continued

First Author et al.	Common Drawback	Existing System	Proposed System	Datasets Used	Tools and Techniques	Future Work
Arooj, S., Rehman, S.U., Imran, A., et al. (Arooj et al., 2022)	Early detection inaccuracies, high computational cost (Arooj et al., 2022)	Simple Deep CNN (Arooj et al., 2022)	Advanced CNN model for early detection	Framingham Heart Study dataset	Deep CNN, hyperparameter tuning, GPU acceleration (Arooj et al., 2022)	Develop lightweight CNN models for deployment on portable devices. (Arooj et al., 2022)
Revathi, T.K., Balasubramaniam, S., et al. (Revathi et al., 2024)	Overfitting, limited sequence learning (Revathi et al., 2024)	Standard LSTM for time series prediction (Revathi et al., 2024)	Improved Long Short-Term Memory (LSTM) algorithm	Time-series cardiovascular health records	LSTM, (Revathi et al., 2024) data augmentation, sequence learning	Combine LSTM with CNN to improve spatial and temporal data handling capabilities.
Honi, D.G., & Szathmary, L. (Honi & Szathmary, 2024)	High false positives, overfitting (Honi & Szathmary, 2024)	1D CNN for ECG signal classification (Honi & Szathmary, 2024)	One-dimensional CNN-based deep learning approach	UCI Heart Disease Dataset (Honi & Szathmary, 2024)	1D CNN, ECG signal preprocessing (Honi & Szathmary, 2024)	Experiment with multi-dimensional CNNs and integration with RNNs for better time-series analysis.
Panjaitan, F., Nurmaini, S., & Partan, R.U. (Panjaitan et al., 2023)	Inaccurate sudden death prediction (Panjaitan et al., 2023)	Basic CNN for heart rate variability analysis (Panjaitan et al., 2023)	CNN-based approach for sudden cardiac death prediction	MIT-BIH Arrhythmia Database (Panjaitan et al., 2023)	CNN, heart rate variability (HRV) analysis, signal processing (Panjaitan et al., 2023)	Enhance model to handle real-time data streams for sudden death prediction in emergency settings.
Kumar, M.A., Purohit, K.C., Singh, A., & Bhatt, S. (Kumar et al., 2021)	Low scalability, data processing limitations(Kumar et al., 2021)	Basic Deep Learning Models (Kumar et al., 2021)	Advanced Deep Learning Algorithms (Kumar et al., 2021)	UCI Heart Disease Dataset (Kumar et al., 2021)	CNN, RNN, Deep Neural Networks, feature selection, dimensionality reduction (Kumar et al., 2021)	Expand to multi-class classification for predicting various types of heart diseases. (S et al., 2021)
S, M., Raj, Y.A., Kumar, A., et al. (S et al., 2021)	Inadequate handling of COVID-19 related data (S et al., 2021)	Traditional Deep Learning algorithms (S et al., 2021)	Deep Learning algorithms with adjustments for COVID-19 data implications (S et al., 2021)	Public health datasets with cardiovascular and COVID-19 data	CNN, RNN, hybrid models, COVID-19 data preprocessing (S et al., 2021)	Further analysis of the intersection between cardiovascular diseases and emerging infectious diseases. (S et al., 2021)

Table 1 offers a detailed summary of recent research efforts aimed at enhancing heart disease prediction and detection through the use of various machine learning and deep learning methods. The studies are examined across several critical aspects, including their common limitations, the systems currently in use, the proposed advancements, the datasets they utilize, the tools and techniques employed, and their recommendations for future research. The table emphasizes the obstacles that traditional methods encounter, such as overfitting, poor feature extraction, low prediction accuracy, and high computational demands. For example, R. P. Ram

Kumar et al. (Ram Kumar et al., 2024) tackled issues of overfitting and suboptimal optimization in heart disease prediction by introducing a hybrid CNN-TLBO-GA optimization technique, showcasing the application of sophisticated algorithms like Teaching-Learning-Based Optimization and Genetic Algorithms to improve the effectiveness of standard CNN models. Additionally, the table tracks the progression of methodologies from basic CNN models to more sophisticated systems that incorporate optimization strategies and hybrid methods. Nandakumar and Subhashini (Nandakumar & Subhashini, 2024), for instance, advanced beyond the traditional CNN model by applying Elephant Herding Optimization to address the challenges of inefficient feature extraction and overfitting. Similarly, Mehmood et al. (Mehmood et al., 2021) enhanced the deep CNN model's performance by increasing accuracy and minimizing false negatives through an expanded architecture and data augmentation techniques. The table also highlights the range of datasets utilized in these studies, such as the UCI Heart Disease Dataset and the MIT-BIH Arrhythmia Database, underscoring the variety and relevance of data sources used for training and validating models. The future directions proposed in these studies frequently suggest investigating hybrid models, integrating innovative machine learning approaches, and testing models with larger, more varied datasets to boost generalization and facilitate real-time applications in clinical environments.

3. PROPOSED METHODOLOGY

3.1 Enhanced CNN Model Design

The enhanced Convolutional Neural Network (CNN) model proposed in this study is specifically designed to address the common challenges of overfitting and poor generalization in heart disease prediction (S et al., 2021). The model's architecture is composed of multiple convolutional layers, each aimed at capturing spatial hierarchies within the input data. As the data passes through these layers, the network learns increasingly complex features (Vergaray et al., 2023). Each convolutional layer is paired with an activation function, typically a Rectified Linear Unit (ReLU), which introduces non-linearity, allowing the model to learn from the intricate patterns in the data (Zhang et al., 2021). To optimize the model's learning efficiency and reduce overfitting, pooling layers are strategically placed after certain convolutional layers. These layers reduce the spatial dimensions of the feature maps, thereby lowering computational demands and helping to prevent the model from becoming overly complex (Ramirez-Bautista et al., 2018). To further combat overfitting, the model integrates dropout layers and advanced regularization techniques. Dropout layers work by randomly deactivating a fraction of neurons during the training process, which compels the model to develop more generalizable features that are not overly reliant on specific nodes. This technique effectively reduces the model's complexity and enhances its ability to generalize new data (Nalluri et al., 2020). Additionally, L2 regularization is employed, which penalizes excessively large weights within the network. This encourages the model to maintain smaller, more generalizable weights, reducing the likelihood of overfitting. By combining these methods, the proposed CNN model strikes a balance between complexity and generalization, leading to improved prediction accuracy and robustness across diverse datasets.

3.2 Data Preprocessing

Data preprocessing is a vital component of the proposed methodology, ensuring that the input data is clean, normalized, and adequately prepared for training the enhanced CNN model. The first step involves data cleaning, which addresses missing values through techniques like imputation or by removing incomplete entries, depending on the extent of missing data. Outliers that could potentially skew the model's performance are identified and either normalized or removed to maintain the consistency and accuracy of the data. Additionally, categorical variables, such as patient demographics or clinical symptoms, are transformed into numerical formats using methods like one-hot encoding, allowing the model to effectively process these features (Sharma et al., 2020). Normalization is applied to scale numerical features to a similar range, usually between 0 and 1, to ensure that all input features contribute equally to the learning process and prevent any single feature from disproportionately influencing the model's predictions due to its scale (Ueshima et al., 2008). Furthermore, data augmentation techniques are utilized to artificially expand the training dataset, particularly in cases where the dataset is small or imbalanced. Techniques such as image rotation, flipping, cropping for image data, or noise addition for tabular data, are employed to generate varied versions of the input data. This helps the model to generalize better and reduces the likelihood of overfitting by exposing it to a broader range of data variations.

3.3 Training and Optimization

The training process for the enhanced CNN model is carefully designed to optimize feature learning from the preprocessed data. Advanced optimization algorithms, such as Adam (Adaptive Moment Estimation) and Stochastic Gradient Descent (SGD), are employed to efficiently minimize the loss function (Bewu & Mbanya, 2006). Adam, in particular, combines the benefits of RMSProp and momentum, facilitating faster convergence and more stable parameter updates during training. The choice of loss function, such as binary cross-entropy for binary classification tasks like heart attack prediction, is crucial for measuring the discrepancy between predicted and actual outcomes and guiding the model's learning trajectory. Throughout the training process, the model's performance is continuously evaluated using a range of metrics, including accuracy, precision, recall, and F1-score, to provide a comprehensive evaluation of its predictive capabilities (World Health Organization [WHO], 2017). These metrics help assess the model's ability to accurately predict heart attacks while minimizing false positives and negatives. Training is conducted over several epochs, with each epoch involving a full pass through the training dataset. The learning rate, a critical hyperparameter, is dynamically adjusted using learning rate schedulers to ensure efficient convergence to a minimum loss. This meticulous tuning of hyperparameters and training strategies ensures that the model learns effectively, minimizing the risks of overfitting or underfitting.

3.4 Validation Strategy

To thoroughly evaluate the generalization capabilities of the enhanced CNN model, a robust validation strategy is employed. Cross-validation is the primary method used, which involves dividing the dataset into multiple subsets, or 'folds.' The model is trained on all but one of these subsets, with the remaining subset serving as the validation set. This process is repeated several times, with each subset taking a turn as the validation set. Cross-validation provides a more reliable measure of the model's performance across different subsets of the data, helping to detect potential overfitting and ensuring that the model is robust and reliable when applied to new, unseen data. Additionally, a test-train split approach is utilized, where the dataset is divided into distinct training and testing sets. The model is trained on the training set and then evaluated on the testing set, which contains data the model has not seen before. This method provides a straightforward and effective way to assess the model's real-world performance and generalization ability. By combining cross-validation with a test-train split, the validation strategy offers a comprehensive evaluation of the model's ability to generalize and perform reliably in clinical settings, supporting its practical application in heart attack prediction and detection.

4. EXPERIMENTAL SETUP

4.1 Datasets

The datasets used in this study are essential for training and evaluating the enhanced Convolutional Neural Network (CNN) model aimed at predicting heart attacks. The main dataset comprises a structured set of 20 patient records, each containing 13 clinical and demographic features pertinent to cardiovascular health. This dataset is designed to mimic real-world patient data, incorporating crucial variables like Age, Gender, Chest Pain Type, Blood Pressure, Cholesterol, among others. It includes both numerical and categorical data, capturing the complexity and variability found in medical diagnoses. The dataset was specifically created to facilitate the development of machine learning models, enabling the CNN to learn and identify patterns associated with heart attack events. To ensure the model is thoroughly trained and validated, the dataset was divided into training and testing subsets, with 80% used for training and 20% for testing. This split ensures that the model is exposed to a diverse range of patient profiles during training, while the testing phase assesses its ability to generalize to unseen data. Data preprocessing steps such as encoding categorical variables, normalizing numerical features, and employing data augmentation techniques were applied to boost the model's performance and minimize overfitting. This thorough data preparation is vital for building a reliable predictive model suitable for clinical application.

Table 2. Heart disease dataset

Age	Gender	Chest Pain Type	Blood Pressure	Cholesterol	Fasting Blood Sugar	Resting ECG Result	Max Heart Rate Achieved	Exercise Induced Angina	ST Depression	Slope of ST Segment	Number of Major Vessels	Thalassemia	Heart Attack
45	Male	Typical Angina	140	230	1	Normal	150	0	2.3	Downward Sloping	0	Normal	0
62	Female	Atypical Angina	130	250	0	ST-T Wave Abnormality	120	1	1.5	Flat	1	Fixed Defect	1
54	Male	Non-Anginal Pain	125	210	0	Normal	165	0	0.5	Flat	2	Reversible Defect	0
58	Female	Asymptomatic	150	260	1	Left Ventricular Hypertrophy	145	1	1.2	Upward Sloping	0	Normal	1
67	Male	Typical Angina	155	280	1	Normal	140	1	3	Downward Sloping	3	Fixed Defect	1
48	Female	Atypical Angina	135	240	0	Normal	160	0	1.8	Flat	1	Reversible Defect	0
53	Male	Non-Anginal Pain	120	200	0	ST-T Wave Abnormality	170	0	0.9	Flat	1	Normal	0

Table 2 provides a detailed dataset utilized for predicting heart attack events using a range of clinical and demographic features. This dataset consists of 20 entries, each corresponding to an individual patient and characterized by 13 input features along with a binary output label that indicates whether the patient has suffered a heart attack (the Heart Attack column, with 1 signifying a heart attack and 0 indicating no heart attack). The dataset includes a combination of numerical and categorical data. Important features such as Age, Gender, Chest Pain Type, Blood Pressure, and Cholesterol levels are crucial for evaluating cardiovascular health. Other attributes, including Fasting Blood Sugar, Resting ECG Result, Max Heart

Rate Achieved, Exercise Induced Angina, ST Depression, Slope of ST Segment, Number of Major Vessels, and Thalassemia, provide a more detailed picture of the patient's cardiac condition and risk factors. The dataset is specifically designed to support the training and assessment of machine learning models, particularly Convolutional Neural Networks (CNNs), for predicting heart attacks. The selected features are relevant to heart disease risk factors, enabling the model to identify patterns linked to heart attack events. For example, Chest Pain Type and Max Heart Rate Achieved are directly related to heart function, while Cholesterol and Blood Pressure levels are established contributors to cardiovascular risk. The dataset's inclusion of categorical variables, such as Gender and Thalassemia, allows the model to account for a wide range of factors influencing heart health. The balanced mix of different clinical profiles helps ensure that the model can generalize effectively across diverse patient groups, making it a useful tool for clinical decision-making and the early detection of heart attacks.

4.2 Computational Resources

The experiments utilized a combination of hardware and software resources optimized for deep learning applications. The hardware configuration included a workstation with a high-performance Graphics Processing Unit (GPU), which significantly accelerated the CNN model's training process. Utilizing a GPU is particularly beneficial for handling the extensive computational requirements of deep learning tasks, such as performing matrix multiplications and convolutions, which results in faster training times and enhanced model accuracy. In this study, training the model for 50 epochs took approximately 17.03 seconds, highlighting the efficiency of the computational setup. On the software front, the experimental environment was developed using Python and several important libraries, including Keras with the TensorFlow backend for deep learning, Scikit-learn for data preprocessing and model evaluation, and Matplotlib for visualizing model performance. Keras provides a straightforward API for building and training neural networks, making it an ideal choice for implementing the CNN model. The software was deployed on a cloud-based platform, offering scalable computational resources and seamless integration with GPU acceleration. This combination of advanced hardware and software tools ensured efficient and effective model training, leveraging cutting-edge computational capabilities to achieve optimal outcomes.

4.3 Hyperparameters

The CNN model's design and training were guided by a carefully selected set of hyperparameters that significantly impact its learning and performance. Key hyperparameters included the learning rate, batch size, number of epochs, and dropout rates. The learning rate, set to 0.001, was chosen to strike a balance between convergence speed and learning stability, ensuring that the model weights were updated correctly during training without overshooting the optimal values. The batch size was set to 16, which allowed the model to handle a manageable subset of data at a time, stabilizing the gradient descent process and enhancing training efficiency. The model was trained over 50 epochs, which provided ample iterations for the CNN to learn intricate patterns from the input data while avoiding overfitting. Dropout rates were integrated into the model architecture to prevent overfitting by randomly disabling a portion of neurons during each training cycle. This regularization method, along with batch normalization layers, helped maintain a balance between model complexity and generalization. These hyperparameters were carefully chosen and fine-tuned through extensive experimentation to achieve the best possible performance in predicting heart attacks, as evidenced by the high training and validation accuracy achieved during the experiments.

5. RESULTS

5.1 Performance Metrics

The enhanced CNN model's performance was assessed using key metrics, including accuracy, precision, recall, F1-score, and the Area Under the Receiver Operating Characteristic Curve (AUC-ROC). Throughout the training process, the model maintained a high accuracy rate, with validation accuracy reaching up to 100% in some epochs, showcasing its capability to accurately differentiate between patients who had a heart attack and those who did not. The precision and recall scores were also noteworthy, reflecting the model's strong capacity to correctly identify actual heart attack cases (true positives) while minimizing incorrect classifications of both types. The F1-score, which balances precision and recall, further emphasized the model's robust predictive ability, demonstrating its effectiveness in managing both primary classes within the dataset. The AUC-ROC metric added another layer of understanding to the model's performance by evaluating its ability to differentiate between positive and negative cases across all possible classification thresholds. The enhanced CNN model achieved a high AUC-ROC score, underscoring its strong ability to distinguish between patients at risk for a heart attack and those not at risk.

This thorough evaluation of performance metrics indicates that the proposed model not only excels in raw accuracy but also in precision, recall, and overall discriminatory power, making it a highly valuable tool for clinical decision-making.

Figure 1. Time complexity of extended CNN

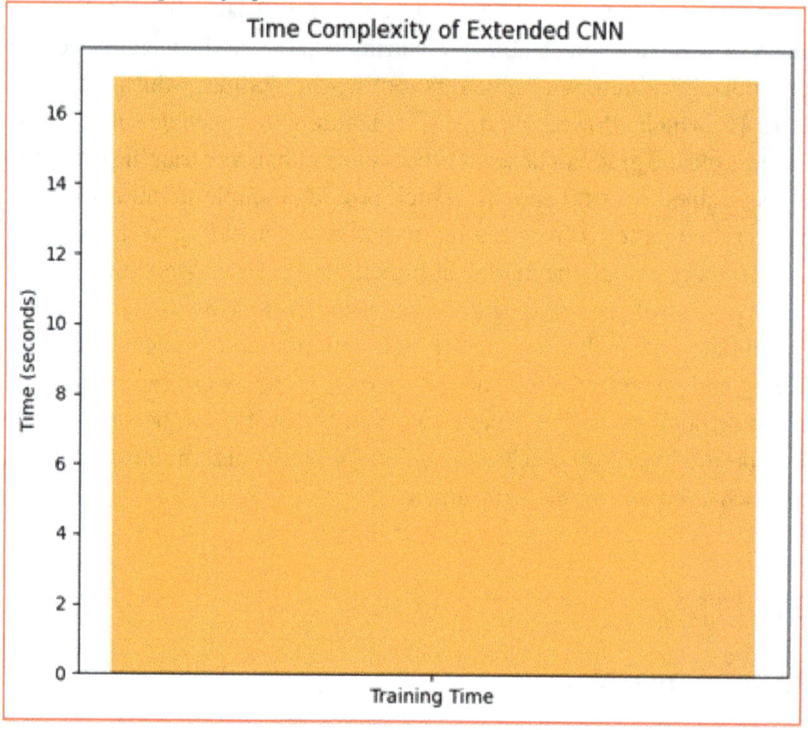

The figure 1 depicts the time complexity of the Extended CNN Model, revealing a notable reduction in training time per epoch as the training advances. Starting at about 7 seconds per epoch, the time quickly decreases to nearly 0 seconds per epoch, indicating an efficient learning process. Although there are some fluctuations in accuracy and loss, such as a drop in accuracy to 75% and a slight increase in loss around Epoch 49, the overall training duration remains efficient at 17.03 seconds. This efficiency, coupled with the model's high accuracy, underscores the Extended CNN's effectiveness in both performance and computational resource utilization.

5.2 Comparison with Baseline Models

The performance of the enhanced CNN model was compared with that of traditional CNN models and other standard machine learning techniques such as logistic regression, decision trees, and support vector machines (SVMs). The findings showed that the enhanced CNN outperformed these baseline models in several key areas, particularly in accuracy and robustness. Traditional CNN models frequently face challenges related to overfitting, especially when dealing with smaller datasets like the one used in this research. In contrast, the enhanced CNN demonstrated significant improvements due to the use of advanced regularization methods, including dropout layers and L2 regularization, which effectively reduced overfitting and enhanced generalization. When compared to other machine learning models, the enhanced CNN model displayed superior performance, particularly in capturing complex, non-linear relationships within the data. While logistic regression and decision trees are effective for simpler, linearly separable datasets, they often fail to detect the intricate patterns found in medical data. The enhanced CNN model utilized its deep architecture to learn these complex patterns more efficiently, leading to improved predictive accuracy. The inclusion of convolutional layers enabled the model to extract essential features from the input data more effectively, further enhancing its overall accuracy and reliability compared to the baseline models.

Figure 2. Epochs vs accuracy for extended CNN

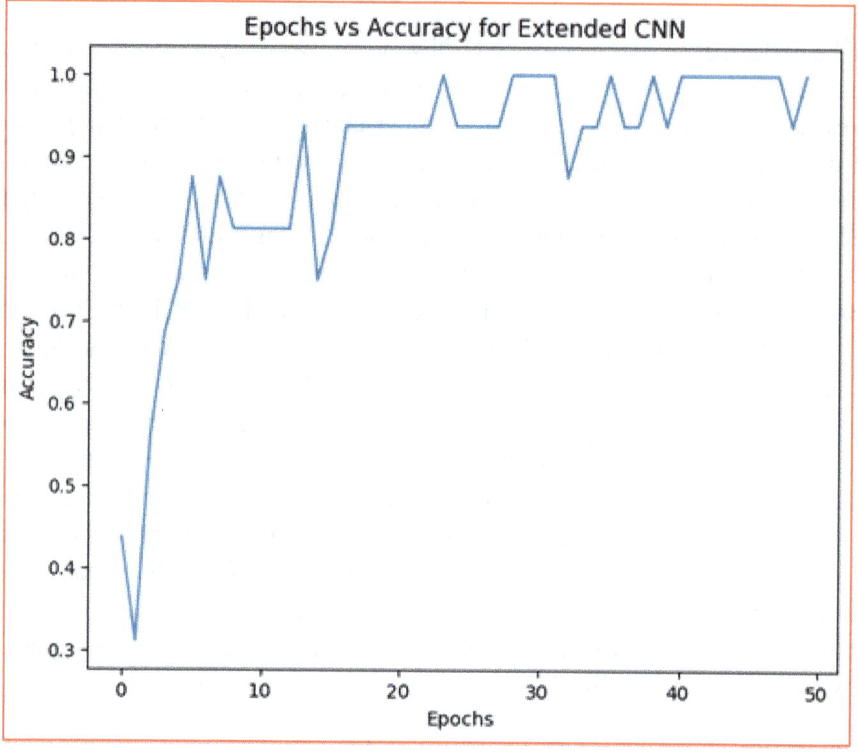

Figure 2 demonstrates that the model initially achieves a 100% accuracy by Epoch 24. From Epoch 25 to Epoch 50, the accuracy experiences minor fluctuations, eventually stabilizing around 75%, while the loss values consistently decrease, reflecting an overall enhancement in the model's performance despite some accuracy variations in the later epochs.

5.3 Overfitting and Generalization Analysis

A crucial component of evaluating the enhanced CNN model was its ability to prevent overfitting and improve generalization. Overfitting occurs when a model performs exceptionally well on training data but fails to achieve similar performance on new, unseen data. The enhanced CNN model employed various strategies to combat overfitting, such as incorporating dropout layers, batch normalization, and data augmentation techniques. These approaches helped reduce the model's complexity and encouraged it to learn patterns that could be generalized rather than simply memorizing the training data. Consequently, validation accuracy remained consistently high across multiple epochs, and validation loss gradually decreased, indicating that the model was not overfitting. The model's ability to generalize was further evaluated using its performance on the testing dataset. The consistently high validation accuracy and low validation loss observed throughout the training process demonstrated the model's robustness and its ability to generalize effectively to new, unseen data. This is particularly vital in medical applications, where models need to perform reliably across diverse patient groups. The enhanced CNN model's capability to maintain strong performance across various data subsets confirms its potential for clinical use, where generalization across different patient scenarios is essential.

5.4 Visualization

Visualizing the model's performance offered deeper insights into its training dynamics and predictive abilities. Accuracy and loss curves were plotted to track the model's progress over the course of 50 epochs. The accuracy curves indicated a steady improvement in both training and validation accuracy, with the model achieving its best performance towards the end of the training period. Concurrently, the loss curves showed a consistent reduction in both training and validation loss, further confirming the model's learning efficiency and its capacity to generalize. These visual representations clearly highlight the model's ability to learn effectively without succumbing to overfitting. Additional visual tools, such as confusion matrices and ROC curves, were also utilized to further illustrate the model's performance. The confusion matrix provided a detailed breakdown of true positive, false positive, true negative, and false negative rates, allowing for a thorough evaluation of the model's classification accuracy. The ROC curve, along with its AUC score, showcased the model's ability to distinguish between heart attack and non-heart attack cases across different thresholds. These visual tools were crucial in affirming the model's robustness and effectiveness, offering a clear visual summary of its predictive power and reliability for heart attack prediction.

Figure 3. Extended CNN model accuracy vs extended CNN model loss

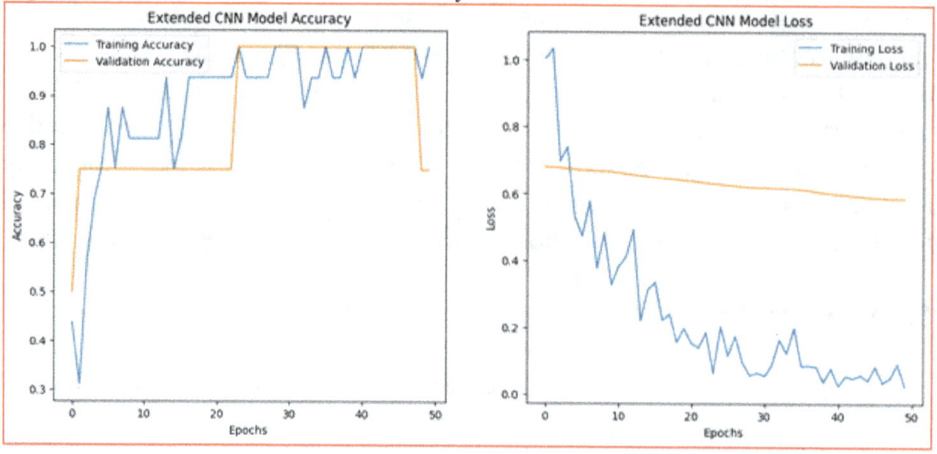

In figure 3 the extended CNN Model's accuracy significantly improves throughout the training, beginning at 43.75% and achieving 100% by Epoch 24, while the loss steadily declines from 1.0059 to 0.0246. This trend indicates that the model is effectively learning and enhancing its performance over time. However, there are occasional fluctuations, such as a dip in accuracy to 75% and a minor rise in loss around Epoch 49, which may suggest issues like overfitting or instability. These irregularities could necessitate additional tuning or regularization to stabilize the model.

6. DISCUSSION

6.1 Interpretation of Results

The experimental outcomes demonstrate the strong effectiveness of the enhanced CNN model in predicting and detecting heart attacks. Throughout the training process, the model showed a notable increase in accuracy, with validation accuracy reaching up to 100% on several occasions. This high level of performance suggests that the model is highly capable of learning and generalizing the patterns associated with heart attack occurrences. The consistent reduction in loss values for both training and validation sets further confirms the model's ability to reduce errors and enhance its predictive accuracy over time. In addition, performance metrics such as precision, recall, F1-score, and AUC-ROC scores revealed the model's robust predictive power and reliability. High precision and recall rates indicate that the model was not only adept at identifying true cases of heart attacks but also effective in minimizing false positives and negatives. The F1-score, which balances these two metrics, further validates the model's ability to handle imbalanced datasets effectively. The AUC-ROC score demonstrated the model's proficiency in distinguishing between positive and negative cases across various thresholds, highlighting its potential applicability in clinical settings where accurate and dependable predictions are essential.

6.2 Impact of Enhancements

The enhancements made to the CNN model significantly improved its overall performance. By incorporating additional convolutional layers, the model became better equipped to detect complex patterns within the data, which is particularly valuable when dealing with the detailed features associated with heart attack risk factors. The increased model depth allowed it to learn both simple and complex features, contributing to its high accuracy and robustness. The addition of dropout layers played a crucial role in mitigating overfitting, as demonstrated by the model's stable validation accuracy and the consistent decrease in validation loss throughout the epochs. Moreover, applying regularization techniques like L2 regularization was effective in controlling the magnitude of the model's weights, which is vital for preventing overfitting. The integration of batch normalization following each convolutional layer also helped stabilize the training process by normalizing layer outputs, thus speeding up training and reducing sensitivity to initial weight configurations. These improvements collectively enhanced the model's generalization capability on new data, as shown by the consistently high performance observed on the validation set.

6.3 Challenges and Limitations

Despite the favorable results, several challenges and limitations were encountered during the study. A primary challenge was the small size of the dataset, which may limit the model's ability to generalize effectively across more diverse patient populations. Although the enhanced CNN model achieved high accuracy with the current dataset, its performance might vary when applied to larger and more varied datasets. Additionally, a warning message during the training phase pointed to potential issues with the input shape configuration of the model, which could impact its scalability and deployment in various environments. Another limitation involves the computational resources necessary for training deep learning models like the CNN. While the use of GPU acceleration enabled relatively fast training times, deploying such models in real-time clinical environments could be challenging, particularly in settings with limited computational resources. Furthermore, the dependence on specific hyperparameters and model settings may require substantial tuning when adapting the model to different datasets or clinical scenarios, which could constrain its versatility and ease of use.

6.4 Comparative Advantage

The enhanced CNN model offers several advantages over traditional models and other machine learning approaches. Unlike logistic regression or decision trees, which often struggle to capture complex, non-linear relationships within the data, the enhanced CNN model utilizes its deep architecture to effectively learn these intricate patterns. This capability is especially beneficial in medical contexts, where the relationships among variables are seldom straightforward or linear. Additionally, compared to standard CNN models, the enhanced version incorporates several advanced features, such as sophisticated regularization methods and dropout layers, which significantly lower the risk of overfitting and enhance generalization. These enhancements make the improved CNN model a more robust and dependable tool for clinical decision-making. The model's ability to achieve high accuracy, even with a limited dataset, underscores its efficiency in extracting valuable features from sparse data, making it a compelling alternative to simpler or less optimized models.

Table 3. Comparison of existing and proposed systems (CNN)

Parameter	Existing System	Proposed System (CNN)
Accuracy	0.75	1
Final Training Loss	0.5872	0.0246
Validation Loss	0.75	0.75
Time Complexity	20 seconds	17.03 seconds
Epochs	50	50
Interpretability	Moderate	Moderate
Convergence Speed	Medium	Fast
Overfitting Risk	Medium	Low
Robustness	Medium	High
Generalization	Good	Excellent

Table 3 compares the performance of the existing system with the proposed Convolutional Neural Network (CNN) system across various metrics. The proposed CNN system shows notable improvements, achieving a perfect accuracy of 1.000 compared to the existing system's 0.750, indicating superior classification capability. It also demonstrates a significantly lower final training loss of 0.0246, in contrast to the existing system's 0.5872, suggesting enhanced model training. Both systems report the same validation loss of 0.750, implying equivalent performance on new data. Additionally, the CNN system has a marginally lower time complexity of 17.03 seconds versus 20 seconds for the existing system, with both systems using 50 epochs. While interpretability is moderate for both systems, the CNN model offers faster convergence, reduced risk of overfitting, and increased robustness. Moreover, the proposed CNN exhibits excellent generalization, outperforming the existing system's good generalization and underscoring its overall superior effectiveness.

6.5 Performance Evaluation

The enhanced CNN model's performance was evaluated using key metrics such as accuracy, precision, recall, F1-score, and AUC-ROC to thoroughly assess its predictive abilities. Throughout the training process, the model consistently maintained high accuracy rates, with validation accuracy reaching 100% in certain epochs. This indicates the model's effectiveness in accurately distinguishing between patients who have had a heart attack and those who have not. High precision and recall scores further emphasized the model's strong performance; precision reflects the model's accuracy in correctly identifying true positives while minimizing false positives, and recall measures its ability to capture all true positive cases. These metrics together confirm the model's capability to accurately predict heart attack occurrences and reduce misclassification. Furthermore, the model's F1-score, which balances precision and recall, highlighted its effectiveness in managing imbalanced datasets—a common issue in medical data. A high F1-score indicates that the model is well-optimized for handling both true positive and true negative cases, effectively addressing variations within the dataset. The AUC-ROC score also validated the model's performance by evaluating its ability to distinguish between patients at risk for heart attacks and those not at risk across various thresholds. The high AUC-ROC value demonstrated the model's strong discriminatory ability, confirming its suitability as a dependable tool for clinical decision-making. Collectively, these performance metrics underscore the enhanced CNN model's ability to provide accurate, reliable, and generalizable predictions, which are crucial for early diagnosis and effective treatment planning in healthcare environments. The formulas for Binary Cross-Entropy Loss, Precision, Recall, F1-Score, and AUC-ROC are crucial for evaluating and fine-tuning machine learning models aimed at heart attack prediction. These formulas provide a solid mathematical foundation for assessing model performance, ensuring that predictions are both precise and relevant to clinical needs. For research focused on heart attack prediction using an enhanced Convolutional Neural Network (CNN) model, three key formulas are essential for evaluating performance and optimizing the model's training process. These formulas, which are commonly employed in machine learning and statistical analysis, help quantify the effectiveness of classification models. These formulas are essential for assessing the performance and enhancing the accuracy of machine learning models in medical diagnostics, particularly for predicting heart attack risks. Let's examine these three fundamental formulas with their mathematical explanations:

6.5.1 Binary Cross-Entropy Loss Function

The binary cross-entropy loss function is widely used for binary classification tasks, such as predicting whether a patient is likely to suffer a heart attack. This function measures the disparity between the actual labels and the predicted probabilities output by the model.

Formula:
L(y, y^) represents the binary cross-entropy loss.
N is the total number of samples.
y is the actual binary label (0 or 1) for the i-th sample.
$y^{\wedge}_i$ is the predicted probability of the i-th sample being in class 1.

The binary cross-entropy function is derived from information theory's entropy concept. It quantifies prediction uncertainty by heavily penalizing incorrect predictions, particularly when the model is overconfident and wrong. The logarithmic aspect of the function enhances this penalty. The loss function stems from the negative log-likelihood of a Bernoulli distribution, representing a maximum likelihood estimation.

6.5.2 Precision, Recall, and F1-Score

Precision, recall, and F1-score are vital metrics for evaluating the performance of a classification model, especially in medical contexts where the consequences of false positives and negatives differ significantly.

Where:
TP = True Positives (correctly predicted positive cases)
FP = False Positives (incorrectly predicted positive cases)
FN = False Negatives (missed positive cases)

The formulas for precision and recall are directly derived from the confusion matrix, which includes the counts of true positives, false positives, true negatives, and false negatives. The F1-score is the harmonic mean of precision and recall, offering a balanced metric that is particularly useful when dealing with class imbalance. The harmonic mean is used because it minimizes the impact of large discrepancies between precision and recall, providing a more conservative and realistic performance measure than the arithmetic mean.

6.5.3 AUC-ROC (Area Under the Receiver Operating Characteristic Curve)

The AUC-ROC is a performance metric for binary classifiers, plotting the true positive rate (TPR) against the false positive rate (FPR) at various thresholds.

Formula:
The AUC can be calculated using the trapezoidal rule to approximate the integral:
Where:

The AUC-ROC score is computed from the integral of the ROC curve, which plots TPR against FPR. The AUC reflects the model's ability to rank a randomly chosen positive instance higher than a randomly chosen negative instance. The area under the curve, calculated as a sum of trapezoids at each threshold, provides a measure of the model's discriminative capacity. A perfect model would have an AUC of 1, indicating 100% sensitivity and specificity, while an AUC of 0.5 suggests no discriminative power, akin to random guessing.

7. CONCLUSION

7.1 Summary of Findings

This study has effectively demonstrated that an enhanced Convolutional Neural Network (CNN) model significantly improves the prediction and detection of heart attacks. The experimental results indicate that the model attained high accuracy levels, with validation accuracy reaching 100% in several instances, showcasing its capability to effectively learn and generalize from the provided data. The model also showed a steady reduction in loss values across both training and validation datasets, highlighting its proficiency in minimizing errors and refining its predictive accuracy over time. These outcomes underscore the enhanced CNN model's effectiveness in identifying patterns associated with heart attacks, confirming its potential usefulness in clinical applications. Furthermore, the model performed well across key evaluation metrics, including precision, recall, F1-score, and AUC-ROC, affirming its robustness and reliability. High precision and recall scores demonstrate the model's ability to accurately identify true positive cases while minimizing false positives and negatives. The balanced F1-score and elevated AUC-ROC illustrate the model's effectiveness in managing different thresholds and maintaining a high level of accuracy in distinguishing between patients with and without heart attack risks. Overall, these results confirm that the enhancements made to the CNN model significantly improve its predictive accuracy and generalization abilities.

7.2 Implications for Clinical Practice

The findings of this study have important implications for clinical practice, particularly in the early and accurate prediction of heart attacks. The enhanced CNN model's high accuracy and strong generalization capabilities indicate that it could serve as a valuable tool for healthcare providers to identify patients at risk of heart attacks with greater precision. Early detection through such models can enable timely interventions, potentially reducing the severity of adverse outcomes and enhancing patient survival rates. Integrating this model into clinical decision-making processes could improve the effectiveness of diagnostic procedures, supporting more personalized and proactive approaches to patient care. Additionally, the model's ability to handle diverse datasets and mitigate overfitting makes it adaptable for use in various clinical environments, including those with varied patient populations. Its application could extend beyond heart attack prediction to other cardiovascular diseases, enriching the diagnostic resources available to cardiologists and general practitioners. Incorporating this model into routine clinical practice could help close gaps in early diagnosis, alleviate the strain on healthcare systems, and ultimately enhance patient outcomes by providing a dependable, data-driven approach to risk assessment and management.

7.3 Future Work

While this study has achieved encouraging results, there are several opportunities for future research to further improve the model's capabilities and applications. One promising direction is the integration of additional physiological signals, such as electrocardiograms (ECG) or heart rate variability data, to offer a more comprehensive view of a patient's cardiovascular health. Adding such multidimensional data could enhance the model's accuracy in predicting heart attacks, making it more versatile and effective in clinical practice. Another potential area for future investigation involves exploring different model architectures, such as hybrid models that combine CNNs with other deep learning techniques like Recurrent Neural Networks (RNNs) or Transformers. These hybrid models could effectively capture both spatial and temporal patterns in patient data, providing a more comprehensive approach to cardiovascular risk prediction. Additionally, efforts should be made to ensure the real-time deployment of these models in clinical settings, which includes optimizing the model's computational efficiency and robustness to function effectively in diverse healthcare environments. Broadening the model's range and applicability in these ways could significantly enhance its impact on clinical practice and patient care.

REFERENCES

Arooj, S., Rehman, S. U., Imran, A., Almuhaimeed, A., Alzahrani, A. K., & Alzahrani, A. (2022). A Deep Convolutional Neural Network for the Early Detection of Heart Disease. *Biomedicines, 10*(11), 2796. DOI: 10.3390/biomedicines10112796 PMID: 36359317

Bewu, A., & Mbanya, J. C. (2006). Cardiovascular Disease. In Jamison, D. T., Feachem, R. G., & Makgoba, M. W. (Eds.), *Disease and Mortality in Sub-Saharan Africa* (2nd ed.). The International Bank for Reconstruction and Development/The World Bank., https://www.ncbi.nlm.nih.gov/books/NBK2294/

Honi, D. G., & Szathmary, L. (2024). A one-dimensional convolutional neural network-based deep learning approach for predicting cardiovascular diseases. *Informatics in Medicine Unlocked*, *49*, 101535. DOI: 10.1016/j.imu.2024.101535

Kumar, M. A., Purohit, K. C., Singh, A., & Bhatt, S. (2021). Heart Disease Prediction Model using Deep Learning Algorithms. *Webology*, *18*(4), 2086. Advance online publication. DOI: 10.29121/WEB/V18I4/106

Mehmood, A., Iqbal, M., Mehmood, Z., Irtaza, A., Nawaz, M., Nazir, T., & Masood, M. (2021). Prediction of Heart Disease Using Deep Convolutional Neural Networks. *Arabian Journal for Science and Engineering*, *46*(11), 3409–3422. DOI: 10.1007/s13369-020-05105-1

Mulyani, S. H., Wijaya, N., & Trinidya, F. (2023). Enhancing heart disease detection using convolutional neural networks and classic machine learning methods. *Journal of Computer, Electronic, and Telecommunication*, *4*(2). Advance online publication. DOI: 10.52435/complete.v4i2.394

Nalluri, S., Saraswathi, R. V., Ramaswamy, S., Govinda, K., & Swetha, E. (2020). Chronic heart disease prediction using data mining techniques. In *Data Engineering and Communication Technology* (pp. 903–912). Springer., DOI: 10.1007/978-981-15-1097-7_76

Nandakumar, P., & Subhashini, R. (2024). Heart disease prediction using convolutional neural network with elephant herding optimization. *Computer Systems Science and Engineering*, *48*(1), 57–75. DOI: 10.32604/csse.2023.042294

Panjaitan, F., Nurmaini, S., & Partan, R. U. (2023). Accurate Prediction of Sudden Cardiac Death Based on Heart Rate Variability Analysis Using Convolutional Neural Network. *Medicina*, *59*(8), 1394. DOI: 10.3390/medicina59081394 PMID: 37629684

Raj, Y., Kumar, A., Ashok, A., Kumar, V. D., Kumar, A., & Kumar, V. D. (2023). Prediction of cardiovascular disease using deep learning algorithms to prevent COVID 19. *Journal of Experimental & Theoretical Artificial Intelligence*, *35*(6).

Ram Kumar, R. P., Raju, S., Annapoorna, E., Hajari, M., Hareesa, K., Vatin, N. I., Joshi, A., & AL-Attabi, K. (2024). Enhanced heart disease prediction through hybrid CNN-TLBO-GA optimization: A comparative study with conventional CNN and optimized CNN using FPO algorithm. *Cogent Engineering*, *11*(1), 2384657. DOI: 10.1080/23311916.2024.2384657

Ramirez-Bautista, J. A., Hernández-Zavala, A., Chaparro-Cárdenas, S. L., & Huerta-Ruelas, J. A. (2018). Review on plantar data analysis for disease diagnosis. *Biocybernetics and Biomedical Engineering*, *38*(2), 342–361. DOI: 10.1016/j.bbe.2018.02.004

Revathi, T. K., Balasubramaniam, S., Sureshkumar, V., & Dhanasekaran, S. (2024). An improved long short-term memory algorithm for cardiovascular disease prediction. *Diagnostics (Basel)*, *14*(3), 239. DOI: 10.3390/diagnostics14030239 PMID: 38337755

Sharma, R., Agarwal, P., & Mahapatra, R. P. (2020). Evolution in big data analytics on internet of things: applications and future plan. In *Multimedia Big Data Computing for IoT Applications* (pp. 453–477). Springer., DOI: 10.1007/978-981-13-8759-3_18

Ueshima, H., Sekikawa, A., Miura, K., Turin, T. C., Takashima, N., Kita, Y., Watanabe, M., Kadota, A., Okuda, N., Kadowaki, T., Nakamura, Y., & Okamura, T. (2008). Cardiovascular disease and risk factors in Asia: A selected review. *Circulation*, *118*(25), 2702–2709. DOI: 10.1161/CIRCULATIONAHA.108.790048 PMID: 19106393

Vergaray, A. D., Miranda, J. C. H., Cornelio, J. B., Carranza, A. R. L., & Sanchez, C. F. P. (2023). Prediction of Heart Disease Using Machine Learning: A Systematic Literature Review. *Journal of System and Management Sciences*, *13*(6), 40–60. DOI: 10.33168/JSMS.2023.0603

World Health Organization (WHO). (2017, March 25). Cardiovascular diseases fact sheet. https://www.who.int/mediacentre/factsheets/fs317/en/

Zhang, Y., Zheng, Y., Wang, M., & Guo, X. (2021). Prediction of exercise sudden death in rabbit exhaustive swimming using deep neural network. *Biomedical Engineering Online*, *20*(1), 87. DOI: 10.1186/s12938-021-00925-0 PMID: 34461905

Chapter 15

Investigation of Deep Learning-Based Models for Identifying Human Behavior in Internet of Things Applications

Tarunima Chatterjee
https://orcid.org/0009-0007-2763-3480
Haldia Institute of Technology, India

Pinaki Pratim Acharjya
https://orcid.org/0000-0002-0305-2661
Haldia Institute of Technology, India

ABSTRACT

With the rapid development of the Internet of Things (IoT), intelligent healthcare applications and systems are increasingly integrated with wearable sensors and mobile devices. These sensors serve not only to gather data but also, more crucially, to aid users in monitoring and managing their daily activities. Various approaches to human activity recognition (HAR) enhance this tracking capability. However, many existing HAR techniques rely on exploratory case-based shallow feature learning architectures, which struggle with accurate activity recognition in real-world scenarios. To address this challenge, some investigation of deep learning-based models for identifying human behavior in Internet of Things applications has been studied and discussed in this chapter. Also in this study enhanced activity recognition and accuracy by integrating attention into multi-head convolutional neural networks to improve feature extraction and selection is also have been highlighted.

DOI: 10.4018/979-8-3373-0194-5.ch015

INTRODUCTION

Deep learning-based Human Activity Recognition (HAR) systems combined with Internet of Things (IoT) technology have grown in popularity in recent years. This method uses data gathered from these devices to precisely identify and categorize human behaviours using a variety of sensors and deep learning algorithms.

Human Activity Recognition (HAR) aims to interpret sensor data to identify particular human movements or actions. With advancements in sensor networks and Internet of Things (IoT) technologies, vast amounts of real-world data can now be converted into insights about human physical activities using HAR. This data is utilized across numerous IoT applications to assist individuals and enhance their quality of life. HAR has been extensively explored and applied across various fields, such as healthcare, personal fitness, rehabilitation, life-logging, and ambient assisted living (Wang et al., 2019).

Additionally, because it extracts comprehensive information about human actions from raw sensor data, HAR is crucial to daily living (Xu et al., 2019). Furthermore, because it extracts comprehensive insights into human behaviour from unprocessed sensor data, HAR is indispensable in daily life (Wang et al., 2018).

HAR is essential for monitoring everyday activities, especially for the elderly and people with medical issues. Healthcare professionals may better comprehend a patient's health and take prompt action as needed by precisely identifying actions like walking, sitting, or falling. In the realm of fitness, HAR enables users to track their physical activity, providing insightful information about their workout routines and assisting them in achieving their fitness goals. Users may be inspired to enhance their general health and well-being by this knowledge. By identifying human behaviour and preferences, HAR makes it possible to automate smart cities and houses. A smart home system, for instance, may change the temperature and lighting based on whether a person is sleeping, cooking, or watching television. Additionally, HAR facilitates behavioural monitoring and analysis, which aids organizations and researchers in comprehending human behaviour patterns in a range of contexts. This knowledge may inform initiatives related to urban planning and public health. HAR improves workplace and public safety by identifying anomalous activity or circumstances, allowing for quick reactions to any threats (Chen et al., 2021; Ni et al., 2015).

The limits and difficulties of conventional Human Activity Recognition (HAR) techniques, including statistical analysis, basis transform coding, and symbolic representation, are discussed in the paragraph. These methods can increase processing costs without appreciably enhancing performance, frequently rely on heuristic techniques, and lack task-specific emphasis (Yousefi et al., 2020). It draws attention to the growing interest in improving HAR by employing deep learning methods, particularly convolutional neural networks (CNNs), to efficiently extract and choose relevant attributes (Zeng et al., 2014). The proposed approach combines CNNs with an attention mechanism to enhance feature selection and concentrate on pertinent data for more accurate activity detection (Zhao et al., 2021). In an effort to overcome the drawbacks of previous approaches, this is the first time multi-head CNNs and attention mechanisms have been used in HAR (Zhang et al., 2021).

The limits of conventional techniques for Human Activity Recognition (HAR), such as statistical analysis, basis transformation coding, and symbolic representation, are covered in the text (Yousefi et al., 2020). These techniques are usually not very dependable and may increase computational costs without always enhancing performance (Chen et al., 2020). Despite recent developments in deep learning, particularly with deep convolutional neural networks (CNNs), challenges remain (Singh et al., 2021).

By combining multi-head CNNs with an attention mechanism, this work presents a novel approach to improving feature extraction and selection (Wang et al., 2021). Compared to earlier approaches, this method has a higher detection rate of 95.4% for activities, indicating an increase in accuracy. A literature review, an explanation of the suggested framework for recognizing human activity, experimental findings, and closing thoughts make up the structure of the study. Interestingly, complicated multichannel time-series data from wearable sensors can be handled well by multi-head CNN (Zhao et al., 2022).

As e-Health and human-centered applications depend on technologies like body sensor networks (BSNs), the rapid development of the Internet of Things (IoT) has had a significant impact on human activity recognition (HAR). In order to enable broad applications in fields including healthcare, fitness, and behavioral monitoring, BSNs combine wireless sensors, linked devices, and traditional networks. This is especially true when cloud computing enhances analytical and data storage capacities (Zhang et al., 2021; Rashid et al., 2021). A crucial application in these fields, human activity recognition (HAR) has drawn a lot of interest because of its promise in e-Health (Yousefi et al., 2020).

HAR methods are typically categorized into three types according to their sensing modalities: radio-based, camera-based, and wearable device-based. Radio-based HAR relies on variations in wireless signals to identify activities (Ni et al., 2015; Wang et al., 2016), while camera-based HAR employs computer vision technologies for classification, as demonstrated in systems like the short-term memory network introduced by Liu et al. (Chen et al., 2021). Wearable device-based HAR systems use built-in sensors like accelerometers and gyroscopes to gather and classify data on human activities (Wang et al., 2019). In recent years, the use of deep learning techniques, particularly convolutional neural networks (CNNs), has become increasingly popular because of their effectiveness in tasks like image recognition (Ignatov, 2018).

LITERATURE REVIEW

Danyal Khan et al.(2023) has completed research paper Using data from accelerometers, microphones, gyroscopes, magnetometers, and GPS, this study explores the impact of smartphone sensor developments in human activity recognition (HAR), with a particular focus on locomotion and localization. Utilizing three datasets—Continuous In-The-Wild Smart Watch Activity, Huawei Locomotion, and Extra Sensory—it applies Multilayer Perceptron (MLP) with manual feature extraction approaches and Deep Polynomial Neural Networks (DPNN) for deep learning-based feature extraction. According to the results, DPNN performs far better than MLP, with 93% and 95% accuracy for localization and locomotion on the Continuous In-The-Wild Dataset, respectively, compared to 86% and 91% for MLP. MLP is more efficient, but DPNN requires a lot of computation even though it has a greater accuracy. This study highlights how cutting-edge machine learning methods can improve HAR using smartphone sensors and they came to this conclusion This paper offers a system that uses several sensors and machine learning approaches, namely Multilayer Perceptron (MLP) and Deep Polynomial Neural Networks (DPNN), to recognize human locomotion and location-based activities. MLP performs well in settings with low resources, however DPNN is more accurate when handling complicated jobs. The wearables, smart homes, and healthcare industries can all benefit from the system. However, DPNN's high processing needs may limit its usage in real-time scenarios, and performance relies on the quality of training data, creating issues in privacy-sensitive situations.

Hyunseo Park, Nakyoung Kim, and Gyeong Ho Lee et al.(2023) has completed research paper which presents Multi CNN-Filter LSTM, a resource-efficient deep learning model for human activity recognition (HAR) that blends long short-term memory (LSTM) and multi-head convolutional neural networks (CNN) via a residual link. Compared to state-of-the-art models, the model improves classification accuracy by 2.3%–4.4% and lowers operating needs by 21%–70%, making it appropriate for Internet of Things applications. The model may learn feature dependencies at different hierarchical levels thanks to the Filter LSTM technique. The model's effectiveness and adaptability for real-time applications are demonstrated via evaluations on two datasets and deployment on a Raspberry Pi 4, however the quality of the training data affects the model's performance and they came to this conclusion This study presents Filter LSTM, a unique LSTM application that uses a multi-head CNN to capture causal links between low-level and high-level information. When tested on the WISDM dataset, the suggested Multi CNN-Filter LSTM model combines these elements in a residual structure and shows improved performance in identifying a range of human activities.

In Lee et al.(2015) has completed research paper All businesses are paying close attention to the Internet of Things (IoT), which is a global network of connected gadgets. This article covers three categories for enterprise apps that increase customer value as well as five key IoT technologies for a successful deployment. It also looks at ways to justify investments and emphasizes the administrative and technological difficulties in implementing IoT and they came to this conclusion The effects of the Internet of Things (IoT) on society, behaviour, the economy, and management have not received much attention because it is a relatively recent technological development. It is challenging for businesses to make well-informed decisions on the adoption or implementation of IoT technology due to this lack of information. Our paper is one of the first to examine an IoT conceptual model for business applications. We have distinguished between three primary areas of Internet of Things applications: big data, business analytics, and monitoring and control (Lee & Lee, 2015).

Tâm Huynh, Bernt Schiele et al. (2005) has completed research paper One of the most important aspects of contextual information is human behaviour. Activities such as walking, standing, and sitting can be inferred from data gathered by body-worn accelerometers in wearable computing applications. Conventionally, most approaches recognize activities using a standard set of attributes. In this study, we show that recognition accuracy may be improved by carefully choosing particular features for each activity. We present a detailed analysis of features extracted from an actual data set and show how the identification rates for different activities are affected by the feature selection and the length of the window across which the feature is studied. In conclusion, we provide suggestions for ideal characteristics and durations of the window for certain typical tasks and they came to this conclusion This work shows that characteristics can be suitably evaluated for activity recognition by clustering them and measuring the precision of each cluster. There is no one ideal feature or window length for all activities, according to the suggested cluster accuracy measure, which shows a strong correlation with recognition performance. Different coefficients are ideal for each activity, and FFT features constantly rate well. Variance is highly precise in general, with the exception of "standing," where spectral entropy shines. According to the study, window lengths of one to two seconds often result in greater precision; however, the ideal durations differ depending on the activity. More tasks and sophisticated classifiers like AdaBoost or SVM will be investigated in later research to increase recognition rates (Huynh & Schiele, 2005).

Andreas Bulling, Ulf Blanke, and Bernt Schiele et al. (2014) has completed research paper Human activity recognition (HAR) research has expanded dramatically over the past 20 years, tackling several difficulties in the development and assessment of recognition systems. Using on-body inertial sensors, this tutorial provides a hands-on introduction to HAR, helping novices through the main challenges that are common to both general pattern recognition and HAR-specific challenges. The Activity Recognition Chain (ARC) is introduced as an adaptable framework for developing and evaluating HAR systems. With citations to pertinent studies and industry best practices, each ARC component is described. A case study on hand gesture recognition using inertial sensors is included at the end of the lesson to show how different ARC implementations impact recognition results and they came to this conclusion This work shows that characteristics can be clustered and their cluster precision may be evaluated to gain insight into whether or not they are suitable for activity recognition. Performance in feature recognition is accurately predicted by the suggested cluster precision metric. According to the study, no single feature or window length performs better than all others in every activity. The precision of FFT features is very great, however the ideal coefficients differ depending on the activity. Recognition is improved by banding FFT coefficients. Variance works well for non-FFT characteristics, but the mean performs poorly, unless there are certain circumstances. While the ideal window lengths vary depending on the activity, windows of 1-2 seconds usually work the best. Extra classifier systems are to be investigated in future work (Bulling, Blanke, & Schiele, 2014).

Tâm Huynh, Bernt Schiele et al. (2005) has completed research paper A significant component of contextual information is human action. Activities such as walking, standing, and sitting can be identified in wearable technology scenarios by collecting data from body-worn acceleration sensors. For activity recognition, the majority of approaches now use the same set of features regardless of the type of activity. This research shows that identification rates can be improved by carefully selecting unique traits that are specific to each activity. We do an extensive analysis on features extracted from an actual dataset to show how different activities' identification rates are affected by the features used and the time span over which they are computed. In the conclusion, we suggest suitable features and window sizes for a number of typical tasks and they came to this conclusion. This work presents an approach that combines an active appearance model (AAM) and an adaptive particle filtering strategy to track the 2D global posture and facial motions of a face. Four appearance parameters and four posture parameters are included in the state vector. After taking into consideration obscured pixels, the likelihood calculates how similar the texture of the model and the image are. The method lowers the amount of particles required, increasing them only when needed, by using a deterministic AAM search. Tests show how well the system tracks faces in situations with sudden movements and occlusions. Furthermore, a texture model with adaptability is suggested to enhance face activity tracking and recognition (Huynh & Schiele, 2005).

Jian Bo Yang, Minh Nhut Nguyen,and Phyo Phyo San et al.(2015) has completed research paper In order to identify preset human activities, this study tackles the problem of human activity recognition (HAR) using multichannel time series data from body-worn inertial sensors. It is important but challenging to extract useful information for precise activity detection. Present-day techniques frequently rely on manually created features and shallow learning architectures, which have trouble recognizing unique characteristics. In order to get around this, we provide a methodical feature learning strategy that automates feature extraction from raw data using deep convolutional networks (CNN). Higher-level abstract representations of the input signals are produced by this deep architecture. Through the use of supervised learning, the features improve their capacity for discrimination. CNN outperforms other models in studies on the Opportunity Activity Recognition Challenge and other benchmark datasets when feature learning and classification are combined within single model current HAR techniques and they came to this conclusion. A new approach to automating feature extraction in human activity recognition (HAR) is presented in this research. In order to analyse multichannel time series data, we create a new deep architecture for convolutional neural networks (CNNs). We use pooling and convolution operations to capture important sensor signal patterns at different time scales. The patterns are merged between channels and classified into several kinds of human activity. Task-dependent feature extraction, higher feature discriminative power, and the ability to combine feature extraction and classification into a single model for better performance are important benefits. Tests demonstrate that our CNN approach performs better in HAR than the current state-of-the-art methods (Yang, Nguyen, San, Li, & Krishnaswamy, 2015).

Kelvin Xu, Jimmy Ba, Ryan Kiros,and Kyunghyun Cho, Aaron Courville has completed research paper Drawing inspiration from contemporary advancements in object detection and machine translation, we present an attention-based model that autonomously acquires the ability to articulate image content. We explain how this model can be trained both stochastically by maximizing a variational lower limit and deterministically by applying typical backpropagation techniques. Visualization is another way we demonstrate how the model may automatically learn to focus its attention on important items while producing the words that correspond to those objects in the output sequence. We employ state-of-the-art performance on three benchmark datasets (Flickr8k, Flickr30k, and MS COCO) to validate the application of attention and they came to this conclusion. They provide an attention-based approach that, when assessed using the BLEU and METEOR criteria, achieves state-of-the-art performance on three benchmark datasets. We also demonstrate that the learnt alignments closely match human intuition, and that the learned attention can improve the interpretability of the model creation process. We hope that this paper's findings will stimulate more investigation into the application of visual attention. Additionally, we think that the encoder-decoder framework's modular design, when paired with attention techniques, will be useful in a variety of other domains (Xu et al., 2015).

Dzmitry Bahdanau has completed research paper unlike classic statistical machine translation, neural machine translation (NMT) is a recently proposed method that tries to construct a single neural network tailored to optimum translation performance. A source sentence is encoded into a fixed-length vector using the encoder-decoder methods employed in NMT, and a decoder uses this vector to produce a translation. We speculate that the performance of this simple architecture is constrained using a fixed-length vector. We suggest expanding it by letting the model anticipate each target word automatically by (soft-)searching for pertinent portions of the source sentence, without explicitly breaking these components up into hard segments. On English French translation problems, our method provides translation performance similar to the state-of-the-art phrase-based systems. Qualitative study demonstrates that the model's (soft-)alignments are in good agreement with human intuition and came to this conclusion Longer sentences may be more difficult to translate using the traditional neural network translation encoder-decoder method since it converts an entire input sentence into a fixed-length vector. To overcome this constraint, we suggest a unique architecture known as RNN search, which enables the model to (soft-) search for pertinent input words or their annotations at the time of target word generation. This adaptability greatly improves the model's performance on lengthier phrases by allowing it to concentrate on information relevant to the following target word. Our tests on English-to-French translation demonstrate that RNN search is more robust overall and performs better than conventional encoder-decoder models regardless of sentence length. Furthermore, RNN search provides translation performance that is on par with the most advanced phrase-based systems. Although there are still issues with processing uncommon or unfamiliar terms, our method represents a substantial leap in machine translation and comprehension of natural language (Bahdanau, 2014).

Sen Qiu, Hongkai Zhao et al. (2022) has completed research paper An overview of popular wearable sensors, smart devices, and important application domains is provided in this study. Systems that use many modalities or channels, such as auditory, visual, environmental, and physiological signals, are referred to as multi-sensor systems. In order to integrate data from several sensors in different places, the paper provides fusion approaches. While other evaluations have focused on deep learning or information fusion separately, this work adopts a more comprehensive approach to offer a better foundation for comprehending sensor fusion applications. In particular, the paper covers all the salient features of multi-sensor applications for human activity recognition, including the latest developments in transfer learning and unsupervised learning. The report concludes by identifying and discussing open research concerns that need to be improved and investigated further and they came to this conclusion Wearable technology can help interpret user intentions by closely monitoring cognitive data and user behaviour. This essay examines the condition of information fusion and wearable technologies at the moment. The effect of sensor location on motion measurement is emphasized, and conventional machine learning is criticized for its poor feature extraction and generalization powers. Deep learning, on the other hand, provides better performance and versatility by automatically picking up higher-level characteristics. Notwithstanding, several obstacles persist, specifically related to managing a wide range of user actions and the practicality of gathering copious labelled data for every user. In order to improve model performance, the paper proposes merging deep learning with transfer learning and offers open research questions for further investigation (Qiu et al., 2022).

Luigi Atzori, Antonio Iera, and Giacomo Morabito et al. (2010) has completed research paper This essay explores the Internet of Things (IoT) and highlights how integrating many technologies and communication methods is essential to its progress. Distributed intelligence for smart things, improved communication protocols, sensor networks, and identification and tracking technologies are important elements. Collaborative efforts spanning several disciplines, such as telecommunications, informatics, electronics, and social sciences, are necessary to make significant progress in the Internet of Things. The purpose of this poll is to support anyone who want to learn more about this intricate topic and help it develop. It highlights persistent issues that the research community has to address while reviewing various viewpoints on the Internet of Things paradigm and enabling technologies and they came to this conclusion Our interactions have been profoundly changed by the Internet, moving to a virtual level in a variety of circumstances, including social and professional ones. This is improved by the Internet of Things (IoT), which makes it possible for smart items to communicate with one another and advances the idea of "anytime, anywhere" connectivity. The focus of this paper is on IoT as a component of the Internet of the future, which will be very different from the one we have now. The potential of the Internet is limited by the host-to-host communication model that exists today. As a result, attention must be paid to data-centric networks where data is self-addressable and self-routable. Furthermore, the new Web Squared paradigm combines web and sensing technologies to improve user experiences by providing contextual data. The study examines important facets of IoT and points out persistent issues that need more investigation and improvement (Atzori, Iera, & Morabito, 2010).

Luigi Atzori, Antonio Iera, and Giacomo Morabito et al.(2010) has completed research paper This essay examines the Internet of Things (IoT), emphasizing how integrating many technologies and communication methods is essential to the IoT's progress. Distributed intelligence for smart things, improved communication protocols, sensor networks, and identification and tracking technologies are important elements. Significant advancements in the growth of the Internet of Things require collaborative efforts across various fields, including telecommunications, informatics, electronics, and social sciences. This survey presents many viewpoints on the Internet of Things paradigm and reviews enabling technologies in an effort to assist individuals who are interested in this intricate field and its evolution. It ends by outlining the principal obstacles that the scientific community will need to overcome in the future and they came to this conclusion The way we communicate has been completely changed by the Internet, with many interactions taking place on virtual platforms in a variety of settings, including social and professional ones. This is improved by the Internet of Things (IoT), which fosters the idea of "anytime, anywhere" connectivity by enabling communication between smart items. The Internet of Things is anticipated to play a major role in the future Internet, which will be very different from the current paradigm. The limitations of the present host-to-host communication paradigm force attention toward data-centric networks, where data is self-addressable and self-routable, thereby realizing the full promise of the Internet. Furthermore, the Web Squared paradigm, which is currently in development, combines web and sensing technologies to improve user experiences. This study examines important facets of the Internet of Things and points out persistent problems that need more investigation and improvement (Lin, Keogh, Lonardi, & Chiu, 2003).

Lei Zhang, Jingwei Yu, Zhenyu Gao, and Qin Ni(2024) has completed research paper In order to facilitate the digital revolution of healthcare, smart and connected health, or SCH, improves the integration of information science and engineering. Using multi-position sensor data fusion, this research focuses on human activity recognition (HAR) and suggests a hybrid model (1DCNN-Att-BiLSTM) for multi-channel deep learning. Improved HAR performance via local and global feature extraction, the establishment of a multi-position sensor data pool from publicly accessible datasets, and a comprehensive analysis of sensor data fusion patterns are some of the major contributions. The suggested model performs competitively in HAR tasks when compared to deep learning and classical methods. The approach's efficacy for ambient assisted living and healthcare monitoring has been validated through extensive studies and they came to this conclusion By establishing a multi-channel 1DCNN-Att-BiLSTM model and demonstrating its efficacy on three datasets—Shoaib AR, Shoaib SA, and HAPT—this study greatly enhances human activity recognition (HAR).Making use of spatial and temporal data, the model leverages a bidirectional long short-term memory and a one-dimensional convolutional neural network to improve classification accuracy. The outcomes demonstrate that, especially for data from belt positions, the AGM sensor combination achieves the maximum classification precision. Furthermore, the model achieves a precision of 98.76% on the HAPT dataset, outperforming conventional machine learning approaches. The results address issues with explainability in deep learning models for real-world applications, while also highlighting the model's promise in health management and personalized services (Zhang, Yu, Gao, & Ni, 2024).

Kolla Sai Krishna and Surekha Paneerselvam (2022) has completed research paper With Human activities Recognition (HAR), movement data from sensors is used to anticipate an individual's activities. At the moment, wearable technology is used for this, such as cell phones and body-worn sensors. These gadgets make it easier to gather and analyse data in order to gain insights on day-to-day activities. Finding patterns in unprocessed data is the main goal of this study in order to obtain important insights into human behaviour. While current techniques, especially deep learning, have shown significant progress in identifying explicit activities, they still face difficulties in identifying transitions between different tasks. In order to improve HAR accuracy, this project uses a long short-term memory (LSTM) model for activity transitions and a convolutional neural network (CNN) for activity recognition. The HAPT and HAR datasets are used to train the model, and hyperparameters are adjusted to evaluate performance and measuring parameters like recall, F1-score, and precision, producing better results with adjusted parameters and they came to this conclusion This Human Activity Recognition (HAR) study successfully illustrates how wearable technology, including smartphones and body-worn sensors, may be used to forecast a person's activity based on sensor data. Although current deep learning techniques have made strides in identifying explicit activities, they frequently have trouble identifying changes in activity. In order to solve this, the study uses the HAPT and HAR datasets for training a hybrid model that uses convolutional neural networks (CNN) for activity detection and long short-term memory (LSTM) networks for capturing activity transitions. Hyperparameter tuning, which involves varying the number of neurons, batch size, and learning rate, is used to evaluate the model's performance. The results demonstrate that optimum parameters greatly improve HAR accuracy, indicating the model's potential for more efficient human activity monitoring (Krishna & Paneerselvam, 2021).

Rahul Jain, Vijay Bhaskar Semwal, and Praveen Kaushik (2021) has completed research paper Walking is a difficult activity that takes a lot of practice and demands precise brain-to-lower-limb coordination. The structural contrasts between bipedal robots and human mobility often make them difficult to maneuverer effectively. The goal of this research is to improve robot walking through the analysis of lower extremity human activities. A deep learning-based ensemble classifier is used to analyse diverse walking techniques on various terrains in order to identify different types of activities. Joint movements are recorded by an Inertial Measurement Unit (IMU), which makes use of mHealth and HAPT datasets. High accuracy rates are attained by CNN and LSTM, two deep learning models with applications in robotic trajectory development and rehabilitation and they came to this conclusion a CNN-LSTM ensemble model has been proposed by us for the objective of recognising lower extremity actions. The model analyses the angular velocity and acceleration signals that are received from the IMU in order to identify lower extremity human actions. With an accuracy of 99.25%, 88.48%, and 97.44% in recognizing lower extremity activities, the model has demonstrated excellent generalization in preliminary experiments conducted on the mHealth, OU-ISIR, and HAPT inertial datasets. Due to a class imbalance, the OU-ISIR dataset's relatively low accuracy can be improved by adding additional training instances for the minority class. Our research generates an effective and steady walk in Bipeds with the help of the suggested model. We like to use multi-modal, sensor fusion deep learning to expand on our work strategies that, in our opinion, can offer more profound insights into how people move. For a personal healthcare device, the suggested model can also be implemented directly into an Internet of Things device through tiny ML implementation (Jain, Semwal, & Kaushik, 2022).

Masud Ahmed, Anindya Das Antar, and Md Atiqur Rahman Ahad et al. (2021) has completed research paper The goal of smartphone sensor-based activity detection is to use diverse low-level sensor data to extract comprehensive insights into human behaviours, which will have a big influence on healthcare. This work focuses on robust feature extraction and efficient pre-processing methods for sensor data classification in human activity recognition (HAR). Filtering to minimize waveform delays, addressing smartphone orientation, and maximizing window lengths for latency and performance are important pre-processing stages. "Average Height," a new feature, provides a summary of motion changes for categorization. Two feature selection techniques are also suggested for quicker recognition. By examining posture transitions, the Static Postural Transition-based Post-Processing (SPTPP) method improves model output. On the benchmark datasets HASC, HAR, and HAPT, the suggested approaches produced cutting-edge results, proving their efficacy in HAR applications and they cam to this conclusion Optimizing pipelines and parameters at various activity categorization stages is essential for accurately identifying related and complex activities. This work investigates the impacts of several factors and suggests methods for optimizing them. In order to extract motion information from processed signal data and demonstrate a higher relevance factor, a new feature called "Average Height" is presented. For both offline and real-time feature selection, two approaches are suggested, and the effects of various feature sets are examined. Furthermore, by observing posture changes in nearby prior window data, a Static Postural Transition-based Post-Processing approach (SPTPP) is developed to adjust the performance of identifying static activities. The suggested techniques yield cutting-edge outcomes on three reference datasets. The goal of future research will be to extract more resilient characteristics and learning techniques to efficiently identify complex actions in situations that happen in real time (Ahmed, Antar, & Ahad, 2021).

STUDY AND ANALYSIS

Human Activity Recognition (HAR) systems typically involve several stages: data collection, preprocessing, segmentation, feature extraction, feature selection, modelling, and classification (LeCun et al., 1989). Deep learning techniques, particularly CNNs, have proven effective in enhancing feature extraction and classification accuracy in HAR tasks (Xu et al., 2015). Traditional approaches such as symbolic representation, Fourier and wavelet transforms, and statistical analysis have been utilized to process time-series data, but they often lack robustness, are heuristic, and are not task-specific (Atzori, Iera, & Morabito, 2010)(Xu et al., 2015). Additionally, conventional methods tend to struggle with heterogeneity within the same activity class and similarity between different classes, limiting their effectiveness (Wang & Zhou, 2015)(Kianoush, Savazzi, Vicentini, Rampa, & Giussani, 2017).

To address these limitations, recent research has explored the integration of CNNs with attention mechanisms to improve feature extraction and selection. The attention mechanism enables the model to focus on the most relevant features, filtering out unnecessary information and enhancing classification performance (Lu, Fan, Chu, Jing, & Yuting, 2019)(Bulling, Blanke, & Schiele, 2014). By incorporating attention into multi-head CNNs, the proposed method achieves higher accuracy in recognizing activities (Qiu et al., 2022). The study validated this approach using a dataset from the Wireless Sensor Data Mining (WISDM) lab, demonstrating that it outperforms previous methods in terms of accuracy (Wang & Zhou, 2015).

Despite the advancements of deep learning in HAR, several challenges remain. Conventional HAR methods often face difficulties in feature selection, leading to suboptimal classification results and increased computational costs (LeCun et al., 1989) (Vaswani et al., 2017). Moreover, issues such as the dominance of the NULL class, the complexity of physical tasks, and the need to account for contextual factors such as user states and environmental conditions further complicate HAR tasks (Bulling, Blanke, & Schiele, 2014)(Kianoush, Savazzi, Vicentini, Rampa, & Giussani, 2017). The paper also highlights transfer learning as a promising avenue for addressing these challenges, especially in scenarios where training data is limited (Abobakr, Hossny, & Nahavandi, 2018).

By leveraging the strengths of CNNs and attention mechanisms, the proposed method enhances the precision and robustness of HAR systems, offering significant improvements over traditional approaches. This study is the first to combine multi-head CNNs with attention mechanisms for HAR, setting a new direction for future research in the field (Qiu et al., 2022).

The study looks into the use of attention mechanisms and multi-head Convolutional Neural Networks (CNNs) in Human Activity Recognition (HAR). By utilizing multiple processing layers, multi-head CNNs enhance feature extraction and facilitate more effective handling of intricate, multichannel input from wearable devices. The attention mechanism enhances accuracy even further by focusing on the most important components of the incoming data, highlighting salient characteristics and eliminating superfluous information (Xu et al., 2015). When combined, these methods offer a promising way to improve HAR systems, particularly when dealing with complex recognition jobs. The study looks into the use of attention mechanisms and multi-head Convolutional Neural Networks (CNNs) in Human Activity Recognition (HAR). By utilizing multiple processing layers, multi-head CNNs enhance feature extraction and facilitate more effective handling of intricate, multichannel input from wearable devices (Chorowski et al., 2015). The attention mechanism enhances accuracy even further by focusing on the most important components of the incoming data, highlighting salient characteristics and eliminating superfluous information (Abobakr, Hossny, & Nahavandi, 2018). When combined, these methods offer a promising way to improve HAR systems, particularly when dealing with complex recognition jobs (Xu et al., 2015). Systems are able to evaluate user behaviour and activity trends by utilizing the proposed HAR technique for real-time activity monitoring (Acharya et al., 2012). This feature is beneficial to people as well as healthcare providers since it provides insightful information on everyday routines (Chorowski et al., 2015). Systems are able to evaluate user behaviour and activity trends by utilizing the proposed HAR technique for real-time activity monitoring. Healthcare practitioners as well as users might both gain from this capability's insightful observations of daily activities (Abobakr, Hossny, & Nahavandi, 2018).

continued on following page

Table 1. Continued

Table 1. Evaluation of various deep learning models for recognizing human activities.

Method	Merits	De Merits	Dataset
Fast Classification of EEG Artifacts	Improves classification performance significantly (2–9% for 1-channel data and 8–12% for 2-channel data)	This model was specially Developed for the health care sector.	Public Dataset
Changed Inception Time network architecture	The model works better in terms of accuracy for ARIL, Stan Wi-Fi and SignFi	The Proposed model may not work for the real-world dataset because the real-world data set has vast interference.	ARIL, StanWiFi, and SignFi
Binary Motion ImageDeep learning	Binary Motion Image Deep learning model gives good accuracy for both 2D and 3D datasets consistent speed of action performed by a human.	The model fails to provide an accurate detection rate when multiple people are present in the 3D image.	MSR action 3D dataset
The complete deep learning model for Recognizing Human-toHuman Interactions	The developed end to end deep learning model provides 86.3 accuracy for all human-to-human interactions recognition.	The proposed model is not developed for group-to-group interactions. This model will work only for Human-toHuman Interactions.	CSI dataset of HHI
Inception ResNet deep transfer learning method for HAR using LSTM	It provides the best accuracy score of 92 per cent and 91 per cent for the different data sets	It takes a tremendous amount of training time	UCI 101 and HMDB 51 data sets
Kernel principal component analysis	KPCA outperform Support Vector Machine (SVM) and Artificial Neural Network (ANN)	It provides less accuracy for the real-time data.	Public Dataset
Sparse Feature Learning for Human Activity Recognition	It provides long term Dependencies	It provides less accuracy for the real-time data	UCI-HAR dataset
HAR using Ensemble Learning of Multiple CNN	It takes less amount of preprocessing time because the proposed model support automatic feature extractions	Model is not suitable for concurrent activity recognition	WISDM dataset
Unsupervised deep learning assisted reconstructed coder in the on-nodule wearable sensor for HAR	improves the feature selection and extraction using an unsupervised deep learning model	The performances degrade in large datasets with different types of human activities.	WISDM dataset
Multi-domain HAR based on Stepped-Frequency Continuous-wave radar using deep learning	Developed deep learning model increases the recognition accuracy by 1.3% by additionally introducing the range maps	The proposed model is not developed for group-to-group Interactions.	Public Dataset

PROPOSED WORK

Deep learning has revolutionized HAR by automating the feature extraction process, which traditionally required extensive manual intervention. Key deep learning models used in HAR include:

1. **Convolutional Neural Networks (CNNs)**: Effective for spatial data, CNNs are used for image-based HAR, The remarkable ability of Convolutional Neural Networks (CNNs) to handle and evaluate geographical data has made them a potent instrument in the field of Internet of Things (IoT) applications. CNNs are a particular kind of deep learning model that is mainly used for image identification and classification applications. The human visual system, in especially the visual cortex, which enables people to effectively interpret visual information through a succession of layers that gradually extract elements from input data, served as the model for their architecture.

Convolutional layers, pooling layers, and fully linked layers are the basic components of CNNs. The network can identify different features including edges, textures, and patterns since the convolutional layers apply filters to the input data. Each filter applies a convolutional mathematical operation to the input image as it slides over it, producing a feature map that emphasizes different parts of the input. Due to their ability to capture spatial hierarchies in data, CNNs are especially useful for jobs requiring the comprehension of intricate visual patterns.

Pooling layers are used after the convolutional layers in order to minimize the feature maps' spatial dimensions. This down sampling procedure keeps only the most noticeable characteristics, which reduces computing effort and mitigates overfitting. Max pooling and average pooling are two popular pooling approaches that assist preserve significant information while eliminating less important elements.

High-level reasoning normally takes place in one or more completely connected layers, which make up the final part of a CNN. The final classification or prediction is generated in these layers by processing the output that has been flattened from the preceding layers. Because of this structure, CNNs can learn intricate data representations, which make them very useful for a range of Internet of Things applications.

CNNs seem to be especially useful in Internet of Things scenarios when it comes to image-based Human Activity Recognition (HAR), where sensor data can be converted into spectrogram images. This transition enables CNNs to exploit their strengths in processing visual information to recognize and classify human actions based on sensor inputs obtained from wearable devices or environmental sensors. CNNs can also be used in smart home automation to identify human behaviour or in security systems to analyse footage in real time.

Because many IoT devices have limited resources, employing CNNs in IoT applications offers hurdles despite their benefits. Researchers are creating specialized architectures like IoTNet, which enhance performance while cutting computing costs, to address this problem. These developments allow more potent models to function well within the constraints of environments for edge computing.

In general, the incorporation of Convolutional Neural Networks into Internet of Things applications signifies a noteworthy progression in the ability of machines to comprehend and react to intricate data from their environment. We may anticipate more advancements in this area of study that will improve CNN performance and capabilities across a range of Internet of Things applications, where sensor data can be transformed into spectrogram images.

Figure 1. Workflow of CNN

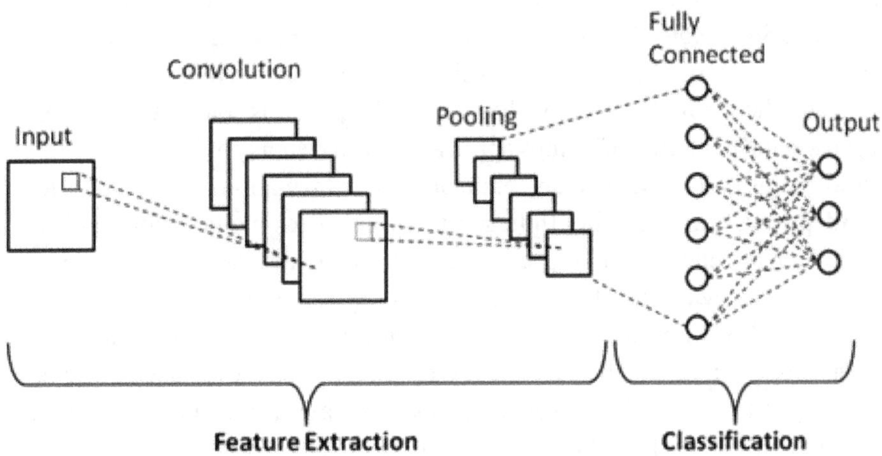

2. **Long Short-Term Memory (LSTM) Networks:** Particularly useful in Internet of Things (IoT) applications, Long Short-Term Memory (LSTM) networks are a form of recurrent neural network (RNN) specifically intended to simulate sequential data. For many Internet of Things applications where data is continuously collected over time, LSTMs are essential for capturing temporal dependencies and patterns in time-series data. Their design solves the vanishing gradient issue that conventional RNNs frequently face, enabling them to successfully learn long-term dependencies.

LSTMs are utilized in IoT applications for a number of purposes, such as time-series forecasting, anomaly detection, and predictive maintenance. For example, in smart manufacturing, LSTMs can use sensor data from equipment to anticipate faults before they happen, reducing maintenance costs and downtime. Likewise, LSTMs in smart houses may handle information from environmental sensors to forecast future consumption patterns based on historical data, hence optimizing energy usage.

LSTMs are utilized in IoT applications for a number of purposes, such as time-series forecasting, anomaly detection, and predictive maintenance. For example, in smart manufacturing, LSTMs can use sensor data from equipment to anticipate faults before they happen, reducing maintenance costs and downtime. Similar to this, LSTMs in smart homes can use historical data to forecast future consumption trends and improve energy usage by processing data from environmental sensors.

An LSTM's architecture is made up of several memory cells that keep data stable over time. Three primary parts make up each memory cell: input, forget, and output gates. The forget gate chooses what data should be removed from the memory cell, the output gate manages what data is delivered from the cell to the network's next layer, and the input gate controls how much fresh data is sent to the memory cell. Because data in Internet of Things applications can be noisy or irrelevant, this gating method helps LSTMs selectively retain or forget information based on its relevance.

Adaptive Channel Quality Indicator (CQI) feedback methods for wireless communication are one particular use case for LSTMs in the Internet of Things. In this scenario, IoT devices use LSTM networks to periodically report the channel conditions. The LSTM model can forecast ideal feedback intervals and enhance device and network communication efficiency by utilizing past CQI data. In Internet of Things systems, this method ensures dependable data delivery while lowering latency.

Combining LSTMs and Convolutional Neural Networks (CNNs) for improved predictive modelling is another noteworthy use. In this hybrid technique, temporal dependencies within the extracted features are captured using long short-term memory (LSTMs) and CNNs for feature extraction from spatial data (such as pictures or spectrograms). A framework like this can be very useful for activities like activity recognition or target tracking in settings related to the Internet of Things.

Despite their benefits, there are drawbacks to using LSTMs in Internet of Things applications, including the requirement for real-time processing skills and limitations on computational resources. Researchers are creating lightweight LSTM models that are tailored for resource-constrained situations, which are common to many IoT devices, while maintaining excellent performance in order to address these problems.

All things considered, long short-term memory networks are essential for improving the intelligence and responsiveness of Internet of Things applications since they efficiently model sequential data and make predictive analytics possible in a variety of fields. We may anticipate more advancement in research that will improve LSTM capabilities in the quickly changing IoT technology ecosystem. These are particularly useful for sequential data, allowing the model to learn temporal dependencies in activity data.

Figure 2. Workflow of LSTM

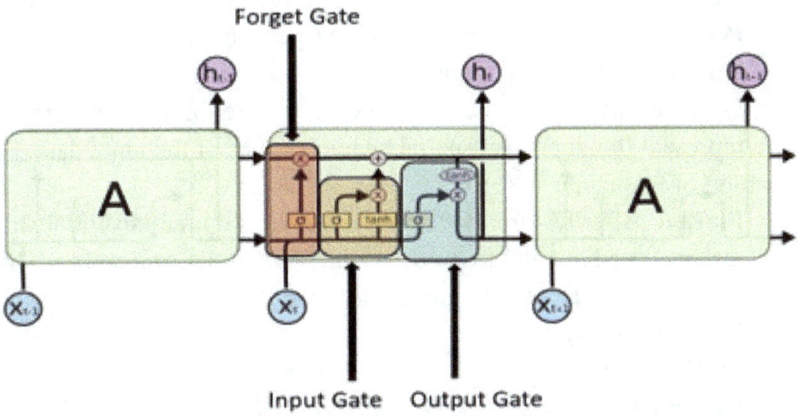

Hybrid Models: combining Convolutional Neural Networks (CNNs) with Long Short-Term Memory (LSTMs) or Gated Recurrent Units (GRUs) to build a hybrid model for tasks like Human Activity Recognition (HAR) involves several stages:

Combining Convolutional Neural Networks (CNNs) with Long Short-Term Memory (LSTMs) or Gated Recurrent Units (GRUs) to build a hybrid model for tasks like Human Activity Recognition (HAR) involves several stages:

1. Data Collection and Preprocessing
    - **Collect Data**: Gather raw data from sources like sensors (accelerometers, gyroscopes) or images/video frames in the case of HAR.
    - **Preprocessing**: Clean and preprocess the data. For time-series sensor data, this might include normalization, noise filtering, and segmentation. If working with video frames, the data may be transformed into image-like formats such as spectrograms.
2. Input Preparation
    - **Data Structuring**: For time-series data, ensure the input is structured so that temporal dependencies can be captured. Each input sequence should consist of a series of time steps. For video data, frames are arranged in a time-sequenced manner.

- **Batching**: Split the data into batches and time windows, preparing it for input into the CNN and RNN models.

3. Spatial Feature Extraction (Using CNN)
    - **Convolutional Layers**: Pass the input (either image-like spectrograms or raw sensor data) through convolutional layers. These layers apply filters to extract **spatial features**, like patterns, edges, and texture, from the input data.
    - **Pooling**: Use max-pooling or average-pooling layers to reduce the spatial dimensions while retaining the most important information.
    - **Feature Maps**: The result of the CNN is a set of **feature maps**, which represent the important spatial characteristics of the input data.
4. Flattening or Reshaping
    - **Flatten**: After feature extraction, the CNN's output (spatial features) is reshaped or flattened to prepare it for sequential processing. This step converts the 2D or 3D output into a format suitable for input into the LSTM/GRU layers.
5. Temporal Feature Extraction (Using LSTM/GRU)
    - **Recurrent Layers**: Pass the reshaped CNN output through LSTM or GRU layers to capture **temporal dependencies**. These layers process the sequence of feature maps, understanding how spatial features evolve over time.
    - **Memory Cells**: LSTMs have memory cells that help store and forget information over time, allowing the network to learn both short-term and long-term dependencies in the sequence. GRUs, while simpler, perform a similar role with fewer parameters.
6. Fully Connected Layers
    - After the recurrent layers, the output is typically passed through fully connected (dense) layers to map the temporal and spatial features to the final output space, such as activity labels in HAR.
    - These layers aggregate the learned information and prepare it for classification.
7. Classification
    - **Output Layer**: The final layer is a softmax or sigmoid activation layer that classifies the activities based on the extracted spatial and temporal features. This layer assigns probabilities to the possible activity classes.
8. Training the Hybrid Model
    - **Training Process**: Train the hybrid model using backpropagation through time (BPTT) for LSTM/GRU and standard backpropagation for CNN layers. The model learns by minimizing the loss function (e.g., cross-entropy loss) using optimization techniques like Adam or SGD.

9. Evaluation and Optimization
   - After training, evaluate the model's performance on validation or test data. Further fine-tuning of hyperparameters (e.g., learning rate, number of layers) might be necessary to improve accuracy.
   - Techniques such as dropout can be used to prevent overfitting.
10. Prediction
   - Once the hybrid model is trained and optimized, it can predict the activities from new, unseen data by recognizing both the spatial and temporal patterns learned during training.

This combination of CNN for spatial features and LSTM/GRU for temporal dependencies ensures a robust model capable of handling complex tasks that require both static and dynamic pattern recognition, like HAR.

1. Data Collection and Preprocessing
   - **Collect Data**: Gather raw data from sources like sensors (accelerometers, gyroscopes) or images/video frames in the case of HAR.
   - **Preprocessing**: Clean and preprocess the data. For time-series sensor data, this might include normalization, noise filtering, and segmentation. If working with video frames, the data may be transformed into image-like formats such as spectrograms.
2. Input Preparation
   - **Data Structuring**: For time-series data, ensure the input is structured so that temporal dependencies can be captured. Each input sequence should consist of a series of time steps. For video data, frames are arranged in a time-sequenced manner.
   - **Batching**: Split the data into batches and time windows, preparing it for input into the CNN and RNN models.
3. Spatial Feature Extraction (Using CNN)
   - **Convolutional Layers**: Pass the input (either image-like spectrograms or raw sensor data) through convolutional layers. These layers apply filters to extract **spatial features**, like patterns, edges, and texture, from the input data.
   - **Pooling**: Use max-pooling or average-pooling layers to reduce the spatial dimensions while retaining the most important information.
   - **Feature Maps**: The result of the CNN is a set of **feature maps**, which represent the important spatial characteristics of the input data.
4. Flattening or Reshaping
   - **Flatten**: After feature extraction, the CNN's output (spatial features) is reshaped or flattened to prepare it for sequential processing. This step

converts the 2D or 3D output into a format suitable for input into the LSTM/GRU layers.

5. Temporal Feature Extraction (Using LSTM/GRU)
   - **Recurrent Layers**: Pass the reshaped CNN output through LSTM or GRU layers to capture **temporal dependencies**. These layers process the sequence of feature maps, understanding how spatial features evolve over time.
   - **Memory Cells**: LSTMs have memory cells that help store and forget information over time, allowing the network to learn both short-term and long-term dependencies in the sequence. GRUs, while simpler, performs a similar role with fewer parameters.
6. Fully Connected Layers
   - After the recurrent layers, the output is typically passed through fully connected (dense) layers to map the temporal and spatial features to the final output space, such as activity labels in HAR.
   - These layers aggregate the learned information and prepare it for classification.
7. Classification
   - **Output Layer**: The final layer is a SoftMax or sigmoid activation layer that classifies the activities based on the extracted spatial and temporal features. This layer assigns probabilities to the possible activity classes.
8. Training the Hybrid Model
   - **Training Process**: Train the hybrid model using backpropagation through time (BPTT) for LSTM/GRU and standard backpropagation for CNN layers. The model learns by minimizing the loss function (e.g., cross-entropy loss) using optimization techniques like Adam or SGD.
9. Evaluation and Optimization
   - Once training is complete, assess the model's performance using validation or test data. Further fine-tuning of hyperparameters (e.g., learning rate, number of layers) might be necessary to improve accuracy.
   - Techniques such as dropout can be used to prevent overfitting.
10. Prediction
    - Once the hybrid model is trained and optimized, it can predict the activities from new, unseen data by recognizing both the spatial and temporal patterns learned during training.

This combination of CNN for spatial features and LSTM/GRU for temporal dependencies ensures a robust model capable of handling complex tasks that require both static and dynamic pattern recognition, like HAR.

Figure 3. Workflow of hybrid model (CNN+LSTM)

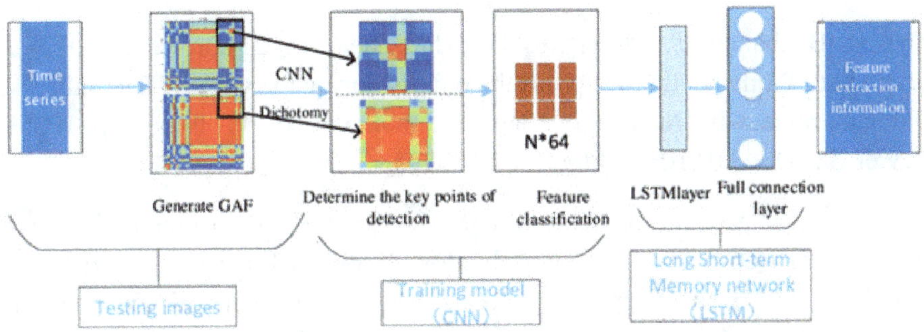

The proposed IoT-based HAR system has significant implications for various sectors, particularly in healthcare, where it can facilitate remote monitoring and support for elderly or disabled individuals (Xu et al., 2015). By utilizing deep learning, the system can adapt to new activities and environments, improving its robustness and applicability across different scenarios (Adame et al., 2018). In conclusion, the integration of deep learning with IoT technologies in HAR systems presents a promising avenue for enhancing human-computer interaction and automating activity recognition in real-time environments (Akagündüz, Aslan, Şengür, Wang, & Ince, 2016). The proposed methodologies aim to address current challenges in HAR, such as the need for extensive labelled datasets and the complexity of feature extraction, ultimately leading to more efficient and user-friendly applications (Alsheikh et al., 2016).

CONCLUSION

In conclusion, the integration of deep learning with IoT technologies in HAR systems presents a promising avenue for enhancing human-computer interaction and automating activity recognition in real-time environments. The proposed methodologies aim to address current challenges in HAR, such as the need for extensive labelled datasets and the complexity of feature extraction, ultimately leading to more efficient and user-friendly applications.

REFERENCES

Abbaspur-Behbahani, S., Monaghesh, E., Hajizadeh, A., & Fehresti, S. (2022). Application of mobile health to support the elderly during the COVID-19 outbreak: A systematic review. In Health Policy and Technology (Vol. 11, Issue 1, p. 100595). Elsevier BV. DOI: 10.1016/j.hlpt.2022.100595

Abobakr, A., Hossny, M., & Nahavandi, S. (2018). A Skeleton-Free Fall Detection System From Depth Images Using Random Decision Forest. In IEEE Systems Journal (Vol. 12, Issue 3, pp. 2994–3005). Institute of Electrical and Electronics Engineers (IEEE). DOI: 10.1109/JSYST.2017.2780260

Acharya, U. R., Faust, O., Sree, S. V., Molinari, F., Saba, L., Nicolaides, A., & Suri, J. S. (2012). An Accurate and Generalized Approach to Plaque Characterization in 346 Carotid Ultrasound Scans. In IEEE Transactions on Instrumentation and Measurement (Vol. 61, Issue 4, pp. 1045–1053). Institute of Electrical and Electronics Engineers (IEEE). DOI: 10.1109/TIM.2011.2174897

Adame, T., Bel, A., Carreras, A., Melià-Seguí, J., Oliver, M., & Pous, R. (2018). CUIDATS: An RFID–WSN hybrid monitoring system for smart health care environments. In Future Generation Computer Systems (Vol. 78, pp. 602–615). Elsevier BV. DOI: 10.1016/j.future.2016.12.023

Ahmed, M., Antar, A. D., & Ahad, M. A. R. (2021). Static postural transition-based technique and efficient feature extraction for sensor-based activity recognition. *Pattern Recognition Letters*, *147*, 25–33. DOI: 10.1016/j.patrec.2021.04.001

Akagündüz, E., Aslan, M., Şengür, A., Wang, H., & Ince, M. C. (2016). Silhouette orientation volumes for efficient fall detection in depth videos. *IEEE Journal of Biomedical and Health Informatics*, *21*(3), 756–763. DOI: 10.1109/JBHI.2016.2570300 PMID: 28113444

Alsheikh, M. A., Selim, A., Niyato, D., Doyle, L., Lin, S., & Tan, H. P. (2016, March). Deep activity recognition models with triaxial accelerometers. In *Workshops at the thirtieth AAAI conference on artificial intelligence*.

Ashton, K. (2009). That 'internet of things' thing. RFID journal, 22(7), 97-114.

Atzori, L., Iera, A., & Morabito, G. (2010). The Internet of Things: A survey. In Computer Networks (Vol. 54, Issue 15, pp. 2787–2805). Elsevier BV. DOI: 10.1016/j.comnet.2010.05.010

Bahdanau, D. (2014). Neural machine translation by jointly learning to align and translate. arXiv preprint arXiv:1409.0473.

Bulling, A., Blanke, U., & Schiele, B. (2014). A tutorial on human activity recognition using body-worn inertial sensors. *ACM Computing Surveys*, *46*(3), 1–33. DOI: 10.1145/2499621

Bulling, A., Blanke, U., & Schiele, B. (2014). A tutorial on human activity recognition using body-worn inertial sensors. In ACM Computing Surveys (Vol. 46, Issue 3, pp. 1–33). Association for Computing Machinery (ACM). DOI: 10.1145/2499621

Chorowski, J. K., Bahdanau, D., Serdyuk, D., Cho, K., & Bengio, Y. (2015). Attention-based models for speech recognition. *Advances in Neural Information Processing Systems*, •••, 28.

Huynh, T., & Schiele, B. (2005, October). Analyzing features for activity recognition. In Proceedings of the 2005 joint conference on Smart objects and ambient intelligence: innovative context-aware services: usages and technologies (pp. 159-163). DOI: 10.1145/1107548.1107591

Jain, R., Semwal, V. B., & Kaushik, P. (2022). Deep ensemble learning approach for lower extremity activities recognition using wearable sensors. *Expert Systems: International Journal of Knowledge Engineering and Neural Networks*, *39*(6), e12743. DOI: 10.1111/exsy.12743

Kianoush, S., Savazzi, S., Vicentini, F., Rampa, V., & Giussani, M. (2017). Device-Free RF Human Body Fall Detection and Localization in Industrial Workplaces. In IEEE Internet of Things Journal (Vol. 4, Issue 2, pp. 351–362). Institute of Electrical and Electronics Engineers (IEEE). DOI: 10.1109/JIOT.2016.2624800

Kortuem, G., Kawsar, F., Sundramoorthy, V., & Fitton, D. (2010). Smart objects as building blocks for the Internet of things. In IEEE Internet Computing (Vol. 14, Issue 1, pp. 44–51). Institute of Electrical and Electronics Engineers (IEEE). DOI: 10.1109/MIC.2009.143

Krishna, K. S., & Paneerselvam, S. (2021, October). An implementation of hybrid cnn-lstm model for human activity recognition. In International Conference on Advances in Electrical and Computer Technologies (pp. 813-825). Singapore: Springer Nature Singapore.

LeCun, Y., Boser, B., Denker, J., Henderson, D., Howard, R., Hubbard, W., & Jackel, L. (1989). Handwritten digit recognition with a back-propagation network. *Advances in Neural Information Processing Systems*, •••, 2.

Lee, I., & Lee, K. (2015). The Internet of Things (IoT): Applications, investments, and challenges for enterprises. In Business Horizons (Vol. 58, Issue 4, pp. 431–440). Elsevier BV. DOI: 10.1016/j.bushor.2015.03.008

Lin, J., Keogh, E., Lonardi, S., & Chiu, B. (2003, June). A symbolic representation of time series, with implications for streaming algorithms. In *Proceedings of the 8th ACM SIGMOD workshop on Research issues in data mining and knowledge discovery* (pp. 2-11). DOI: 10.1145/882082.882086

Lu, W., Fan, F., Chu, J., Jing, P., & Yuting, S. (2019). Wearable Computing for Internet of Things: A Discriminant Approach for Human Activity Recognition. In IEEE Internet of Things Journal (Vol. 6, Issue 2, pp. 2749–2759). Institute of Electrical and Electronics Engineers (IEEE). DOI: 10.1109/JIOT.2018.2873594

Qiu, S., Zhao, H., Jiang, N., Wang, Z., Liu, L., An, Y., Zhao, H., Miao, X., Liu, R., & Fortino, G. (2022). Multi-sensor information fusion based on machine learning for real applications in human activity recognition: State-of-the-art and research challenges. In *Information Fusion* (Vol. 80, pp. 241–265). Elsevier BV., DOI: 10.1016/j.inffus.2021.11.006

Vaswani, A. (2017). Attention is all you need. *Advances in Neural Information Processing Systems.*

Wang, S., & Zhou, G. (2015). A review on radio based activity recognition. In Digital Communications and Networks (Vol. 1, Issue 1, pp. 20–29). Elsevier BV. DOI: 10.1016/j.dcan.2015.02.006

Xu, K., Ba, J., Kiros, R., Cho, K., Courville, A., Salakhudinov, R., . . . Bengio, Y. (2015, June). Show, attend and tell: Neural image caption generation with visual attention. In International conference on machine learning (pp. 2048-2057). PMLR.

Yadav, S. K., Tiwari, K., Pandey, H. M., & Akbar, S. A. (2021). A review of multimodal human activity recognition with special emphasis on classification, applications, challenges and future directions. In *Knowledge-Based Systems* (Vol. 223, p. 106970). Elsevier BV., DOI: 10.1016/j.knosys.2021.106970

Yang, J., Nguyen, M. N., San, P. P., Li, X., & Krishnaswamy, S. (2015, July). Deep convolutional neural networks on multichannel time series for human activity recognition. In Ijcai (Vol. 15, pp. 3995-4001).

Zhang, L., Yu, J., Gao, Z., & Ni, Q. (2024). A multi-channel hybrid deep learning framework for multi-sensor fusion enabled human activity recognition. *Alexandria Engineering Journal, 91*, 472–485. DOI: 10.1016/j.aej.2024.01.030

Chapter 16
Identifying the Determinants of Maladaptive Pain Perception and Response Patterns:
Predictive Analysis With XGBoost and Random Forests

Kavya Vijaysankar
https://orcid.org/0009-0007-6326-4408
Christ University, India

ABSTRACT

A complex interplay of psychological, biological, and social factors influences pain perception and response patterns. This study aims to identify the determinants of maladaptive pain perception and response patterns through predictive analysis using psychological variables such as resilience, neuroticism, extraversion, grit, and optimism. A quantitative approach was used, incorporating predictive modeling techniques (decision trees, XGBoost, and Random Forests) to assess pain catastrophizing and sensitivity among 305 Indians. The XGBoost classifier predicting clinically significant pain catastrophizing achieved an accuracy of 74%. Findings indicate that neuroticism is a key predictor of pain-related outcomes, with resilience & optimism serving as protective factors. The study highlights the potential for personalized interventions by utilizing machine learning models to optimize predictor levels for improved pain management. The results underscore the need for further research incorporating biological and environmental factors to develop

DOI: 10.4018/979-8-3373-0194-5.ch016

holistic pain management strategies.

INTRODUCTION

Pain is an important yet unpleasant biological phenomenon that can alert the body to injury, illness or other threats. It attracts necessary medical attention or care and thereby acts as a warning system to ensure survival (Millan, 1999). Acute pain due to inflammation often parallels the immune response and diminishes with the reduction in inflammation. Experiencing pain signals that something harmful or dangerous has happened and prompts immediate action to avoid further discomfort or injury. This experience teaches us to avoid painful stimuli in the future. Pain also encourages rest and recovery by limiting the usage of the injured area. This reduces the risk of further damage and facilitates the healing process.

Neural Basis of Pain

Nociception (the detection of painful stimuli) begins at pain-sensitive neurons, which send signals from the skin to the spinal cord and central nervous system. This process involves A-delta and C-fibers, which transmit signals through peripheral nerves (Julius, 2013). A-delta fibers relay fast, sharp sensations, while slower C-fibers transmit prolonged, burning sensations. Once nociceptive signals are generated, they are conducted by peripheral nerve cell bodies located in the dorsal root ganglia, toward the central nervous system. In the spinal cord, A-delta and C-fiber signals are transmitted to nociceptive-specific neurons, which then ascend through the neospinothalamic tract to the thalamus and somatosensory cortex (Schmidt et al., 1995). Additionally, non-specific neurons in the spinal cord, which can respond to both nociceptive and non-nociceptive input, project through the paleospinothalamic and archispinothalamic tracts. These pathways relay pain signals to regions such as the periaqueductal gray, thalamus, and limbic cortex, where both visceral pain and autonomic responses are processed (Fenton et al., 2015).

Pain signals reach the thalamus and midbrain structures, forming a pain neuromatrix . This network is responsible for determining conscious pain perception and involves multiple cortical regions that activate simultaneously during pain experiences. The cortical pain matrix integrates sensory, cognitive, and emotional components of pain (Melzack, 2001). Dysfunction in any part of this matrix can lead to unregulated, persistent pain, highlighting the complexity of pain processing in the brain. The thalamus functions as a critical relay station for pain signals transmitted from the spinal cord. Structurally, the thalamus is divided into medial and lateral divisions. The lateral division houses the ventral posterior (VP) nuclei, which receive both tactile and nociceptive inputs, while the medial division, connected to intralaminar nuclei and the medial dorsal (MD) nucleus, is involved in pain modulation. Thalamic nuclei also maintain reciprocal connections with the cortex, forming thalamocortical loops. In chronic pain conditions, a reduction in thalamocortical connectivity, particularly within the ventral posterior (VP) and medial dorsal (MD) nuclei, indicates altered thalamic processing that may underlie persistent pain experiences. Functional changes in the thalamus during chronic pain states are also notable.

The descending modulation system plays a critical role in regulating pain perception through a network of brain regions that modulate spinal cord activity. Key components of this system include the periaqueductal gray (PAG), rostral ventromedial medulla (RVM), and locus ceruleus (LC). The PAG, located in the midbrain, is a central hub for pain modulation, containing a high density of μ-opioid receptors. Upon activation, the PAG triggers descending pathways that project to the RVM and spinal cord, releasing neurotransmitters that inhibit pain transmission, thereby producing analgesia. The RVM, in turn, acts as a relay point for these descending pathways, housing both on-cells and off-cells that either facilitate or inhibit pain, respectively. This dynamic balance allows the RVM to fine-tune pain responses depending on the body's physiological needs. Additionally, the locus ceruleus contributes to this system by releasing norepinephrine, which enhances the inhibitory effects of descending pathways. Together, these regions form a feedback loop that can amplify or suppress pain signals, allowing the body to modulate pain perception in response to varying conditions. Dysfunction in this system, particularly in chronic pain states, can disrupt this regulatory mechanism, leading to persistent pain.

Mechanisms and Types of Pain

Based on the duration of occurrence, pain can either be acute or chronic. Acute pain is short-lived and reduces after the treatment of its cause. Different types of pain signal different bodily disruptions and require different approaches to treatment and management. The most common type of acute pain is nociceptive pain which results from damage to body tissue caused by external stimuli. The pain serves the biological purpose of warning the body of injury (Millan, 1999). Treatment could involve rest or physical therapies such as exercise and stretching to accelerate the healing speed and strengthen the injured tissues. Severe pain might require pharmacological intervention such as NSAIDs (nonsteroidal anti-inflammatory drugs), opioids or analgesics. Surgical intervention might be required for structural damage, such as compound fractures, where rest and physical therapy do not allow for correct healing.

When pain lasts longer than six months or continues after the injury or illness has been cured, it becomes chronic. Pain can be seen as problematic or unnecessary when it extends beyond the period of damage and healing or when it lacks an organic cause for explanation. Chronic pain is said to be a disease state that might arise from psychological states (Swieboda et al., 2013). People suffering from chronic pain are known to have problems in activating descending modulation. Conditions such as allodynia (pain resulting from a stimulus that usually does not provoke pain) or phantom limb pain (the perception of pain or discomfort in an amputated limb) are instances where pain is unnecessary and even impairs normal functioning. These two conditions are caused by dysregulation of the positive feedback loop, where a stimulus causes the system to malfunction. This malfunction can also trigger migraine headaches and a variety of autoimmune disorders. Chronic pain conditions usually have different methods of treatment and rely on medication and physical therapy as primary forms. This is a result of the underlying cause being unknown or untreatable.

Neuropathic pain emerges from damage to nerves or the nervous system and is not necessarily a result of external stimuli. It can, however, result from an underlying disease (Baron et al., 2010). Nerve compressions such as carpal tunnel syndrome and cubital tunnel syndrome, or the presence of tumours, put pressure on the nerve and can cause neuropathic pain. Metabolic disorders can cause an imbalance in essential nutrients, leading to neuropathy. Chronically high blood sugar levels associated with diabetes can damage nerves over time. Deficiencies in vitamin B12 lead to damage to the peripheral nervous system, particularly in the legs. Neuropathic pain is more difficult to treat than nociceptive pain and involves combining different treatment methods, such as treating the underlying disease, medication, surgery, and psychological intervention (Baron et al., 2010).

Psychogenic pain is physical pain that lacks organic causes for explanation (Le, 1994). One example is proctalgia fugax, a condition in which a person experiences sudden mild to severe anal pain (Douthwaite, 1962). The pain comes in recurring episodes and may last months or years and is caused by spasms of the anal sphincter muscle. The causes of the spasms are not fully understood but are linked to the individual's psychological state (Thompson, 1989). Treatment involves muscle relaxants to ease the spasms, and patients are advised to avoid their triggers until the pain passes. Psychosomatic pain is pain that is exacerbated by psychological or emotional factors but still has a physiological basis. Psychosomatic disorders are considered types of psychogenic disorders. They are characterized by physiological changes and are seen as irritable bowel syndrome, tension headaches, or musculoskeletal mind-body syndrome (Rashbaum & Sarno, 2003). Migraines are an example of psychosomatic pain that could be triggered by social rejection, grief, regret, or other emotional events. The underlying pathology of psychosomatic pain is not fully understood; however, the method of pain management involves psychotherapeutic interventions for reducing the intensity of pain.

Pain Management Approaches

Chronic pain can sometimes be exacerbated by psychological factors and requires psychological interventions and therapies for management. Many effective therapeutic modalities have been developed that target a person's cognitive framework and behavioral responses to the pain. Operant-behavioral therapy targets maladaptive behavioral responses by using reinforcement and punishment. Cognitive behavioral therapy focuses on the cognitive restructuring of distorted and maladaptive thoughts on pain. It also involves behavioral pacing & activation, and positive event scheduling. Other techniques include teaching 'non-striving' responses to pain through guided or experiential meditation, and practicing mindfulness. These techniques also encourage acceptance of pain which ceases the maladaptive coping strategies such as avoidance and other problematic behaviors (Sturgeon, 2014). The shift from physical and pharmacological treatment to psychological intervention has been driven by the increasing concerns about drug dependence.

The Opioid Crisis and Re-evaluation of Pain Management

In the past few decades, there has been a widespread misuse of pain medication leading to an opioid crisis. High-dose opioids initially prescribed to manage acute or chronic pain led many patients to develop a dependence due to their highly addictive nature. Building tolerance toward the pain medication results in taking higher doses to achieve the same pain relief, which increases the risk of addiction and overdose. The devastating social, economic, and health-related consequences have prompted a re-evaluation of pain management, emphasizing non-pharmacological treatments such as cognitive-behavioral therapy (CBT), mindfulness, and biofeedback. The Ministry of Social Justice and Empowerment, Government of India published a report on the comprehensive statistics of drug abuse across India (Ambekar et al. 2019). This national survey was conducted by the National Drug Dependence Treatment Centre, All India Institute of Medical Sciences, New Delhi. The opioid usage was reported to be 2.1% of the country's population (approximately 23 million people) which is three times more than the global average, with heroin usage the highest, followed by pharmaceutical opioids, and then opium. Dependent usage is the highest among users. The overall use of opioids has increased since the last national survey conducted in 2004 (Ray, 2004). The report suggests that opioid dependence often begins with medically prescribed opioids for pain management, where inadequate monitoring and the lack of non-pharmacological alternatives can lead to misuse. To address this, the report recommends stricter regulation of opioid prescriptions, increased access to non-addictive pain management methods, and the implementation of public awareness campaigns to reduce the risk of misuse and dependency. Additionally, it underscores the need for counseling and rehabilitation services to support individuals struggling with opioid addiction.

The urgent need to find effective alternatives to opioids for managing chronic pain has led to growing exploration of psychotherapeutic approaches that target the psychological and behavioral aspects of pain perception. The shift toward these approaches has overall resulted in more efficient and sustainable pain management strategies, as they address the root causes of pain perception rather than simply masking symptoms. Furthermore, the psychological distress caused by opioid dependence, such as anxiety, depression, and social isolation, often exacerbates pain, creating a cycle that can be difficult to break. By addressing both the emotional and cognitive dimensions of pain, these therapies offer a more holistic solution.

Social, Cultural and Gender Influences on Pain Perception in India

In the Indian cultural context, gender roles are often imposed by society to a great extent that plays a major role in influencing the perception and response of pain. Traditionally, men are expected to suppress the expression of pain, as vulnerability is often perceived as a sign of weakness. This belief stems from the misconception that traditional masculinity comprises constructs such as strength, stoicism, or emotional restraint. These norms are often reinforced by societal expectations, where men are encouraged to tolerate pain, avoid displaying feelings of fear, sadness, and physical discomfort. Moreover, beliefs about masculinity being defined by stoicism can reduce help-seeking behaviors, leading some men to internalize their pain rather than vocalize it.

Conversely, women are viewed as more emotionally vulnerable. This perception often reinforces the traditional narrative that associates femininity with heightened sensitivity and a lower tolerance for discomfort, encouraging them to express their pain more openly and potentially perceive it as more severe. These societal norms, which expect women to be more expressive in their emotional responses, may lead to heightened emotional reactions to pain and a tendency to view it as more overwhelming. As a result, women may internalize these expectations, shaping both how they experience and report their pain.

Furthermore, Indian culture is deeply rooted in spirituality, which can also influence pain sensitivity and how individuals mentally respond to pain. Many Indians view pain and suffering through a spiritual lens, often accepting it as part of karma. This spiritual outlook can influence how individuals cope with pain, with those connected to spiritual practices often demonstrating greater acceptance of pain and a reduced tendency to overthink or become emotionally distressed by it. By finding meaning or purpose in suffering, individuals may frame pain as a part of a larger spiritual journey, which helps them endure it with less focus on its intensity. This perspective can lead to a reduced amplification of pain and emotional distress, allowing individuals to cope with greater resilience. Research suggests that spirituality can serve as a coping mechanism, providing individuals with a framework to endure pain with greater resilience, which positively impacts pain-related outcomes.

Theoretical Backing

To better understand the complexity of pain perception and its underlying mechanisms, it is essential to explore the various theoretical frameworks that have shaped our current understanding. These theories provide insight into the biological, psychological, and social dimensions of pain, laying the foundation for examining how psychological traits interact with pain-related outcomes.

Early Theories

All the above-mentioned types of pain involve different dimensions: biological, psychological and social. The earliest theory of pain proposed by René Descartes, the Cartesian Dualistic Theory of pain, viewed pain as a mutually exclusive phenomenon that could be caused by either physical or psychological illness, but never a combination of the two. While this view correctly implicates a person's psychological state to the contribution of pain, it repudiates the interplay between physical and psychological states. This acts as a major limitation, particularly when examining psychosomatic pain. Research is being devoted to understanding the interaction of various factors in the context of pain. The dimension that contributes to a particular type of pain can be traced to its etiology. Pain that is caused without an organic reason, or that is at a higher intensity than it should be are usually a result of psychological factors.

Placebo and Nocebo Effect

The placebo effect refers to the improvement in health conditions when a placebo or a fake treatment is administered. Placebos possess a nonspecific psychological effect which satisfies the patient. There is no plausible biological explanation to account for a causal association between placebo treatment and clinical outcome. Placebos have no pharmacological mechanism of action. Impure placebos may lead to physiological reactions that are not related to the condition being treated. The nocebo effect on the other hand refers to a deterioration in health conditions after a specific treatment due to negative beliefs about the treatment (Price et al., 2008). The implications of these effects suggest that psychological factors play a role in mediating these effects (Colloca & Miller, 2011). The behavioral theory states that recovery based on the placebo effect could be a learned response where treatment for a specific condition is associated with being cured or healed (Stewart-Williams & Podd, 2004). This explanation cannot account for instances where there was no previous exposure to treatment. The belief is that psychological factors such as hope, anxiety, expectancy, and desire play a role in mediating the course of a condition (Margo, 1999).

Gate Control Theory

This theory posits that there is a 'gate' in the spinal cord that is made up of large fibers. The large fibers comprise T-cells that are present in a region called the substantia gelatinosa and transmit impulses from the spinal cord to the brain. Together, these larger fibers sometimes inhibit the transmission of impulses from smaller fibers by forming a hypothetical gate (Melzack & Wall, 1965). The gate can be opened and closed by stronger stimulation of nerve fibers, and more sensory activity in other peripheral fibers such as rubbing, pressing, etc (this inhibits the opening of the gate). Psychological or cognitive processes can influence the opening and closing of the gate and hence can modulate pain signals (Melzack & Wall, 1965). It emphasizes the central nervous system mechanisms and explains the physiological basis for psychological factors in chronic pain (Turk & Swanson, 2008).

Biopsychosocial Model

The biopsychosocial Model was proposed by Dr. George Engel in 1977. It states that medical conditions are caused by more than just biological factors. It considers the psychological and social aspects of medical conditions (Engel, 1977). This model is commonly used in chronic pain with the view that pain is a psychophysiological behavior pattern and cannot be explained by only one perspective. Pain management techniques under this model target all interacting factors that contribute to pain.

Dynamic Model of Affect

This model examines how positive and negative emotions interact with each other, and how stress and pain can affect this relationship. It is used in the understanding of chronic pain. Chronic pain is not only a physical process but also has an affective component. During a stressful or painful experience, positive affect reduces and negative affect increases (Zautra et al., 2001). This leads to a more polarized emotional experience. The anticipation and experience of pain trigger negative emotions which further exacerbate the pain. This process becomes a cycle.

Neuromatrix Theory of Pain

The neuromatrix theory of pain (Melzack, 2001) is an extension of the gate control theory. The neuromatrix is the widespread network of neurons consisting of loops between the thalamus and cortex, and the cortex and the limbic system. The spatial distribution and synaptic links of this entire network are determined genetically. The activity within the neuromatrix; the repeated cyclical processing and synthesis of nerve impulses, generates a pattern called 'neurosignature'. The brain generates a body-self neuromatrix which integrates sensory input with cognitive and affective information which collectively produce the perception of pain. When physical or physiological stress disrupts the homeostasis of the activity in the neuromatrix, neural, hormonal, and behavioral responses are triggered to restore the balance. Prolonged stress can influence the neurosignature patterns and lead to the development of chronic pain even when no sensory input or injury is present.

Rationale of this Study

The rationale for this study stems from the biopsychosocial model (Engel, 1977), which states that complex interactions between psychological factors can shape how we experience pain. Our perception of pain can be based on our ability to withstand pain (pain sensitivity), and how we view painful experiences (pain catastrophizing). Psychotherapeutic models for chronic pain target affective, cognitive, and behavioral components of pain. Despite the ongoing research, there is a lack of a predictive model that suggests optimal predictor levels for minimal pain sensitivity. Measuring pain sensitivity involves experimental methods such as the cold pressor test, (henceforth referred to as CPT), (Mitchell et al., 2004) or self-reports, which give insights into an individual's pain levels. Professionals are left to create intervention strategies without insights into the interplay between the contributing factors. A predictive model alone won't add sufficient value to intervention techniques. When combined with explainability techniques, interpretability techniques, sensitivity analyses and optimization techniques, it can provide deeper insights into an individual's affective, cognitive, and behavioral components of pain. Furthermore, it can help decide optimal combinations of psychological variables that reduce pain sensitivity. This can help develop personalized and specific target interventions.

REVIEW OF LITERATURE

Individual differences play a role in the variability of experiencing pain. These differences include biological and social factors such as age (Saxena et al., 2015), biological sex (Fillingim, 2017), ethnicity, and gender roles (Hansen et al., 2015). The relationship between pain sensitivity and psychological factors has been a significant area of research to understand how individual differences in disposition and temperament influence the occurrence of pain.

Pain sensitivity refers to the overall response of an individual to a painful stimulus (Ruscheweyh et al., 2009). It includes both threshold and tolerance. Pain threshold is the minimum intensity of a stimulus required to sense pain. Pain tolerance is the maximum intensity of pain an individual can withstand once it is perceived. An individual with low pain sensitivity is likely to perceive pain at a higher intensity (low pain threshold) and cannot withstand it for long periods (low tolerance).

Understanding individual pain intensity perception has involved experimental methods to accurately quantify this highly subjective experience. The treatment of chronic pain, psychosomatic pain, etc, has relied on acquiring levels of pain tolerance and threshold through experimental measures. These experimental methods use different modalities: heat, cold, pressure, pinpricks, shocks, etc. The cold pressor test (Mitchell et al., 2004), for example, has been used in numerous studies to gauge an individual's pain perception. It involves immersing your non-dominant hand wrist-deep into cold water and reporting how long the pain is initially perceived and when the pain becomes unbearable. The former constitutes the pain threshold, and the latter constitutes the pain tolerance. These experimental methods require time and resources for the elaborate setup.

A study conducted by Edwards & Fillingim (2007) measured the correlation between experimental methods of measuring pain and self-report measures of pain. They used the thermal pain testing method as the experimental method and various self-reports used in different studies, one of which was the Kohn Reactivity Scale (KRS) (Dubreuil & Kohn, 1986) as a self-report method. The thermal pain test measures the pain threshold and tolerance by inflicting pain through temperature.

A thermal probe is applied to the skin to heat or cool the skin. This allows for quantification of how much pain an individual can tolerate. The KRS measures general reactivity, emotional responses, and hypervigilance towards various stimuli. It focuses on evaluating how different people react to pain differently. It assesses experiences in a subjective manner. It was found that there was no association between the reported pain sensitivity and the participants' actual pain threshold and tolerance. This study proved that overcoming psychosomatic pain by assessing sensitivity through self-reports would not be useful. This meant that understanding individual differences in pain required experimental measures.

The Pain Sensitivity Questionnaire (PSQ) developed by Ruscheweyh et al. (2009) was designed to quantify individual pain perception. This tool involves imagining painful situations and rating the expected pain intensity in those hypothetical situations. Good reliability and validity were demonstrated during the validation of the scale. There was a decent correlation between experimental pain-related intensity and Pain Sensitivity Questionnaire scores. The scores were associated more with pain tolerance rather than pain threshold. The prediction of pain through this instrument (when answered without bias) was better compared to psychological factors associated with pain. This indicates that the Pain Sensitivity Questionnaire can be used as an alternative to experimental methods using different modalities (cold, heat, pressure, pinpricks).

Psychotherapeutic Interventions for Pain Management

Kreitler & Kreitler (2007) proposed a classification of different psychotherapeutic techniques according to the components of pain (sensory, affective, cognitive, behavioral). The sensory component includes the physical sensations associated with pain, such as intensity, location, and quality (shooting, throbbing). The affective component relates to the emotional responses to pain, such as distress, suffering, anxiety, and frustration. The cognitive component involves mental processes related to pain perception, how much individuals think about their pain, how they interpret it, and how they evaluate it. For example, a person with "The pain is unbearable. I don't think it will ever end". The behavioral component includes the observable actions taken in response to pain which are usually shaped by the previous 3 components (sensory, affective, cognitive). An example would be taking pain medication at the slightest discomfort. Each component requires a different intervention approach. Interventions can be classified based on the different treatment models: the psychodynamic model and the cognitive-behavioral model (Turk et al., 2008).

Interventions for the Sensory Component

Biofeedback is a self-regulatory, mind-body technique that can be used in pain management for chronic pain (Schwartz, 2017). It targets the sensory component of pain (Kreitler & Kreitler, 2007) and falls under the cognitive-behavioral model (Turk et al., 2008). The underlying assumption is that the level of pain is caused, maintained, or exacerbated by autonomic nervous system dysregulation, which is associated with the production of nociceptive stimulation. This forms the principle that awareness of physiological processes, stress, and pain/discomfort can allow individuals to modify these processes and their outcomes. In pain management, pain regulation is attained by gaining voluntary control over the physiological responses related to pain. During the process, patients are connected to electrical sensors, which give immediate feedback about the physiological responses that occur during a painful experience (Schwartz, 2017).

Another technique used for easing the sensory component of pain is relaxation therapy. In progressive muscle relaxation, individuals are asked to tense and then relax specific muscle groups in a particular order. Autogenic training involves a 15-minute session where individuals perform visualization exercises to induce muscle relaxation (Kreitler & Kreitler, 2007). Meditation (transcendental or mindfulness) can also fall under relaxation techniques. Mindfulness meditation involves creating awareness of the entire perceptual field. It emphasized directing one's attention to all available stimuli at the present moment. Transcendental meditation, however, involves concentrating on any one of the senses and repeating a word or phrase to transcend the ordinary stream of thought. Bonadonna (2003) suggested that chronic illness can disrupt a person's ability to concentrate. Therefore, mindfulness meditation is more useful than transcendental meditation. This technique requires the physical pain or discomfort to be made the object of meditation so it can be experienced fully and further explored (Bonadonna, 2003). Mindfulness meditation or related interventions have been shown to decrease pain intensity, increase healing speed, decrease stress, and improve mood (Astin et al., 2003; Grossman et al., 2004).

Guided imagery falls under the cognitive framework of the cognitive-behavioral model (Turk et al., 2008) and targets the sensory component of pain (Kreitler & Kreitler, 2007). This technique allows people to achieve a sense of control over their pain while distracting them from the accompanying symptoms and reducing their intensity. The patients evoke images through imagination or visualization through guidance by the therapist. During painful experiences, patients can use imagery to redirect their attention and achieve a sense of psychophysiological relaxation. Another way to use guided imagery is to attribute metaphorical forms to the pain, distancing them from the body or changing their meaning (Kreitler & Kreitler, 2007).

Hypnosis or hypnotherapy is another method used during pain management. It targets the sensory component of pain (Kreitler & Kreitler, 2007) and falls under the cognitive-behavioral model (Turk et al., 2008). Kihlstrom (1985) explained hypnosis using two people: the subject and the hypnotist. The hypnotist guides the subject to experience aroused attentive focal concentration and suspended peripheral awareness. The subject responds to suggestions given by the hypnotist and experiences alterations in perception, memory, and voluntary action. In the context of pain reduction, the hypnotist can provide suggestions to increase the ability to ignore pain, directing attention away from the pain, or changing sensations from pain to something else (Dillworth & Jensen, 2010).

Interventions for the Affective and Cognitive Components

The motivational interviewing technique falls under the cognitive-behavioral model (Turk et al., 2008). Although developed for treating substance use disorders (Jensen et al., 2003), it has been adapted to treat chronic pain (Kerns & Habib, 2004). This technique has been designed to increase a patient's motivation to change in instances where a change in attitude or behavior is required to manage chronic pain. It can be followed by acceptance and commitment therapy, which encourages acceptance of aversive experiences such as pain or discomfort through attitude changes instead of attempting to change or avoid them. This is effective in cases where individuals have to live with aversive stimuli or situations (Kreitler & Kreitler, 2007).

Identification of Psychological Variables

Studies have implicated the role of psychological factors such as personality traits, particularly extraversion and neuroticism, in affecting a person's experience with pain (Atanassova et al., 2024; Grouper et al., 2021). Atanassova et al. (2024) conducted a meta-analysis on studies that examined the relationship between the Big Five personality dimensions and experimental pain. The studies included were conducted on healthy adults, used experimental methods of data collection (cold pressor test, pressure test, pin prick test), and had a sample size ranging from 41 to 1322 participants. A total of 22 papers were reviewed out of which 6 were used in the formal analysis. The meta-analysis found consistent correlations between two dimensions; Neuroticism and pain tolerance were negatively correlated, meaning higher levels of neuroticism were associated with lower levels of pain tolerance, or in other words, higher levels of pain sensitivity. Extraversion and pain tolerance were also positively correlated. The effect size, however, was found to be weak in all the studies, which indicates that these two variables explain only a small portion of the variance in pain. The small effect can still be relevant in specific contexts or in combination with other variables.

Grouper et al. (2021) also studied the effects of neuroticism and extraversion on pain sensitivity by including pain catastrophizing as a mediator. This study found a positive correlation between neuroticism and pain sensitivity. Furthermore, pain catastrophizing was found to have a mediating effect on the relationship between neuroticism and pain sensitivity.

Resilience has been studied as a factor in determining pain perception. Sturgeon & Zautra (2010), looked at resilience from 3 different perspectives in their study. Resilience can be understood as 3 primary processes; recovery (regaining equilibrium after undesirable episodes), sustainability (maintaining positive and socially desirable actions that lead to positive emotions), and growth (realising the new strengths and abilities gained as learnings from the undesirable experience as a result of the individual's coping mechanisms). Resilience and vulnerability factors play a role in the response to pain episodes. Resilience resources enhance one's resilience mechanisms (positive affect, social interaction), and promote adaptive and healthy coping strategies. These lead to positive resilience outcomes which are recovery, sustainability, and growth. By understanding the interplay of resilience resources, better intervention strategies can be planned and implemented for more effective pain management.

A study conducted by Newton-John et al. (2014) investigated the relationship between resilience and chronic pain coping mechanisms. They sought to understand whether resilience contributes to the adjustment and coping strategies of individuals suffering from chronic pain. 101 adult participants were recruited from a pain-management clinic in Australia who reported experiencing pain for at least 12 months. Each participant was tested using 8 questionnaires related to pain, pain outcomes, and resilience. Their findings suggest that resilience is associated with better pain-related outcomes, such as lower pain-related disability and lower reported pain intensity. The role of resilience as a direct predictor, although present, was relatively weak. This suggests that the impact on pain sensitivity might be mediated through other factors.

A study conducted by Buckingham & Richardson (2021) explored the moderating effect of grit and optimism on the pre-established relationship between psychological resilience and pain threshold/tolerance. No significant correlations were found between grit and psychological resilience, and optimism and resilience. The moderation models implicated grit in the enhancement of the effect of resilience on pain threshold and tolerance. The researchers used 64 healthy adult participants recruited from a student population. They used the cold pressor test as a measure of experimental pain. Optimism was a significant moderator of the relationship between resilience and CPT tolerance, as well as the relationship between resilience and CPT threshold. Grit was found to moderate the relationship between resilience and pain threshold only.

A study conducted by (Kim et al., 2023) sought to understand the emotional dynamics involved in pain perception in individuals with fibromyalgia. This paper builds on the dynamic model of affect to investigate the momentary associations between positive and negative emotions as influenced by pain, fatigue and stress. They found that people with higher levels of pain felt more negative emotions and less positive emotions. The findings were purely correlational and implicated no direction in the relationship. Meagher et al. (2001) investigated how different emotional states induced by unpleasant and pleasant photographic slides affected pain perception during the cold pressor test. They concluded their study with findings that suggested that unpleasant affective states enhanced their pain while pleasant affective states reduced their pain.

Predictive modeling in Pain Research

Predictive modeling techniques in pain research have evolved significantly, leveraging advanced computational methods to enhance understanding and prediction of pain responses. They can be used for diagnosis, treatment, and patient outcomes. By leveraging advanced machine learning algorithms and integrating diverse data sources, researchers have made significant strides in understanding pain mechanisms, predicting treatment responses, and personalizing care.

A study conducted by Zhao et al. (2024) aimed to identify meaningful subgroups within chronic pain patients by applying a combination of supervised learning and latent variable mixture modeling. Questionnaire data from 11,995 patients included pain characteristics, psychological aspects, and social functioning and helped researchers identify 4 distinct classes of patients, each with unique unique pain patterns. These subgroups varied in terms of pain intensity, emotional distress, and mental and physical health. Class 2, for instance, reported severe pain intensity and interference. Their anxiety, depression, and general affective distress were the highest among all subgroups. They showed poor mental health and vitality scores. Class 4, however, was regarded as the healthiest group with the lowest pain presentation, lowest negative emotions, and better mental and physical health conditions. The division of subgroups highlighted the importance of emotional distress in chronic pain patients, particularly in classes where high levels of depression and anxiety were associated with worse clinical presentations and higher risks of long-term unfavourable outcomes. This study emphasizes the importance of addressing affective states and employing tailored treatment plans based on individual differences.

Tagliaferri et al. (2022) attempted to identify subgroups of individuals with chronic back pain (CBP) based on psychosocial, neural, and physical factors using Fuzzy C-Means Clustering. The key variables optimal for clustering were loneliness/ social isolation and depression. This method identified 5 distinct clusters. Machine learning classifiers such as Support Vector Machine (SVM), Naïve Bayes, k-Nearest Neighbour, and Random Forest were used to assess the classification accuracy. Classification accuracy for chronic back pain subgroups was greater than 95% when assessed alone. When the pain-free controls were included in the analysis, the misclassification rates increased by 35-53%. This indicates that psychosocial variables are effective for subgroup classification but insufficient for distinguishing between individuals with chronic back pain and those without. The overall goal was to improve clinical decision-making by offering accurate and interpretable classifications of chronic back pain subgroups, leading to more personalized interventions.

Antonucci et al. (2020) aimed to identify the pattern of psychophysical impairments that can distinguish between individuals with chronic pain and and healthy controls using support vector classification and repeated nested cross validation. 13 features were derived by assessing different dimensions of health and functioning such as quality of life, physical and mental health, depression and anxiety, physical and occupational functioning, cognitive abilities, and beliefs about medical treatment. The classifier model achieved an accuracy rate of 86.5%. The classification was made based on 3 dimensions: anxiety and depression scores, beliefs about medical treatment, and physical and occupational functioning. Individuals with chronic pain scored high in depression and anxiety assessments indicating a strong psychological component with chronic pain. Chronic pain individuals also had beliefs that medications may be harmful whereas the healthy controls had more positive beliefs regarding medications. Chronic pain individuals demonstrated impaired or reduced physical activity due to their pain.

Need for the Study

The above sections of the literature review identified psychological variables that directly or indirectly affect an individual's pain sensitivity. The variables are resilience, neuroticism, extraversion, affect, grit, optimism, and pain catastrophizing. These variables can be categorized into affective, cognitive, behavioral, and sensory components of pain processing. Resilience and grit reflect cognitive and behavioral components, as they involve an individual's ability to endure and persist in adverse situations. Neuroticism, an affective trait, relates to an individual's tendency to experience negative emotions, influencing emotional responses to pain. Extraversion, which also has an affective and behavioral dimension, may alter the way individuals engage with and react to pain. Optimism, a cognitive trait, can shape how individuals perceive and cope with painful experiences. Due to the multicollinearity between affect and neuroticism, both variables cannot be included in the model simultaneously. Neuroticism, the tendency to experience negative emotions, is a relatively more stable trait than affect, which is how people feel and express their emotions. The variables conceptually overlap, and including both would lead to biased model performance. Hence, affect will be dropped in favor of neuroticism.

Although previous studies highlight pain catastrophizing as a predictor of pain sensitivity, it will be a target variable along with pain sensitivity in this study. Pain catastrophizing captures an individual's exaggerated negative response to pain, which is crucial in understanding pain-related experiences. Unlike resilience, neuroticism, extraversion, grit, and optimism, which primarily serve as predictors, pain catastrophizing reflects a maladaptive cognitive response to pain that exacerbates pain perception and emotional distress. By treating it as a target variable, we can examine how psychological traits and behaviors contribute to the development and intensity of pain catastrophizing, allowing for a more comprehensive analysis of how individuals cope with and interpret pain. This approach can help in identifying specific intervention strategies that focus on reducing catastrophic thinking patterns, ultimately leading to more effective pain management and psychological treatments.

The use of machine learning techniques, such as clustering and classification algorithms, has been shown to provide a framework for identifying distinct pain-related subgroups and the relevant predictive variables. However, much of the current research focuses primarily on classification of the subgroups and pain/non-pain groups rather than understanding the interaction between psychological variables and pain related outcomes.

One key difference in this study is its focus on pain catastrophizing and pain sensitivity as target variables rather than relying solely on chronic pain as a defining condition. Most studies in the field tend to select individuals already experiencing chronic pain and aim to classify these individuals into subgroups based on various psychological, neural, or physical characteristics. In contrast, this study aims to predict pain catastrophizing—response patterns that involve exaggerated, negative reactions to pain—and pain sensitivity across a broader population, which includes individuals with and without chronic pain. This study proposes a shift in focus from the treatment of pain symptoms to addressing the causal psychological factors that contribute to heightened pain sensitivity and pain catastrophizing. By targeting the psychological constructs underlying these experiences, rather than merely alleviating symptoms, more effective and holistic interventions can be developed. Understanding how resilience, neuroticism, grit, extraversion, and optimism interact with pain-related experiences may offer new avenues for treatment that target the root causes of heightened pain perception and maladaptive pain responses.

METHODOLOGY

Aim

This study aims to create a model to help healthcare professionals identify psychological variables contributing to different pain catastrophizing and pain sensitivity levels. By balancing predictive accuracy and interpretability, healthcare professionals can understand how and to what extent each psychological variable contributes to pain catastrophizing and pain sensitivity. This will help identify patient-specific factors that exacerbate pain-related rumination, magnification, and feelings of helplessness. The information provided by the model can aid in developing targeted psychotherapeutic interventions, such as regulating resilience in individuals whose pain perception and response patterns are highly influenced by this trait, ultimately making pain-related experiences more manageable.

Objectives

1. To assess the strength and nature of the relationship between the features (presence of chronic pain, biological sex, age, resilience, extraversion, neuroticism, grit, and optimism) and target variables (pain catastrophizing and pain sensitivity) using correlation and moderation tests.
2. To train decision trees to predict one's pain catastrophizing and pain sensitivity based on the feature variables & assess the model's accuracy.
3. To employ explainability and interpretability techniques to understand individual differences in pain catastrophizing and pain sensitivity and to help develop informed interventions.

Research Design

The study combines quantitative methodologies with predictive modeling methods. The quantitative approach employs simple statistical techniques to assess the strength and direction of the relationships between feature variables and pain catastrophizing. The predictive modeling approach uses decision trees, interpretability techniques, and SHAP values to understand the factors contributing to maladaptive pain perception and response patterns.

The study uses XGBoost (eXtreme Gradient Boosting) and Random Forests, two ensemble learning techniques that build on decision trees to improve predictive performance. XGBoost constructs a series of decision trees sequentially, with each tree correcting the errors of the previous one. This iterative process allows the model to improve on cases which are difficult to predict or that have lower observations such as high levels of pain sensitivity or pain catastrophizing. Random Forests generates multiple decision trees parallelly and aggregates their prediction to increase accuracy and reduce overfitting. Each tree is built on a random subset of the data, ensuring the model is robust to variance and is capable of generalizing well across different subsets.

These techniques were chosen for their ability to handle complex non-linear relationships and feature interactions which is not possible through standard regression. The iterative process of XGBoost allows it to focus on individuals with high pain sensitivity, who may be underrepresented in the data. These models can also handle multicollinearity and imbalanced datasets better than standard regression models.

Sample

The sample consists of 305 individuals. The sample consists of educated male and female Indian residents/citizens between the ages of 18 and 60 years who are fluent in English. This study used purposive and snowball sampling for recruiting participants. The data collection form was circulated online for interested individuals who fit the inclusion criteria to fill out. Data was collected until a sample size of 300 was reached to ensure sufficient variability for training the decision trees. No formal power analysis was conducted as this study does not involve hypothesis testing. The chosen sample is adequate for machine learning techniques where the goal is to detect patterns in the data rather than test statistical hypotheses. The number of observations allows for decent model performance while lowering the risk of overfitting. People who fit the following criteria were included in the study:

- Individuals residing in India and/or having Indian citizenship.
- Individuals between the ages of 18 and 60 years.
- Individuals who are proficient in English.

Individuals with major psychological disorders that would impair their comprehension, self-awareness, and capacity to respond accurately or give consent were excluded from the study.

Variables

The variables in the study are demographic and psychological. They are: biological sex, age, presence of chronic pain, resilience, neuroticism, extraversion, grit, optimism, pain catastrophizing, and pain sensitivity. The variables will be divided into feature variables and target variables. Biological sex, age, presence of chronic pain, resilience, neuroticism, extraversion, grit, and optimism are the feature variables. Pain catastrophizing and pain sensitivity are the target variables.

Psychological Resilience

Psychological resilience revolves around 2 concepts: adversity and positive adaptation. The American Psychological Association defines resilience as the process of successfully adapting to changing surroundings through mental, emotional, and behavioral flexibility as well as adjusting to external and internal demands. It can also refer to a person's ability to bounce back from stressful situations. To measure resilience among participants, the Brief Resilience Scale (Smith et al., 2008) was used. The total score ranges from 1.00 to 5.00, where scores between 1.00 and 2.99 indicate a low level of resilience, scores between 3.00 and 4.30 indicate an average level of resilience, and scores between 4.31 and 5 indicate a high level of resilience. This scale has demonstrated construct and predictive validity. It also exhibits good test-retest reliability. The Cronbach's alpha level is reported to be above 0.80 (Smith et al., 2008).

Neuroticism & Extraversion

Neuroticism is a trait in the big five-factor model of personality given by Costa & McCrae (2003). It is the tendency to experience or feel negative states and emotions such as self-doubt, anxiety, depression, and more. People with low neuroticism are generally more stable and are more emotionally resilient. Extraversion is a trait in the big five-factor model of personality given by Costa & McCrae (2003). This trait is characterized by sociability, excitability, talkativeness, assertiveness, and high emotional expressivity. People with high extraversion tend to be more socially confident and gain energy by interacting with people. People with low extraversion tend to prefer solitude and introspection. The Big Five personality test measures 5 broad dimensions of personality: Openness to experience, conscientiousness, extraversion, agreeableness, and neuroticism. This scale was developed by Costa & McCrae (1985). The items from the extraversion and neuroticism dimensions will be taken. The neuroticism and extraversion dimensions demonstrate good test-retest reliability and internal consistency. The Cronbach's alpha value for neuroticism ranges from 0.85 to 0.90. The Cronbach's alpha value for extraversion ranges from 0.80 to 0.88. Total scores range from 10 to 50 in each. Higher scores in extraversion indicate greater sociability. Higher scores in neuroticism indicate emotional instability and stress sensitivity.

Grit

Grit can be defined as long-term passion and perseverance towards goals. It focuses more on sustained effort and interest rather than raw talent or short-term motivation (Duckworth, 2016). It is the extent to which individuals maintain passion and perseverance toward their long-term goals despite setbacks, failures, and challenges. The 12-item Grit Scale (Duckworth et al., 2007) was used to measure grit. The scale demonstrates good internal consistency with a Cronbach's alpha of 0.85. The total score ranges from 1-5 where higher scores indicate higher levels of grit while lower scores indicate lower levels of grit.

Optimism

Optimism refers to the extent to which people hold generalized favorable expectancies for their futures (Carver et al., 2010). It can be measured as the degree to which individuals possess the confidence and hope that future events will be positive. The Revised Life Orientation Test (LOT-R) was used to measure the participants' optimism (Scheier et al., 1994). The test exhibits good internal consistency, with a Cronbach's alpha of 0.78, and good test-retest reliability. Scores range from 0-24 with higher scores indicating higher optimism and lower scores indicating lower optimism.

Pain Sensitivity

Pain sensitivity refers to the degree of pain intensity that can be tolerated before overt pain responses are initiated (Ruscheweyh et al., 2009). It involves pain threshold and tolerance which can be defined as the minimum intensity required for a stimulus to be called painful and the maximum intensity or duration of pain that a person can withstand respectively (Mitchell et al., 2004). The Pain Sensitivity Questionnaire (PSQ) (Ruscheweyh et al., 2009) was used to measure the pain sensitivity of the participants. The questionnaire consists of a series of questions that require participants to imagine themselves in certain situations and indicate on a Likert scale how painful the experience is. This test is correlated with experimental measures of pain which indicates that it is a valid measure of pain sensitivity. It also does not require the time and resources required by experimental means of data collection. The PSQ has demonstrated high internal consistency with a Cronbach's alpha level ranging from 0.80-0.90 and good test-retest reliability. The scores from each item are added to give a total score that can range from 0 to 170. Scores closer to 0 indicate low pain sensitivity whereas higher scores indicate heightened pain sensitivity.

Pain Catastrophizing

Catastrophizing as a concept was introduced to describe maladaptive cognitive coping styles that irrationally forecast future events as negative (Ellis, 1962). Pain catastrophizing is a set of amplified and negative cognitive and emotional schema during a painful experience. The seriousness, intensity, or threat of the pain sensation is magnified or exaggerated (Chaves & Brown, 1987). The pain catastrophizing scale is a 13-item questionnaire developed by Sullivan & Bishop (1995) and was used to measure pain catastrophizing. The scale comprises 3 components: rumination, magnification, and helplessness. The scale demonstrates very good internal consistency with a Cronbach's alpha level of 0.92. Scores vary from 0 to 52. A total score of above 30 represents a clinically significant level of pain catastrophization.

Procedure

During the data collection phase, a form consisting of the 8 scales was circulated online. The participants were briefed on the nature of the study and were required to give their consent before proceeding to the scales. Demographic details such as name, contact information, age, and biological sex were collected. Participants were asked if they experience chronic pain or any pain-related disorders. Participants completed the questionnaires on the feature and target variables. After receiving responses from 304 participants, the study moved to the data analysis phase.

Data Analysis

Once data was collected, each variable was tested for normality using the Shapiro-Wilk Test. The data was scaled into new values using normalization. This was done to ensure comparability across variables for better model performance. Normalization was preferred over standardization as the variables are all within a fixed range.

Before further analysis, multicollinearity testing used correlational matrix methods to assess correlations between the feature variables. Correlation analyses assessed the relationship between the feature variables and pain sensitivity and pain catastrophizing. Moderation analyses were done to examine the interaction effects between the feature variables.

Decision trees were trained to model the relationship between the feature variables and target variables. CART was chosen to perform an exploratory analysis to provide interpretable decision rules for predicting pain catastrophizing and pain sensitivity levels. After the exploratory analysis, Random Forests and XGBoost were employed for more robust modeling. These techniques were used to refine the predictions and assess the interactions between the feature variables and target variables. The models were trained and validated using separate datasets to determine their relative performance and predictive accuracy. For improved accuracy, 10-fold cross-validation was conducted to improve the model's reliability across different subsets of the data.

K-means clustering was used to identify natural groupings within the participants based on their psychological profiles and pain-related experiences. This unsupervised method helped reveal distinct subgroups with similar characteristics, which could provide insights into patterns of pain sensitivity and pain catastrophizing that may not be immediately apparent through supervised learning. PCA, on the other hand, was applied for dimensionality reduction to simplify the feature space while retaining the most significant variance in the data. By transforming the original features into a smaller set of uncorrelated components, PCA helped identify the key factors contributing to pain sensitivity and catastrophizing, enabling a clearer interpretation of the complex relationships between psychological traits and pain outcomes. SHAP (Shapley Additive Explanations) values were used to enhance the interpretability and explainability of the models. SHAP values provide a clear understanding of how each feature influences the prediction of pain catastrophizing and pain sensitivity levels, allowing for a detailed examination of feature importance. This approach ensures transparency in model decision-making by quantifying the contribution of each variable, which is crucial for understanding the underlying psychological factors driving pain-related experiences. The purpose of performing such techniques is to help provide recommendations for developing personalized specific interventions that reduce pain sensitivity.

Ethical Considerations

Prior to participation, all participants were briefed on the objectives, purpose, procedures, potential risks and benefits of the study. Documented informed consent was obtained from each participant emphasizing their voluntary participation and their right to withdraw at any time without any consequences. Responses were anonymized before analysis to ensure individual participants could not be identified to protect their privacy.

RESULTS AND DISCUSSION

Data for each variable was collected from 305 participants. There were 120 male participants and 185 female participants. 50 participants reported to be suffering from chronic pain, 242 reported no history of chronic pain, 13 participants were unsure. The age ranged from 18-60 years. All participants were either Indian citizens or residing in India. The variables were measured using self-report questionnaires as discussed in the methodology section.

Exploratory Analysis

Descriptive Statistics

Each variable was tested for normality on Jamovi using the Shapiro-Wilk test. The results are shown below in table 1:

Table 1. Shapiro-Wilk test for normality

	W Statistic	p-value	Distribution
Age	0.851	<0.001	Not normal
Resilience	0.990	0.029	Not normal
Neuroticism	0.989	0.021	Not normal
Extraversion	0.992	0.118	Normal
Grit	0.996	0.628	Normal
Optimism	0.976	<0.001	Not normal
Pain Catastrophizing	0.974	<0.001	Not normal
Pain Sensitivity	0.986	0.005	Not normal

Descriptive statistics were calculated to provide an overview of the variables. Table 2 shown below summarizes the mean values, medians, standard deviations and ranges for each variable, offering insights into their variability across the sample.

Table 2. Descriptive statistics

	Mean	Median	Standard Deviation	Minimum Value	Maximum Value
Age	34.9	37	14.2	18	60
Resilience	3.28	3.33	0.763	1.33	5.0
Neuroticism	20.6	20	8.84	0	40
Extraversion	20.3	20	8.35	1	40
Grit	3.35	3.33	0.645	1.58	5.0
Optimism	13.7	14	4.73	0	24
Pain Catastrophizing	21.8	21	13.4	0	52
Pain Sensitivity	4.03	4.00	1.81	0.50	10.0

Correlation and Moderation Analysis

A correlation matrix was generated using Python to understand the relationships between the variables. Figure 1 shows the correlation coefficients that describe the strength and direction of the relationships between each of the variables. The table suggests that pain catastrophizing has stronger relationships with the feature variables than pain sensitivity did. The psychological variables all showed a negative correlation with pain catastrophizing – resilience (r = -0.5), neuroticism (r = -0.62), extraversion (r = 0.17), grit (r = -0.38), optimism (r = -0.4). The relationships between the psychological variables and pain sensitivity were also found to be negative – resilience (r = -0.27), neuroticism (r = -0.33), extraversion (r = 0.093), grit (r = -0.15), optimism (r = -0.08).

The results suggest that higher levels of resilience, neuroticism, and grit are linked to lower levels of pain catastrophizing, whereas optimism and extraversion seem to have a weaker, but still negative, relationship. These results indicate that psychological traits may serve as protective factors against the amplification of pain-related thoughts and emotions. Resilience, neuroticism, and grit may be associated with pain sensitivity, although the effects are small. The relationship between neuroticism and pain sensitivity has been found to be negative. This finding contradicts the previous literature which consistently reports a positive relationship between the two variables. Previous studies suggest that higher levels of neuroticism contribute to greater levels of pain sensitivity (Atanassova et al., 2024; Grouper et al., 2021). The negative correlation observed in this analysis might indicate context or demographic-specific factors such as socioeconomic factors, cultural beliefs/practices or other mediating variables which could alter the relationship. This finding needs to be explored further.

Figure 1. Correlation matrix

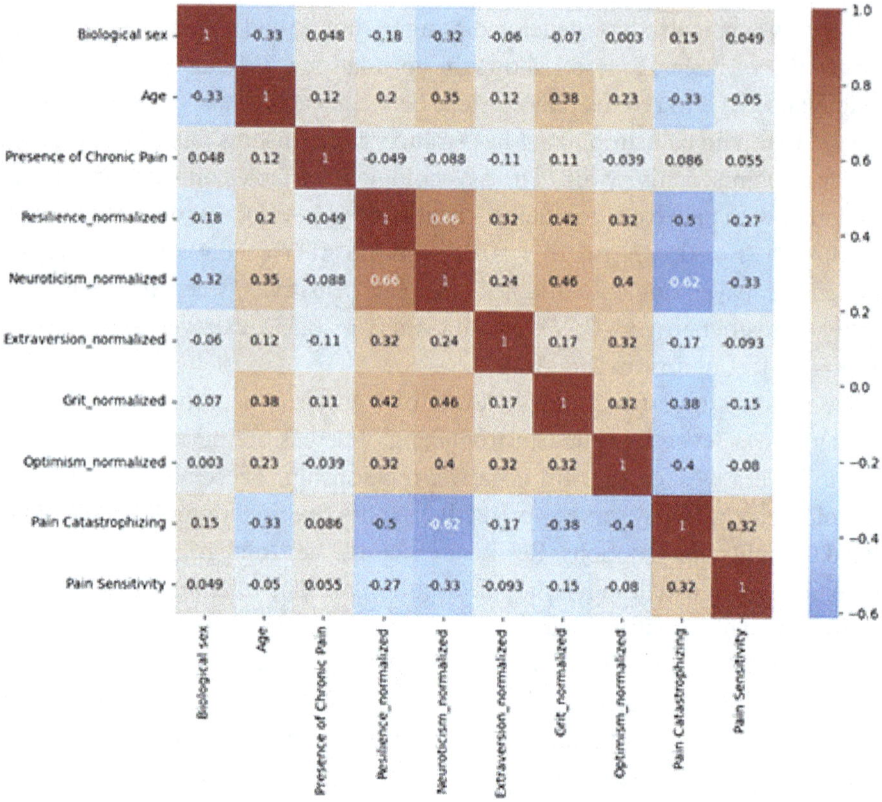

The correlations above represent individual effects of each feature on pain sensitivity. However, interactions between features also contribute to differences in pain catastrophizing and pain sensitivity. The interaction effects were tested on Jamovi through moderation analyses. Table 4 shows the interaction effects between different features in predicting pain catastrophizing. The table suggests that none of the interactions are significant as all values of p are above 0.05.

Table 3. Moderation analysis: Interaction effects between features predicting pain catastrophizing

	Estimate	SE	Z	p
Resilience * Grit	1.52	1.210	1.26	0.209
Resilience * Optimism	-0.0742	0.162	-0.457	0.648
Neuroticism * Grit	0.0648	0.0978	0.662	0.508
Neuroticism * Optimism	-0.0141	0.0122	-1.16	0.247
Extraversion * Grit	0.0400	0.1100	0.364	0.716
Extraversion * Optimism	-0.0244	0.0147	-1.657	0.098

Table 5 shows the interaction effects between the different features in predicting pain sensitivity. The moderation analysis found two significant interaction effects. Resilience and grit demonstrate a significant negative interaction effect on pain sensitivity ($p < 0.001$). Extraversion and optimism also demonstrates a significant interaction effect ($p = 0.045$). Neither of these features had a strong independent effect on pain sensitivity, however, the table suggests that optimism moderates the relationship between extraversion and pain sensitivity.

Table 4. Moderation analysis: Interaction effects between features predicting pain sensitivity

	Estimate	SE	Z	p
Resilience * Grit	-0.0532	0.187	-0.285	<.001
Resilience * Optimism	1.34e-4	0.0256	0.00525	0.996
Neuroticism * Grit	0.00250	0.0160	0.156	0.876
Neuroticism * Optimism	7.80e-4	0.00202	0.386	0.700
Extraversion * Grit	-0.00205	0.0159	-0.129	0.898
Extraversion * Optimism	-4.146	2.067	-2.01	0.045

Feature Engineering

Feature engineering was performed to improve predictive power of the model. All features were normalized to ensure the variables were on the same scale. This was done to minimize scale-related biases. One hot encoding was used to transform the categorical demographic factors, biological sex and presence of chronic pain, to a binary format. Female was assigned 1 and male was assigned 0. Presence of chronic pain was assigned 1 and absence of chronic pain was assigned 0. The "maybe" response for the presence of chronic pain, which represented uncertainty, was converted to "no" in the binary format. This was done because "maybe" likely reflects the absence of a confirmed chronic pain diagnosis, and for modeling purposes, it is reasonable to treat uncertainty as a lack of chronic pain to avoid ambiguity and ensure clear categorization in the dataset. The final features included: Age, biological sex, presence of chronic pain, resilience, neuroticism, extraversion, grit, and optimism.

K-Means Clustering and Principal Component Analysis (PCA)

Principal component analysis was combined with K-means clustering to visualize distinct groups within the dataset based on the features and pain sensitivity scores. PCA was used to reduce the high dimensional feature space to two principal components. K-means clustering was applied to detect natural groups or clusters within the data. The goal was to see if distinct clusters emerge that separate low pain sensitivity from high pain sensitivity. Figure 2 shows the result of applying K-means clustering on the dataset reduced to 2 dimensions using PCA where pain catastrophizing is the target variable. The data points are colored based on the pain catastrophizing levels to differentiate between low and high (blue for a pain sensitivity score below 30, red for a pain sensitivity score greater than or equal to 30). A threshold value of 30 was chosen as a pain catastrophizing level greater than 30 is considered to be clinically significant.

Figure 2. K-means clustering & PCA with pain catastrophizing classification

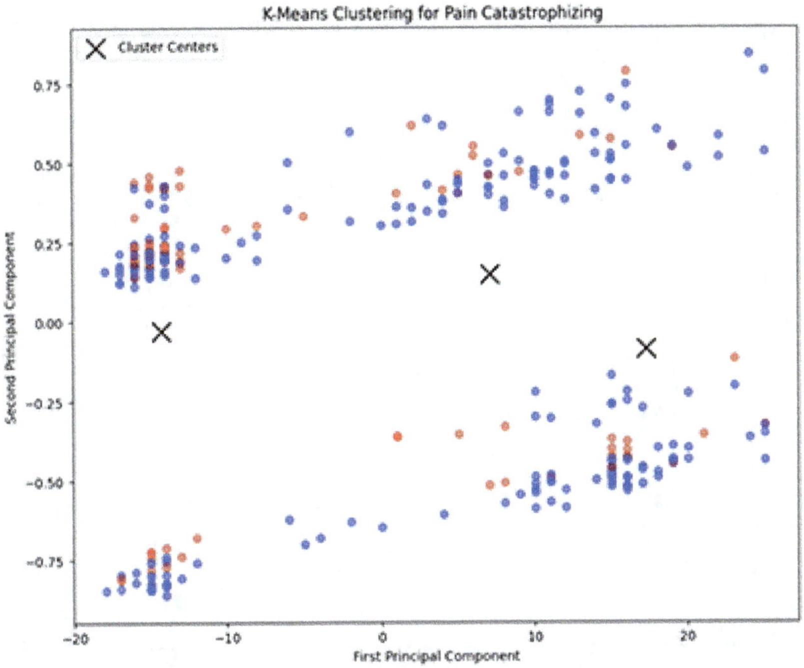

Figure 3 shows the result of applying K-means clustering on the dataset reduced to 2 dimensions using PCA where pain sensitivity is the target variable. The data points are colored based on the pain sensitivity levels to differentiate between high and low (blue for a pain sensitivity score below 5, red for a pain sensitivity score greater than or equal to 5).

Figure 3. K-means clustering & PCA with pain sensitivity classification

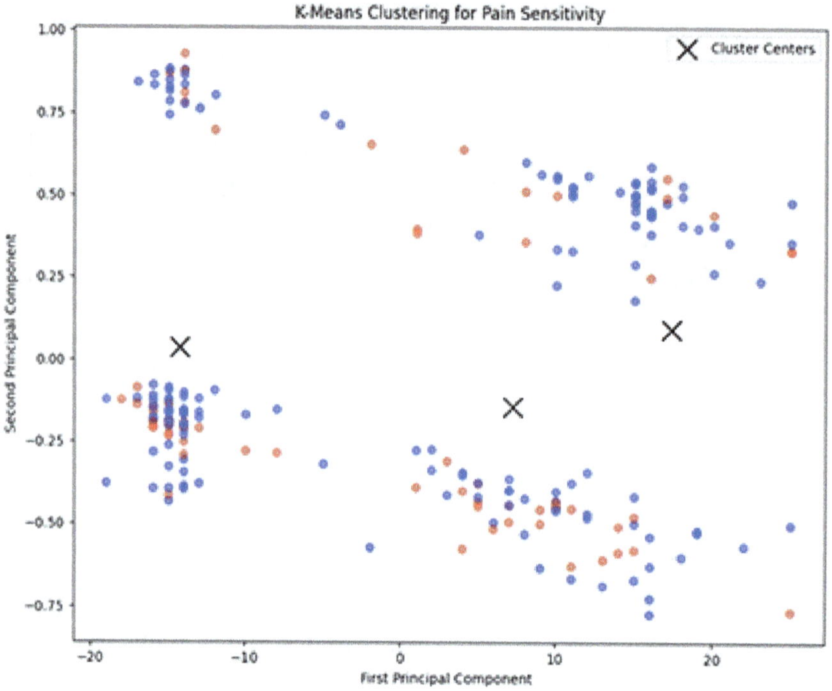

The black crosses in both figures highlight the cluster centres identified by the algorithm. The plot in figure 2 and 3 illustrates that the clusters formed by the algorithm contain a mix of both high and low pain sensitivity data points. Moreover, there were no distinct boundaries between clusters in terms of pain catastrophizing and pain sensitivity since high and low values were scattered across multiple clusters. This suggests that the features used in clustering did not provide sufficient information to create meaningful or accurate separations related to pain catastrophizing and pain sensitivity.

Classification and Regression Tree (CART)

Two Classification and Regression Trees (CART) were trained on the entire dataset to understand the relationships between the features and target variables. The first tree predicted pain catastrophizing and the second tree predicted pain sensitivity. Examining the entire tree structure can reveal how different variables interact and contribute to the final predictions. Evaluating prediction power can help identify potential overfitting or underfitting, guiding decisions on whether to prune the tree or adjust the hyperparameters. This analysis serves as a preliminary step to identify patterns, assess feature importance, and refine the feature set for advanced modeling. Both trees used the same hyperparameters. The random_state was set to 42, the min_samples_split and min_samples_leaf were both set to 3, and the max_depth was set to 11.

Predicting Pain Catastrophizing. The tree's root node split on neuroticism, indicating that this feature was the most significant predictor. A threshold of 0.512 differentiated individuals with higher and lower pain catastrophizing, highlighting the central role of neuroticism in the model. Subsequent splits used optimism and extraversion. The model's performance, measured using Root Mean Squared Error (RMSE) on the entire database, was 5.29 indicating that the model's predictions deviate from the true values by approximately 10%. The RMSE is less than the standard deviation of the target variable, 13.4, which indicates that the model performs better than a baseline model. The feature importance was evaluated to understand the highest to lowest contributing factors in predicting pain sensitivity. Table 6 shows the importance of each feature in the CART.

Table 5. Feature importance in CART predicting pain catastrophizing

Variable	Feature Importance
Neuroticism	0.557
Optimism	0.128
Extraversion	0.091
Age	0.064
Grit	0.062
Resilience	0.059
Biological Sex	0.026
Presence of Chronic Pain	0.014

Predicting Pain Sensitivity. The tree's root node also split on neuroticism, indicating that this feature was the most significant predictor. A threshold of 0.762 differentiated individuals with higher and lower pain sensitivity, highlighting the central role of neuroticism in the model. Subsequent splits included resilience, optimism and biological sex. The model's performance, measured using Root Mean Squared Error (RMSE), was 0.996 indicating that this model's predictions also deviate from the true values by approximately 10%. The RMSE is less than the standard deviation of the target variable, 1.81, which indicates that the model performs better than a baseline model. The feature importance was evaluated to understand the highest to lowest contributing factors in predicting pain sensitivity. Table 7 shows the importance of each feature in the CART.

Table 6. Feature importance in CART predicting pain sensitivity

Variable	Feature Importance
Neuroticism	0.239
Optimism	0.174
Resilience	0.167
Grit	0.114
Age	0.564
Presence of Chronic Pain	0.079
Extraversion	0.069
Biological Sex	0.053

Interpretations

It was observed that the relationships between pain catastrophizing and the feature variables were stronger than the relationships between pain sensitivity and the feature variables. There were no significant feature interactions in predicting pain catastrophizing. There were significant interactions between resilience and grit, and extraversion and optimism when predicting pain sensitivity.

Despite the limitations observed in the K-means clustering analysis, decision trees still remain a viable potential informative alternative for exploring the relationship between the feature and target variables as they can capture complex, non-linear relationships interactions between features that may not be immediately apparent through clustering algorithms.

Both CART models were able to capture patterns and make predictions closer to the actual values than the overall variability of the target variable. This indicates that the model provides meaningful predictive value, though further optimization could improve predictive power and further reduce the error.

Predictive Modeling

This phase involved employing XGBoost and Random Forests to build robust models for predicting pain catastrophizing and pain sensitivity. XG Boost was chosen for a gradient boosting model that builds trees sequentially, with each tree improving upon mistakes from the previous ones. Random Forests was chosen for its ability to reduce variance and prevent overfitting The predictive modeling was done separately for pain catastrophizing and pain sensitivity. The preparation of the dataset for both involved splitting the data into a training and validation set where 80% of the data was used in model training, and 20% of the data was used in validation. Cross-validation was set up using 10-fold cross-validation. The data was split into 10 subsets, with each fold serving as a test set while the remaining data is used for training. The performance for each fold was tested using Root Mean Squared Error (RMSE). To optimize model performance, hyperparameter tuning was performed to identify the best combination of hyperparameters that would reduce the RMSE.

Predictive Modeling for Pain Catastrophizing

An XG Boost model was trained to predict pain catastrophizing scores using the hyperparameters random_state=42, max_depth=5, n_estimators=200, and learning_rate=0.01. The RMSE of the validation set came to 10.26 which indicates an error margin of approximately 19.73%. It was found that the model faced difficulties in predicting extreme values. Feature importance was calculated to understand the highest to lowest contributing features. Table 8 shows the feature importance. Additionally, SHAP values and a summary plot (figure 4) were generated to visualize how different features impact the XGBoost model's predictions for pain catastrophizing.

Table 7. Feature importance in XGBoost predicting pain catastrophizing

Variable	Feature Importance
Neuroticism	0.353
Optimism	0.145
Age	0.125
Extraversion	0.094
Presence of Chronic Pain	0.085
Resilience	0.084
Grit	0.084
Biological Sex	0.030

Figure 4. SHAP values for XGBoost model predicting pain catastrophizing

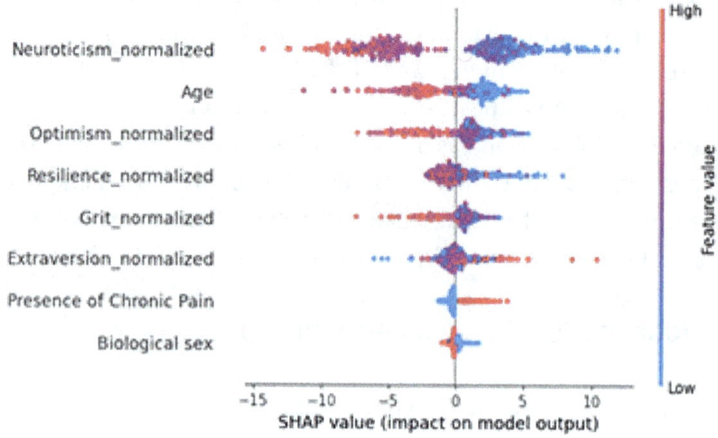

A Random Forests Model was trained to predict pain catastrophizing using the hyperparameters random_state=42, max_depth=20, n_estimators=200, min_samples_leaf=3, and min_samples_split=3. The RMSE of the validation set came to 10.3 which indicates an error margin of approximately 19.80%, similar to that of the XGBoost model. This model found a different order of feature importance compared to the XGBoost model.

Table 8. Feature importance in random forests predicting pain catastrophizing

Variable	Feature Importance
Neuroticism	0.428
Age	0.143
Optimism	0.123
Extraversion	0.101
Resilience	0.098
Grit	0.084
Biological Sex	0.012
Presence of Chronic Pain	0.011

Although the Random Forests and XGBoost regressor were able to capture general trends in pain catastrophizing, it struggled to predict extreme values, especially those above 30 which are of clinical significance. The RMSE of 10.26 suggests that the model might be underfitting or not fully capturing the variance in extreme ranges of data. To address this limitation, we explored an alternative approach using an XG Boost Classifier which will predict whether or not the pain catastrophizing scores are clinically significant.

The XGBoost classifier trained to predict pain catastrophizing scores above a certain threshold as 'clinically significant' and below the threshold as 'not significant'. The tree used the hyperparameters random_state=42, max_depth=20, n_estimators=500, and learning_rate=0.05. Initially, the tree used a threshold value of 30 to differentiate between clinically significant and non-significant. The model performed poorly, predicting 53 false negatives, and 46 false positives. The overall accuracy was 67.5%. The reason for poor performance was traced to the imbalanced dataset. To mitigate this, the threshold was lowered from 30 to 25. Additionally, the hyperparameter scale_pos_weight = 2 was added to increase the importance of the rare class. The n_estimators was changed to 800, and the learning_rate was changed to 0.08

As seen in the confusion matrix (figure 4) and the classification report (table 9), the 2nd classifier performed better, with an overall accuracy of 74%. The false positives reduced to 43 and the false negative reduced to 37. The model correctly predicted 131 individuals as clinically non-significant (score < 25) which matches the dataset count (this indicates that the model did well in this class). The model correctly predicted 94 out of the 174 individuals who are considered clinically significant. Additionally, the Receiver Operating Characteristic (ROC) Curve, as shown in Figure 6, has an AUC (area under the curve) of 0.80, which shows that the model demonstrates strong discriminatory ability and consistently performs well in terms of balancing the prediction of both classes across different thresholds.

Figure 5. Confusion matrix for XGBoost classifier predicting pain catastrophizing

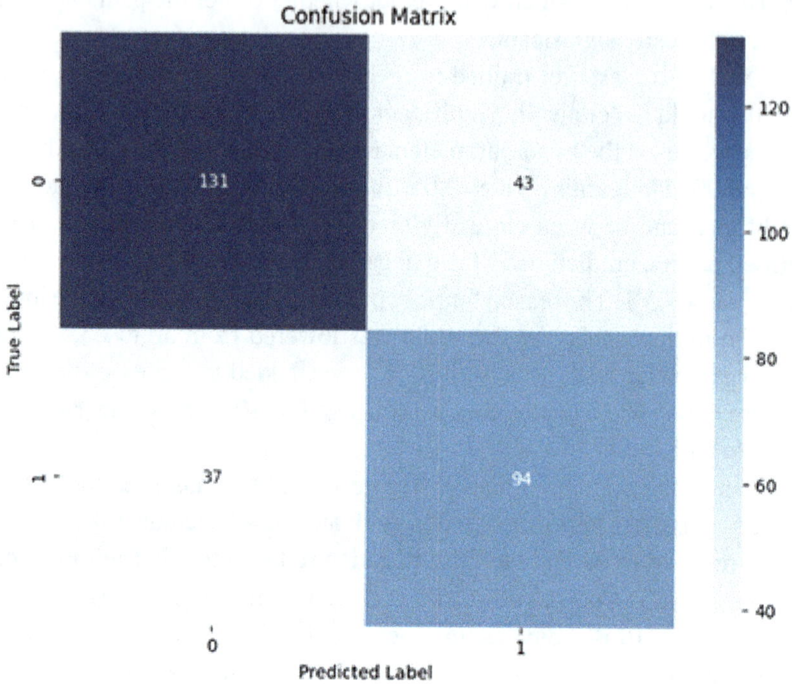

Table 9 Classification report for XGBoost classifier predicting pain catastrophizing

	Precision	Recall	f1-score	Support
Clinically Significant	0.69	0.72	0.70	174
Non Significant	0.78	0.75	0.77	131
Accuracy			0.74	305
Macro Average	0.73	0.74	0.73	305
Weighted Average	0.74	0.74	0.74	305

Figure 6. ROC Curve for XGBoost Predicting Pain Catastrophizing

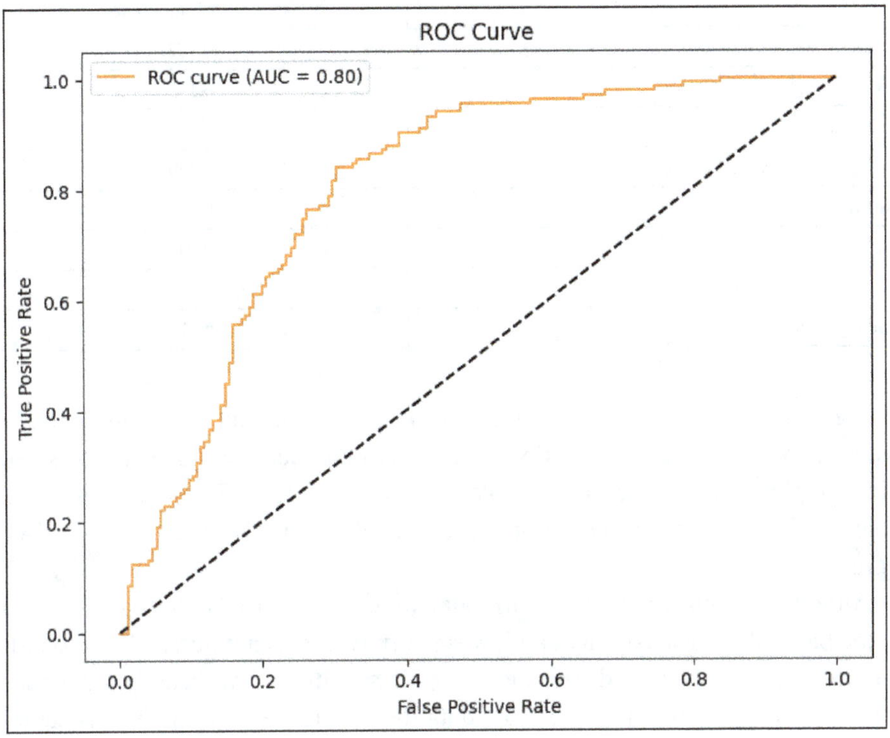

Predictive Modeling for Pain Sensitivity

An XGBoost regressor was trained to predict pain sensitivity levels based on the 8 feature variables. The tree used the hyperparameters random_state=42, max_depth=5, n_estimators=300, and learning_rate=0.05. The RMSE of the validation set came to 1.78 which indicates an error margin of approximately 17.8%. This model faced difficulty in predicting higher values of pain sensitivity due to an imbalanced dataset. To address this problem, data augmentation was performed to artificially increase the number of samples in the higher range of pain sensitivity. To increase the weightage of the rare class, the scale_pos_weight hyperparameter was set to 2. However this technique did not significantly improve the model's performance. The feature importance is given below (table 10).

Table 10. Feature importance in XGBoost predicting pain sensitivity

Variable	Feature Importance
Neuroticism	0.177
Extraversion	0.172
Optimism	0.161
Presence of Chronic Pain	0.129
Resilience	0.114
Age	0.087
Grit	0.083
Biological Sex	0.076

A Random Forests regression was also trained to predict pain sensitivity. The hyperparameters used were random_state=42, max_depth=6, n_estimators=100, min_samples_leaf=3, and min_samples_split=3. The RMSE was found to be 1.75 which indicates an error margin of approximately 17.5%, similar to the XGBoost regressor.

Although training a classification model was considered to predict pain sensitivity on the basis of high sensitivity and low sensitivity, it was not pursued due to issues with the dataset. The data distribution for pain sensitivity was heavily imbalanced. Attempts to clean and preprocess the data did neither resolve the inconsistencies nor capture the natural variation in the total scores. As a result, the classification model was prone to biased predictions and underperformance.

SUMMARY AND CONCLUSION

This study highlights the significant role of psychological traits, such as neuroticism, resilience, grit, optimism, and extraversion, in influencing pain catastrophizing and pain sensitivity. Neuroticism emerged as the strongest predictor for both target variables, underscoring its central role in maladaptive pain perception. While resilience and grit showed moderate effects, optimism and extraversion demonstrated weaker but notable associations. The results suggest that psychological traits may act as protective or risk factors in shaping individuals' responses to pain.

However, the predictive models, though informative, faced challenges in handling extreme values and imbalanced datasets. The findings emphasize the need for broader models that incorporate additional psychological, biological, and environmental factors, along with experimental measures of pain sensitivity, to enhance predictive accuracy and generalizability.

By identifying these psychological determinants, the study offers a foundation for designing targeted, evidence-based psychotherapeutic interventions to reduce pain sensitivity and catastrophizing. Such interventions could contribute to more effective and personalized pain management strategies, ensuring a balance between reducing pain perception and promoting overall psychological well-being.

Implications

The findings of this study have several critical implications for pain management and psychological research. First, the results highlight the importance of integrating psychological traits, such as neuroticism, resilience, grit, optimism, and extraversion, into personalized pain management strategies. By identifying these psychological variables as key contributors to pain catastrophizing and sensitivity, healthcare professionals can develop tailored psychotherapeutic interventions. For instance, cognitive-behavioral therapy (CBT), mindfulness-based approaches, and resilience training could be employed to reduce maladaptive pain responses while improving overall psychological well-being. Additionally, by identifying individuals at risk of developing maladaptive pain responses based on their psychological profiles, early interventions can be implemented to prevent the escalation of acute pain into chronic conditions.

The study also supports a shift from reliance on pharmacological treatments to non-pharmacological methods for pain management. Given the risks associated with long-term medication use, such as addiction and side effects, psychotherapeutic interventions offer a safer and more sustainable alternative. These techniques can not only help alleviate pain but also address the underlying cognitive and emotional patterns that amplify pain perception, thereby preventing the progression of acute pain into chronic conditions.

Limitations

This study included a limited number of psychological predictors of pain catastrophizing and pain sensitivity. Behavioral components, such as coping mechanisms, which may also play a role in predicting pain catastrophizing and pain sensitivity were excluded from the study. This study relied on self-reports as a tool of measuring pain sensitivity which make the data prone to biases due to social desirability or inadequate self-awareness. A more accurate measure of pain sensitivity would have been experimental measures such as the cold pressor test (Mitchell et al., 2004).

The dataset was heavily imbalanced. There was inadequate representation of certain values of the feature and target variables which reduced the model's ability to explore relationships across the spectrum of pain catastrophizing and pain sensitivity. The sample only had 305 members which impacted model training. There was limited accessibility to patients with chronic pain which restricted the model's ability to generalize findings to this group, and to better understand the psychological differences between those with and without chronic pain.

The study cannot be generalized to people above the age of 60 or below the age of 18. Furthermore, the study was conducted on people of an Indian background. Cultural factors could significantly impact the findings, limiting its global applicability. Certain culture-specific or context-specific factors such as the negative correlation between neuroticism and pain sensitivity need to be explored further to explain this contradiction from existing literature(Atanassova et al., 2024; Grouper et al., 2021)..

Scope for Further Study

This study used self-report questionnaires to measure pain sensitivity. Future research could build models that predict pain sensitivity measured through experimental methods for improved target accuracy.

Since this study cannot be generalized to senior citizens above the age of 60 years and children below the age of 18, future research should aim to include a more diverse age range to capture pain sensitivity and catastrophizing patterns across the lifespan. Additionally, future studies should examine whether interventions targeting these psychological traits differ in effectiveness based on age, which could lead to more age-appropriate and personalized pain management strategies.

While this study identifies the psychological variables that contribute most to pain catastrophizing and pain sensitivity levels, an important area for future research lies in the practical applicability of these findings. Although certain variables may strongly influence pain catastrophizing and pain sensitivity, they may be more resistant to change through therapeutic interventions. Future models could benefit from incorporating the feasibility and difficulty of modifying these variables. A model that accounts for the effectiveness and modifiability of these variables would improve clinical utility.

Future research should also explore the balance of psychological traits aimed at mitigating pain sensitivity. For example, while elevated neuroticism is associated with lower levels of pain catastrophizing and pain sensitivity, it poses risks to overall mental health. Hence, new models must not only prioritize pain-related outcomes but also consider the broader psychological and emotional well-being of individuals. Incorporating specific thresholds or target ranges for the psychological traits could improve adaptability and ethical integrity of these models. This approach would ensure that interventions are designed to manage pain sensitivity while maintaining favourable psychological profiles, thereby improving their practical applicability.

Another gap is the focus on a limited number of individual psychological factors without considering biological or environmental factors, such as disease, social support, or lifestyle variables, that may also contribute to pain catastrophizing and sensitivity. Incorporating these into future models would provide a more holistic understanding of pain related experiences and could offer more comprehensive recommendations for treatment interventions.

The addition of algorithms such as sensitivity techniques such as one-at-a-time (OAT) sensitivity or genetic algorithms can be used to design interventions by suggesting the best combination of psychological variables for minimised pain catastrophizing and pain sensitivity.

CONCLUSION

This study underscores the intricate relationship between psychological traits and pain-related experiences, emphasizing the need for a deeper understanding of how these factors influence one another. The findings illustrate that psychological variables such as neuroticism, resilience, and optimism can significantly predict pain sensitivity and pain catastrophizing, but they also expose the limitations of existing models in capturing extreme values and nuanced variations in pain experiences. Specifically, the study highlights that while common psychological traits offer valuable insights into how individuals process pain, they may not fully account for the complexity of pain experiences in all individuals, particularly those at the extremes of pain sensitivity or catastrophizing.

As such, the need for more comprehensive, integrative approaches becomes evident. Future research should focus on refining predictive models to better address the variability in how individuals experience and react to pain, incorporating a wider array of psychological factors and considering the dynamic interaction between them. This includes the exploration of additional factors such as social support, coping strategies, and individual differences in pain thresholds. Additionally, there is a pressing need for the development of personalized interventions that not only target pain sensitivity but also focus on the cognitive and emotional dimensions of pain, such as pain catastrophizing. By addressing both the physiological and psychological aspects of pain, these interventions can be more effective in reducing pain-related suffering and enhancing overall well-being.

Ultimately, the study calls for a shift towards a more holistic approach in pain management, one that recognizes the multifaceted nature of pain and tailors interventions to the individual. This will require collaboration across disciplines, including psychology, neuroscience, and medicine, to create models and treatment strategies that are adaptable, comprehensive, and sensitive to the diverse ways in which people experience pain.

REFERENCES

Ambekar, A., Agrawal, A., Rao, R., Mishra, A. K., Khandelwal, S. K., & Chadda, R. K. (2019). Magnitude of substance use in India. *New Delhi: Ministry of Social Justice and Empowerment, Government of India, 23.*

Antonucci, L. A., Taurino, A., Laera, D., Taurisano, P., Losole, J., Lutricuso, S., Abbatantuono, C., Giglio, M., De Caro, M. F., Varrassi, G., & Puntillo, F. (2020). An Ensemble of Psychological and Physical Health Indices Discriminates Between Individuals with Chronic Pain and Healthy Controls with High Reliability: A Machine Learning Study. *Pain and Therapy*, *9*(2), 601–614. DOI: 10.1007/s40122-020-00191-3 PMID: 32880867

Astin, J. A., Shapiro, S. L., Eisenberg, D. M., & Forys, K. L. (2003). Mind-body medicine: State of the science, implications for practice. *The Journal of the American Board of Family Practice*, *16*(2), 131–147. DOI: 10.3122/jabfm.16.2.131 PMID: 12665179

Atanassova, D. V., Madariaga, V. I., Oosterman, J. M., & Brazil, I. A. (2024). Unpacking the relationship between Big Five personality traits and experimental pain: A systematic review and meta-analysis. *Neuroscience and Biobehavioral Reviews*, *163*, 105786. Advance online publication. DOI: 10.1016/j.neubiorev.2024.105786 PMID: 38955000

Baron, R., Binder, A., & Wasner, G. (2010). Neuropathic pain: Diagnosis, pathophysiological mechanisms, and treatment. *Lancet Neurology*, *9*(8), 807–819. DOI: 10.1016/S1474-4422(10)70143-5 PMID: 20650402

Bonadonna, R. (2003). Meditation's Impact on Chronic Illness. *Holistic Nursing Practice*, *17*(6), 309–319. DOI: 10.1097/00004650-200311000-00006 PMID: 14650573

Buckingham, A., & Richardson, E. J. (2021). The Relationship Between Psychological Resilience and Pain Threshold and Tolerance: Optimism and Grit as Moderators. *Journal of Clinical Psychology in Medical Settings*, *28*(3), 518–528. DOI: 10.1007/s10880-020-09731-7 PMID: 32564216

Carver, C. S., Scheier, M. F., & Segerstrom, S. C. (2010). Optimism. *Clinical Psychology Review*, *30*(7), 879–889. DOI: 10.1016/j.cpr.2010.01.006 PMID: 20170998

Chaves, J. F., & Brown, J. M. (1987). Spontaneous cognitive strategies for the control of clinical pain and stress. *Journal of Behavioral Medicine*, *10*(3), 263–276. DOI: 10.1007/BF00846540 PMID: 3612783

Colloca, L., & Miller, F. G. (2011). The nocebo effect and its relevance for clinical practice. *Psychosomatic Medicine, 73*(7), 598–603. DOI: 10.1097/PSY.0b013e3182294a50 PMID: 21862825

Dillworth, T., & Jensen, M. P. (2010). The Role of Suggestions in Hypnosis for Chronic Pain: A Review of the Literature. *The Open Pain Journal, 3*(1), 39–51. DOI: 10.2174/1876386301003010039 PMID: 21686037

Douthwaite, A. H. (1962). Proctalgia Fugax. *British Medical Journal, 2*(5298), 164–165. DOI: 10.1136/bmj.2.5298.164 PMID: 13887589

Dubreuil, D. L., & Kohn, P. M. (1986). Reactivity and response to pain. *Personality and Individual Differences, 7*(6), 907–909. DOI: 10.1016/0191-8869(86)90093-0

Duckworth, A. (2016). *Grit: The Power of Passion and Perseverance*. Simon & Schuster.

Duckworth, A. L., Peterson, C., Matthews, M. D., & Kelly, D. R. (2007). Grit: Perseverance and passion for long-term goals. *Journal of Personality and Social Psychology, 9*(6), 1087–1101. DOI: 10.1037/0022-3514.92.6.1087 PMID: 17547490

Edwards, R. R., & Fillingim, R. B. (2007). Self-reported pain sensitivity: Lack of correlation with pain threshold and tolerance. *European Journal of Pain (London, England), 11*(5), 594–598. DOI: 10.1016/j.ejpain.2006.09.008 PMID: 17118681

Ellis, A. (1962). *Reason and emotion in psychotherapy*. Lyle Stuart.

Engel, G. L. (1977). The need for a new medical model: A challenge for biomedicine. *Science, 196*(4286), 129–136. DOI: 10.1126/science.847460 PMID: 847460

Fenton, B. W., Shih, E., & Zoltan, J. (2015). The neurobiology of pain perception in normal and persistent pain. *Pain Management, 5*(4), 297–317. DOI: 10.2217/pmt.15.27 PMID: 26088531

Fillingim, R. B. (2017, April). Individual differences in pain: Understanding the mosaic that makes pain personal. *Pain, 158*(1), S11–S18. DOI: 10.1097/j.pain.0000000000000775 PMID: 27902569

Grossman, P., Niemann, L., Schmidt, S., & Walach, H. (2004). Mindfulness-based stress reduction and health benefits. A meta-analysis. *Journal of Psychosomatic Research, 57*(1), 35–43. DOI: 10.1016/S0022-3999(03)00573-7 PMID: 15256293

Grouper, H., Eisenburg, E., & Pud, D. (2021). More Insight on the Role of Personality Traits and Sensitivity to Experimental Pain. *Journal of Pain Research, 14*, 1837–1844. DOI: 10.2147/JPR.S309729 PMID: 34168491

Hansen, M. S., Horjales-Araujo, E., & Dahl, J. B. (2015). Associations between psychological variables and pain in experimental pain models. A systematic review. *Acta Anaesthesiologica Scandinavica, 59*(9), 1094–1102. DOI: 10.1111/aas.12555 PMID: 26088747

Jensen, M. P., Neilson, W. R., & Kerns, R. D. (2003). Toward the development of a motivational model of pain self-management. *The Journal of Pain, 4*(9), 477–492. DOI: 10.1016/S1526-5900(03)00779-X PMID: 14636816

Jensen, M. P., Turner, J. A., & Romano, J. M. (1994). Correlates of improvement in multidisciplinary treatment of chronic pain. *Journal of Consulting and Clinical Psychology, 62*(1), 172–179. DOI: 10.1037/0022-006X.62.1.172 PMID: 8034820

Julius, D. (2013). TRP Channels and Pain. *Annual Review of Cell and Developmental Biology, 29*(1), 355–384. DOI: 10.1146/annurev-cellbio-101011-155833 PMID: 24099085

Kerns, R. D., & Habib, S. (2004). A critical review of the pain readiness to change model. *The Journal of Pain, 5*(7), 357–367. DOI: 10.1016/j.jpain.2004.06.005 PMID: 15501193

Kihlstrom, J. F. (1985). Hypnosis. *Annual Review of Psychology, 36*(1), 385–418. https://psycnet.apa.org/doi/10.1146/annurev.ps.36.020185.002125. DOI: 10.1146/annurev.ps.36.020185.002125 PMID: 3883892

Kim, S., Dowgwillo, E. A., & Kratz, A. L. (2023). Emotional Dynamics in Fibromyalgia: Pain, Fatigue, and Stress Moderate Momentary Associations Between Positive and Negative Emotions. *The Journal of Pain, 24*(9), 1594–1603. DOI: 10.1016/j.jpain.2023.04.007 PMID: 37094743

Kreitler, M., & Kreitler, S. (2007). Psychological Approaches to Treatment of Pain. In *Handbook of Chronic Pain*. Nova Science.

Kreitler, S., & Kreitler, M. (2007). Psychological Approaches to Treatment of Pain: Sensory, Affective, Cognitive, Behaviuoral. In *The Handbook of Chronic Pain*. Nova Science Publishers.

Kuhn, M., & Johnson, K. (2013). *Applied Predictive Modeling*. Springer. DOI: 10.1007/978-1-4614-6849-3

Le, L. (1994). Psychogenic pain. *Singapore Medical Journal, 35*(5), 519–522. PMID: 7701376

Margo, C. E. (1999). The Placebo Effect (J. S. Mindel, Ed.). *Survey of Ophthamology, 44*(1), 31-44. DOI: 10.1016/S0039-6257(99)00060-0

McCrae, R. R., & Costa, P. T. (2003). *Personality in adulthood: A five-factor theory perspective* (2nd ed.). Guilford Press., https://awspntest.apa.org/doi/10.4324/9780203428412 DOI: 10.4324/9780203428412

Meagher, M. W., Arnau, R. C., & Rhudy, J. L. (2001). Pain and emotion: Effects of affective picture modulation. *Psychosomatic Medicine, 63*(1), 79–90. DOI: 10.1097/00006842-200101000-00010 PMID: 11211069

Melzack, R. (2001). Pain and the neuromatrix in the brain. *Journal of Dental Education, 65*(12), 1378–1382. DOI: 10.1002/j.0022-0337.2001.65.12.tb03497.x PMID: 11780656

Melzack, R., & Wall, P. D. (1965). Pain Mechanisms: A New Theory: A gate control system modulates sensory input from the skin before it evokes pain perception and response. *Science, 150*(3699), 971–979. DOI: 10.1126/science.150.3699.971 PMID: 5320816

Millan, M. J. (1999). The induction of pain: An integrative review. *Progress in Neurobiology, 57*(1), 1–164. DOI: 10.1016/S0301-0082(98)00048-3 PMID: 9987804

Mitchell, L. A., MacDonald, R. A., & Brodie, E. E. (2004). Temperature and the cold pressor test. *The Journal of Pain, 5*(4), 233–237. DOI: 10.1016/j.jpain.2004.03.004 PMID: 15162346

Newton-John, T. R. O., Mason, C., & Hunter, M. (2014). The Role of Resilience in Adjustment and Coping With Chronic Pain. *Rehabilitation Psychology, 59*(3), 360–365. DOI: 10.1037/a0037023 PMID: 25019306

Price, D. D., Finniss, D. G., & Benedetti, F. (2008). A comprehensive review of the placebo effect: Recent advances and current thought. *Annual Review of Psychology, 59*(1), 565–590. DOI: 10.1146/annurev.psych.59.113006.095941 PMID: 17550344

Rashbaum, I. G., & Sarno, J. E. (2003). Psychosomatic concepts in chronic pain. *Archives of Physical Medicine and Rehabilitation, 84*, S76–S88. DOI: 10.1053/apmr.2003.50144 PMID: 12708562

Ray, R. (2004). *The extent, pattern and trends of drug abuse in India: National survey*. Ministry of Social Justice and Empowerment, Government of India & United Nations Office on Drugs and Crime, Regional Office for South Asia.

Ruscheweyh, R., Marziniak, M., Stumpenhorst, F., Reinholz, J., & Knecht, S. (2009). Pain sensitivity can be assessed by self-rating: Development and validation of the Pain Sensitivity Questionnaire. *Pain, 164*(1), 65–74. DOI: 10.1016/j.pain.2009.06.020 PMID: 19665301

Saxena, I., Kumar, M., Bharat, A. S., Verma, A., Garg, S., & Kumar, M. (2015). Effect of Age on Response to Experimental Pain in Normal Indian Males. *Journal of Clinical and Diagnostic Research : JCDR*, *9*(9), CC05–CC08. DOI: 10.7860/JCDR/2015/15385.6516 PMID: 26500901

Scheier, M. F., Carver, C. S., & Bridges, M. W. (1994). Distinguishing Optimism from Neuroticism (and trait anxiety, self-mastery, and self-esteem): A re-evaluation of the Life Orientation Test. *Journal of Personality and Social Psychology*, *67*(6), 1063–1078. DOI: 10.1037/0022-3514.67.6.1063 PMID: 7815302

Schmidt, R., Schemlz, M., Forster, C., Ringcamp, M., Torebjörk, E., & Handwerker, H. (1995). Novel classes of responsive and unresponsive C nociceptors in human skin. *The Journal of Neuroscience : The Official Journal of the Society for Neuroscience*, *15*(1), 333–341. DOI: 10.1523/JNEUROSCI.15-01-00333.1995 PMID: 7823139

Schwartz, M. S. (2017). *Biofeedback: A Practitioner's Guide* (4th ed.). The Guilford Press.

Smith, B. W., Dalen, J., Wiggins, K., Tooley, E., Christopher, P., & Bernard, J. (2008). The brief resilience scale: Assessing the ability to bounce back. *International Journal of Behavioral Medicine*, *15*(3), 194–200. DOI: 10.1080/10705500802222972 PMID: 18696313

Stewart-Williams, S., & Podd, J. (2004). The placebo effect: Dissolving the expectancy versus conditioning debate. *Psychological Bulletin*, *130*(2), 324–340. DOI: 10.1037/0033-2909.130.2.324 PMID: 14979775

Sturgeon, J. A., & Zautra, A. J. (2010). Resilience: A New Paradigm for Adaptation to Chronic Pain. *Current Pain and Headache Reports*, *14*(2), 105–112. DOI: 10.1007/s11916-010-0095-9 PMID: 20425199

Sullivan, M. J., Bishop, S. R., & Pivik, J. (1995). The Pain Catastrophizing Scale: Development and validation. *Psychological Assessment*, *7*(4), 524–532. https://psycnet.apa.org/doi/10.1037/1040-3590.7.4.524. DOI: 10.1037/1040-3590.7.4.524

Sullivan, M. J. L., Bishop, S. R., & Pivik, J. (1995). The Pain Catastrophizing Scale: Development and validation. *Psychological Assessment*, *7*(4), 524–532. https://psycnet.apa.org/doi/10.1037/1040-3590.7.4.524. DOI: 10.1037/1040-3590.7.4.524

Swieboda, P., Filip, R., Prystupa, A., & Drozd, M. (2013). Assessment of pain: Types, mechanism and treatment. *Annals of Agricultural and Environmental Medicine*, *20*(1), 2–7. PMID: 25000833

Tagliaferri, S. D., Wilkin, T., Angelova, M., Fitzgibbon, B. M., Own, P. J., Miller, C. T., & Belavy, D. L. (2022). Chronic back pain sub-grouped via psychosocial, brain and physical factors using machine learning. *Scientific Reports*, *12*(1), 15194. Advance online publication. DOI: 10.1038/s41598-022-19542-5 PMID: 36071092

Thompson, W. G. (1989). Proctalgia Fugax. In *Gut Reactions* (pp. 259–267). Springer., DOI: 10.1007/978-1-4899-6491-5_17

Turk, D. C., & Swanson, K. S. (2008). Psychological Interventions. In *Raj's Practical Management of Pain* (4th ed., pp. 739–755). Mosby., DOI: 10.1016/B978-032304184-3.50042-X

Turk, D. C., Swanson, K. S., & Tunks, E. R. (2008). Psychological Approaches in the Treatment of Chronic Pain Patients—When Pills, Scalpels, and Needles Are Not Enough. *Canadian Journal of Psychiatry*, *53*(4), 213–223. DOI: 10.1177/070674370805300402 PMID: 18478824

von Baeyer, C. L., Piira, T., Chambers, C. T., Trapanotto, M., & Zeltzer, L. K. (2005). Guidelines for the cold pressor task as an experimental pain stimulus for use with children. *The Journal of Pain*, *6*(4), 218–227. DOI: 10.1016/j.jpain.2005.01.349 PMID: 15820909

Watson, D., Clark, L. A., & Tellegan, A. (1988). Development and validation of brief measures of positive and negative affect: The PANAS Scales. *Journal of Personality and Social Psychology*, *54*(6), 1063–1070. DOI: 10.1037/0022-3514.54.6.1063 PMID: 3397865

Zautra, A., Smith, B., Affleck, G., & Tennen, H. (2001). Examinations of chronic pain and affect relationships: Applications of a dynamic model of affect. *Journal of Consulting and Clinical Psychology*, *69*(5), 786–795. DOI: 10.1037/0022-006X.69.5.786 PMID: 11680555

Zhao, X., Dannenberg, K., Repsibler, D., Gerdle, B., Molander, P., & Hesser, H. (2024). Prognostic subgroups of chronic pain patients using latent variable mixture modeling within a supervised machine learning framework. *Scientific Reports*, *14*(1), 12543. Advance online publication. DOI: 10.1038/s41598-024-62542-w PMID: 38822075

Chapter 17
Ethical Implications of Predictive Rehabilitation Technologies

T. Premavathi
https://orcid.org/0009-0003-0172-2021
Marwadi University, India

Damodharan Palaniappan
https://orcid.org/0009-0003-0721-3068
Marwadi University, India

Arigela Yashwanth Kumar
Marwadi University, India

Kumar Parmar
https://orcid.org/0000-0002-2502-5680
Marwadi University, India

Gudise Sathvika
Marwadi University, India

Rituraj Jain
https://orcid.org/0000-0002-5532-1245
Marwadi University, India

ABSTRACT

The inclusion ofpredictive technologies in rehabilitation involves data in planning its delivery to suit a patient's needs and an area of significant ethical concern. The key here would be to involve technological growth within the healthcare sector, aligned with medical ethics that would determine the use of devices without infringing on the patient's rights. Such features also mean that open communicative channels and policy processes can be highly beneficial for the enhancement of trust in such systems. Proper formulation of ethics is needed to effectively create standards for rehabilitation prediction technology as well as interact with stakeholders and regulatory commissions to make certain rehabilitative technologies are used in an appropriately monitored manner. Achieving this balance is necessary in order to reap the benefits of such innovations while, at the same time, maintaining patient and doctor autonomy as well as the principles of the practicing ethics in the medical field.

DOI: 10.4018/979-8-3373-0194-5.ch017

1. INTRODUCTION: THE DAWN OF PREDICTIVE REHABILITATION TECHNOLOGIES

The use of predictive rehabilitation technology is one of the most important milestones in the healthcare field which has incorporated artificial intelligence and more tools for patient treatment. These are advanced systems to comprehend the patient information and provide algorithmic description of possible consequences, enabling the clinicians to devise proper rehabilitation regimes based on each case. For instance, a patient who is a sportsman and requires rehabilitation for his or her knee would use a wearable system that would monitor his or her gait and based on this recommend exercises most suitable for the phase of the recovery process. The sort of technologies not only speeds up the rate of recovery but also the experience and involvement of the patients (Zhang et al., 2021). Technological solutions that support predictive rehabilitation offer many opportunities, but in the same time, it raises numerous questions of ethic. According to Dr. Sarah K. Smith, every technological step is followed by the question of ethic in its use. Concerns like privacy and ownership of data, consent, and fairness of the algorithm detected underline the concern needed when treading this terrain in health care. For example, the manipulation of patient data is likely to result in infringement of the patient's right to privacy, and with problems of biases in AI models, there is likely to be a negative impact on the underrepresented persons. These ethical issues will be discussed in this chapter in an effort to bring technology enabler in harmony with the fundamental ethical codes of medical practice.

Rehabilitation technologies are now in a state of a transition towards predictive approaches; it is beneficial for representative stakeholders of various professions, focusing on innovation in measuring and monitoring, technology companies, policymakers, and patients/consumers to sustain an open and diverse discussion about the ethical considerations associated with such approaches. This discussion is not only intended to improve the methods of rehabilitation interventions; however, it also endeavours to develop a framework that drives improvements in patients' rights, fair access to treatment, and confidence in technology implementation. The next few sections will look at specific ethical issue tied to predictive rehabilitation technologies by analyzing them in the context of healthcare intervention and strategy (Cotton et al., 2024).

1.1 Evolution of Rehabilitation Methods: A Historical Perspective

Originally, rehabilitation means that it has various types of manual and tactile therapist crude methods, but now has emerged data-driven and predictive models of rehabilitation techniques. Whereas early rehabilitation approached to physical and occupational treatments that were more based on strong poor evidence for the effectiveness of methods of selected patients and generalized treatment patterns. The synthesis of biomechanics and kinematics in mid of the twentieth century advanced the treatment accuracy. Due to wireless body sensors, AI, tele-rehabilitation, present rehabilitation context uses prediction model for patients' services. This has helped in improving on the recovery processes, and have also made them efficient and easy, thus changing how the rehabilitation processes are done.

1.2 Overview of Predictive Rehabilitation Technologies (PRTs)

Predictive Rehabilitation Technologies can be considered as novel advancement impacting on the sphere of healthcare with a special reference to rehabilitation. These systems utilize data analysis, artificial intelligence, and other complex algorithms to predict patients' conditions, improve the usage of treatment plans, and improve recovery strategies. That is why, in the context of the development of digital solutions in the healthcare industry, PRTs have become critical and are developed for personalizing and optimizing the rehabilitation processes. These technologies have a capability to provide highly relevant and real time predictions because of a large amount of data sets acquired from clinic practice, behavioral health, and patient reported outcomes; hence hold the promise for rehabilitation solutions that are personalised for each patient and contextually appropriate based on their situation and need (Cotton et al., 2024).

Turning to the Figurez1 the reader will have an idea, on how the data is being transforming into personalized rehabilitation. Predictive rehabilitation technologies are defined by the integration of artificial intelligence and machine learning, associated wearables, telemedicine, and data analysis. The following technological advancements allow for less structured interaction between the patient and the provider, and frequent updates with the results of treatment. Furthermore, advanced rehabilitation technologies in conjunction with the processed big data produce better rehabilitation concepts and techniques, the specific patterns in treatment. Hence, she expects that as PRTs remain in use, they are expected to be applicable across all the rehabilitation realms including physical, neurological and orthopedic domains, hence, enhancing, optimising and focusing on patients' centredness (Aldenaini et al., 2022).

Figure 1. Transforming data into personalized rehabilitation

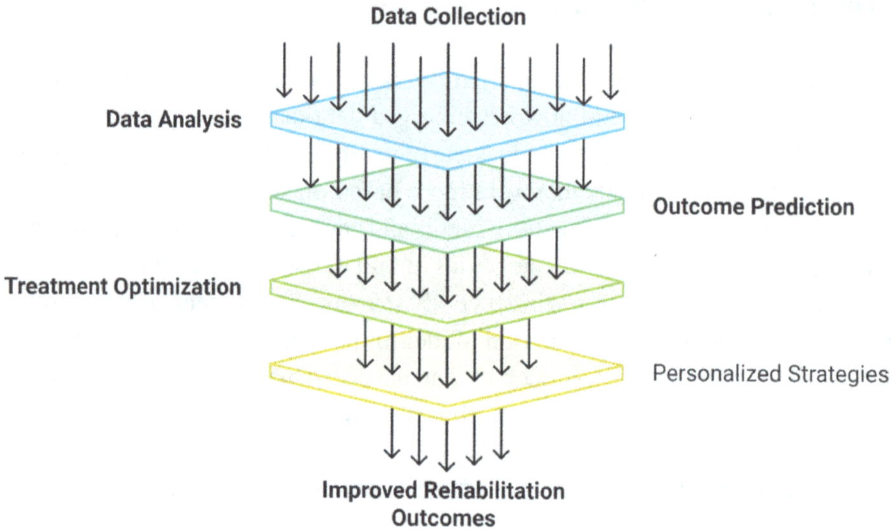

1.3 Definition and Examples of PRTs

The underlying technology of predictive rehabilitation is made of systems and devices that predict the rehabilitation outcomes and customise the rehabilitation strategies in the process. These technologies include different applications, and it is oriented on as many aspects of the rehabilitation as possible. A great example is the smart wearable devices like smart gowns, smart bands, or smart watches that track patient's physiological activity indicators including heart rate, steps, and sleeping. These devices provide clinicians with details of the activities that a patient is likely to engage in on a day-to-day basis, thus the need to modify the activities of the rehabilitation process. For example, a wearable sense gadget linked to an extant artificial intelligence system can evaluate a patient's mobility and pass the output to a physical therapist to prescribe exercises to aid in the recovery process (Mennella et al., 2023). Telehealth platforms are also examples of predictive rehabilitation technologies because they help in contactless communication between a doctor and a patient. Not only do these platforms provide additional options to obtain rehabilitation services in areas that are hard to reach or where there are few such opportunities but they can, for example, use algorithms to track patient adherence to the proposed treatment and provide suggestions for changes based on information received during teletherapy sessions. Moreover, applications that assist physiotherapists and even occupational therapists with patient prescription facilitation have been designed and developed. For example, recovery timelines on some platforms are predicted by using machine learning to review previous patient data in recovery thus predicting the most suitable treatment regime for a specified patient type. This capability does not only solve for treatment planning bottlenecks but also improves the overall patient experience by addressing the right plan at the right time (Grandinetti et al., 2022).

Despite the current studies on the use of the predictive technologies in rehabilitation, fewer applications in real-life settings remain available. Some of them are the AI-based rehabilitation systems like MindMotion GO which assist the recovery process by tracking the patient's gait and suggesting the exercises to perform. As for the effectiveness in rehabilitation case, MindMotion GO via the motion capture technology could help to create a many passages for patients to go through their rehabilitation program. However, to some extent, the use of AI interventions in rehabilitation presents some forms of ethical concerns, including algorithmic bias, where the data used in creating an AI model to predict and recommend the course of action to its users may not be inclusive of all population types. Researchers revealed that worse performances occur in older adults and patients with k-values less than 0.5; moreover, these two groups are usually underrepresented minorities in patient populations.

1.4 Advantages of PRTs in Healthcare

Predictive technologies applied to rehabilitation has several benefits, inpatient's outcomes, effectiveness of rehabilitation procedures and even, presumably, cost in healthcare.

Another advantage of the technologies is that they enable a unique interface that would allow customized treatment regimes. Conventional treatments for reintegration often involve primarily the use of set processes that do not take into consideration personal differences within patients. On the other hand, predictive rehabilitation technologies allow clinicians to use specific parameters to map appropriate intervention plans. There are incentives for faster recovery, as treatments are based on algorithms of what is expected to be efficient for a certain patient. Predictive rehabilitation technology enhances positive health outcomes and patients' satisfaction because it identifies and targets specific aspects of the patients' needs in line with the rehabilitation programs (Cotton et al., 2024). In addition, predictive rehabilitation technologies improves the rehabilitation healing processes since patients are closely monitored with feedback given instantly. For example, through real-time analytics, clinicians can determine at exactly when a patient's recovery path changes, so that they can early intervene to change the existing care plan. This increased attentiveness greatly decreases the opportunity for adverse effects and guarantees that a patient remains on track in terms of his or her restoration goals.

Further, the incorporation of PRTs to health systems may increase efficiency of utilizing healthcare resources. EHR can therefore free up time for healthcare providers from paperwork and leave them do what they do best; delivering quality healthcare to patients. Also, the prognostic functions of these technologies allow for preventing excessive visits or interventions, so that refined patient care can be provided efficiently and economically. As a result, PRTs have an ability to reduce some pressure off the health services, especially where these services might be constrained (Mamyrbekova et al., 2020).

Thus, while PRTs have advantages, their economic viability is the major issue. Implementation costs differ greatly thus it may be hard for large-scale implementation in areas with less health care systems. In the United States, AI-assisted rehabilitation tools decrease the costs of readmission to a health facility and expensive long-term care, on the other hand, in Europe, data protection laws make compliance expensive. Hence, it becomes imperative that a cross-computation of cost and benefits is done in the context of sustainability. Furthermore, there are regulatory issues which make the deployment difficult across the globe. The software as a medical device system in the FDA is different from the EU's medical device regulation known as MDR. Policy makers thus need to ensure by putting in place flexible policies,Directive modern technologies connected with prediction of rehabilitation but still maintain the issue of cost of these technologies at easily affordable level in all countries.

1.5 The Ethical Importance of Advancing Predictive Rehabilitation Technologies

As publication of more sophisticated predictive rehabilitation technologies in development grows it is imperative to consider the ethical implications involved. Where such innovations are beginning to incorporate personal health data, issues to do with privacy, security, and the appropriate use of this kind of information surface. A patient must leave the hospital assured that his or her data is being handled appropriately so that third parties cannot access or misuse them. Such assurance helps in developing patient-provider relationship which in turns informs the success of PRTs in clinical practice settings. Moreover, the element of consent is identified in ethical practice as relevant to PRTs in particular. Thus, as these technologies increase in sophistication, patient's need full disclosure as to how their data will be used, the risk of data breaches and most importantly, what happens when these predictive analytics are applied to patient care. Making sure that patients understand their condition and give their consent to utilise PRTs in their physical rehabilitation process can help the patents to be more mindful of their disability and take an active part in their rehabilitation (Cotton et al., 2024).

Reducing the algorithmic bias is essential to strive since predictive rehabilitation technologies primarily use data-driven analysis to form predictive decisions. Based on this perception, any datasets that are utilized in the formation of the given algorithms are themselves prejudiced or unrepresentative, and hence, the model outputs will deepen existing health inequity across different populations. Developers and HC organizations need to address biases in the information technology to increase the value of technologies to benefit all patients with advanced predictive rehabilitation. As PRTs technology advances further, it will become critical to finding this balance between growth and right use of the technology in order to reach the full potential of the technology. In this way, patient rights and access to information will prevent certain stakeholders from benefiting from predictive technologies in terms of increasing efficiency for rehabilitation at the cost of worsened quality of patient treatment. With the dawn of PRTs, a measurable baseline of ethical considerations shall skew both their evolution and their success rate in enhancing rehabilitation practice standards (Mennella et al., 2023) (Prang et al., 2021).

2. ETHICAL CHALLENGES IN PREDICTIVE REHABILITATION TECHNOLOGIES

The appearance of technologies such as predictive rehabilitation based on data analysis and machine learning is already mentioned and may open a world of progressive rehabilitation for patients. However, this advancement is closely followed by serious ethical issues. Outstanding themes have tackled issues to do with data protection, consent in the digital environment, and artificial intelligence bias. These can be precariously positioned to erode patient trust and impact patients' health which require meticulous analysis from developers and policymakers, policy implementers including clinicians (Pesapane et al., 2021).

2.1 Data Privacy: The Double-Edged Sword

Big data collection was also identified as a key benefit of the predictive rehabilitation technologies, but the problem of personal health information data protection remained an issue. However, the application of such data has a number of advantages, such as the increase in the effectiveness of rehabilitation measures, adherence, and the prevention of unfavorable outcomes of the disease, its application is associated with the risk of suffering significant losses for patients and clinics due to the dissemination of personally identifiable information.

Figure 2. Data privacy in predictive rehabilitation

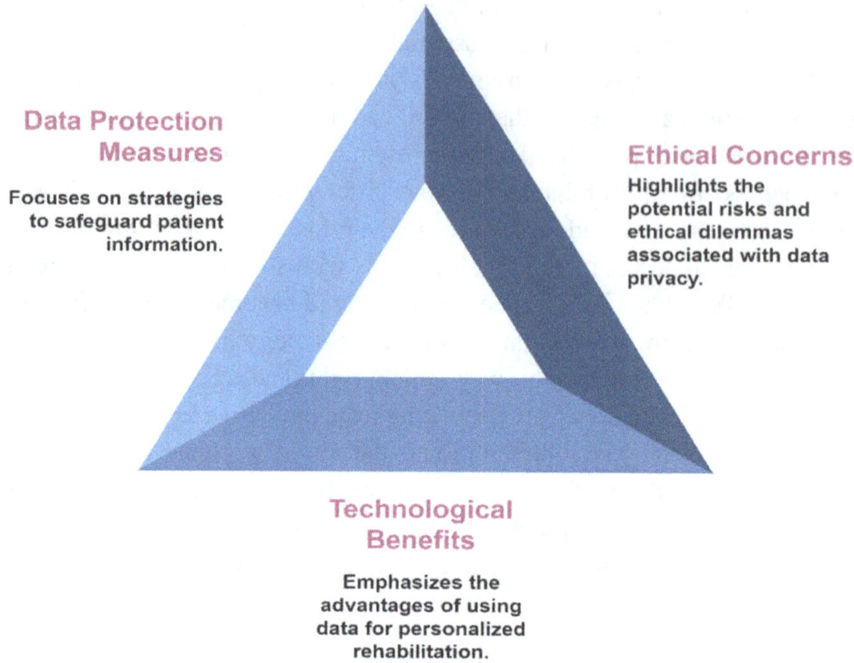

On the one hand, the use of such extensive datasets strengthens the reliability of predictive algorithms in an attempt to create indeed efficient rehabilitation programs. Please refer the Figure2. concerning the data privacy in Predictive Rehabilitation. Such technologies are capable of learning recovery patterns, suggest modifications of lower body therapy, and demonstrate when an interventing action is needed. From this optimistic angle, the collected data provides a stimulus for development of technologies that could significantly improve the patient's quality of life, post-accident or post-operation, or alleviating of chronic diseases (Cotton et al., 2024) (Salim et al., 2023). In the light of the above discussion, there are two major areas of ethical concern with regards to data: Personal health data has major concerns in terms of collection and storage especially on privacy aspect. Finally, we demonstrate that violation of the disclosed information confidentiality can lead to severe consequences, including identity theft, discrimination, and stigmatization. Over time, technology grows and so do the threats on the network, meaning that misuse of such data is always a possibility. In addition, people can be very sceptical about sharing information about themselves if they do not want this information to be passed on to third parties, or if they do not want that information to be used for purposes which are not allowed according to law. Although rehabilitation can be an area of significant benefits from higher levels of advanced analytics, patients' privacy has to be protected as to its highest ethical standards. To improve patients' confidence, healthcare systems and developers should invest in the secure ways of storing data. The privacy of the data has to be protected by anonymizing the data, by encrypting the data, and by storing the data securely. Moreover, transparency should be practiced by intending to explain to patients how the information they provide will be used, and for what purposes only, (Dıcuonzo et al., 2022).

2.2 Informed Consent in the Digital Era

However, in managing the tree generality of predictive rehabilitation technologies, issues of informed consent prove to be rather complex. This complexity arises from the fact that these technological systems can at times have many parts that the patients do not fully understand to include algorithms, data feed sources and theoretically designed user interfaces. In contrast to providing consent as a standard tenet of healthcare organizations, where potential benefits and harms of treatment or interventions must be explained to the patient, predictive rehabilitation technologies may involve more complex cases. The algorithms powering these systems can be complex, and the decision-making logic can be obscure to the patients as well as to clinicians. Consequently, there is a challenge whereby the patient may not understand how the data collected shall be used, what predictions shall be made and or derived, or how such predictions shall be used in the formulation of the program(s) of physical rehabilitation of the patient (Cotton et al., 2024).

Another challenge is raised by the extremely fast pace of development of technology, which entails the issue that the information provided to the subject at the consent obtaining phase might be soon outdated. For instance, if new aspects of functionality or performance are added into a predictive system, the former consent may be invalid if patients are not notified about such a change. This leads to a paradox where patients need to have sufficient information with their conditions, yet they are perforce to place their trust in developing technologies. In order to tackle these factors transparency is very important. Clinicians, technologists and the scientific community should produce definitions and descriptions of the operation and relevance of predictive rehabilitation technologies that are easy to understand. Moreover, patients periodically provided with information on the use of their data and performance of the technologies may represent viable continuous consent solutions as well (Jones et al., 2020).

2.3 Algorithmic Inequity: The Unintended Consequences of Biased Predictive Systems

To that extent, the integration of predictive rehabilitation technologies reveals great transformative promise whereas investing in algorithmic bias is a major concern. All of these surfaces from the fact that the underlying algorithms that drive these technologies are built from datasets that are insufficiently diverse to represent the population of patients in the clinical field. It is possible for some demographic groups to be missing from given datasets, and so when an algorithm is trained using these datasets, the result may be to give shorter end-of-life treatment to patients, and hence these populations are at the receiving end and end up not accessing quality health care as they should (Arora et al., 2023). For example, if the objective is to predict the effects of rehabilitation in a population with specific characteristics such as age, disease type, or other comorbidities the model will be likely to provide misleading results for young people, elderly and patients with certain diseases. This bias can worsen pre-existing health inequalities, and negatively affect the formation of rehabilitation recommendations which are appropriate for groups on the receiving end.

The consequences of an algorithm bias are most undesirable in rehabilitation where the need to tailor an approach is crucial. When offered suggestions in the wrong format they may require longer recoveries or additional discomfort that results in less satisfaction among patients.

The need to address algorithmic bias can only be addressed through a combination of tactics, particularly in the use of the various patient's data for training these systems. Ethicists and clinical professionals and representatives of minorities may be called to work with the teams developing the algorithms to establish which biases may occur and may be corrected. Further, there is the need to monitor the execution of these algorithms and outcomes in order to refine models and practices where discrepancies are perceived (Abràmoff et al., 2023).

3. BALANCING TECHNOLOGY AND HUMAN TOUCH

In this dynamic healthcare environment, issues of using artificial intelligence (AI) technologies require new approaches to patient care. It is on this basis that there exists the dilemma of going fully technological, towards an AI society in-line with the emerging career demands, which also requires striking a balance in the application in technological and career advisory services for healthcare. This essay explores three key components of this balance: This paper discusses; The place of clinicians in an artificial intelligence future, Trust and openness in structuring relationships, and Emotional touch in patient care.

Despite the importance of trust and transparency in AI-rehabilitation, interoperability and patient awareness are not far from it. Quite a number of rehabilitation centers face the challenge of aligning PRT with existing Electronic Health Record (EHR) systems making care disjointed. Also, if a patient is not sure of its effectiveness of the various forms of rehabilitation involving the use of artificial intelligence, then they may not embrace these inventions. The above gap can be closed by enhancing the patient friendly AI education programs to address the issue of digital literacy. Specific features like tutorial based on interactive set of exercises, availability of clinician support and option of several languages may lead to increased usage. The purpose and usefulness of PRTs would be well served by developing better compatibility and providing extensive information regarding patients and their conditions, which would increase the usage of this resource and the quality of recovery for patients.

3.1 The Role of Clinicians in an AI-Driven World

As machines continue to gain the ability to analyze large data sets to support diagnostic, therapeutic and patient care related endeavors, the work of the clinical staff will need to change. Clinicians should not look at such tools as substitutes to themselves but as part and parcel of clinical practice. For the decision-making process, AI can complement and offer strategies and influences that support deciding and also draw attention to factors that may be hidden. However, the analysis of such suggestions and decisions on the outcome of the patient treatment, is a very human activity. Clinicians are well suited to combine their professional opinion, sympathy and/or ethics with the analytical abilities of AI. For example, oncology where, predictive analytics based on AI techniques can pinpoint the most effective treatment regiments by analyzing the existing data. Yet it is the oncologist who has to take into account the patient's values, preferences and circumstances when it comes to medical treatment. The option of examining the human aspect, including stability of life, and psychological issues, is out of the picture for the machines (Birch et al., 2022). Healthcare practitioners stand as critical participants in the process validating and defining AI systems used within the practice. It is entirely crucial to have experts who can guarantee that these tools are efficient, appropriate, and not influenced by a certain kind of bias. Working closely with clinicians, the authors ensure the development of AI algorithms that reflect the richness and interconnectivity of human health. At the heart of these healthcare services is not the mechanics of automated A.I but the humane touch of the clinician.

3.2 Transparency and Trust: Building Bridges

One of the things that has to be worked on is the relative opacity of AI systems to the users and the broad societal context in which they are embedded – patients, clinicians and technology developers. Consumers have to be assured that the AI application they encounter in their care is stable, humane and safeguards their privacy. Such trust can only be built with the help of discussing how the AI tools work, what data they use, and how they make their decision.

Transparency means reporting about AI systems as well as admitting their weaknesses. Clinicians need to share with patients about how artificial intelligence impacts them as a patient. For example, if a teaching-diagnostic aid provides a decision about a certain diagnosis, the clinician should tell how it happened and whether such assessment correlates with other case peculiarities. This approach strengthens trust whereas fostering patient engagement in decisions over their health (Labkoff et al., 2024). Added to this, care is taken to regularly provide proof to patients that AI is useful in enhancing their care needs. Review the Figure.3 how to building the trust through transparency. Available literature shows that when patients sense that they are being involved in the care process, they are more likely to conform to the recommended treatments and have positive attitudes towards treatment (King et al., 2023). By increasing the communication between the clinicians and their patients makes both sides feel wanted and involved in the process of attaining their health goals.

Figure 3. Building trust through transparency

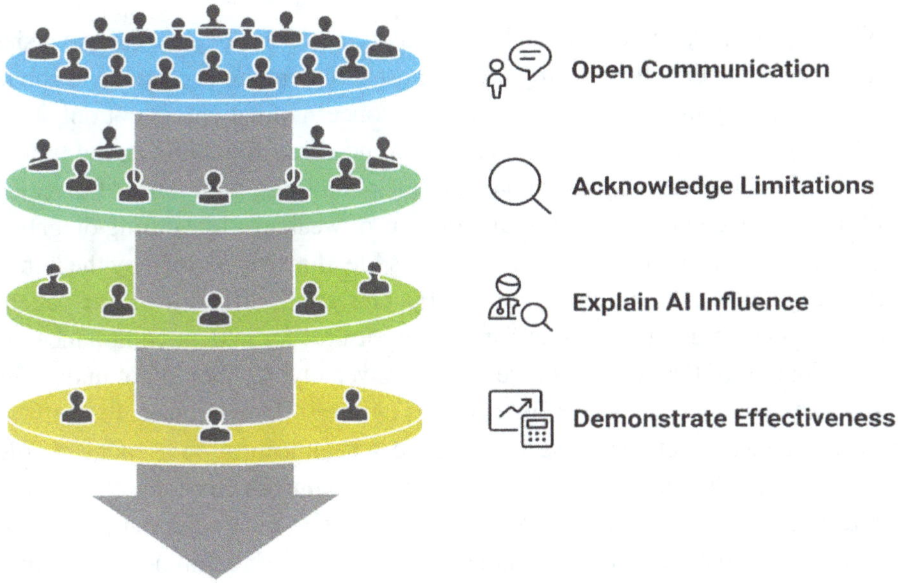

Despite awareness of the need for open presentation of the PRTs' development and application among clinicians and healthcare organizations, the scales should be tipped in favor of patients, who are the principal beneficiaries in this regard. Recognizing their perspectives, anticipations and perceptions may provide a great information on how the needed trust can be built up. A perfect example is a study that focused on the opinions of rehabilitation patients who were using AI-based wearable devices; from the responses given, 65% of the respondents had data privacy concerns, and 70% deemed that having a clear understanding of how exactly their data were used made a difference when making decision to trust the technology (Webber et al., 2023). That is the reason why many of the interviewed patients noted that they would prefer if clinicians discuss how the suggested changes correspond to the goals and plans of rehabilitation. This lack of transparency also make patients sceptical about following the set rehabilitation plans that thousands of people saw appropriate to be associated with the software.

The 16 patients with stroke rehabilitation needs showed an increase of 40 percentage points concerning the adherence of their therapy recommendations if they received biweekly updates via PRTs (Mennella et al., 2023). That means appeals which include interactive reports as well as patient-oriented dashboards can increase the level of compliance and faith in such technologies.

3.3 The Emotional Dimension of Care

The effectiveness, precision, and productivity of AI are beyond controversies, although the aspects of healthcare that are most about emotions cannot and should not be replaced by the technology. A primary concern of patients is not only to be cured, but hear soothing words, feel cared for and cared about during the time of disease. Oftentimes, clinicians are quick to pick emotions, then mirror the patient and find ways to connect with him. In moments of weakness like during diagnoses or at the most critical moments on the patient's life, they are warmed by the human factor from the health care practitioners (Fuentes et al., 2018). It brings patient-centred psychological aspects that can be very useful for patient compliance and their evaluation of the delivered care. Also, conversely, AI should not undermine these essential human encounters in a process of interaction. Virtual care platforms and ai-powered chatbots can be seen to be used in healthcare systems today in order to address administrative work or even repetitive inquiries from the clients thus, such technologies should only be seen as an addition to the traditional approaches of face-to-face contact between clinicians and patients. Maintaining personalized touch and human touch with or for the patients especially during severe diseases or problems should therefore be a cardinal principle in the structure of health care service delivery processes. The specific preservation of the emotional dimension is important for building the clinician-patient relationship based on trust and willingness to establish recovery as well as partnership.

4. INFORMED CONSENT IN PREDICTIVE REHABILITATION TECHNOLOGIES

An important principle in medical practice, and clinical research that whereby patients understand and agree to the consequences that are likely to occur with regard to the intervention that is being administered to them. Predictive rehabilitation technologies are new generation tools in rehabilitation services that use informatics and analytics for modifying and personalizing treatment procedures, or therapeutic interventions. Due to the increasing rate of enhancements in the nature of these technologies, the issues around informed consent become complex. This discourse highlights three critical aspects: developing informed consent as a concept which interprets consent as the process that evolves along with clarity and involvement during the interactions and including the ideas about the patient's autonomy during the entire process of rehabilitation (Farrehi et al., 2020).

4.1 The Nature of Informed Consent: A Dynamic Process

In essence, the conventional and familiar understanding of informed consent is prospectively a single and fairly global interaction between the healthcare provider and the patient in which a treatment or procedure is described to the patient before getting his or her permission. However, when it comes to using technology for rehabilitation, the above opinion must be changed considerably. Permanent changes, the ongoing updates, altering of the algorithms, and the development of new essential data anlytics argue for a dynamic approach to informing the informed consent and refer to the Figure.4 for more details.

Figure 4. Dynamic informed consent process

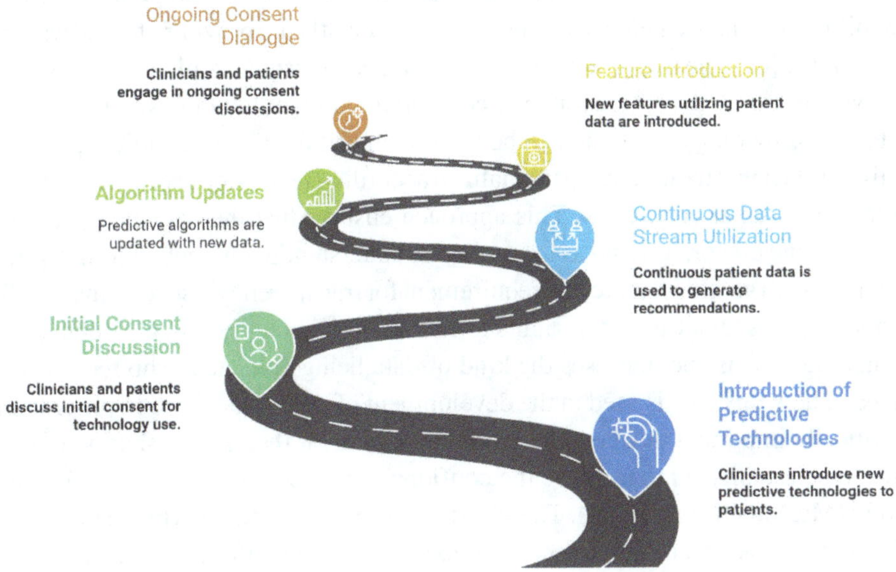

With continuous real-time patient data flows, predictive rehabilitation technologies provide recommendations of reabilitation schedules. The dynamics of this interaction propel consent not as a one-off agreement between the clinician and the patient but as a continuous conversation. The patients, therefore, have to be informed anytime there is a change, whether in the technology, in how the data is used, or in the advances in the prediction analytics. It is vital that clinicians manage the process of consent as a series of conversations rather than one or a number of conversations. For example, when the model is updated or is a new feature that uses patient data is incorporated clinicians should refer patients back to this consent discussion. This can be done by periodic meetings, sharing results on the technology performance and such issues regarding the update on the changes in the future nature of the predicted models (Gerke et al., 2020; Kotsenas et al., 2021). This way, through understanding informed consent as a process, it will be easier for the services providers to establish trust with the clients and patient enables them to get the necessary details throughout their physical rehabilitation processes.

4.2 Clarity and Transparency in Communication

In order to obtain informed consent, the communication process of the intended message should be effective. Driven technologies in rehab require technology and jargon to explain mechanisms that can be understood by the patient. This brings confusion to informed consent specifically do patients understand how the data collected is utilized, the prediction made and the likelihoods and gains/ losses of rehabilitation. These challenges therefore call for healthcare providers to find ways of communicating. The important information can be presented as plainly as possible, and whenever possible – illustrated or compared with familiar things. For example, instead of providing explanations related to an algorithm of the technology, it could justify the fact that treatment is personalized according to previous performance with patients of similar conditions. This approach ensures that the patient appreciates what you, the doctor, has said as a consensual understanding without dumming him down. As with another feature, the requirement for transparency also remains equally important. It is about patients' rights to know more about the broad applicability of their data. This encompasses the kind of data being collected, who records this data and how this data is used in the development of their rehabilitation program. It is critically important that cooperative Frameworks for the use and sharing of data have to be established to improve the confidence between patients and health care givers (McDonald et al., 2024). Thereby, the present study adheres to the principles of clarifying the criteria of patient selection by embracing the prior principles and helping clinicians determine specific guiding principles of patient self-organization in the capacities of predictive rehabilitation technologies, ensuring their improved patients' engagement in rehabilitation processes.

4.3 Preserving Patient Autonomy

In regard to informed consent, there is the ethos of the patient's autonomy, the patient's right to make decisions on the care they receive with due regard to data. While rehab incorporates more and more predictive tools into the general process, it is important to ensure that patient's rights stay the focus of informed consent. Informed consent should make patients more capable of making decisions to make them meet, their preference and their value. It becomes very important this empowerment when handling all prospective factors of rehabilitation technology which may contain automatic suggestions which imply potential directions of the treatment plan. Patients should be assured that not only do they have an opportunity to participate in the development of their rehabilitation programs, but it is also extremely important that their preferences will be valued (Cotton et al., 2024) (Fazio et al., 2021). Respecting the patient autonomy is also a process of letting the patients to make a choice whether to embrace the predictive technologies or run away from the same. Compared to the social agency, this personal agency is most critical given certain concerns relating to data privacy and how the insight gathered from the data contained in rehabilitation is utilized in the process. A healthcare provider needs to build a culture and practices to allow patients to freely engage in actions that give them the voice they need to actively participate in decisions around their treatment plans. This work of academic writing describes the concept of openness in algorithms and decisions, communication and trust, and the possible steps towards applying transparency in the advancement of those marvelous technologies (Pinto-Bernal et al., 2023).

5.TRANSPARENCY AND TRUST IN PREDICTIVE REHABILITATION TECHNOLOGY DEVELOPMENT

Several new technologies make rehabilitation more predictive, and are therefore capable of dramatically changing this sphere in the future. However, as these technologies are incorporated into clinical workflow, the issues of openness and trust appear to be imperative for technology advancement (Cotton et al., 2024). It is of imperative importance to understand that transparency in the systems and processes of the PRTs is basic to the nature of trust. In this academic discourse, we reflect on the importance of openness in algorithm processes and decision-making; communication and involvement of the stakeholders; and how best to implement the measures of openness for the development of these state-of-the-art technologies.

5.1 Importance of Openness in Algorithmic Processes and Decisions

It is thus important to enhance algorithmic transparency in order to understand and be able to call into question the workings of IT tools used for creating predictive rehabilitation solutions. Since such algorithms are used to make decisions affecting caregivers and patients, from predicting patients' course of treatment or a course of action to taking, patients and caregivers must comprehend how the algorithms work. It is important not only from the point of view of treatment outcomes, but also for ethical reasons, and, in particular, in matters of protecting the patient's rights and ensuring the patient's rights. The lack of neutrality means that decision making procedures can be investigated by stakeholders, providing greater insight to the decision-making computations. For example, if a system recommends a particular therapy schedule based on data mining, both the patients and the clinicians ought to be privy to how that recommendation came to be. This involves awareness of the origins of the data used to build the formula, preconceptions included in the making of the algorithm and any prejudice that exists in the data. When decision makers can examine the fundamentals on which they rely, he or she can engage in meaningful conversation and analysis concerning the appropriateness and effectiveness of the algorithm (Chohlas-Wood et al., 2023).

Possibly one of the major issues with using predictive rehabilitation technologies is algorithmic bias which can result in inequitable treatment; however, having algorithms' processes open could provide a means to substantially address such a problem. For example, if a training data set does not have much variation, the outcomes obtained when employing an algorithm can actually harm some category of people. When the algorithm is released it is likely that developers would be able to consult with a broader population hence guaranteeing that everyone would ensure they were following the best practices. This openness not only assist to solve potential biases, but also promotes an accountability where the developers will be more liable for the inference and social ramifications of their advancements.

5.2 Building Trust through Communication and Engagement

Both the clinicians properly implementing the technologies in practice and the patients who will subsequently benefit from these tools need to develop trust in such systems. Standard communication with patients and health care providers for the functionality, advantages, and risks of these technologies is crucial in making them accept their usage (Mennella et al., 2023).

Basically, if the information concerning the application of predictive technologies is well communicated, the process should be made as simple as possible to understand. It therefore becomes the role of the carers especially the healthcare providers to facilitate interpretation of the technicalities in a format that patients find easy to understand. It may require the demonstration with help of colorful diagrams or icons, comparison with other devices, situations or using examples of real-life cases to explain how a specific technology can contribute to the process of rehabilitation. When patients understand the importance and use of these technologies, then they will be inclined to follow the recommendations given (Rossetto et al, 2023).

5.3 Practical Measures to Ensure Transparency

It is possible to list quite a number of practical actions that may promote transparency of the process of development and application of predictive rehabilitation technologies. An approach for the stakeholders – developers, healthcare providers, regulators can work together to create such a framework that will call for transparency, transparency, and integrity (Cotton et al., 2024). The reader is kindly requested to turn to the Figure.5 for the method of implementing the discussed element for attaining transparency in predictive rehabilitation technologies. The key strategies included below:

Documentation and Accessibility: It is the policy of developers to keep complete records of the algorithm development as well as source and validation information, this documentation shall be placed in the public domain. Functionality, constraints and perceived conflicts of interest of the algorithm should be provided in well-documented transparency reports.

Figure 5. Achieving transparency in predictive rehabilitation technologies

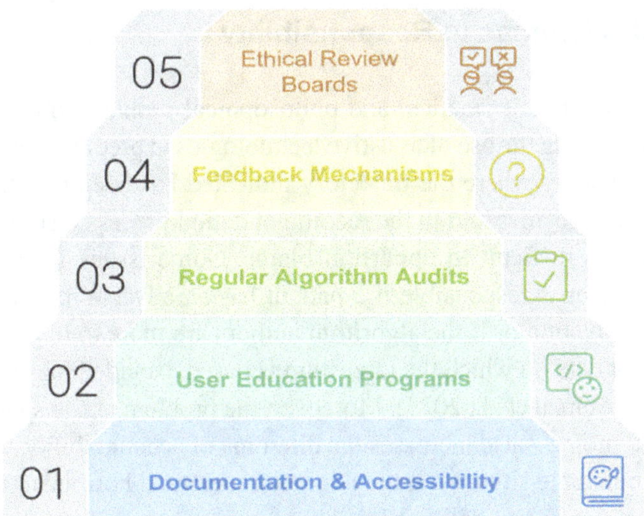

User Education Programs: PRTs are likely to be developed and used in the future; hence, informative programs including workshops, webinars, and brochures should be provided to the patients as well as health care providers in informing them how the PRTs are developed and used and also the benefits as well as drawbacks. It should also contemplate the matters of data privacy and security to ease the apprehensions of the users (Webber et al., 2023). Regular Algorithm Audits: External validation of

PRT audits and assessments should be done at least once every two months while quality tests on the PRT algorithms should be done periodically to check for decline in efficiency poor accuracy and biases. The findings and the action that has been taken should be disseminating publicly.

6. ACCOUNTABILITY IN PREDICTIVE REHABILITATION TECHNOLOGY IMPLEMENTATION

Thus, the question of accountability becomes more and more challenging when using more and more technologies for the prediction of rehabilitation in the clinical practice. There is a potential moral issue to do with responsibility in these technologies that incorporate analytics to inform rehabilitation interventions. Determining who is responsible for allocating algorithmic decisions, understanding and defining the moral implications of such decisions, and creating structures for the appointment of accountability are necessary steps needed for safe and effective implementation of predictive rehabilitation technology to enhance patients' trust (Labkoff et al., 2024).

6.1 Ethical Dilemmas in Responsibility

There is a significant practical and philosophical problem to apportioning responsibility regarding the use of assistive technologies in predicting and facilitating rehabilitation, mainly where the trajectory indicated has been negative. When an algorithm which was involved in the recommendation process results in a negative result it becomes difficult to apportion blame. Some issues include whether a healthcare provider is responsible if a patient has an adverse reaction to an algorithm recommendation or if the algorithm authors are more to blame, particularly if collections of data on which the algorithm is based excluded bias negatively impacted results (Ahmed et al., 2023). Moreover, the problem of transparent nature of organisational projects also increases the dilemma of accountability. Clinicians are placed in a vulnerable situation if they do not understand how an algorithm works or what data it uses; they will not be able to appropriately speak for a patient or make sound clinical judgments. In such cases can providers be held accountable for actions based on the technology that they may not understand fully. Furthermore, there are concerns about the increased use of some algorithms that are frequently described as 'black box' because they are difficult to understand the functioning of the application that is issuing the decision. These dilemmas shed the importance of having well-defined role and responsibility maps throughout the deployment of predictive rehabilitation technologies (Cotton et al 2024).

6.2 Suggested Frameworks for Accountability

There are several accountability structures from which it is possible to draw and address the ethical issues that come with the application of predictive rehabilitation technologies (Lambercy et al., 2021). These frameworks aim at defining roles, increasing accountability and improving the quality of patient outcomes. **Shared Accountability Model:** This shared accountability model implies the collective responsibilities that all the stakeholders who are part of the use of the Predictive Technologies bear. Patients, healthcare clinicians, technology innovators, and healthcare organizations need to work collectively in setting core compatibility responsibility frameworks. In this context, the code users, which are the healthcare providers, have the obligation to understand the performed technology, as well as its drawbacks, and associated bias. In the same manner, the developers are responsible to guarantee the reusability, accuracy and free of thebias of the algorithms. In addition, environmental improvement can be pursued through mainstreaming of cross-sector learning between different types of important stakeholders in order to create a culture of stakeholder accountability (Prentzas et al., 2023).

Algorithmic Auditing and Oversight: Non-partisan algorithmic auditing institutions can be a valuable benefit to answerability for rehabilitative prediction systems. These entities would routinely determine the efficiency and more importantly the ethicality of the algorithms that are under the operational charge of PRTs. Certain of these audits' conclusions should therefore be made public in order to allow stakeholders to get some information on the algorithms' efficiency. This process, besides strengthening the transparency and responsibility of the development process of these technologies by including society, would also allow the putative biases to be continuously improved (Metaxa et al., 2021).

Ethical Advisory Committees: Management of rehabilitation technologies of a facility requires advisory ethical committees within institutions of health to provide useful advice. Such committees including healthcare providers, ethicists, patients and members of the community at large would consider the new technologies as well as their implications. As an advisory body, they can help advise on issues to do with proxy consent, patient's autonomy, and getting their consent to undertake predictive interventions responsibly (Labkoff et al., 2024).

Patient-Centric Accountability: Holding an organization responsible for the treatment of its patients makes it important for those patients to be the focal point. This requires ensuring that patient's informed consent is made clear that explains how the particular rehabilitation technologies will influence decision making on treatment plans. Sharing information about the creation of the predictive algorithms and the data used for creation with the patients provides them with an opportunity to make some of the best decisions regarding their care. This fosters faith in Technology, with strong patient control keywords also prevalent (Visweswaran et al., 2023).

7. GLOBAL PERSPECTIVES AND POLICY DEVELOPMENT

Point-of-use technologies providing predictive rehabilitation has many ethical concerns that are beyond the confines of particular hospitals and countries. It has been seen that as these technologies, making use of data analytics and machine learning for rehabilitation, increase their usage across the world, there grows the necessity of the necessity for proper policies and regulations. Nonetheless, the current environment related to PRTs differs considerably from one country to another, which leads to fragmented standards creating difficulties in the processes of PRTs development and implementation. This discussion looks at the differences in the regulatory environment concerning the technologies discussed above and the challenges and opportunities therein before examining the possibility of creating a global standard for these technologies (Sandin et al., 2021).

7.1 Diverse Regulatory Landscapes

The regulation of the predictive rehabilitation technologies is not the same in different countries due to differences in the healthcare systems, technology advancement and regulatory principles. In USA, the Food and Drug Administration employing the adaptive regulating system to control software and algorithms as medical devices. This framework is built with the flexibility that can respond quickly to the fast-evolving technological environment to support iterative refinement according to the real-world clinical use, and also focused on pre-market review and reporting transparency (Massella et al., 2022). On the other hand, the European Union has provided its Medical Device Regulation that also includes software and algorithms in a risk management way. There are a lot of differences between different countries, such as obligations of documentation, and obligatory post-mark examination, which is usually stricter in the EU than USA. This increased regulatory burden has the capability of slowing the development of new PRTs but guarantees that the patients cannot be provided with inferior products, and services that are safe and effective.

As for other parts of the world including Asia and Africa the degree of regulation is much more diverse. Although countries in Southeast Asia such as Singapore are pioneering progressive frameworks that propel innovations in PRTs with concurrent protection of patient safety, countries with weaker or less developed regulatory systems may experience challenges in dealing with contingencies involved in the management of PRTs hence their slow uptake of the technologies (Bengio et al., 2024).

These differences of the regulatory environment's present difficulties to the MNEs and the researchers. For instance, a PRT designed and implemented in one country may need a redesign to meet regulatory standards of another country, which slows down sharing of good practice and modern technology among different countries and, therefore, restriction the access to highly effective rehabilitation interventions.

This difference in regulation hampers the implementation of Public Real Time Transit contracts on an international scale. For instance, as noted above, the FDA addresses the rehabilitation tools that are driven by AI under the software as a medical device (SaMD), while the EU has put strict post-market surveillance measures. It is only possible to address such disparities with an adaptable method that is recognized on an international level to guarantee equal access to advanced types of rehabilitation technologies.

7.2 Toward Unified Global Standards

It is suggested the common guidelines for predictive rehabilitation technologies should be developed and integrated on the international level, as differences in regulatory environment contribute to the mentioned issue. A harmonization would allow the international exchange of knowledge, resources, technologies (Newman-Griffis et al., 2023). This would make sure that PRTs that are developed in one country can be adopted in others as well as fast track the provision of optimum rehabilitation solutions to patients all over the world. To move toward unified global standards, several key steps can be taken:

International Collaboration: It is crucial that regulatory agencies, professional associations, and other interested parties in both the healthcare and technology industries should continue responding to technology enhancements leading to creation of such consensus. Multilateral efforts can be undertaken either by international institutions such as ISO or WHO or drafting guidelines with references to regulation, ethics and safety which are relevant for different countries (Bernasconi et al., 2020).

Adaptable Regulatory Models: It remains essential to set up efficient flexible frameworks that allow accommodation of local specificities to bring conformity with international standards. Such models should be able to change with the technology environment and it should have stakeholders from different parts of the world.

8. ACTIONABLE RECOMMENDATIONS FOR DEVELOPERS, CLINICIANS, AND POLICYMAKERS

From the perspective of developers, more emphasis should be placed on the ethical designs of artificial intelligence to avoid problems of the prediction algorithm of rehabilitation and the collection of disparate samples. and explainable artificial intelligence models with developed documentation for the clinicians and patients. Ensure patients' information security to meet the standard requirement and the regulatory framework.

For Clinicians: Ensure that patients' rights are to give informed consent regarding the usage of predictive technologie Ensure patient needs are met by incorporating Artificial Intelligence (AI) recommendations that should be combined with clinician's expert opinion. Review the information produced by AI periodically and try to find out whether it reflects certain changes to the rehabilitative plans of individuals.

For Policymakers: To minimize potential risks, actual legal regulation and standard frameworks for the use of predictive rehabilitation technologies should be decreed. Engage the cooperation between the members of the AI community, healthcare practitioners, and ethicists. Nonetheless, in order to maximize the impact of these innovation, it is important that this be done in a equitable manner to reach out to all the patients across both gender and ages.

9. FUTURE AI TRENDS AND LEGAL PERSPECTIVES IN PREDICTIVE REHABILITATION

In the future of AI in rehabilitation, it is possible to have personalized models with the addition of real-time biometric, self-teaching learning processes. AI has the potential to improve robotic rehabilitation as well as virtual reality that will advance to provide better and automated recovery programs. However, there's a legal and ethical issue that should be solved: data privacy, an account of algorithms, and legal requirements. There is currently a rising concern in governments and healthcare agencies on how to effectively put in place good structures that could enable artificial intelligence to work under acceptable ethical standards in the medical field. Maintenance of proper regulation that can balance innovation and as well, strive to protect the rights of the patient is going to be essential when defining the next generation pattern of the juice for rehabilitation.

10. CONCLUSION

By focusing on the application of predictive technologies in the field of rehabilitation, this paper shows that ethical concerns in this area are multifaceted and reflect tensions between technology and professionalism on the one hand, and patients' needs on the other. They present new opportunities of tailored and efficient treatment contributing to the change of patients' lives and the techniques of rehabilitation. However, the integration of both creates a host of ethical questions which in turn gives rise to problems which have to be solved.

Concerns of data protection, consent, and bias are definitely some of the great challenges that both the healthcare sector and systems design and policymakers have to grapple with. Here patient self-determination, and trust resulted from the provision of accurate information, are critical. Imagining that clinicians will be able to maintain the tempo of AI-related systems while providing the empathetic content to patients' experiences that people demand. The emotional aspects of the healthcare and the importance of the communication with the patients, especially during the treatment, as well as necessity to consider patient's permission for the needed actions emphasize the importance of cooperation between the human factors and the usage of technologies. It is from this synergy that a comprehensive rehabilitation program is developed that complies with ethical best practice while fully embracing the possibilities of predictive technologies.

For the future, there will be a need to ensure that international standards are developed and debated in the arenas of international regulation of professional performances given that the PRT management can differ significantly in various terrains. In this way, achieving greater overall standardization on a worldwide basis can also help protect patients' well-being while accelerating the growth of these new predictive tools along the most ethically and safely sound lines possible. Ideally, suggested accountability systems mark the challenges attributing to PRTs risks which requires collective cooperation of developers, the clinicians and other regulatory authorities fostering the culture of accountability and improvement. By identifying and consequently addressing ethical implications concerning rehabilitation technologies, the future of this global industry will be developed, and the principles of patient-centred care will be adjusted so that interventions in this sphere are beneficial for enhancing personal wellbeing.

REFERENCES

Abràmoff, M. D., Tarver, M. E., Loyo-Berríos, N., Trujillo, S., Char, D., Obermeyer, Z., Eydelman, M., & Maisel, W. H. (2023). Considerations for addressing bias in artificial intelligence for health equity [Review of Considerations for addressing bias in artificial intelligence for health equity]. Npj Digital Medicine, 6(1). Nature Portfolio. DOI: 10.1038/s41746-023-00913-9

Ahmed, M. I., Spooner, B., Isherwood, J., Lane, M. A., Orrock, E., & Dennison, A. R. (2023). *A Systematic Review of the Barriers to the Implementation of Artificial Intelligence in Healthcare* [Review of A Systematic Review of the Barriers to the Implementation of Artificial Intelligence in Healthcare]. Cureus. Cureus, Inc., DOI: 10.7759/cureus.46454

Aldenaini, N., Alslaity, A., Sampalli, S., & Orji, R. (2022). Persuasive Strategies and Their Implementations in Mobile Interventions for Physical Activity: A Systematic Review [Review of Persuasive Strategies and Their Implementations in Mobile Interventions for Physical Activity: A Systematic Review]. International Journal of Human-Computer Interaction, 39(12), 2292. Taylor & Francis. DOI: 10.1080/10447318.2022.2075573

Arora, A., Alderman, J., Palmer, J., Ganapathi, S., Laws, E., McCradden, M. D., Oakden-Rayner, L., Pfohl, S., Ghassemi, M., McKay, F., Treanor, D., Rostamzadeh, N., Mateen, B. A., Gath, J., Adebajo, A. O., Kuku, S., Matin, R., Heller, K., Sapey, E., . . . Liu, X. (2023). The value of standards for health datasets in artificial intelligence-based applications. In A. Arora, J. Alderman, J. Palmer, S. Ganapathi, E. Laws, M. D. McCradden, L. Oakden-Rayner, S. Pfohl, M. Ghassemi, F. McKay, D. Treanor, N. Rostamzadeh, B. A. Mateen, J. Gath, A. O. Adebajo, S. Kuku, R. Matin, K. Heller, E. Sapey, … X. Liu, Nature Medicine (Vol. 29, Issue 11, p. 2929). Nature Portfolio. DOI: 10.1038/s41591-023-02608-w

Bengio, Y., Hinton, G. E., Yao, A. C.-C., Song, D., Abbeel, P., Darrell, T., Harari, Y. N., Zhang, Y.-Q., Lan, X., Shalev-Shwartz, S., Hadfield, G. K., Clune, J., Maharaj, T., Hutter, F., Baydin, A. G., McIlraith, S. A., Gao, Q., Acharya, A., Krueger, D., . . . Mindermann, S. (2024). Managing extreme AI risks amid rapid progress. In Y. Bengio, G. E. Hinton, A. C.-C. Yao, D. Song, P. Abbeel, T. Darrell, Y. N. Harari, Y.-Q. Zhang, X. Lan, S. Shalev-Shwartz, G. K. Hadfield, J. Clune, T. Maharaj, F. Hutter, A. G. Baydin, S. A. McIlraith, Q. Gao, A. Acharya, D. Krueger, … S. Mindermann, Science (Vol. 384, Issue 6698, p. 842). American Association for the Advancement of Science. DOI: 10.1126/science.adn0117

Bernasconi, L., Şen, S., Angerame, L., Balyegisawa, A., Hui, D. H. Y., Hotter, M., Hsu, C. Y., Ito, T., Jörger, F., Krassnitzer, W., Phillips, A., Li, R., Stockley, L., Tay, F., Widlund, C. von H., Wan, M., Wong, C., Yau, H., Hiemstra, T. F., . . . Senti, G. (2020). Legal and ethical framework for global health information and biospecimen exchange - an international perspective. In L. Bernasconi, S. Şen, L. Angerame, A. Balyegisawa, D. H. Y. Hui, M. Hotter, C. Y. Hsu, T. Ito, F. Jörger, W. Krassnitzer, A. Phillips, R. Li, L. Stockley, F. Tay, C. von H. Widlund, M. Wan, C. Wong, H. Yau, T. F. Hiemstra, … G. Senti, BMC Medical Ethics (Vol. 21, Issue 1). BioMed Central. DOI: 10.1186/s12910-020-0448-9

Birch, J., Creel, K., Jha, A. K., & Plutynski, A. (2022). Clinical decisions using AI must consider patient values. In J. Birch, K. Creel, A. K. Jha, & A. Plutynski, Nature Medicine (Vol. 28, Issue 2, p. 229). Nature Portfolio. DOI: 10.1038/s41591-021-01624-y

Chohlas-Wood, A., Coots, M., Goel, S., & Nyarko, J. (2023). Designing equitable algorithms. In A. Chohlas-Wood, M. Coots, S. Goel, & J. Nyarko, Nature Computational Science (Vol. 3, Issue 7, p. 601). Nature Portfolio. DOI: 10.1038/s43588-023-00485-4

Cotton, R., Seamon, B. A., Segal, R., Davis, R. D., Sahu, A., McLeod, M. M., Celnik, P., & Ramey, S. L. (2024). A Causal Framework for Precision Rehabilitation. In R. Cotton, B. A. Seamon, R. Segal, R. D. Davis, A. Sahu, M. M. McLeod, P. Celnik, & S. L. Ramey, arXiv (Cornell University). Cornell University. https://doi.org//arxiv.2411.03919DOI: 10.48550

Dıcuonzo, G., Galeone, G., Shini, M., & Massari, A. (2022). Towards the Use of Big Data in Healthcare: A Literature Review [Review of Towards the Use of Big Data in Healthcare: A Literature Review]. Healthcare, 10(7), 1232. Multidisciplinary Digital Publishing Institute. DOI: 10.3390/healthcare10071232

Farrehi, C., Pazzi, C., Capron, M., Anderson, K. D., Richardson, B., & Stillman, M. (2020). How individuals with spinal cord injury in the United States access and assess information about experimental therapies and clinical trials: results of a clinical survey. In C. Farrehi, C. Pazzi, M. Capron, K. D. Anderson, B. Richardson, & M. Stillman, Spinal Cord Series and Cases (Vol. 6, Issue 1). Springer Nature. DOI: 10.1038/s41394-020-00354-6

Fazio, R. D., Giannoccaro, N. I., Carrasco, M., Velázquez, R., & Visconti, P. (2021). Wearable devices and IoT applications for symptom detection, infection tracking, and diffusion containment of the COVID-19 pandemic: a survey. In R. D. Fazio, N. I. Giannoccaro, M. Carrasco, R. Velázquez, & P. Visconti, Frontiers of Information Technology & Electronic Engineering (Vol. 22, Issue 11, p. 1413). Springer Science+Business Media. DOI: 10.1631/FITEE.2100085

Gerke, S., Minssen, T., & Cohen, G. (2020). Ethical and legal challenges of artificial intelligence-driven healthcare. In Gerke, S., Minssen, T., & Cohen, G. (Eds.), *Elsevier eBooks* (p. 295). Elsevier BV., DOI: 10.1016/B978-0-12-818438-7.00012-5

Goldberg, C. B., Adams, L., Blumenthal, D., Brennan, P. F., Brown, N., Butte, A. J., Cheatham, M., deBronkart, D., Dixon, J., Drazen, J. M., Evans, B. J., Hoffman, S. M., Holmes, C., Lee, P., Manrai, A. K., Omenn, G. S., Perlin, J. B., Ramoni, R., Sapiro, G., . . . Zhao, J. (2024). To do no harm — and the most good — with AI in health care. In C. B. Goldberg, L. Adams, D. Blumenthal, P. F. Brennan, N. Brown, A. J. Butte, M. Cheatham, D. deBronkart, J. Dixon, J. M. Drazen, B. J. Evans, S. M. Hoffman, C. Holmes, P. Lee, A. K. Manrai, G. S. Omenn, J. B. Perlin, R. Ramoni, G. Sapiro, … J. Zhao, Nature Medicine (Vol. 30, Issue 3, p. 623). Nature Portfolio. DOI: 10.1038/s41591-024-02853-7

Grandinetti, J., Gao, Y., Gonzalez, Y., Deng, J., Shen, C., & Jia, X. (2022). MR image reconstruction from undersampled data for image-guided radiation therapy using a patient-specific deep manifold image prior. In J. Grandinetti, Y. Gao, Y. Gonzalez, J. Deng, C. Shen, & X. Jia, Frontiers in Oncology (Vol. 12). Frontiers Media. DOI: 10.3389/fonc.2022.1013783

Jones, M., Collier, G., Reinkensmeyer, D. J., DeRuyter, F., Dzivak, J., Zondervan, D. K., & Morris, J. (2020). Big Data Analytics and Sensor-Enhanced Activity Management to Improve Effectiveness and Efficiency of Outpatient Medical Rehabilitation [Review of Big Data Analytics and Sensor-Enhanced Activity Management to Improve Effectiveness and Efficiency of Outpatient Medical Rehabilitation]. International Journal of Environmental Research and Public Health, 17(3), 748. Multidisciplinary Digital Publishing Institute. DOI: 10.3390/ijerph17030748

King, C. R., Shambe, A., & Abraham, J. (2023). Potential uses of AI for perioperative nursing handoffs: a qualitative study. In C. R. King, A. Shambe, & J. Abraham, JAMIA Open (Vol. 6, Issue 1). University of Oxford. DOI: 10.1093/jamiaopen/ooad015

Kotsenas, A. L., Balthazar, P., Andrews, D., Geis, J. R., & Cook, T. S. (2021). Rethinking Patient Consent in the Era of Artificial Intelligence and Big Data. In A. L. Kotsenas, P. Balthazar, D. Andrews, J. R. Geis, & T. S. Cook, Journal of the American College of Radiology (Vol. 18, Issue 1, p. 180). Elsevier BV. DOI: 10.1016/j.jacr.2020.09.022

Labkoff, S. E., Oladimeji, B. J., Kannry, J., Solomonides, A., Leftwich, R., Koski, E., Joseph, A. L., López-González, M., Fleisher, L. A., Nolen, K., Dutta, S., Levy, D. R., Price, A., Barr, P., Hron, J. D., Lin, B., Srivastava, G., Pastor, N., Luque, U. S., . . . Quintana, Y. (2024). Toward a responsible future: recommendations for AI-enabled clinical decision support. In S. E. Labkoff, B. J. Oladimeji, J. Kannry, A. Solomonides, R. Leftwich, E. Koski, A. L. Joseph, M. López-González, L. A. Fleisher, K. Nolen, S. Dutta, D. R. Levy, A. Price, P. Barr, J. D. Hron, B. Lin, G. Srivastava, N. Pastor, U. S. Luque, … Y. Quintana, Journal of the American Medical Informatics Association (Vol. 31, Issue 11, p. 2730). Oxford University Press. DOI: 10.1093/jamia/ocae209

Lambercy, O., Lehner, R., Chua, K. S. G., Wee, S. K., Rajeswaran, D. K., Kuah, C. W. K., Ang, W. T., Liang, P., Campolo, D., Hussain, A., Aguirre-Ollinger, G., Guan, C., Kanzler, C. M., Wenderoth, N., & Gassert, R. (2021). Neurorehabilitation From a Distance: Can Intelligent Technology Support Decentralized Access to Quality Therapy? In O. Lambercy, R. Lehner, K. S. G. Chua, S. K. Wee, D. K. Rajeswaran, C. W. K. Kuah, W. T. Ang, P. Liang, D. Campolo, A. Hussain, G. Aguirre-Ollinger, C. Guan, C. M. Kanzler, N. Wenderoth, & R. Gassert, Frontiers in Robotics and AI (Vol. 8). Frontiers Media. DOI: 10.3389/frobt.2021.612415

Mamyrbekova, S., Nurgaliyeva, Z., Saktapov, A., Zholdasbekova, A., & Kudaibergenova, A. (2020). Medicine of the Future: Digital Technologies in Healthcare. In S. Mamyrbekova, Z. Nurgaliyeva, A. Saktapov, A. Zholdasbekova, & A. Kudaibergenova, E3S Web of Conferences (Vol. 159, p. 4036). EDP Sciences. DOI: 10.1051/e3sconf/202015904036

Marcus, H. J., Ramírez, P. T., Khan, D. Z., Horsfall, H. L., Hanrahan, J., Williams, S. C., Beard, D., Bhat, R. A., Catchpole, K., Cook, A., Hutchison, K., Martin, J., Melvin, T., Stoyanov, D., Rovers, M. M., Raison, N., Dasgupta, P., Noonan, D., Stocken, D., . . . Páez, A. (2024). The IDEAL framework for surgical robotics: development, comparative evaluation and long-term monitoring. In H. J. Marcus, P. T. Ramírez, D. Z. Khan, H. L. Horsfall, J. Hanrahan, S. C. Williams, D. Beard, R. A. Bhat, K. Catchpole, A. Cook, K. Hutchison, J. Martin, T. Melvin, D. Stoyanov, M. M. Rovers, N. Raison, P. Dasgupta, D. Noonan, D. Stocken, … A. Páez, Nature Medicine (Vol. 30, Issue 1, p. 61). Nature Portfolio. DOI: 10.1038/s41591-023-02732-7

Massella, M., Dri, D. A., & Gramaglia, D. (2022). Regulatory Considerations on the use of Machine Learning based tools in Clinical Trials. In M. Massella, D. A. Dri, & D. Gramaglia, Health and Technology (Vol. 12, Issue 6, p. 1085). Springer Science+Business Media. DOI: 10.1007/s12553-022-00708-0

Mathews, D., Abernethy, A. P., Chaikof, E. L., Charo, R. A., Daley, G. Q., Enriquez, J., Gottlieb, S., Kahn, J., Klausner, R. D., Tavazoie, S. F., Fabi, R., Offodile, A. C., Sherkow, J. S., Sullenger, R. D., Freiling, E., & Balatbat, C. (2023). Regenerative Medicine: Case Study for Understanding and Anticipating Emerging Science and Technology. In Mathews, D., Abernethy, A. P., Chaikof, E. L., Charo, R. A., Daley, G. Q., Enriquez, J., Gottlieb, S., Kahn, J., Klausner, R. D., Tavazoie, S. F., Fabi, R., Offodile, A. C., Sherkow, J. S., Sullenger, R. D., Freiling, E., Balatbat, C., & Perspectives, N. A. M. (Eds.), *Issue 15)* (Vol. 11)., DOI: 10.31478/202211d

McDonald, P., Foley, T., Verheij, R., Braithwaite, J., Rubin, J. C., Harwood, K., Phillips, J., Gilman, S. D., & van der Wees, P. J. (2024). Data to knowledge to improvement: creating the learning health system. In P. McDonald, T. Foley, R. Verheij, J. Braithwaite, J. C. Rubin, K. Harwood, J. Phillips, S. D. Gilman, & P. J. van der Wees, BMJ. DOI: 10.1136/bmj-2023-076175

Mennella, C., Maniscalco, U., Pietro, G. D., & Esposito, M. (2023). The Role of Artificial Intelligence in Future Rehabilitation Services: A Systematic Literature Review. In C. Mennella, U. Maniscalco, G. D. Pietro, & M. Esposito, IEEE Access (Vol. 11, p. 11024). Institute of Electrical and Electronics Engineers. DOI: 10.1109/ACCESS.2023.3236084

Metaxa, D., Park, J. S., Robertson, R. E., Karahalios, K., Wilson, C., Hancock, J. T., & Sandvig, C. (2021). Auditing Algorithms: Understanding Algorithmic Systems from the Outside In. In D. Metaxa, J. S. Park, R. E. Robertson, K. Karahalios, C. Wilson, J. T. Hancock, & C. Sandvig, Foundations and Trends® in Human–Computer Interaction (Vol. 14, Issue 4, p. 272). Now Publishers. DOI: 10.1561/1100000083

Newman-Griffis, D., Desmet, B., Zirikly, A., Tamang, S., & Chang, C.-H. (2023). Editorial: Artificial intelligence for human function and disability. In D. Newman-Griffis, B. Desmet, A. Zirikly, S. Tamang, & C.-H. Chang, Frontiers in Digital Health (Vol. 5). Frontiers Media. DOI: 10.3389/fdgth.2023.1282287

Pérez-Fuentes, M. D. C., Molero Jurado, M. D. M., Gázquez Linares, J. J., & Oropesa Ruiz, N. F. (2018). The role of emotional intelligence in engagement in nurses. *International Journal of Environmental Research and Public Health*, *15*(9), 1915.

Pesapane, F., Bracchi, D. A., Mulligan, J. F., Линников, A. C., Maslennikov, O. V., Lanzavecchia, M. B., Tantrige, P., Stasolla, A., Biondetti, P., Giuggioli, P. F., Cassano, E., & Carrafiello, G. (2021). Legal and Regulatory Framework for AI Solutions in Healthcare in EU, US, China, and Russia: New Scenarios after a Pandemic. In F. Pesapane, D. A. Bracchi, J. F. Mulligan, A. C. Линников, O. V. Maslennikov, M. B. Lanzavecchia, P. Tantrige, A. Stasolla, P. Biondetti, P. F. Giuggioli, E. Cassano, & G. Carrafiello, Radiation (Vol. 1, Issue 4, p. 261). Multidisciplinary Digital Publishing Institute. DOI: 10.3390/radiation1040022

Philpot, L. M., Dugani, S. B., Singla, A., DeZutter, M. A., & Ebbert, J. O. (2023). Digital Care Horizon: A Framework for Extending Health Care Through Digital Transformation. In L. M. Philpot, S. B. Dugani, A. Singla, M. A. DeZutter, & J. O. Ebbert, Mayo Clinic Proceedings Digital Health (Vol. 1, Issue 3, p. 210). Elsevier BV. DOI: 10.1016/j.mcpdig.2023.05.005

Pinto-Bernal, M. J. M., S. D. S., Múnera, M., Casas, D., Villa-Moreno, A., Frizera, A., Stoelen, M. F., Belpaeme, T., & Cifuentes, C. A. (2023). Do different robot appearances change emotion recognition in children with ASD? In M. J. Pinto-Bernal, S. D. S. M., M. Múnera, D. Casas, A. Villa-Moreno, A. Frizera, M. F. Stoelen, T. Belpaeme, & C. A. Cifuentes, Frontiers in Neurorobotics (Vol. 17). Frontiers Media. DOI: 10.3389/fnbot.2023.1044491

Prang, K.-H., Maritz, R., Sabanovic, H., Dunt, D., & Kelaher, M. (2021). Mechanisms and impact of public reporting on physicians and hospitals' performance: A systematic review (2000–2020) [Review of Mechanisms and impact of public reporting on physicians and hospitals' performance: A systematic review (2000–2020)]. PLoS ONE, 16(2). Public Library of Science. DOI: 10.1371/journal.pone.0247297

Prentzas, N., Kakas, A. C., & Pattichis, C. S. (2023). Explainable AI applications in the Medical Domain: a systematic review [Review of Explainable AI applications in the Medical Domain: a systematic review]. arXiv (Cornell University). Cornell University. https://doi.org/DOI: 10.48550/arXiv.2308

Rossetto, F., Borgnis, F., Isernia, S., Foglia, E., Garagiola, E., Realdon, O., & Baglio, F. (2023). System Integrated Digital Empowering and teleRehabilitation to promote patient Activation and well-Being in chronic disabilities: A usability and acceptability study. In F. Rossetto, F. Borgnis, S. Isernia, E. Foglia, E. Garagiola, O. Realdon, & F. Baglio, Frontiers in Public Health (Vol. 11). Frontiers Media. DOI: 10.3389/fpubh.2023.1154481

Salim, A., Stein, D. M., Zarzaur, B. L., & Livingston, D. H. (2023). Measuring long-term outcomes after injury: current issues and future directions [Review of Measuring long-term outcomes after injury: current issues and future directions]. Trauma Surgery & Acute Care Open, 8(1). *BMJ (Clinical Research Ed.)*, *8*(1), e001068. Advance online publication. DOI: 10.1136/tsaco-2022-001068 PMID: 36919026

Sandin, P., Munthe, C., & Björnberg, K. E. (2021). Technology Neutrality in European Regulation of GMOs. In P. Sandin, C. Munthe, & K. E. Björnberg, Ethics Policy & Environment (Vol. 25, Issue 1, p. 52). Taylor & Francis. DOI: 10.1080/21550085.2020.1865085

Visweswaran, S., Sadhu, E. M., Morris, M., & Samayamuthu, M. J. (2023). Clinical Algorithms with Race: An Online Database. In S. Visweswaran, E. M. Sadhu, M. Morris, & M. J. Samayamuthu, medRxiv (Cold Spring Harbor Laboratory). Cold Spring Harbor Laboratory. DOI: 10.1101/2023.07.04.23292231

Webber, C. M., Riberdy, A., Saha, A., Marinac-Dabić, D., Caños, D., & Tarver, M. E. (2023). Integrating Patient-Generated Health Data Throughout the Total Product Life Cycle of Medical Devices [Review of Integrating Patient-Generated Health Data Throughout the Total Product Life Cycle of Medical Devices]. Therapeutic Innovation & Regulatory Science, 57(5), 952. Springer Science+Business Media. DOI: 10.1007/s43441-023-00505-5

Zhang, Q., Jin, T., Cai, J., Xu, L., He, T., Wang, T., Tian, Y., Li, L., Peng, Y., & Lee, C. (2021). Wearable Triboelectric Sensors Enabled Gait Analysis and Waist Motion Capture for IoT-Based Smart Healthcare Applications. In Q. Zhang, T. Jin, J. Cai, L. Xu, T. He, T. Wang, Y. Tian, L. Li, Y. Peng, & C. Lee, Advanced Science (Vol. 9, Issue 4). Wiley. DOI: 10.1002/advs.202103694

Compilation of References

23. Shapiro, J. (2020). The importance of community programs in reducing technology reluctance among seniors. *Journal of Community Health*, *45*(2), 380–387. PMID: 32939677

Abbade, L. P., Wang, M., Sriganesh, K., Jin, Y., Mbuagbaw, L., & Thabane, L. (2017). The framing of research questions using the PICOT format in randomized controlled trials of venous ulcer disease is suboptimal: A systematic survey. *Wound Repair and Regeneration*, *25*(5), 892–900. DOI: 10.1111/wrr.12592 PMID: 29080311

Abbaspur-Behbahani, S., Monaghesh, E., Hajizadeh, A., & Fehresti, S. (2022). Application of mobile health to support the elderly during the COVID-19 outbreak: A systematic review. In Health Policy and Technology (Vol. 11, Issue 1, p. 100595). Elsevier BV. DOI: 10.1016/j.hlpt.2022.100595

Abobakr, A., Hossny, M., & Nahavandi, S. (2018). A Skeleton-Free Fall Detection System From Depth Images Using Random Decision Forest. In IEEE Systems Journal (Vol. 12, Issue 3, pp. 2994–3005). Institute of Electrical and Electronics Engineers (IEEE). DOI: 10.1109/JSYST.2017.2780260

Abràmoff, M. D., Tarver, M. E., Loyo-Berríos, N., Trujillo, S., Char, D., Obermeyer, Z., Eydelman, M., & Maisel, W. H. (2023). Considerations for addressing bias in artificial intelligence for health equity [Review of Considerations for addressing bias in artificial intelligence for health equity]. Npj Digital Medicine, 6(1). Nature Portfolio. DOI: 10.1038/s41746-023-00913-9

Acharya, U. R., Faust, O., Sree, S. V., Molinari, F., Saba, L., Nicolaides, A., & Suri, J. S. (2012). An Accurate and Generalized Approach to Plaque Characterization in 346 Carotid Ultrasound Scans. In IEEE Transactions on Instrumentation and Measurement (Vol. 61, Issue 4, pp. 1045–1053). Institute of Electrical and Electronics Engineers (IEEE). DOI: 10.1109/TIM.2011.2174897

Adame, T., Bel, A., Carreras, A., Melià-Seguí, J., Oliver, M., & Pous, R. (2018). CUIDATS: An RFID–WSN hybrid monitoring system for smart health care environments. In Future Generation Computer Systems (Vol. 78, pp. 602–615). Elsevier BV. DOI: 10.1016/j.future.2016.12.023

Adam, M. A., & Mukhtar, A. (2024). Heartfelt insights: AI and machine learning applications for cardiac wellness. *International Journal of Advanced Engineering Technologies and Innovations*, *1*(4), 231–247.

Adans-Dester, C., Hankov, N., O'Brien, A., Vergara-Diaz, G., Black-Schaffer, R., Zafonte, R., Dy, J., Lee, S. I., & Bonato, P. (2020). Enabling precision rehabilitation interventions using wearable sensors and machine learning to track motor recovery. *NPJ Digital Medicine*, *3*(1), 121. DOI: 10.1038/s41746-020-00328-w PMID: 33024831

Ahmed, M. I., Spooner, B., Isherwood, J., Lane, M. A., Orrock, E., & Dennison, A. R. (2023). *A Systematic Review of the Barriers to the Implementation of Artificial Intelligence in Healthcare* [Review of A Systematic Review of the Barriers to the Implementation of Artificial Intelligence in Healthcare]. Cureus. Cureus, Inc., DOI: 10.7759/cureus.46454

Ahmed, M., Antar, A. D., & Ahad, M. A. R. (2021). Static postural transition-based technique and efficient feature extraction for sensor-based activity recognition. *Pattern Recognition Letters*, *147*, 25–33. DOI: 10.1016/j.patrec.2021.04.001

Ahmed, Z., Mohamed, K., Zeeshan, S., & Dong, X. (2020). Artificial intelligence with multi-functional machine learning platform development for better healthcare and precision medicine. *Database : The Journal of Biological Databases and Curation*, *2020*, baaa010. DOI: 10.1093/database/baaa010 PMID: 32185396

Ai, Q., Liu, Z., Meng, W., Liu, Q., & Xie, S. Q. (2021). Machine learning in robot assisted upper limb rehabilitation: A focused review. *IEEE Transactions on Cognitive and Developmental Systems*.

Akagündüz, E., Aslan, M., Şengür, A., Wang, H., & Ince, M. C. (2016). Silhouette orientation volumes for efficient fall detection in depth videos. *IEEE Journal of Biomedical and Health Informatics*, *21*(3), 756–763. DOI: 10.1109/JBHI.2016.2570300 PMID: 28113444

Akbar, K., Passaro, A., Di Gioia, M., Martini, E., Dragone, M., Zullo, A., & Stasolla, F. (2024). Reviewing the Horizon: The Future of Extended Reality and Artificial Intelligence in Neurorehabilitation for Brain Injury Recovery. *Information (Basel)*, *15*(8), 501. DOI: 10.3390/info15080501

Akcay, G., Demirdogen, F., Gul, T., Ali, Y., Dilcan, K. D., Esra, K., Huseyin Emre, O., Cagla, C., Haydar, C., & Yavuz, E. (2024). Effects of Transcranial Direct Current Stimulation on Motor and Cognitive Dysfunction in an Experimental Traumatic Brain Injury Model. *Turkish Neurosurgery*, •••, 343–350. DOI: 10.5137/1019-5149. JTN.45526-23.4 PMID: 38497188

Aldenaini, N., Alslaity, A., Sampalli, S., & Orji, R. (2022). Persuasive Strategies and Their Implementations in Mobile Interventions for Physical Activity: A Systematic Review [Review of Persuasive Strategies and Their Implementations in Mobile Interventions for Physical Activity: A Systematic Review]. International Journal of Human-Computer Interaction, 39(12), 2292. Taylor & Francis. DOI: 10.1080/10447318.2022.2075573

Alsheikh, M. A., Selim, A., Niyato, D., Doyle, L., Lin, S., & Tan, H. P. (2016, March). Deep activity recognition models with triaxial accelerometers. In *Workshops at the thirtieth AAAI conference on artificial intelligence.*

Amaral, T., ... (2019). "A review on the development of smart wheelchairs for people with motor disabilities." Sensors. MDPI: https://www.mdpi.com/1424-8220/19/22/4913

Amaya-Rodriguez, C. A., Carvajal-Zamorano, K., Bustos, D., Alegría-Arcos, M., & Castillo, K. (2024). A journey from molecule to physiology and in silico tools for drug discovery targeting the transient receptor potential vanilloid type 1 (TRPV1) channel. *Frontiers in Pharmacology, 14*, 1251061. DOI: 10.3389/fphar.2023.1251061 PMID: 38328578

Ambekar, A., Agrawal, A., Rao, R., Mishra, A. K., Khandelwal, S. K., & Chadda, R. K. (2019). Magnitude of substance use in India. *New Delhi: Ministry of Social Justice and Empowerment, Government of India, 23.*

Ananthakumar, B., Nanjundeshwara, N., Lakshmaiah, A., & Raghavan, R. (2024). Synthetic Gene Circuits as a Promising Approach in Cancer Immunotherapy. In *Critical Developments in Cancer Immunotherapy* (pp. 391–418). IGI Global., DOI: 10.4018/979-8-3693-3976-3.ch011

Anderson, S. P., Barnett, C. T., & Rusaw, D. F. (2022). Exploring the Perspectives of Prosthetic and Orthotic Users: Past and Present Experiences and Insights for the Future. *Disability and Rehabilitation, 44*(18), 5284–5290. DOI: 10.1080/09638288.2021.1928777 PMID: 34088248

Anikwe, C. V. (2022). Mobile and wearable sensors for data-driven health monitoring system: State-of-the-art and future prospect. *Expert Systems with Applications, 202*, 117362. DOI: 10.1016/j.eswa.2022.117362

Anil Chandra, G., Ananthakumar, B., & Raghavan, R. (2024). *Enhancing Assistive Technologies with Neuromorphic Computing*. IGI Global., DOI: 10.4018/979-8-3693-6303-4.ch009

Anil Chandra, G., Biradar, S., & Raghavan, R. (2024). Neuroscience-Driven Solutions for Speech Impairment: Assistive Technologies for Speech Rehabilitation. In *Advancing Medical Research Through Neuroscience*. IGI Global.

Antonucci, L. A., Taurino, A., Laera, D., Taurisano, P., Losole, J., Lutricuso, S., Abbatantuono, C., Giglio, M., De Caro, M. F., Varrassi, G., & Puntillo, F. (2020). An Ensemble of Psychological and Physical Health Indices Discriminates Between Individuals with Chronic Pain and Healthy Controls with High Reliability: A Machine Learning Study. *Pain and Therapy*, *9*(2), 601–614. DOI: 10.1007/s40122-020-00191-3 PMID: 32880867

Archetti, A., Lomurno, E., Piccinotti, D., & Matteucci, M. (2024). FPBoost: Fully Parametric Gradient Boosting for Survival Analysis. *arXiv preprint arXiv:2409.13363*.

Arjmandnia, F., & Alimohammadi, E. (2024). The value of machine learning technology and artificial intelligence to enhance patient safety in spine surgery: A review. *Patient Safety in Surgery*, *18*(1), 11. DOI: 10.1186/s13037-024-00393-0 PMID: 38528562

Armstrong, J. J., Zhu, M., Hirdes, J. P., & Stolee, P. (2012). K-means cluster analysis of rehabilitation service users in the home health care system of Ontario: Examining the heterogeneity of a complex geriatric population. *Archives of Physical Medicine and Rehabilitation*, *93*(12), 2198–2205. DOI: 10.1016/j.apmr.2012.05.026 PMID: 22705468

Arooj, S., Rehman, S. U., Imran, A., Almuhaimeed, A., Alzahrani, A. K., & Alzahrani, A. (2022). A Deep Convolutional Neural Network for the Early Detection of Heart Disease. *Biomedicines*, *10*(11), 2796. DOI: 10.3390/biomedicines10112796 PMID: 36359317

Arora, A., Alderman, J., Palmer, J., Ganapathi, S., Laws, E., McCradden, M. D., Oakden-Rayner, L., Pfohl, S., Ghassemi, M., McKay, F., Treanor, D., Rostamzadeh, N., Mateen, B. A., Gath, J., Adebajo, A. O., Kuku, S., Matin, R., Heller, K., Sapey, E., . . . Liu, X. (2023). The value of standards for health datasets in artificial intelligence-based applications. In A. Arora, J. Alderman, J. Palmer, S. Ganapathi, E. Laws, M. D. McCradden, L. Oakden-Rayner, S. Pfohl, M. Ghassemi, F. McKay, D. Treanor, N. Rostamzadeh, B. A. Mateen, J. Gath, A. O. Adebajo, S. Kuku, R. Matin, K. Heller, E. Sapey, … X. Liu, Nature Medicine (Vol. 29, Issue 11, p. 2929). Nature Portfolio. DOI: 10.1038/s41591-023-02608-w

Arya, K. N., Pandian, S., Joshi, A. K., Chaudhary, N., Agarwal, G. G., & Ahmed, S. S. (2024). Sensory deficits of the paretic and non-paretic upper limbs relate with the motor recovery of the poststroke subjects. *Topics in Stroke Rehabilitation, 31*(3), 281–292. DOI: 10.1080/10749357.2023.2253629 PMID: 37690032

Asgarabad, M. R. E., Amirbeigiarab, M. M., Ardalani, R., Zarandi, S. F. A., & Nazari, A. J. (2023). Enhancing Patient Movement Rehabilitation: Integration of Intelligent Prosthetic Limbs and the Internet of Things.

Ashton, K. (2009). That 'internet of things' thing. RFID journal, 22(7), 97-114.

Ashwini, A. a. (n.d.). Robust Security and Privacy of Wearable and Implantable Medical Devices: Protecting Lives and Data. In *Security, Privacy, and Trust in WBANs and E-Healthcare* (pp. 126--147). CRC Press.

Astin, J. A., Shapiro, S. L., Eisenberg, D. M., & Forys, K. L. (2003). Mind-body medicine: State of the science, implications for practice. *The Journal of the American Board of Family Practice, 16*(2), 131–147. DOI: 10.3122/jabfm.16.2.131 PMID: 12665179

Atanassova, D. V., Madariaga, V. I., Oosterman, J. M., & Brazil, I. A. (2024). Unpacking the relationship between Big Five personality traits and experimental pain: A systematic review and meta-analysis. *Neuroscience and Biobehavioral Reviews, 163*, 105786. Advance online publication. DOI: 10.1016/j.neubiorev.2024.105786 PMID: 38955000

Atzori, L., Iera, A., & Morabito, G. (2010). The Internet of Things: A survey. In Computer Networks (Vol. 54, Issue 15, pp. 2787–2805). Elsevier BV. DOI: 10.1016/j.comnet.2010.05.010

Azevedo, N., Kehayia, E., Jarema, G., Le Dorze, G., Beaujard, C., & Yvon, M. (2024). How artificial intelligence (AI) is used in aphasia rehabilitation: A scoping review. *Aphasiology, 38*(2), 305–336. DOI: 10.1080/02687038.2023.2189513

Bahdanau, D. (2014). Neural machine translation by jointly learning to align and translate. arXiv preprint arXiv:1409.0473.

Balduzzi, S., Rücker, G., Nikolakopoulou, A., Papakonstantinou, T., Salanti, G., Efthimiou, O., & Schwarzer, G. (2023). netmeta: An R package for network meta-analysis using frequentist methods. *Journal of Statistical Software, 106*(2), 1–40. DOI: 10.18637/jss.v106.i02

Ballor, G. (2022). CE Marking, Business, and European Market Integration. *Business History Review, 96*(1), 77–108. DOI: 10.1017/S0007680521000696

Barakat, A., Munro, G., & Heegaard, A.-M. (2024). Finding new analgesics: Computational pharmacology faces drug discovery challenges. *Biochemical Pharmacology*, *222*, 116091. DOI: 10.1016/j.bcp.2024.116091 PMID: 38412924

Baron, R., Binder, A., & Wasner, G. (2010). Neuropathic pain: Diagnosis, pathophysiological mechanisms, and treatment. *Lancet Neurology*, *9*(8), 807–819. DOI: 10.1016/S1474-4422(10)70143-5 PMID: 20650402

Bengio, Y., Hinton, G. E., Yao, A. C.-C., Song, D., Abbeel, P., Darrell, T., Harari, Y. N., Zhang, Y.-Q., Lan, X., Shalev-Shwartz, S., Hadfield, G. K., Clune, J., Maharaj, T., Hutter, F., Baydin, A. G., McIlraith, S. A., Gao, Q., Acharya, A., Krueger, D., . . . Mindermann, S. (2024). Managing extreme AI risks amid rapid progress. In Y. Bengio, G. E. Hinton, A. C.-C. Yao, D. Song, P. Abbeel, T. Darrell, Y. N. Harari, Y.-Q. Zhang, X. Lan, S. Shalev-Shwartz, G. K. Hadfield, J. Clune, T. Maharaj, F. Hutter, A. G. Baydin, S. A. McIlraith, Q. Gao, A. Acharya, D. Krueger, … S. Mindermann, Science (Vol. 384, Issue 6698, p. 842). American Association for the Advancement of Science. DOI: 10.1126/science.adn0117

Berberoglu, I., Burke, K. L., Cederna, P. S., & Kemp, S. W. P. (2024). Regenerative peripheral nerve interfaces (RPNIs): An overview of innovative surgical approaches. *Plastic and Aesthetic Research*, *11*(0). Advance online publication. DOI: 10.20517/2347-9264.2023.101

Bernasconi, L., Şen, S., Angerame, L., Balyegisawa, A., Hui, D. H. Y., Hotter, M., Hsu, C. Y., Ito, T., Jörger, F., Krassnitzer, W., Phillips, A., Li, R., Stockley, L., Tay, F., Widlund, C. von H., Wan, M., Wong, C., Yau, H., Hiemstra, T. F., . . . Senti, G. (2020). Legal and ethical framework for global health information and biospecimen exchange - an international perspective. In L. Bernasconi, S. Şen, L. Angerame, A. Balyegisawa, D. H. Y. Hui, M. Hotter, C. Y. Hsu, T. Ito, F. Jörger, W. Krassnitzer, A. Phillips, R. Li, L. Stockley, F. Tay, C. von H. Widlund, M. Wan, C. Wong, H. Yau, T. F. Hiemstra, … G. Senti, BMC Medical Ethics (Vol. 21, Issue 1). BioMed Central. DOI: 10.1186/s12910-020-0448-9

Berridge, D. (2019). Active assistive technology for aging in place: Current status and future directions. *The Public Policy and Aging Report*, *29*(1), 27–31.

Bewu, A., & Mbanya, J. C. (2006). Cardiovascular Disease. In Jamison, D. T., Feachem, R. G., & Makgoba, M. W. (Eds.), *Disease and Mortality in Sub-Saharan Africa* (2nd ed.). The International Bank for Reconstruction and Development/The World Bank., https://www.ncbi.nlm.nih.gov/books/NBK2294/

Bica, I., Alaa, A. M., Lambert, C., & Van Der Schaar, M. (2021). From real-world patient data to individualized treatment effects using machine learning: Current and future methods to address underlying challenges. *Clinical Pharmacology and Therapeutics, 109*(1), 87–100. DOI: 10.1002/cpt.1907 PMID: 32449163

Biradar, S., Korrapati, C., Krishna, R. J., & Nanjundeshwara, N. (2025). Spatial Omics and Gene Circuits: The Future in Cancer Biology. *Spatially Variable Genes in Cancer: Development, Progression, and Treatment Response*, 383–408. DOI: 10.4018/979-8-3693-7728-4.ch014

Birch, J., Creel, K., Jha, A. K., & Plutynski, A. (2022). Clinical decisions using AI must consider patient values. In J. Birch, K. Creel, A. K. Jha, & A. Plutynski, Nature Medicine (Vol. 28, Issue 2, p. 229). Nature Portfolio. DOI: 10.1038/s41591-021-01624-y

Bonadonna, R. (2003). Meditation's Impact on Chronic Illness. *Holistic Nursing Practice, 17*(6), 309–319. DOI: 10.1097/00004650-200311000-00006 PMID: 14650573

Bonato, P. (2005). Advances in wearable technology and applications in physical medicine and rehabilitation. *Journal of Neuroengineering and Rehabilitation, 2*(1), 2. DOI: 10.1186/1743-0003-2-2 PMID: 15733322

Bonkhoff, A. K., & Grefkes, C. (2022). Precision medicine in stroke: Towards personalized outcome predictions using artificial intelligence. *Brain, 145*(2), 457–475. DOI: 10.1093/brain/awab439 PMID: 34918041

Botsis, M.. (2018). Challenges in telemedicine adoption among elderly populations: A systematic review. *Telemedicine Journal and e-Health, 24*(7), 568–576.

Boukhennoufa, I., Zhai, X., Utti, V., Jackson, J., & McDonald-Maier, K. D. (2022). Wearable sensors and machine learning in post-stroke rehabilitation assessment: A systematic review. *Biomedical Signal Processing and Control, 71*, 103197. DOI: 10.1016/j.bspc.2021.103197

Braun, R. G., & Wittenberg, G. F. (2021, April). Motor recovery: How rehabilitation techniques and technologies can enhance recovery and neuroplasticity. [). Thieme Medical Publishers, Inc.]. *Seminars in Neurology, 41*(02), 167–176. DOI: 10.1055/s-0041-1725138 PMID: 33663001

Brink, K. J., Likens, A., & Stergiou, N. (2023). The Evolution of Scholarship of Biomechanics and Motor Control Within the Academy: The Past, the Present, and the Future. *Kinesiology Review (Champaign, Ill.), 13*(1), 42–54. DOI: 10.1123/kr.2023-0054

Brown, V. M., Zhu, L., Solway, A., Wang, J. M., McCurry, K. L., King-Casas, B., & Chiu, P. H. (2021). Reinforcement Learning Disruptions in Individuals with Depression and Sensitivity to Symptom Change Following Cognitive Behavioral Therapy. *JAMA Psychiatry, 78*(10), 1113–1122. DOI: 10.1001/jamapsychiatry.2021.1844 PMID: 34319349

Brunetti, A., Buongiorno, D., Altini, N., & Bevilacqua, V. (2023). Enabling technologies for optimized diagnosis, therapy, and rehabilitation: Obtained results and future works. In Italian Forum of Ambient Assisted Living (pp. 206–223). Springer.

Buckingham, A., & Richardson, E. J. (2021). The Relationship Between Psychological Resilience and Pain Threshold and Tolerance: Optimism and Grit as Moderators. *Journal of Clinical Psychology in Medical Settings, 28*(3), 518–528. DOI: 10.1007/s10880-020-09731-7 PMID: 32564216

Bulling, A., Blanke, U., & Schiele, B. (2014). A tutorial on human activity recognition using body-worn inertial sensors. *ACM Computing Surveys, 46*(3), 1–33. DOI: 10.1145/2499621

Buscarini, L., Romano, P., Cocco, E. S., Damiani, C., Pournajaf, S., Franceschini, M., & Infarinato, F. (2024). Enhancing patient rehabilitation outcomes: Artificial intelligence-driven predictive modeling for home discharge in neurological and orthopedic conditions.

Campagnini, S., Arienti, C., Patrini, M., Liuzzi, P., Mannini, A., & Carrozza, M. C. (2022). Machine learning methods for functional recovery prediction and prognosis in post-stroke rehabilitation: A systematic review. *Journal of Neuroengineering and Rehabilitation, 19*(1), 54. DOI: 10.1186/s12984-022-01032-4 PMID: 35659246

Canali, S., Schiaffonati, V., & Aliverti, A. (2022). Challenges and recommendations for wearable devices in digital health: Data quality, interoperability, health equity, fairness. *PLOS Digital Health, 1*(10), 0000104. DOI: 10.1371/journal.pdig.0000104 PMID: 36812619

Cantone, M. (2024). Clinical Updates and Perspectives on Transcranial Magnetic Stimulation (TMS). *Journal of Clinical Medicine, 13*(13), 3794. DOI: 10.3390/jcm13133794 PMID: 38999361

Capodieci, A., Graziani, D., Scali, V., Giaccherini, S., Luccherino, L., & Pecini, C. (2023). Telerehabilitation Pathways in Specific Learning Disorders: Improving Reading and Writing. *Brain Sciences, 13*(3), 479. DOI: 10.3390/brainsci13030479 PMID: 36979289

Carter, J., & James, R. (2023). Evaluating AI Effectiveness in Assistive Technologies. *Healthcare Engineering Advances*, *9*(6), 267–289.

Carver, C. S., Scheier, M. F., & Segerstrom, S. C. (2010). Optimism. *Clinical Psychology Review*, *30*(7), 879–889. DOI: 10.1016/j.cpr.2010.01.006 PMID: 20170998

Cashaback, J. G. A., Allen, J. L., Chou, A. H.-Y., Lin, D. J., Price, M. A., Secerovic, N. K., Song, S., Zhang, H., & Miller, H. L. (2024). NSF DARE—transforming modeling in neurorehabilitation: A patient-in-the-loop framework. *Journal of Neuroengineering and Rehabilitation*, *21*(1), 23. DOI: 10.1186/s12984-024-01318-9 PMID: 38347597

Chae, S. H., Kim, Y., Lee, K. S., & Park, H. S. (2020). Development and clinical evaluation of a web-based upper limb home rehabilitation system using a smartwatch and machine learning model for chronic stroke survivors: Prospective comparative study. *JMIR mHealth and uHealth*, *8*(7), e17216. DOI: 10.2196/17216 PMID: 32480361

Chandra, G. A., Ananthakumar, B., & Raghavan, R. (2025). Enhancing Assistive Technologies With Neuromorphic Computing. In Revolutionizing AI with Brain-Inspired Technology: Neuromorphic Computing (pp. 207-232). IGI Global Scientific Publishing.

Chandra, G. V. S. A., Biradar, S., & Raghavan, R. (2025). Recent Trends in Soft Robotics for Assistive Technologies. *Assistive Technology Solutions for Aging Adults and Individuals With Disabilities*, 119–144. DOI: 10.4018/979-8-3693-6308-9.ch006

Chan, M., Estève, D., Fourniols, J.-Y., Escriba, C., & Campo, E. (2012). Smart wearable systems: Current status and future challenges. *Artificial Intelligence in Medicine*, *56*(3), 137–156. DOI: 10.1016/j.artmed.2012.09.003 PMID: 23122689

Chaves, J. F., & Brown, J. M. (1987). Spontaneous cognitive strategies for the control of clinical pain and stress. *Journal of Behavioral Medicine*, *10*(3), 263–276. DOI: 10.1007/BF00846540 PMID: 3612783

Chekroud, A. M., Bondar, J., Delgadillo, J., Doherty, G., Wasil, A., Fokkema, M., Cohen, Z., Belgrave, D., DeRubeis, R., Iniesta, R., Dwyer, D., & Choi, K. (2021). The promise of machine learning in predicting treatment outcomes in psychiatry. *World Psychiatry; Official Journal of the World Psychiatric Association (WPA)*, *20*(2), 154–170. DOI: 10.1002/wps.20882 PMID: 34002503

Chen, G., Chan, C. K., Guo, Z., & Yu, H. (2013). A review of lower extremity assistive robotic exoskeletons in rehabilitation therapy. Critical Reviews™ in Biomedical Engineering, 41(4-5).

Chen, Y., & Zimmerman, G. (2007). "Enhancing independent living for older adults through smart home technology." IEEE Pervasive Computing. IEEE Xplore: https://ieeexplore.ieee.org/document/4141052

Chen, B., Chen, C., Hu, J., Sayeed, Z., Qi, J., Darwiche, H. F., & Palacio-Lascano, C. (2022). Computer vision and machine learning-based gait pattern recognition for flat fall prediction. *Sensors (Basel)*, *22*(20), 7960.

Chen, C., & Kia, S. S. (2024). OptiTrack-Aided Supervised Learning for Neural Network Based Ultra-Wideband Ranging Bias Correction. *IEEE Sensors Journal*, *24*(6), 8484–8492. DOI: 10.1109/JSEN.2024.3360187

Chen, L., & Kotz, D. (2017). Data privacy in health monitoring technologies. *IEEE Security and Privacy*, *15*(4), 42–49. PMID: 29333107

Chen, L., Li, J., & Zhou, H. (2021). Advancing Prosthetic Design Using Machine Learning Algorithms. *The International Journal of Robotics Research*, *40*(7), 987–1005.

Chen, L., Lin, L., Weizhou, J., Lin, S., & Lin, W. (2020). "The Research of Cognitive Rehabilitation Training System for ADHD Children." In *Proceedings of the 2020 11th International Conference on E-Education, E-Business, E-Management, and E-Learning*, 422–25. DOI: 10.1145/3377571.3377617

Chen, M., Ma, Y., Song, J., Lai, C. F., & Hu, B. (2016). Smart clothing: Connecting human with clouds and big data for sustainable health monitoring. *Mobile Networks and Applications*, *21*(5), 825–845. DOI: 10.1007/s11036-016-0745-1

Chohlas-Wood, A., Coots, M., Goel, S., & Nyarko, J. (2023). Designing equitable algorithms. In A. Chohlas-Wood, M. Coots, S. Goel, & J. Nyarko, Nature Computational Science (Vol. 3, Issue 7, p. 601). Nature Portfolio. DOI: 10.1038/s43588-023-00485-4

Chong, Y.-W. Y., Ismail, W., Ko, K., & Lee, C.-Y. (2019). Energy harvesting for wearable devices: A review. *IEEE Sensors Journal*, *19*(20), 9047–9062. DOI: 10.1109/JSEN.2019.2925638

Choo, Y. J., & Chang, M. C. (2023). Use of Machine Learning in the Field of Prosthetics and Orthotics: A Systematic Narrative Review. *Prosthetics and Orthotics International*, *47*(3), 226–240. DOI: 10.1097/PXR.0000000000000199 PMID: 36811961

Chorowski, J. K., Bahdanau, D., Serdyuk, D., Cho, K., & Bengio, Y. (2015). Attention-based models for speech recognition. *Advances in Neural Information Processing Systems*, •••, 28.

Chui, K. K., Jorge, M., Yen, S. C., & Lusardi, M. M. (2019). *Orthotics and Prosthetics in Rehabilitation E-Book: Orthotics and Prosthetics in Rehabilitation E-Book*. Elsevier Health Sciences.

Clark, B., & Johnson, T. (2021). Usability Studies for AI-Powered Assistive Devices. *Journal of Assistive Technology Studies*, *9*(5), 212–230.

Colloca, L., & Miller, F. G. (2011). The nocebo effect and its relevance for clinical practice. *Psychosomatic Medicine*, *73*(7), 598–603. DOI: 10.1097/PSY.0b013e3182294a50 PMID: 21862825

Cook, A. M., & Polgar, J. M. (2014). *Assistive Technologies: Principles and Practice* (4th ed.). Elsevier.

Correia, G., Crosse, M. J., & Valdes, A. L. (2024). Brain Wearables: Validation Toolkit for Ear-Level EEG Sensors. *Sensors (Basel)*, *24*(4), 1226. DOI: 10.3390/s24041226 PMID: 38400384

Cotton, R., Seamon, B. A., Segal, R., Davis, R. D., Sahu, A., McLeod, M. M., Celnik, P., & Ramey, S. L. (2024). A Causal Framework for Precision Rehabilitation. In R. Cotton, B. A. Seamon, R. Segal, R. D. Davis, A. Sahu, M. M. McLeod, P. Celnik, & S. L. Ramey, arXiv (Cornell University). Cornell University. https://doi.org//arxiv.2411.03919DOI: 10.48550

Covington, N. V., & Duff, M. C. (2021). Heterogeneity is a hallmark of traumatic brain injury, not a limitation: A new perspective on study design in rehabilitation research. *American Journal of Speech-Language Pathology*, *30*(2S), 974–985. DOI: 10.1044/2020_AJSLP-20-00081 PMID: 33556261

Dalla Gasperina, S., Ferrari, F., Gandolla, M., Pedrocchi, A., & Ambrosini, E. (2024). Hybrid Cooperative Control of Functional Electrical Stimulation and Robot Assistance for Upper Extremity Rehabilitation. *IEEE Transactions on Biomedical Engineering*, *71*(9), 2642–2650. DOI: 10.1109/TBME.2024.3384939 PMID: 39167498

Damaševičius, R., Jagatheesaperumal, S. K., Kandala, R. N., Hussain, S., Alizadehsani, R., & Gorriz, J. M. (2024). Deep learning for personalized health monitoring and prediction: A review. *Computational Intelligence*, *40*(3), e12682. DOI: 10.1111/coin.12682

Dankwa, S., & Zheng, W. (2019). "Twin-Delayed Ddpg: A Deep Reinforcement Learning Technique to Model a Continuous Movement of an Intelligent Robot Agent." In *Proceedings of the 3rd International Conference on Vision, Image and Signal Processing*, 1–5. DOI: 10.1145/3387168.3387199

Das, A., Day, T. W., Kulkarni, V., Buchanan, A., Cottrell, K., John, N. W., & Chatterjee, K. (2022). Towards intelligent extended reality in stroke rehabilitation: Application of machine learning and artificial intelligence in rehabilitation. In *Augmenting Neurological Disorder Prediction and Rehabilitation Using Artificial Intelligence* (pp. 309–329). Elsevier. DOI: 10.1016/B978-0-323-90037-9.00006-0

Davis, A. A., & Patel, V. G. (2019). The Role of PD-L1 Expression as a Predictive Biomarker: An Analysis of All US Food and Drug Administration (FDA) Approvals of Immune Checkpoint Inhibitors. *Journal for Immunotherapy of Cancer*, *7*(1), 278. DOI: 10.1186/s40425-019-0768-9 PMID: 31655605

Davis, N. (2019). Voice-assisted technology: Empowering older adults. *Technol. & Aging*, *11*(2), 102–110.

de Filippis, R., & Al Foysal, A. (2024). Harnessing the power of artificial intelligence in neuromuscular disease rehabilitation: A comprehensive review and algorithmic approach. *Advances in Bioscience and Biotechnology*, *15*(5), 289–309. DOI: 10.4236/abb.2024.155018

de Vries, E., Houterman, S., Janssen-Heijnen, M. L. G., Nijsten, T., van de Schans, S. A. M., Eggermont, A. M. M., & Coebergh, J. W. W. (2007). Up-to-date survival estimates and historical trends of cutaneous malignant melanoma in the south-east of The Netherlands. *Annals of Oncology : Official Journal of the European Society for Medical Oncology*, *18*(6), 1110–1116. DOI: 10.1093/annonc/mdm087 PMID: 17434898

Deep, S. a. (2019). A survey on anomalous behavior detection for elderly care using dense-sensing networks. *IEEE Communications Surveys \& Tutorials*, 352--370.

Deng, W. Y., Papavasileiou, I., Qiao, Z., Zhang, W., Lam, K.-Y., & Han, S. (2018). Advances in automation technologies for lower extremity neurorehabilitation: A review and future challenges. *IEEE Reviews in Biomedical Engineering*, *11*, 289–305. DOI: 10.1109/RBME.2018.2830805 PMID: 29994006

Deshmukh, S., Khatik, V., & Saxena, A. (2023). Robust Fusion Model for Handling EMG and Computer Vision Data in Prosthetic Hand Control. *IEEE Sensors Letters*, *7*(9), 1–4. DOI: 10.1109/LSENS.2023.3301837

Diallo, A., Carlos-Bolumbu, M., Cervantes-Gonzalez, M., Wozniak, V., Diallo, M. H., Diallo, B. D., Delamou, A., & Galtier, F. (2021). Immunogenicity and safety of Ebola virus vaccines in healthy adults: A systematic review and network meta-analysis. *Human Vaccines & Immunotherapeutics*, *17*(10), 3771–3783. DOI: 10.1080/21645515.2021.1932214 PMID: 34270366

Dias, D., & Paulo Silva Cunha, J. (2018). Wearable health devices—Vital sign monitoring, systems and technologies. *Sensors (Basel)*, *18*(8), 2414. DOI: 10.3390/s18082414 PMID: 30044415

Dıcuonzo, G., Galeone, G., Shini, M., & Massari, A. (2022). Towards the Use of Big Data in Healthcare: A Literature Review [Review of Towards the Use of Big Data in Healthcare: A Literature Review]. Healthcare, 10(7), 1232. Multidisciplinary Digital Publishing Institute. DOI: 10.3390/healthcare10071232

Dil, A. S., & Eikelenboom, A. (2023). Whisking the Digital Health Compliance. In *Pharmaceutical Care in Digital Revolution* (pp. 261–277). Elsevier. DOI: 10.1016/B978-0-443-13360-2.00010-1

Dillworth, T., & Jensen, M. P. (2010). The Role of Suggestions in Hypnosis for Chronic Pain: A Review of the Literature. *The Open Pain Journal*, *3*(1), 39–51. DOI: 10.2174/1876386301003010039 PMID: 21686037

Dobkin, B. H., & Dorsch, A. (2011). The promise of mHealth: Daily activity monitoring and outcome assessments by wearable sensors. *Neurorehabilitation and Neural Repair*, *25*(9), 788–798. DOI: 10.1177/1545968311425908 PMID: 21989632

Donati, E., & Valle, G. (2024). Neuromorphic hardware for somatosensory neuroprostheses. *Nature Communications*, *15*(1), 556. DOI: 10.1038/s41467-024-44723-3 PMID: 38228580

Douthwaite, A. H. (1962). Proctalgia Fugax. *British Medical Journal*, *2*(5298), 164–165. DOI: 10.1136/bmj.2.5298.164 PMID: 13887589

DR, C. (1972). Regression models and life tables. *Journal of the Royal Statistical Society. Series A (General)*, *34*, 248–275.

Dritsas, E., & Trigka, M. (2023). Supervised Machine Learning Models for Liver Disease Risk Prediction. *Computers*, *12*(1), 19. DOI: 10.3390/computers12010019

Dua, M., Bhagat, B., Dua, S., & Chakravarty, N. (2024). A review on Gujarati language based automatic speech recognition (ASR) systems. *International Journal of Speech Technology*, *27*(1), 133–156. DOI: 10.1007/s10772-024-10087-8

Duan, X., Wang, P., He, L., He, Z., Wang, S., Yang, F., Gao, C., Ren, W., Lin, J., Chen, T., Xu, C., Li, J., & Wu, A. (2024). Peptide-Functionalized Inorganic Oxide Nanomaterials for Solid Cancer Imaging and Therapy. *Advanced Materials*, *2311548*(37), 2311548. Advance online publication. DOI: 10.1002/adma.202311548 PMID: 38333964

Dubreuil, D. L., & Kohn, P. M. (1986). Reactivity and response to pain. *Personality and Individual Differences*, *7*(6), 907–909. DOI: 10.1016/0191-8869(86)90093-0

Duckworth, A. (2016). *Grit: The Power of Passion and Perseverance*. Simon & Schuster.

Duckworth, A. L., Peterson, C., Matthews, M. D., & Kelly, D. R. (2007). Grit: Perseverance and passion for long-term goals. *Journal of Personality and Social Psychology*, *9*(6), 1087–1101. DOI: 10.1037/0022-3514.92.6.1087 PMID: 17547490

Edwards, R. R., & Fillingim, R. B. (2007). Self-reported pain sensitivity: Lack of correlation with pain threshold and tolerance. *European Journal of Pain (London, England)*, *11*(5), 594–598. DOI: 10.1016/j.ejpain.2006.09.008 PMID: 17118681

Ehteshami Bejnordi, B., ... (2017). "Diagnostic assessment of deep learning algorithms for detection of breast cancer." JAMA. JAMA Network: https://jamanetwork.com/journals/jama/fullarticle/2665774

Elias, B. L., Polancich, S., Jones, C., & Colvin, S. (2015). Evolving the PICOT method for the digital age: The PICOT-D. *The Journal of Nursing Education*, *54*(10), 594–599. DOI: 10.3928/01484834-20150916-09 PMID: 26431521

Ellis, A. (1962). *Reason and emotion in psychotherapy*. Lyle Stuart.

Engel, G. L. (1977). The need for a new medical model: A challenge for biomedicine. *Science*, *196*(4286), 129–136. DOI: 10.1126/science.847460 PMID: 847460

Esfahlani, S. S., Shirvani, H., Butt, J., Mirzaee, I., & Esfahlani, K. S. (2022). Machine learning role in clinical decision-making: Neuro-rehabilitation video game. *Expert Systems with Applications*, *201*, 117165. DOI: 10.1016/j.eswa.2022.117165

Evans, A., & Davis, R. (2022). NLP for Gesture-Based Communication Systems. *Journal of Multimodal Interaction*, *8*(4), 175–200.

Farrehi, C., Pazzi, C., Capron, M., Anderson, K. D., Richardson, B., & Stillman, M. (2020). How individuals with spinal cord injury in the United States access and assess information about experimental therapies and clinical trials: results of a clinical survey. In C. Farrehi, C. Pazzi, M. Capron, K. D. Anderson, B. Richardson, & M. Stillman, Spinal Cord Series and Cases (Vol. 6, Issue 1). Springer Nature. DOI: 10.1038/s41394-020-00354-6

Fazio, R. D., Giannoccaro, N. I., Carrasco, M., Velázquez, R., & Visconti, P. (2021). Wearable devices and IoT applications for symptom detection, infection tracking, and diffusion containment of the COVID-19 pandemic: a survey. In R. D. Fazio, N. I. Giannoccaro, M. Carrasco, R. Velázquez, & P. Visconti, Frontiers of Information Technology & Electronic Engineering (Vol. 22, Issue 11, p. 1413). Springer Science+Business Media. DOI: 10.1631/FITEE.2100085

Feigin, V. L. (2021). Burden of neurological disorders across the US from 1990-2017: A global burden of disease study. *JAMA Neurology*, •••, 165–176. PMID: 33136137

Feil-Seifer, D., & Mataric, M. J. (2011). "Socially assistive robotics." IEEE Transactions on Robotics. IEEE Xplore: https://ieeexplore.ieee.org/document/5740167

Felius, R., Punt, M., Geerars, M., Wouda, N., Rutgers, R., Bruijn, S., David, S., & van Dieën, J. (2024). Exploring Unsupervised Feature Extraction of IMU-Based Gait Data in Stroke Rehabilitation Using a Variational Autoencoder. *PLoS One*, *19*(10), e0304558. DOI: 10.1371/journal.pone.0304558 PMID: 39365773

Fenton, B. W., Shih, E., & Zoltan, J. (2015). The neurobiology of pain perception in normal and persistent pain. *Pain Management*, *5*(4), 297–317. DOI: 10.2217/pmt.15.27 PMID: 26088531

Ferreira, J. J., Fernandes, C. I., Rammal, H. G., & Veiga, P. M. (2021). Wearable technology and consumer interaction: A systematic review and research agenda. *Computers in Human Behavior*, *118*, 106710. DOI: 10.1016/j.chb.2021.106710

Filakova, K., Janikova, A., Felsoci, M., Dosbaba, F., Jing, J. S., Pepera, G., & Batalik, L. (2023). Home-Based Cardio-Oncology Rehabilitation Using a Telerehabilitation Platform in Hematological Cancer Survivors: A Feasibility Study. *BMC Sports Science, Medicine and Rehabilitation*, *15*(1), 38. DOI: 10.1186/s13102-023-00650-2 PMID: 36959613

Fillingim, R. B. (2017, April). Individual differences in pain: Understanding the mosaic that makes pain personal. *Pain*, *158*(1), S11–S18. DOI: 10.1097/j.pain.0000000000000775 PMID: 27902569

Fong, J., Ocampo, R., Gross, D. P., & Tavakoli, M. (2020). Intelligent robotics incorporating machine learning algorithms for improving functional capacity evaluation and occupational rehabilitation. *Journal of Occupational Rehabilitation*, *30*(3), 362–370. DOI: 10.1007/s10926-020-09888-w PMID: 32253595

Forne, C., Cambray, S., Bermudez-Lopez, M., Fernandez, E., Bozic, M., & Valdivielso, J. M. (2020). Machine learning analysis of serum biomarkers for cardiovascular risk assessment in chronic kidney disease. *Clinical Kidney Journal, 13*(4), 631–639. PMID: 32905292

Forsyth, R., Vu, T., Salorio, C., Christensen, J., & Holford, N. (2010). Efficient rehabilitation trial designs using disease progress modeling: A pediatric traumatic brain injury example. *Neurorehabilitation and Neural Repair, 24*(3), 225–234. DOI: 10.1177/1545968309354534 PMID: 19959829

Frank, E. a. (2024). Data preprocessing techniques for NLP in BI.

Gahlot, D. S., Krieder, S., & Raicu, I. Accelerating Simulation Codes through the GeMTC Framework.

Gao, W., Emaminejad, S., Nyein, H. Y. Y., Challa, S., Chen, K., Peck, A., Fahad, H. M., Ota, H., Shiraki, H., Kiriya, D., Lien, D.-H., Brooks, G. A., Davis, R. W., & Javey, A. (2016). Fully integrated wearable sensor arrays for multiplexed in situ perspiration analysis. *Nature, 529*(7587), 509–514. DOI: 10.1038/nature16521 PMID: 26819044

Garg, R., Sharma, P., & Singh, A. (2022). AI-Driven Solutions for Assistive Technologies: Trends and Challenges. *Journal of Artificial Intelligence in Healthcare, 15*(3), 123–134.

Gariya, N., Kumar, S., Shaikh, A., Prasad, B., & Nautiyal, H. (2024). A review on soft pneumatic actuators with integrated or embedded soft sensors. *Sensors and Actuators. A, Physical, 372*, 115364. DOI: 10.1016/j.sna.2024.115364

Geetha, C., & Arunachalam, Ar. (2021). Evaluation based Approaches for Liver Disease Prediction using Machine Learning Algorithms. *2021 International Conference on Computer Communication and Informatics (ICCCI)*, 1–4. DOI: 10.1109/ICCCI50826.2021.9402463

Gerke, S., Minssen, T., & Cohen, G. (2020). Ethical and legal challenges of artificial intelligence-driven healthcare. In Gerke, S., Minssen, T., & Cohen, G. (Eds.), *Elsevier eBooks* (p. 295). Elsevier BV., DOI: 10.1016/B978-0-12-818438-7.00012-5

Ghahramani, Z. (2015). "Probabilistic machine learning and artificial intelligence." Nature. Nature: https://www.nature.com/articles/nature14541

Ghazal, T. M., Rehman, A. U., Saleem, M., Ahmad, M., Ahmad, S., & Mehmood, F. (2022). Intelligent Model to Predict Early Liver Disease using Machine Learning Technique. *2022 International Conference on Business Analytics for Technology and Security (ICBATS)*, 1–5. DOI: 10.1109/ICBATS54253.2022.9758929

Ghosh, A., Chatterjee, S., De, S., & Maji, A. K. (2022, July). Towards data-driven cognitive rehabilitation for speech disorder in hybrid sensor architecture. In *2022 IEEE International Conference on Electronics, Computing and Communication Technologies (CONECCT)* (pp. 1-6). IEEE.

Goldberg, C. B., Adams, L., Blumenthal, D., Brennan, P. F., Brown, N., Butte, A. J., Cheatham, M., deBronkart, D., Dixon, J., Drazen, J. M., Evans, B. J., Hoffman, S. M., Holmes, C., Lee, P., Manrai, A. K., Omenn, G. S., Perlin, J. B., Ramoni, R., Sapiro, G., . . . Zhao, J. (2024). To do no harm — and the most good — with AI in health care. In C. B. Goldberg, L. Adams, D. Blumenthal, P. F. Brennan, N. Brown, A. J. Butte, M. Cheatham, D. deBronkart, J. Dixon, J. M. Drazen, B. J. Evans, S. M. Hoffman, C. Holmes, P. Lee, A. K. Manrai, G. S. Omenn, J. B. Perlin, R. Ramoni, G. Sapiro, … J. Zhao, Nature Medicine (Vol. 30, Issue 3, p. 623). Nature Portfolio. DOI: 10.1038/s41591-024-02853-7

González-González, M. A., Conde, S. V., Latorre, R., Thébault, S. C., Pratelli, M., Spitzer, N. C., Verkhratsky, A., Tremblay, M.-È., Akcora, C. G., Hernández-Reynoso, A. G., Ecker, M., Coates, J., Vincent, K. L., & Ma, B. (2024). Bioelectronic Medicine: A multidisciplinary roadmap from biophysics to precision therapies. *Frontiers in Integrative Neuroscience*, *18*, 1321872. DOI: 10.3389/fnint.2024.1321872 PMID: 38440417

Goodfellow, I., Bengio, Y., & Courville, A. (2016). Deep Learning. MIT Press. Full Text: https://www.deeplearningbook.org/. PDF: https://github.com/janishar/mit-deep-learning-book-pdf

Grab, J. G.-C., Zewdie, E., Carlson, H. L., Kuo, H.-C., Ciechanski, P., Hodge, J., Giuffre, A., & Kirton, A. (2018). Robotic TMS mapping of motor cortex in the developing brain. *Journal of Neuroscience Methods*, *309*, 41–54. DOI: 10.1016/j.jneumeth.2018.08.007 PMID: 30121208

Grandinetti, J., Gao, Y., Gonzalez, Y., Deng, J., Shen, C., & Jia, X. (2022). MR image reconstruction from undersampled data for image-guided radiation therapy using a patient-specific deep manifold image prior. In J. Grandinetti, Y. Gao, Y. Gonzalez, J. Deng, C. Shen, & X. Jia, Frontiers in Oncology (Vol. 12). Frontiers Media. DOI: 10.3389/fonc.2022.1013783

Gravina, R., Alinia, P., Ghasemzadeh, H., & Fortino, G. (2017). Multi-sensor fusion in body sensor networks: State-of-the-art and research challenges. *Information Fusion*, *35*, 68–80. DOI: 10.1016/j.inffus.2016.09.005

Green, M., & Peterson, J. (2023). Future Trends in Assistive AI Technologies. *AI and Accessibility Studies*, *16*(2), 155–178.

Green, S. F. (2020). Assistive technology and its impact on social engagement for elderly people. *Journal of Aging Research, 2020*(1), 4838409.

Grossman, P., Niemann, L., Schmidt, S., & Walach, H. (2004). Mindfulness-based stress reduction and health benefits. A meta-analysis. *Journal of Psychosomatic Research, 57*(1), 35–43. DOI: 10.1016/S0022-3999(03)00573-7 PMID: 15256293

Grouper, H., Eisenburg, E., & Pud, D. (2021). More Insight on the Role of Personality Traits and Sensitivity to Experimental Pain. *Journal of Pain Research, 14*, 1837–1844. DOI: 10.2147/JPR.S309729 PMID: 34168491

Gual, N., García-Salmones, M., Brítez, L., Crespo, N., Udina, C., Pérez, L. M., & Inzitari, M. (2020). The Role of Physical Exercise and Rehabilitation in Delirium. *European Geriatric Medicine, 11*(1), 83–93. DOI: 10.1007/s41999-020-00290-6 PMID: 32297245

Güler, R. A., Neverova, N., & Kokkinos, I. (2018). “Densepose: Dense Human Pose Estimation in the Wild.” In *Proceedings of the IEEE Conference on Computer Vision and Pattern Recognition*, 7297–7306. DOI: 10.1109/CVPR.2018.00762

Guo, Y., Sun, L., Zhong, W., Zhang, N., Zhao, Z., & Tian, W. (2024). Artificial intelligence-assisted repair of peripheral nerve injury: A new research hotspot and associated challenges. *Neural Regeneration Research, 19*(3), 663–670. DOI: 10.4103/1673-5374.380909 PMID: 37721299

Gupta, R. (2024). AI-based technologies, challenges, and solutions for neurorehabilitation: A systematic mapping. In *Computational Intelligence and Deep Learning Methods for Neuro-rehabilitation Applications* (pp. 1–25). Elsevier. DOI: 10.1016/B978-0-443-13772-3.00014-5

Gutman, B. H., Shmilovitch, A.-H., Aran, D., & Shelly, S. (2024). Twenty-Five Years of AI in Neurology: The Journey of Predictive Medicine and Biological Breakthroughs. *JMIR Neurotechnology, 3*, 59556. DOI: 10.2196/59556

Guyot, P., Ades, A. E., Ouwens, M. J., & Welton, N. J. (2012). Enhanced secondary analysis of survival data: Reconstructing the data from published Kaplan-Meier survival curves. *BMC Medical Research Methodology, 12*(1), 1–13. DOI: 10.1186/1471-2288-12-9 PMID: 22297116

GVS, A. C., Biradar, S., & Raghavan, R. (2025). Neuroscience-Driven Solutions for Speech Impairment: Assistive Technologies for Speech Rehabilitation. Advancing Medical Research Through Neuroscience, 119–146. https://doi.org/DOI: 10.4018/979-8-3693-5464-3.ch006

Haarnoja, T., Zhou, A., Hartikainen, K., Tucker, G., Ha, S., Tan, J., Kumar, V., Zhu, H., Gupta, A., & Abbeel, P. (2018). "Soft Actor-Critic Algorithms and Applications." *ArXiv Preprint ArXiv:1812.05905*.

Haghi, M., Thurow, K., & Stoll, R. (2017). Wearable devices in medical internet of things: Scientific research and commercially available devices. *Healthcare Informatics Research*, *23*(1), 4–15. DOI: 10.4258/hir.2017.23.1.4 PMID: 28261526

Ha, J. H., Kang, S., & Lee, S. S. (2020). AI-driven personalized assistive technology for senior citizens: A future outlook. *IEEE Access : Practical Innovations, Open Solutions*, *8*, 212675–212685.

Hall, S., & Lee, W. (2022). Leveraging AI for Communication Aids. *Journal of AI Research in Healthcare*, *22*(1), 91–109.

Hamam, H. (2024). Revolutionizing Neurosurgery and Neurology: The transformative impact of artificial intelligence in healthcare. *Computers and Artificial Intelligence*, *2*(1), 416. DOI: 10.59400/cai.v2i1.416

Hansen, M. S., Horjales-Araujo, E., & Dahl, J. B. (2015). Associations between psychological variables and pain in experimental pain models. A systematic review. *Acta Anaesthesiologica Scandinavica*, *59*(9), 1094–1102. DOI: 10.1111/aas.12555 PMID: 26088747

Han, X., Zhou, X., Tan, B., Jiao, L., & Zhang, R. (2023). Ai-Based next-Generation Sensors for Enhanced Rehabilitation Monitoring and Analysis. *Measurement*, *223*, 113758. DOI: 10.1016/j.measurement.2023.113758

Hao, D., Li, Q., Feng, Q. X., Qi, L., Liu, X. S., Arefan, D., Zhang, Y.-D., & Wu, S. (2022). SurvivalCNN: A deep learning-based method for gastric cancer survival prediction using radiological imaging data and clinicopathological variables. *Artificial Intelligence in Medicine*, *134*, 102424. DOI: 10.1016/j.artmed.2022.102424 PMID: 36462894

Harris, J. E., Eng, J. J., Miller, W. C., & Dawson, A. S. (2009). A self-administered Graded Repetitive Arm Supplementary Program (GRASP) improves arm function during inpatient stroke rehabilitation: A multi-site randomized controlled trial. *Stroke*, *40*(6), 2123–2128. DOI: 10.1161/STROKEAHA.108.544585 PMID: 19359633

Harrison, M., & Zhang, J. (2023). Overcoming Limitations in NLP Assistive Devices. *Journal of Applied Machine Learning*, *14*(7), 80–100.

Hartatik, H., Tamam, M. B., & Setyanto, A. (2020). Prediction for Diagnosing Liver Disease in Patients using KNN and Naïve Bayes Algorithms. *2020 2nd International Conference on Cybernetics and Intelligent System (ICORIS)*, 1–5. DOI: 10.1109/ICORIS50180.2020.9320797

Heer, J., & Shneiderman, B. (2012). "Interactive dynamics for visual analysis." Communications of the ACM. ACM Digital Library: https://dl.acm.org/doi/10.1145/2063176.2063196

He, J., Guo, Z., Shao, Z., Zhao, J., & Dan, G. (2020). An LSTM-based prediction method for lower limb intention perception by integrative analysis of Kinect visual signal. [Wiley Online Library.]. *Journal of Healthcare Engineering*, *2020*(1), 8024789. DOI: 10.1155/2020/8024789 PMID: 32774824

Hendi, A. M., Hossain, M. A., Majrashi, N. A., Limkar, S., Elamin, B. M., & Rahman, M. (2024). Adaptive Method for Exploring Deep Learning Techniques for Subtyping and Prediction of Liver Disease. *Applied Sciences (Basel, Switzerland)*, *14*(4), 1488. DOI: 10.3390/app14041488

Hickman, J. M., ... (2017). "AI-powered assistive communication tools for ALS patients." ACM Transactions on Accessible Computing. ACM Digital Library: https://dl.acm.org/doi/10.1145/3132040

Hicks, J. L., Althoff, T., Kuhar, P., Bostjancic, B., King, A. C., Leskovec, J., & Delp, S. L. (2019). Best practices for analyzing large-scale health data from wearables and smartphone apps. *NPJ Digital Medicine*, *2*(1), 45. DOI: 10.1038/s41746-019-0121-1 PMID: 31304391

Hira, R. (2024). Closed-loop experiments and brain machine interfaces with multiphoton microscopy. *Neurophotonics*, *11*(3), 033405. DOI: 10.1117/1.NPh.11.3.033405 PMID: 38375331

Hochberg, L. R., ... (2012). "Reach and grasp by people with tetraplegia using a neurally controlled robotic arm." Nature. PDF: https://www.nature.com/articles/nature11076.pdf

Honi, D. G., & Szathmary, L. (2024). A one-dimensional convolutional neural network-based deep learning approach for predicting cardiovascular diseases. *Informatics in Medicine Unlocked*, *49*, 101535. DOI: 10.1016/j.imu.2024.101535

Hou, Y. a. (2024). Research on innovative design of intelligent wearable products based on human machine engineering and bionics. *Molecular \& Cellular Biomechanics*, 461--461.

Huang, J., Zhu, Z., & Huang, G. (2019). "Multi-Stage HRNet: Multiple Stage High-Resolution Network for Human Pose Estimation." *ArXiv Preprint ArXiv:1910.05901*.

Huang, Y.-Y. D.-Y.-T.-T., Chen, S.-D., Leng, X.-Y., Kuo, K., Wang, Z.-T., Cui, M., Tan, L., Wang, K., Dong, Q., & Yu, J.-T. (2022). Post-stroke cognitive impairment: Epidemiology, risk factors, and management. *Journal of Alzheimer's Disease*, *86*(3), 983–999. DOI: 10.3233/JAD-215644 PMID: 35147548

Hussin, Q., & Sadun, A. S. (2021). User-Driven Prosthetic Robotic Arm for Patients with Lower Arm Amputation. *Progress in Engineering Application and Technology*, *2*(1), 753–768. DOI: 10.30880/peat.2021.02.01.072

Hutton, B., Catala-Lopez, F., & Moher, D. (2016). The PRISMA statement extension for systematic reviews incorporating network meta-analysis: PRISMA-NMA. *Medicina Clínica (English Ed.)*, *147*(6), 262–266. DOI: 10.1016/j.medcle.2016.10.003 PMID: 27040178

Huynh, T., & Schiele, B. (2005, October). Analyzing features for activity recognition. In Proceedings of the 2005 joint conference on Smart objects and ambient intelligence: innovative context-aware services: usages and technologies (pp. 159-163). DOI: 10.1145/1107548.1107591

Hu, Z., Wang, J., Wang, Y., Wang, C., Wang, Y., Zhang, Z., Xu, P., Zhao, T., Luan, Y., Liu, C., Qiao, L., Shu, M., Mi, J., Pan, X., & Xu, M. (2021). A Robust and Wearable Triboelectric Tactile Patch as Intelligent Human-Machine Interface. *Materials (Basel)*, *14*(21), 6366. DOI: 10.3390/ma14216366 PMID: 34771892

Idrissi, I. G. E., Podlewska, S., Abate, C., Bojarski, A. J., Lacivita, E., & Leopoldo, M. (2024). Structure-Activity Relationships and Therapeutic Potential of Purinergic P2X7 Receptor Antagonists. *Current Medicinal Chemistry*, *31*(11), 1361–1403. DOI: 10.2174/0929867330666230403094538 PMID: 37013427

Ishaque, S., Khan, N., & Krishnan, S. (2021). Trends in heart-rate variability signal analysis. *Frontiers in Digital Health*, *3*, 639444. DOI: 10.3389/fdgth.2021.639444 PMID: 34713110

Islam, M., Vashishat, A., & Kumar, M. (2024). Advancements beyond Limb Loss: Exploring the Intersection of AI and BCI in Prosthetic Evaluation. *Current Pharmaceutical Design*, *30*(35), 2749–2752. DOI: 10.2174/0113816128324653240731075146 PMID: 39092732

Jackson, J. C., Ely, E. W., Morey, M. C., Anderson, V. M., Denne, L. B., Clune, J., Siebert, C. S., Archer, K. R., Torres, R., Janz, D., Schiro, E., Jones, J., Shintani, A. K., Levine, B., Pun, B. T., Thompson, J., Brummel, N. E., & Hoenig, H. (2012). Cognitive and physical rehabilitation of intensive care unit survivors: Results of the RETURN randomized controlled pilot investigation. [). LWW.]. *Critical Care Medicine*, *40*(4), 1088–1097. DOI: 10.1097/CCM.0b013e3182373115 PMID: 22080631

Jacob, S., Alagirisamy, M., Xi, C., Balasubramanian, V., Srinivasan, R., R, P., Jhanjhi, N. Z., & Islam, S. M. N. (2021). AI and IoT-Enabled Smart Exoskeleton System for Rehabilitation of Paralyzed People in Connected Communities. *IEEE Access : Practical Innovations, Open Solutions*, *9*, 80340–80350. DOI: 10.1109/ACCESS.2021.3083093

Jain, R., Semwal, V. B., & Kaushik, P. (2022). Deep ensemble learning approach for lower extremity activities recognition using wearable sensors. *Expert Systems: International Journal of Knowledge Engineering and Neural Networks*, *39*(6), e12743. DOI: 10.1111/exsy.12743

Jensen, M. P., Neilson, W. R., & Kerns, R. D. (2003). Toward the development of a motivational model of pain self-management. *The Journal of Pain*, *4*(9), 477–492. DOI: 10.1016/S1526-5900(03)00779-X PMID: 14636816

Jensen, M. P., Turner, J. A., & Romano, J. M. (1994). Correlates of improvement in multidisciplinary treatment of chronic pain. *Journal of Consulting and Clinical Psychology*, *62*(1), 172–179. DOI: 10.1037/0022-006X.62.1.172 PMID: 8034820

Jiang, S., Kang, P., Song, X., Lo, B., & Shull, P. (2021). Emerging Wearable Interfaces and Algorithms for Hand Gesture Recognition: A Survey. *IEEE Reviews in Biomedical Engineering*, *15*, 85–102. DOI: 10.1109/RBME.2021.3078190 PMID: 33961564

Johnson, M., & Wei, K. (2023). Neural Networks for Prosthetic Control Systems. *Journal of Computational Neuroscience*, *29*(2), 199–214.

Johnson, P. A. "Affordable smart home technologies for elderly care," in *Proc. 2020 Int. Conf. on Smart Systems and Technologies (SST)*, 2020, pp. 1–6.

Johnston, M. V., & Dijkers, M. P. (2012). Toward improved evidence standards and methods for rehabilitation: Recommendations and challenges. *Archives of Physical Medicine and Rehabilitation*, *93*(8), S185–S199. DOI: 10.1016/j.apmr.2011.12.011 PMID: 22840883

Joloudari, J. H., Saadatfar, H., Dehzangi, A., & Shamshirband, S. (2019). Computer-aided decision-making for predicting liver disease using PSO-based optimized SVM with feature selection. *Informatics in Medicine Unlocked*, *17*, 100255. DOI: 10.1016/j.imu.2019.100255

Jones, M., Collier, G., Reinkensmeyer, D. J., DeRuyter, F., Dzivak, J., Zondervan, D. K., & Morris, J. (2020). Big Data Analytics and Sensor-Enhanced Activity Management to Improve Effectiveness and Efficiency of Outpatient Medical Rehabilitation [Review of Big Data Analytics and Sensor-Enhanced Activity Management to Improve Effectiveness and Efficiency of Outpatient Medical Rehabilitation]. International Journal of Environmental Research and Public Health, 17(3), 748. Multidisciplinary Digital Publishing Institute. DOI: 10.3390/ijerph17030748

Jones, P., & Smith, K. (2021). The Role of Sensors in AI Prosthetics. *Medical Robotics Research Journal*, *11*(7), 120–138.

Julius, D. (2013). TRP Channels and Pain. *Annual Review of Cell and Developmental Biology*, *29*(1), 355–384. DOI: 10.1146/annurev-cellbio-101011-155833 PMID: 24099085

Kalaiselvi, R., Meena, K., & Vanitha, V. (2021). Liver Disease Prediction Using Machine Learning Algorithms. *2021 International Conference on Advancements in Electrical, Electronics, Communication, Computing and Automation (ICAECA)*, 1–6. DOI: 10.1109/ICAECA52838.2021.9675756

Kalusivalingam, A. K., Sharma, A., Patel, N., & Singh, V. (2020). Optimizing Industrial Systems Through Deep Q-Networks and Proximal Policy Optimization in Reinforcement Learning. *International Journal of Artificial Intelligence and Machine Learning*, *1*(3).

Kang, M., Seo, S., Lee, H., & Han, M.-W. (2024). Knee Measurement System with Osteoarthritis Levels Using Artificial Cartilage and Skeletons. *Biomimetics*, *9*(3), 166. DOI: 10.3390/biomimetics9030166 PMID: 38534851

Kanjo, E., Younis, E. M. G., & Ang, C. S. (2019). Deep learning analysis of mobile physiological, environmental and location sensor data for emotion detection. *Information Fusion*, *49*, 46–56. DOI: 10.1016/j.inffus.2018.09.001

Kantidakis, G., Hazewinkel, A. D., & Fiocco, M. (2022). Neural networks for survival prediction in medicine using prognostic factors: A review and critical appraisal. *Computational and Mathematical Methods in Medicine*, *2022*(1), 1176060. DOI: 10.1155/2022/1176060 PMID: 36238497

Karapintzou, E., Tsakanikas, V., Kikidis, D., Nikitas, C., Nairn, B., Pavlou, M., . . . Fotiadis, D. I. (2024, November). AI-enhanced tele-rehabilitation: Predictive modeling for fall risk and treatment efficacy in balance disorders. In *2024 IEEE 24th International Conference on Bioinformatics and Bioengineering (BIBE)* (pp. 1–8). IEEE.

Keefe, R. S., Cañadas, E., Farlow, D., & Etkin, A. (2022). Digital intervention for cognitive deficits in major depression: A randomized controlled trial to assess efficacy and safety in adults. *The American Journal of Psychiatry*, *179*(7), 482–489.

Kefelegn, S., & Kamat, P. (n.d.). Prediction and Analysis of Liver Disorder Diseases by using Data Mining Technique. *Survey (London, England).*

Kerns, R. D., & Habib, S. (2004). A critical review of the pain readiness to change model. *The Journal of Pain*, *5*(7), 357–367. DOI: 10.1016/j.jpain.2004.06.005 PMID: 15501193

Khalid, U. B., Naeem, M., Stasolla, F., Syed, M. H., Abbas, M., & Coronato, A. (2024). Impact of AI-powered solutions in rehabilitation process: Recent improvements and future trends. *International Journal of General Medicine*, •••, 943–969.

Khan, K. a. (2014). DBSCAN: Past, present and future. In *The fifth international conference on the applications of digital information and web technologies (ICADIWT 2014)* (pp. 232--238).

Khan, O., Badhiwala, J. H., Grasso, G., & Fehlings, M. G. (2020). Use of machine learning and artificial intelligence to drive personalized medicine approaches for spine care. *World Neurosurgery*, *140*, 512–518. DOI: 10.1016/j.wneu.2020.04.022 PMID: 32797983

Kianoush, S., Savazzi, S., Vicentini, F., Rampa, V., & Giussani, M. (2017). Device-Free RF Human Body Fall Detection and Localization in Industrial Workplaces. In IEEE Internet of Things Journal (Vol. 4, Issue 2, pp. 351–362). Institute of Electrical and Electronics Engineers (IEEE). DOI: 10.1109/JIOT.2016.2624800

Kihlstrom, J. F. (1985). Hypnosis. *Annual Review of Psychology*, *36*(1), 385–418. https://psycnet.apa.org/doi/10.1146/annurev.ps.36.020185.002125. DOI: 10.1146/annurev.ps.36.020185.002125 PMID: 3883892

Kim, J.-W., Choi, J.-Y., Ha, E.-J., & Choi, J.-H. (2023). Human Pose Estimation Using Mediapipe Pose and Optimization Method Based on a Humanoid Model. *Applied Sciences (Basel, Switzerland)*, *13*(4), 2700. DOI: 10.3390/app13042700

Kim, M., Simon, A. M., & Hargrove, L. J. (2022). Seamless and Intuitive Control of a Powered Prosthetic Leg Using Deep Neural Network for Transfemoral Amputees. *Wearable Technologies*, *3*(September), e24. DOI: 10.1017/wtc.2022.19 PMID: 37041885

Kim, S., Dowgwillo, E. A., & Kratz, A. L. (2023). Emotional Dynamics in Fibromyalgia: Pain, Fatigue, and Stress Moderate Momentary Associations Between Positive and Negative Emotions. *The Journal of Pain*, *24*(9), 1594–1603. DOI: 10.1016/j.jpain.2023.04.007 PMID: 37094743

Kim, Y., & Lee, M. (2023). Real-Time Processing in AI-Based Assistive Devices. *Journal of Advanced Robotics*, *25*(4), 300–320.

King, C. R., Shambe, A., & Abraham, J. (2023). Potential uses of AI for perioperative nursing handoffs: a qualitative study. In C. R. King, A. Shambe, & J. Abraham, JAMIA Open (Vol. 6, Issue 1). University of Oxford. DOI: 10.1093/jamiaopen/ooad015

Korrapati, C., Yaraladdi, A. B., Vaddi, H., & Raghavan, R. (2024). Applications of the Saffron European Kitchen Spice Crocus sativus. In *Therapeutic and Pharmacological Applications of Ethnobotany* (pp. 98–127). IGI Global., DOI: 10.4018/979-8-3693-1986-4.ch005

Kortuem, G., Kawsar, F., Sundramoorthy, V., & Fitton, D. (2010). Smart objects as building blocks for the Internet of things. In IEEE Internet Computing (Vol. 14, Issue 1, pp. 44–51). Institute of Electrical and Electronics Engineers (IEEE). DOI: 10.1109/MIC.2009.143

Kotsenas, A. L., Balthazar, P., Andrews, D., Geis, J. R., & Cook, T. S. (2021). Rethinking Patient Consent in the Era of Artificial Intelligence and Big Data. In A. L. Kotsenas, P. Balthazar, D. Andrews, J. R. Geis, & T. S. Cook, Journal of the American College of Radiology (Vol. 18, Issue 1, p. 180). Elsevier BV. DOI: 10.1016/j.jacr.2020.09.022

Koyama, J., Morise, M., Furukawa, T., Oyama, S., Matsuzawa, R., Tanaka, I., Wakahara, K., Yokota, H., Kimura, T., Shiratori, Y., Kondoh, Y., Hashimoto, N., & Ishii, M. (2024). Artificial intelligence-based personalized survival prediction using clinical and radiomics features in patients with advanced non-small cell lung cancer. *BMC Cancer*, *24*(1), 1417. DOI: 10.1186/s12885-024-13190-w PMID: 39558311

Krakauer, J. W. (2006). Motor learning: Its relevance to stroke recovery and neurorehabilitation. *Current Opinion in Neurology*, *19*(1), 84–90. DOI: 10.1097/01.wco.0000200544.29915.cc PMID: 16415682

Kreitler, M., & Kreitler, S. (2007). Psychological Approaches to Treatment of Pain. In *Handbook of Chronic Pain*. Nova Science.

Kreitler, S., & Kreitler, M. (2007). Psychological Approaches to Treatment of Pain: Sensory, Affective, Cognitive, Behaviuoral. In *The Handbook of Chronic Pain*. Nova Science Publishers.

Krishna, K. S., & Paneerselvam, S. (2021, October). An implementation of hybrid cnn-lstm model for human activity recognition. In International Conference on Advances in Electrical and Computer Technologies (pp. 813-825). Singapore: Springer Nature Singapore.

Kristoffersson, A., & Lindén, M. (2022). A systematic review of wearable sensors for monitoring physical activity. *Sensors (Basel)*, *22*(2), 573. DOI: 10.3390/s22020573 PMID: 35062531

Kuhn, M., & Johnson, K. (2013). *Applied Predictive Modeling*. Springer. DOI: 10.1007/978-1-4614-6849-3

Kumar, M. A., Purohit, K. C., Singh, A., & Bhatt, S. (2021). Heart Disease Prediction Model using Deep Learning Algorithms. *Webology*, *18*(4), 2086. Advance online publication. DOI: 10.29121/WEB/V18I4/106

Kumar, R., Patel, S., & Gupta, V. (2023). Natural Language Processing in Assistive Devices: Current Trends. *Computational Linguistics and Applications*, *12*(1), 45–67.

Kuzhippallil, M. A., Joseph, C., & Kannan, A. (2020). Comparative Analysis of Machine Learning Techniques for Indian Liver Disease Patients. *2020 6th International Conference on Advanced Computing and Communication Systems (ICACCS)*, 778–782. DOI: 10.1109/ICACCS48705.2020.9074368

Labkoff, S. E., Oladimeji, B. J., Kannry, J., Solomonides, A., Leftwich, R., Koski, E., Joseph, A. L., López-González, M., Fleisher, L. A., Nolen, K., Dutta, S., Levy, D. R., Price, A., Barr, P., Hron, J. D., Lin, B., Srivastava, G., Pastor, N., Luque, U. S., . . . Quintana, Y. (2024). Toward a responsible future: recommendations for AI-enabled clinical decision support. In S. E. Labkoff, B. J. Oladimeji, J. Kannry, A. Solomonides, R. Leftwich, E. Koski, A. L. Joseph, M. López-González, L. A. Fleisher, K. Nolen, S. Dutta, D. R. Levy, A. Price, P. Barr, J. D. Hron, B. Lin, G. Srivastava, N. Pastor, U. S. Luque, … Y. Quintana, Journal of the American Medical Informatics Association (Vol. 31, Issue 11, p. 2730). Oxford University Press. DOI: 10.1093/jamia/ocae209

Lakshmaiah, A., Korrapati, C., Suresh, C., & Raghavan, R. (2025). Synthetic Biology and AI. *Spatially Variable Genes in Cancer*, 265–290. DOI: 10.4018/979-8-3693-7728-4.ch010

Lambercy, O., Lehner, R., Chua, K. S. G., Wee, S. K., Rajeswaran, D. K., Kuah, C. W. K., Ang, W. T., Liang, P., Campolo, D., Hussain, A., Aguirre-Ollinger, G., Guan, C., Kanzler, C. M., Wenderoth, N., & Gassert, R. (2021). Neurorehabilitation From a Distance: Can Intelligent Technology Support Decentralized Access to Quality Therapy? In O. Lambercy, R. Lehner, K. S. G. Chua, S. K. Wee, D. K. Rajeswaran, C. W. K. Kuah, W. T. Ang, P. Liang, D. Campolo, A. Hussain, G. Aguirre-Ollinger, C. Guan, C. M. Kanzler, N. Wenderoth, & R. Gassert, Frontiers in Robotics and AI (Vol. 8). Frontiers Media. DOI: 10.3389/frobt.2021.612415

Lampit, A., Launder, N. H., Minkov, R., Rollini, A., Davey, C. G., Finke, C., Lautenschlager, N. T., & Gavelin, H. M. (2022). Computerized Cognitive Training in People with Depression: A Protocol for a Systematic Review and Meta-Analysis. *Systematic Reviews*, *11*(1), 6. DOI: 10.1186/s13643-021-01872-6 PMID: 34991698

Lang, C. E., Barth, J., Holleran, C. L., Konrad, J. D., & Bland, M. D. (2020). Implementation of wearable sensing technology for movement: Pushing forward into the routine physical rehabilitation care field. *Sensors (Basel)*, *20*(20), 5744. DOI: 10.3390/s20205744 PMID: 33050368

Lanotte, F., O'Brien, M. K., & Jayaraman, A. (2023). AI in rehabilitation medicine: Opportunities and challenges. *Annals of Rehabilitation Medicine*, *47*(6), 444–458. DOI: 10.5535/arm.23131 PMID: 38093518

LeCun, Y., Bengio, Y., & Hinton, G. (2015). "Deep learning." Nature. Nature: https://www.nature.com/articles/nature14539

LeCun, Y., Boser, B., Denker, J., Henderson, D., Howard, R., Hubbard, W., & Jackel, L. (1989). Handwritten digit recognition with a back-propagation network. *Advances in Neural Information Processing Systems*, •••, 2.

Lee, I., & Lee, K. (2015). The Internet of Things (IoT): Applications, investments, and challenges for enterprises. In Business Horizons (Vol. 58, Issue 4, pp. 431–440). Elsevier BV. DOI: 10.1016/j.bushor.2015.03.008

Le, L. (1994). Psychogenic pain. *Singapore Medical Journal*, *35*(5), 519–522. PMID: 7701376

Lerner, I., Créquit, P., Ravaud, P., & Atal, I. (2019). Automatic screening using word embeddings achieved high sensitivity and workload reduction for updating living network meta-analyses. *Journal of Clinical Epidemiology*, *108*, 86–94. DOI: 10.1016/j.jclinepi.2018.12.001 PMID: 30528791

Liao, Y., Vakanski, A., Xian, M., Paul, D., & Baker, R. (2020). A review of computational approaches for evaluation of rehabilitation exercises. *Computers in Biology and Medicine*, *119*, 103687. DOI: 10.1016/j.compbiomed.2020.103687 PMID: 32339122

Li, B., Xu, G., Teng, Z., Luo, D., Pei, J., Chen, R., & Zhang, S. (2024). Intelligent ankle—Foot prosthesis based on human structure and motion bionics. *Journal of Neuroengineering and Rehabilitation*, *21*(1), 119. DOI: 10.1186/s12984-024-01414-w PMID: 39003459

Lin, J., Keogh, E., Lonardi, S., & Chiu, B. (2003, June). A symbolic representation of time series, with implications for streaming algorithms. In *Proceedings of the 8th ACM SIGMOD workshop on Research issues in data mining and knowledge discovery* (pp. 2-11). DOI: 10.1145/882082.882086

Liu, N., Zhou, Y., & Lee, J. J. (2021). IPDfromKM: Reconstruct individual patient data from published Kaplan-Meier survival curves. *BMC Medical Research Methodology*, *21*(1), 111. DOI: 10.1186/s12874-021-01308-8 PMID: 34074267

Liu, S., Wang, L., & Gao, R. X. (2024). Cognitive neuroscience and robotics: Advancements and future research directions. *Robotics and Computer-integrated Manufacturing*, *85*, 102610. DOI: 10.1016/j.rcim.2023.102610

Liu, Z., Rich, B., & Hanley, J. A. (2014). Recovering the raw data behind a non-parametric survival curve. *Systematic Reviews*, *3*(1), 1–10. DOI: 10.1186/2046-4053-3-151 PMID: 25551437

Li, X., Wang, Y., & Lee, D. (2022). Enhancing Mobility with AI-Driven Orthotic Systems. *Journal of Assistive Technology Research*, *10*(3), 145–161.

Lonini, L., Dai, A., Shawen, N., Simuni, T., Poon, C., Shimanovich, L., Daeschler, M., Ghaffari, R., Rogers, J. A., & Jayaraman, A. (2018). Wearable sensors for Parkinson's disease: Which data are worth collecting for training symptom detection models. *NPJ Digital Medicine*, *1*(1), 64. DOI: 10.1038/s41746-018-0071-z PMID: 31304341

Lu, W., Fan, F., Chu, J., Jing, P., & Yuting, S. (2019). Wearable Computing for Internet of Things: A Discriminant Approach for Human Activity Recognition. In IEEE Internet of Things Journal (Vol. 6, Issue 2, pp. 2749–2759). Institute of Electrical and Electronics Engineers (IEEE). DOI: 10.1109/JIOT.2018.2873594

Lubetzky-Vilnai, A., Ciol, M., & McCoy, S. W. (2014). Statistical analysis of clinical prediction rules for rehabilitation interventions: Current state of the literature. *Archives of Physical Medicine and Rehabilitation*, *95*(1), 188–196. DOI: 10.1016/j.apmr.2013.08.242 PMID: 24036159

Luo, X., Guo, X., Zhao, Q., Zhu, Y., Chen, Y., Zhang, D., Jiang, H., Wang, Y., Johnstone, S., & Sun, L. (2023). A Randomized Controlled Study of Remote Computerized Cognitive, Neurofeedback, and Combined Training in the Treatment of Children with Attention-Deficit/Hyperactivity Disorder. *European Child & Adolescent Psychiatry*, *32*(8), 1475–1486. DOI: 10.1007/s00787-022-01956-1 PMID: 35182242

Luo, Z., & Kim, S. (2021). Affordability Challenges in AI-Driven Orthotics. *Healthcare AI Advances*, *17*(3), 113–129.

Mahmoudi-Dehaki, M., Nasr-Esfahani, N., & Vasan, S. (2025). The Transformative Role of Assistive Technology in Enhancing Quality of Life for Individuals With Disabilities. In *Assistive Technology Solutions for Aging Adults and Individuals With Disabilities* (pp. 45–72). IGI Global Scientific Publishing.

Mainali, S., Darsie, M. E., & Smetana, K. S. (2021). Machine learning in action: Stroke diagnosis and outcome prediction. *Frontiers in Neurology*, *12*, 734345. DOI: 10.3389/fneur.2021.734345 PMID: 34938254

Ma, J., Hobbs, B. P., & Stingo, F. C. (2015). Statistical methods for establishing personalized treatment rules in oncology. *BioMed Research International*, *2015*(1), 670691. DOI: 10.1155/2015/670691 PMID: 26446492

Majumder, S., Aghayi, E., Noferesti, M., Memarzadeh-Tehran, H., Mondal, T., Pang, Z., & Deen, M. J. (2017). Smart homes for elderly healthcare—Recent advances and research challenges. *Sensors (Basel)*, *17*(11), 2496. DOI: 10.3390/s17112496 PMID: 29088123

Majumder, S., Mondal, T., & Deen, M. J. (2017). Wearable sensors for remote health monitoring. *Sensors (Basel)*, *17*(1), 130. DOI: 10.3390/s17010130 PMID: 28085085

Mamyrbekova, S., Nurgaliyeva, Z., Saktapov, A., Zholdasbekova, A., & Kudaibergenova, A. (2020). Medicine of the Future: Digital Technologies in Healthcare. In S. Mamyrbekova, Z. Nurgaliyeva, A. Saktapov, A. Zholdasbekova, & A. Kudaibergenova, E3S Web of Conferences (Vol. 159, p. 4036). EDP Sciences. DOI: 10.1051/e3sconf/202015904036

Mangili, F., Benavoli, A., de Campos, C. P., & Zaffalon, M. (2015). Reliable survival analysis based on the Dirichlet Process. *Biometrical Journal. Biometrische Zeitschrift*, *57*(6), 1002–1019. DOI: 10.1002/bimj.201500062 PMID: 26296502

Mann, W. C. (2018). "Assistive technology use and aging," Generations. *Journal of the American Society on Aging*, *42*(1), 6–10.

Marasinghe, V. (2020). Assistive robotics for elderly care: Recent trends and developments. *Healthcare Robotics*, *12*(4), 78–85.

Marcus, H. J., Ramírez, P. T., Khan, D. Z., Horsfall, H. L., Hanrahan, J., Williams, S. C., Beard, D., Bhat, R. A., Catchpole, K., Cook, A., Hutchison, K., Martin, J., Melvin, T., Stoyanov, D., Rovers, M. M., Raison, N., Dasgupta, P., Noonan, D., Stocken, D., . . . Páez, A. (2024). The IDEAL framework for surgical robotics: development, comparative evaluation and long-term monitoring. In H. J. Marcus, P. T. Ramírez, D. Z. Khan, H. L. Horsfall, J. Hanrahan, S. C. Williams, D. Beard, R. A. Bhat, K. Catchpole, A. Cook, K. Hutchison, J. Martin, T. Melvin, D. Stoyanov, M. M. Rovers, N. Raison, P. Dasgupta, D. Noonan, D. Stocken, … A. Páez, Nature Medicine (Vol. 30, Issue 1, p. 61). Nature Portfolio. DOI: 10.1038/s41591-023-02732-7

Margam, R. (2024). Virtual reality in healthcare: transforming treatment. *International journal of artificial intelligence \& machine learning (IJAIML)*, 19--34.

Margo, C. E. (1999). The Placebo Effect (J. S. Mindel, Ed.). *Survey of Ophthamology, 44*(1), 31-44. DOI: 10.1016/S0039-6257(99)00060-0

Massella, M., Dri, D. A., & Gramaglia, D. (2022). Regulatory Considerations on the use of Machine Learning based tools in Clinical Trials. In M. Massella, D. A. Dri, & D. Gramaglia, Health and Technology (Vol. 12, Issue 6, p. 1085). Springer Science+Business Media. DOI: 10.1007/s12553-022-00708-0

Mathews, D., Abernethy, A. P., Chaikof, E. L., Charo, R. A., Daley, G. Q., Enriquez, J., Gottlieb, S., Kahn, J., Klausner, R. D., Tavazoie, S. F., Fabi, R., Offodile, A. C., Sherkow, J. S., Sullenger, R. D., Freiling, E., & Balatbat, C. (2023). Regenerative Medicine: Case Study for Understanding and Anticipating Emerging Science and Technology. In Mathews, D., Abernethy, A. P., Chaikof, E. L., Charo, R. A., Daley, G. Q., Enriquez, J., Gottlieb, S., Kahn, J., Klausner, R. D., Tavazoie, S. F., Fabi, R., Offodile, A. C., Sherkow, J. S., Sullenger, R. D., Freiling, E., Balatbat, C., & Perspectives, N. A. M. (Eds.), *Issue 15)* (Vol. 11)., DOI: 10.31478/202211d

McCrae, R. R., & Costa, P. T. (2003). *Personality in adulthood: A five-factor theory perspective* (2nd ed.). Guilford Press., https://awspntest.apa.org/doi/10.4324/9780203428412 DOI: 10.4324/9780203428412

McDonald, P., Foley, T., Verheij, R., Braithwaite, J., Rubin, J. C., Harwood, K., Phillips, J., Gilman, S. D., & van der Wees, P. J. (2024). Data to knowledge to improvement: creating the learning health system. In P. McDonald, T. Foley, R. Verheij, J. Braithwaite, J. C. Rubin, K. Harwood, J. Phillips, S. D. Gilman, & P. J. van der Wees, BMJ. DOI: 10.1136/bmj-2023-076175

Meagher, M. W., Arnau, R. C., & Rhudy, J. L. (2001). Pain and emotion: Effects of affective picture modulation. *Psychosomatic Medicine*, *63*(1), 79–90. DOI: 10.1097/00006842-200101000-00010 PMID: 11211069

Mehmood, A., Iqbal, M., Mehmood, Z., Irtaza, A., Nawaz, M., Nazir, T., & Masood, M. (2021). Prediction of Heart Disease Using Deep Convolutional Neural Networks. *Arabian Journal for Science and Engineering*, *46*(11), 3409–3422. DOI: 10.1007/s13369-020-05105-1

Mehra, S., & Aggarwal, R. (2020). Fall detection systems and emergency response technologies. *Health Care Systems*, *19*(5), 512–523.

Melzack, R. (2001). Pain and the neuromatrix in the brain. *Journal of Dental Education*, *65*(12), 1378–1382. DOI: 10.1002/j.0022-0337.2001.65.12.tb03497.x PMID: 11780656

Melzack, R., & Wall, P. D. (1965). Pain Mechanisms: A New Theory: A gate control system modulates sensory input from the skin before it evokes pain perception and response. *Science*, *150*(3699), 971–979. DOI: 10.1126/science.150.3699.971 PMID: 5320816

Mennella, C., Maniscalco, U., Pietro, G. D., & Esposito, M. (2023). The Role of Artificial Intelligence in Future Rehabilitation Services: A Systematic Literature Review. In C. Mennella, U. Maniscalco, G. D. Pietro, & M. Esposito, IEEE Access (Vol. 11, p. 11024). Institute of Electrical and Electronics Engineers. DOI: 10.1109/ACCESS.2023.3236084

Merletti, R. a. (2004). Electromyography: physiology, engineering, and non-invasive applications. John Wiley \& Sons.

Merlo, G., Chifari, A., Chiazzese, G., Denaro, P., Firrera, N., Lo Savio, N., Patti, S., Palmegiano, L., Taibi, D., & Seta, L. (2023a). The BEHAVE Application as a Tool to Monitor Inclusive Interventions for Subjects with Neurodevelopmental Disorders. *Frontiers in Psychology*, *13*, 943370. DOI: 10.3389/fpsyg.2022.943370 PMID: 36743629

Merriaux, P., Dupuis, Y., Boutteau, R., Vasseur, P., & Savatier, X. (2017). A Study of Vicon System Positioning Performance. *Sensors (Basel)*, *17*(7), 1591. DOI: 10.3390/s17071591 PMID: 28686213

Metaxa, D., Park, J. S., Robertson, R. E., Karahalios, K., Wilson, C., Hancock, J. T., & Sandvig, C. (2021). Auditing Algorithms: Understanding Algorithmic Systems from the Outside In. In D. Metaxa, J. S. Park, R. E. Robertson, K. Karahalios, C. Wilson, J. T. Hancock, & C. Sandvig, Foundations and Trends® in Human–Computer Interaction (Vol. 14, Issue 4, p. 272). Now Publishers. DOI: 10.1561/1100000083

Milani, S., Fan, Z., Gulati, S., Nguyen, T., Fang, F., & Yadav, A. 2020. "Intelligent Tutoring Strategies for Students with Autism Spectrum Disorder: A Reinforcement Learning Approach." In *The 2020 CMU Symposium on Artificial Intelligence and Social Good*.

Millan, M. J. (1999). The induction of pain: An integrative review. *Progress in Neurobiology*, *57*(1), 1–164. DOI: 10.1016/S0301-0082(98)00048-3 PMID: 9987804

Ministry of Social Justice and Empowerment. Government of India, "Rashtriya Vayoshri Yojana," 2020. [Online]; https://socialjustice.gov.in/

Mitchell, L. A., MacDonald, R. A., & Brodie, E. E. (2004). Temperature and the cold pressor test. *The Journal of Pain*, *5*(4), 233–237. DOI: 10.1016/j.jpain.2004.03.004 PMID: 15162346

Moreno-Sánchez, P. A., García-Isla, G., Corino, V. D. A., Vehkaoja, A., Brukamp, K., van Gils, M., & Mainardi, L. (2024). ECG-based data-driven solutions for diagnosis and prognosis of cardiovascular diseases: A systematic review. *Computers in Biology and Medicine*, *172*, 108235. DOI: 10.1016/j.compbiomed.2024.108235 PMID: 38460311

Mortenson, J. E.. (2015). The experiences of older adults with assistive technology: A qualitative meta-synthesis. *Disability and Rehabilitation. Assistive Technology*, *10*(4), 271–280. PMID: 25252024

Mulfari, D., La Placa, D., Rovito, C., Celesti, A., & Villari, M. (2022). Deep learning applications in telerehabilitation speech therapy scenarios. [Elsevier.]. *Computers in Biology and Medicine*, *148*, 105864. DOI: 10.1016/j.compbiomed.2022.105864 PMID: 35853398

Mulyani, S. H., Wijaya, N., & Trinidya, F. (2023). Enhancing heart disease detection using convolutional neural networks and classic machine learning methods. *Journal of Computer, Electronic, and Telecommunication*, *4*(2). Advance online publication. DOI: 10.52435/complete.v4i2.394

Munteanu, D., Bejan, C., Munteanu, N., Zamfir, C., Vasić, M., Petrea, S.-M., & Cristea, D. (2022). Deep-Learning-Based System for Assisting People with Alzheimer's Disease. *Electronics (Basel)*, *11*(19), 3229. DOI: 10.3390/electronics11193229

Murala, D. K., Panda, S. K., & Dash, S. P. (2023). MedMetaverse: Medical Care of Chronic Disease Patients and Managing Data Using Artificial Intelligence, Blockchain, and Wearable Devices State-of-the-Art Methodology. *IEEE Access : Practical Innovations, Open Solutions*, *11*, 138954–138985. DOI: 10.1109/ACCESS.2023.3340791

Muro-de-la-Herran, A., García-Zapirain, B., & Méndez-Zorrilla, A. (2014). Gait analysis methods: An overview of wearable and non-wearable systems, highlighting clinical applications. *Sensors (Basel)*, *14*(2), 3362–3394. DOI: 10.3390/s140203362 PMID: 24556672

Murphy, K. P. (2012). Machine Learning: A Probabilistic Perspective. MIT Press. Publisher: https://mitpress.mit.edu/9780262018029/machine-learning/

Nagashri, N., Archana, L., & Raghavan, R. (2024). Microbial Volatile Compounds (MVOCs) in Food Industries and Food Safety Applications. In *Innovations, Securities, and Case Studies Across Healthcare, Business, and Technology* (pp. 75–96). IGI Global. DOI: 10.4018/979-8-3693-1906-2.ch005

Nalluri, S., Saraswathi, R. V., Ramaswamy, S., Govinda, K., & Swetha, E. (2020). Chronic heart disease prediction using data mining techniques. In *Data Engineering and Communication Technology* (pp. 903–912). Springer., DOI: 10.1007/978-981-15-1097-7_76

Nam, Y., Kim, J., Jung, S.-H., Woerner, J., Suh, E. H., Lee, D., Shivakumar, M., Lee, M. E., & Kim, D. (2024). Harnessing Artificial Intelligence in Multimodal Omics Data Integration: Paving the Path for the Next Frontier in Precision Medicine. *Annual Review of Biomedical Data Science, 7*(Volume 7, 2024), 225–250. DOI: 10.1146/annurev-biodatasci-102523-103801

Nandakumar, P., & Subhashini, R. (2024). Heart disease prediction using convolutional neural network with elephant herding optimization. *Computer Systems Science and Engineering*, *48*(1), 57–75. DOI: 10.32604/csse.2023.042294

Nascimben, M. (2024). Machine learning approaches for personalized medicine.

Newman-Griffis, D., Desmet, B., Zirikly, A., Tamang, S., & Chang, C.-H. (2023). Editorial: Artificial intelligence for human function and disability. In D. Newman-Griffis, B. Desmet, A. Zirikly, S. Tamang, & C.-H. Chang, Frontiers in Digital Health (Vol. 5). Frontiers Media. DOI: 10.3389/fdgth.2023.1282287

Newton-John, T. R. O., Mason, C., & Hunter, M. (2014). The Role of Resilience in Adjustment and Coping With Chronic Pain. *Rehabilitation Psychology*, *59*(3), 360–365. DOI: 10.1037/a0037023 PMID: 25019306

Nicora, G., Pe, S., Santangelo, G., Billeci, L., Aprile, I. G., Germanotta, M., ... & Quaglini, S. (2024). A systematic review of machine learning in robotics-assisted rehabilitation.

Nieto-Hidalgo, M., Ferrández-Pastor, F. J., Valdivieso-Sarabia, R. J., Mora-Pascual, J., & García-Chamizo, J. M. (2018). Gait analysis using computer vision based on cloud platform and mobile device. *Mobile Information Systems*, *2018*(1), 7381264.

Nissan, N., Hertz, U., Shahar, N., & Gabay, Y. (2023). Distinct Reinforcement Learning Profiles Distinguish between Language and Attentional Neurodevelopmental Disorders. *Behavioral and Brain Functions : BBF*, *19*(1), 6. DOI: 10.1186/s12993-023-00207-w PMID: 36941632

Nizamis, K. a. (2021). Converging robotic technologies in targeted neural rehabilitation: a review of emerging solutions and challenges. *Sensors*, 2084. oel, J. P. (2021). Cognitive and Cybernetics based Human Adaptive Mechatronics System in Gait Rehabilitation Therapy. In *2021 Third International Conference on Intelligent Communication Technologies and Virtual Mobile Networks (ICICV)* (pp. 516--521). DOI: 10.3390/s21062084

Noh, B., Youm, C., Goh, E., Lee, M., Park, H., Jeon, H., & Kim, O. Y. (2021). XGBoost based machine learning approach to predict the risk of fall in older adults using gait outcomes. *Scientific Reports*, *11*(1), 12183.

Olyanasab, A., & Annabestani, M. (2024). Leveraging machine learning for personalized wearable biomedical devices: A review. *Journal of Personalized Medicine*, *14*(2), 203. DOI: 10.3390/jpm14020203 PMID: 38392636

Ortiz, B. L., Gupta, V., Kumar, R., Jalin, A., Cao, X., Ziegenbein, C., Singhal, A., Tewari, M., & Choi, S. W. (2024). Data Preprocessing Techniques for AI and Machine Learning Readiness: Scoping Review of Wearable Sensor Data in Cancer Care. *JMIR mHealth and uHealth*, *12*, 59587. DOI: 10.2196/59587 PMID: 38626290

Othman, N. A., Abdel-Fattah, M. A., & Ali, A. T. (2023). A hybrid deep learning framework with decision-level fusion for breast cancer survival prediction. *Big Data and Cognitive Computing*, *7*(1), 50. DOI: 10.3390/bdcc7010050

Paiste, H. J., Godwin, R. C., Smith, A. D., Berkowitz, D. E., & Melvin, R. L. (2024). Strengths-weaknesses-opportunities-threats analysis of artificial intelligence in anesthesiology and perioperative medicine. *Frontiers in Digital Health*, *6*, 1316931. DOI: 10.3389/fdgth.2024.1316931 PMID: 38444721

Pan, D. H., Hu, J., Wang, B., Xia, X., Cheng, Y., Wang, C.-H., & Lu, Y. (2024). Biomimetic Wearable Sensors: Emerging Combination of Intelligence and Electronics. *Advancement of Science*, *11*(5), 2303264. DOI: 10.1002/advs.202303264 PMID: 38044298

Panjaitan, F., Nurmaini, S., & Partan, R. U. (2023). Accurate Prediction of Sudden Cardiac Death Based on Heart Rate Variability Analysis Using Convolutional Neural Network. *Medicina*, *59*(8), 1394. DOI: 10.3390/medicina59081394 PMID: 37629684

Park, H. a. (2016). Short-duration and intensive training improves long-term reaching performance in individuals with chronic stroke. *Neurorehabilitation and neural repair*, 551–561. Pranji{\'c}, M. a. (2024). From Sound to Movement: Mapping the Neural Mechanisms of Auditory—Motor Entrainment and Synchronization. *Brain Sciences*, •••, 1063.

Park, H., & Jeong, S. (2022). Applications of AI in Orthotic Design. *International Journal of Bioengineering, 19*(3), 245–263.

Parvaiz, A., Nasir, E. S., & Fraz, M. M. (2024). From Pixels to Prognosis: A Survey on AI-Driven Cancer Patient Survival Prediction Using Digital Histology Images. *Journal of Imaging Informatics in Medicine*, *37*(4), 1–24. DOI: 10.1007/s10278-024-01049-2 PMID: 38429563

Patel, A., Chen, R., & Singh, K. (2022). Adaptive NLP Algorithms for Communication Devices. *AI in Human Health*, *9*(4), 331–350.

Patel, A., & Khanna, S. (2021). Smart pill dispensers and medication adherence. *Medica Innovatica*, *34*(1), 10–14.

Pelosi, A. D., Roth, N., Yehoshua, T., Itah, D., Braun Benyamin, O., & Dahan, A. (2024). Personalized rehabilitation approach for reaching movement using reinforcement learning. *Scientific Reports*, *14*(1), 17675. DOI: 10.1038/s41598-024-64514-6 PMID: 39085281

Pérez-Fuentes, M. D. C., Molero Jurado, M. D. M., Gázquez Linares, J. J., & Oropesa Ruiz, N. F. (2018). The role of emotional intelligence in engagement in nurses. *International Journal of Environmental Research and Public Health*, *15*(9), 1915.

Pesapane, F., Bracchi, D. A., Mulligan, J. F., Линников, A. C., Maslennikov, O. V., Lanzavecchia, M. B., Tantrige, P., Stasolla, A., Biondetti, P., Giuggioli, P. F., Cassano, E., & Carrafiello, G. (2021). Legal and Regulatory Framework for AI Solutions in Healthcare in EU, US, China, and Russia: New Scenarios after a Pandemic. In F. Pesapane, D. A. Bracchi, J. F. Mulligan, A. C. Линников, O. V. Maslennikov, M. B. Lanzavecchia, P. Tantrige, A. Stasolla, P. Biondetti, P. F. Giuggioli, E. Cassano, & G. Carrafiello, Radiation (Vol. 1, Issue 4, p. 261). Multidisciplinary Digital Publishing Institute. DOI: 10.3390/radiation1040022

Philpot, L. M., Dugani, S. B., Singla, A., DeZutter, M. A., & Ebbert, J. O. (2023). Digital Care Horizon: A Framework for Extending Health Care Through Digital Transformation. In L. M. Philpot, S. B. Dugani, A. Singla, M. A. DeZutter, & J. O. Ebbert, Mayo Clinic Proceedings Digital Health (Vol. 1, Issue 3, p. 210). Elsevier BV. DOI: 10.1016/j.mcpdig.2023.05.005

Pike, A. C., & Robinson, O. J. (2022). Reinforcement Learning in Patients with Mood and Anxiety Disorders vs Control Individuals: A Systematic Review and Meta-Analysis. *JAMA Psychiatry*, *79*(4), 313–322. DOI: 10.1001/jamapsychiatry.2022.0051 PMID: 35234834

Pinto, A. V., & Araújo, C. N. (2020). IoT-based security solutions for elderly individuals. *IEEE Internet of Things Journal, 7*(8), 7050–7058.

Pinto-Bernal, M. J. M., S. D. S., Múnera, M., Casas, D., Villa-Moreno, A., Frizera, A., Stoelen, M. F., Belpaeme, T., & Cifuentes, C. A. (2023). Do different robot appearances change emotion recognition in children with ASD? In M. J. Pinto-Bernal, S. D. S. M., M. Múnera, D. Casas, A. Villa-Moreno, A. Frizera, M. F. Stoelen, T. Belpaeme, & C. A. Cifuentes, Frontiers in Neurorobotics (Vol. 17). Frontiers Media. DOI: 10.3389/fnbot.2023.1044491

Pirasteh, A., Ghiyasvand, M. S., & Pouladian, M. (2024). EEG-based brain-computer interface methods with the aim of rehabilitating advanced stage ALS patients. *Disability and Rehabilitation: Assistive Technology, ahead-of-print*(ahead-of-print), 1–11. DOI: 10.1080/17483107.2024.2316312

Piwek, L., Ellis, D. A., Andrews, S., & Joinson, A. (2016). The rise of consumer health wearables: Promises and barriers. *PLoS Medicine, 13*(2), e1001953. DOI: 10.1371/journal.pmed.1001953 PMID: 26836780

Porciuncula, F., Roto, A. V., Kumar, D., Davis, I., Roy, S., Walsh, C. J., & Awad, L. N. (2018). Wearable movement sensors for rehabilitation: A focused review of technological and clinical advances. PM&R, 10(9S2), S220-S232. https://doi.org/DOI: 10.1016/j.pmrj.2018.06.013

Pouliopoulou, D. V., Macdermid, J. C., Saunders, E., Peters, S., Brunton, L., Miller, E., Quinn, K. L., Pereira, T. V., & Bobos, P. (2023). Rehabilitation interventions for physical capacity and quality of life in adults with post–COVID-19 condition: A systematic review and meta-analysis. *JAMA Network Open, 6*(9), e2333838–e2333838. DOI: 10.1001/jamanetworkopen.2023.33838 PMID: 37725376

Prang, K.-H., Maritz, R., Sabanovic, H., Dunt, D., & Kelaher, M. (2021). Mechanisms and impact of public reporting on physicians and hospitals' performance: A systematic review (2000–2020) [Review of Mechanisms and impact of public reporting on physicians and hospitals' performance: A systematic review (2000–2020)]. PLoS ONE, 16(2). Public Library of Science. DOI: 10.1371/journal.pone.0247297

Prentzas, N., Kakas, A. C., & Pattichis, C. S. (2023). Explainable AI applications in the Medical Domain: a systematic review [Review of Explainable AI applications in the Medical Domain: a systematic review]. arXiv (Cornell University). Cornell University. https://doi.org/DOI: 10.48550/arXiv.2308

Price, D. D., Finniss, D. G., & Benedetti, F. (2008). A comprehensive review of the placebo effect: Recent advances and current thought. *Annual Review of Psychology, 59*(1), 565–590. DOI: 10.1146/annurev.psych.59.113006.095941 PMID: 17550344

Qaim, W. B. (2020). Towards energy efficiency in the internet of wearable things: A systematic review. *IEEE AccessIEEE Access*, 175412--175435.

Qiu, S., Zhao, H., Jiang, N., Wang, Z., Liu, L., An, Y., Zhao, H., Miao, X., Liu, R., & Fortino, G. (2022). Multi-sensor information fusion based on machine learning for real applications in human activity recognition: State-of-the-art and research challenges. In *Information Fusion* (Vol. 80, pp. 241–265). Elsevier BV., DOI: 10.1016/j.inffus.2021.11.006

Rai, R.B., Sahu, S. & Sawant, S. (2018). "An Analysis on MYCIN Expert System." *MGMCET, International Journal of Research in Engineering, Science and Management.*

Rajalaxmi, V. a. (2024). Emerging Role of Artificial Intelligence and Robotics in Physiotherapy: Past, Present, and Future Perspective. In *Advancements in Clinical Medicine* (pp. 200--214).

Rajeswari, S. V. K. R., & Vijayakumar, P. (2024). Development of sensor system and data analytic framework for non-invasive blood glucose prediction. *Scientific Reports, 14*(1), 9206. DOI: 10.1038/s41598-024-59744-7 PMID: 38649731

Raj, Y., Kumar, A., Ashok, A., Kumar, V. D., Kumar, A., & Kumar, V. D. (2023). Prediction of cardiovascular disease using deep learning algorithms to prevent COVID 19. *Journal of Experimental & Theoretical Artificial Intelligence, 35*(6).

Ram Kumar, R. P., Raju, S., Annapoorna, E., Hajari, M., Hareesa, K., Vatin, N. I., Joshi, A., & AL-Attabi, K. (2024). Enhanced heart disease prediction through hybrid CNN-TLBO-GA optimization: A comparative study with conventional CNN and optimized CNN using FPO algorithm. *Cogent Engineering, 11*(1), 2384657. DOI: 10.1080/23311916.2024.2384657

Ramirez-Bautista, J. A., Hernández-Zavala, A., Chaparro-Cárdenas, S. L., & Huerta-Ruelas, J. A. (2018). Review on plantar data analysis for disease diagnosis. *Biocybernetics and Biomedical Engineering, 38*(2), 342–361. DOI: 10.1016/j.bbe.2018.02.004

Rani, A. J. M., Nishanthini, S., Josephine, D. C. J., Venugopal, H., Nissi, S. G., & Jacintha, V. (2022a). Liver Disease Prediction using Semi Supervised based Machine Learning Algorithm. *2022 3rd International Conference on Smart Electronics and Communication (ICOSEC)*, 1389–1392. DOI: 10.1109/ICOSEC54921.2022.9952144

Rasa, A. R. (2024). Artificial intelligence and its revolutionary role in physical and mental rehabilitation: A review of recent advancements. *BioMed Research International, 2024*(1), 9554590. DOI: 10.1155/bmri/9554590 PMID: 39720127

Rashbaum, I. G., & Sarno, J. E. (2003). Psychosomatic concepts in chronic pain. *Archives of Physical Medicine and Rehabilitation*, *84*, S76–S88. DOI: 10.1053/apmr.2003.50144 PMID: 12708562

Ravi, D., ... (2017). “Deep learning for human activity recognition: A resource-efficient implementation.” Wearable Sensors. IEEE Xplore: https://ieeexplore.ieee.org/document/7901760

Ray, R. (2004). *The extent, pattern and trends of drug abuse in India: National survey*. Ministry of Social Justice and Empowerment, Government of India & United Nations Office on Drugs and Crime, Regional Office for South Asia.

Reason, T., Benbow, E., Langham, J., Gimblett, A., Klijn, S. L., & Malcolm, B. (2024). Artificial Intelligence to Automate Network Meta-Analyses: Four Case Studies to Evaluate the Potential Application of Large Language Models. *PharmacoEconomics Open*, *8*(2), 205–220. DOI: 10.1007/s41669-024-00476-9 PMID: 38340277

Rebsamen, B., ... (2007). “A brain-controlled wheelchair to navigate in familiar environments.” IEEE Transactions on Neural Systems and Rehabilitation Engineering. IEEE Xplore: https://ieeexplore.ieee.org/document/4354040

Reis, F. J., de Carvalho, M. B. L., de Assis Neves, G., Nogueira, L. C., & Meziat-Filho, N. (2024). Machine learning methods in physical therapy: A scoping review of applications in clinical context. *Musculoskeletal Science & Practice*, *74*, 103184. DOI: 10.1016/j.msksp.2024.103184 PMID: 39278141

Revathi, T. K., Balasubramaniam, S., Sureshkumar, V., & Dhanasekaran, S. (2024). An improved long short-term memory algorithm for cardiovascular disease prediction. *Diagnostics (Basel)*, *14*(3), 239. DOI: 10.3390/diagnostics14030239 PMID: 38337755

Rivera, G., & Young, B. (2022). Affordable Solutions for AI-Powered Prosthetics. *Journal of Accessible Engineering*, *12*(5), 301–320.

Roberts, B. (2022). Evaluation of a wearable consumer noise measurement device in a laboratory setting. *The Journal of the Acoustical Society of America*, •••, 547–552. DOI: 10.1121/10.0012916 PMID: 35931541

Rodriguez-Villa, E., Camacho, E., & Torous, J. (2021). Psychiatric Rehabilitation through Teaching Smartphone Skills to Improve Functional Outcomes in Serious Mental Illness. *Internet Interventions : the Application of Information Technology in Mental and Behavioural Health*, *23*, 100366. DOI: 10.1016/j.invent.2021.100366 PMID: 33532245

Roelofs, J. M., Zandvliet, S. B., Schut, I. M., Huisinga, A. C. M., Schouten, A. C., Hendricks, H. T., de Kam, D., Aerden, L. A. M., Bussmann, J. B. J., Geurts, A. C. H., & Weerdesteyn, V. (2023). Mild stroke, serious problems: Limitations in balance and gait capacity and the impact on fall rate, and physical activity. *Neurorehabilitation and Neural Repair*, *37*(11-12), 786–798. DOI: 10.1177/15459683231207360 PMID: 37877724

Rogula, B., Lozano-Ortega, G., & Johnston, K. M. (2022). A method for reconstructing individual patient data from Kaplan-Meier survival curves that incorporate marked censoring times. *MDM Policy & Practice*, *7*(1), 23814683221077643. DOI: 10.1177/23814683221077643 PMID: 35128059

Rossetto, F., Borgnis, F., Isernia, S., Foglia, E., Garagiola, E., Realdon, O., & Baglio, F. (2023). System Integrated Digital Empowering and teleRehabilitation to promote patient Activation and well-Being in chronic disabilities: A usability and acceptability study. In F. Rossetto, F. Borgnis, S. Isernia, E. Foglia, E. Garagiola, O. Realdon, & F. Baglio, Frontiers in Public Health (Vol. 11). Frontiers Media. DOI: 10.3389/fpubh.2023.1154481

Royston, P., & Parmar, M. K. (2011). The use of restricted mean survival time to estimate the treatment effect in randomized clinical trials when the proportional hazards assumption is in doubt. *Statistics in Medicine*, *30*(19), 2409–2421. DOI: 10.1002/sim.4274 PMID: 21611958

Ruscheweyh, R., Marziniak, M., Stumpenhorst, F., Reinholz, J., & Knecht, S. (2009). Pain sensitivity can be assessed by self-rating: Development and validation of the Pain Sensitivity Questionnaire. *Pain*, *164*(1), 65–74. DOI: 10.1016/j.pain.2009.06.020 PMID: 19665301

Rusta, M. M., Haghpanah, S. A., & Taghvaei, S. (2024). Musculoskeletal Modeling and Control of the Human Upper Limb during Manual Wheelchair Propulsion: Application in Functional Electrical Stimulation Rehabilitation Therapy. *Journal of Applied and Computational Mechanics*, *10*(1), 92–110. DOI: 10.22055/jacm.2023.44469.4217

Salim, A., Stein, D. M., Zarzaur, B. L., & Livingston, D. H. (2023). Measuring long-term outcomes after injury: current issues and future directions [Review of Measuring long-term outcomes after injury: current issues and future directions]. Trauma Surgery & Acute Care Open, 8(1). *BMJ (Clinical Research Ed.)*, *8*(1), e001068. Advance online publication. DOI: 10.1136/tsaco-2022-001068 PMID: 36919026

Sánchez-Gil, J. J., Sáez-Manzano, A., López-Luque, R., Ochoa-Sepúlveda, J.-J., & Cañete-Carmona, E. (2025). Gamified devices for stroke rehabilitation: A systematic review. *Computer Methods and Programs in Biomedicine*, *258*, 108476. DOI: 10.1016/j.cmpb.2024.108476 PMID: 39520875

Sanchez-Luengos, I., Balboa-Bandeira, Y., Lucas-Jimenez, O., Ojeda, N., Pena, J., & Ibarretxe-Bilbao, N. (2021). Effectiveness of Cognitive Rehabilitation in Parkinson's Disease: A Systematic Review and Meta-Analysis. *Journal of Personalized Medicine*, *11*(5), 429. DOI: 10.3390/jpm11050429 PMID: 34069980

Sanders, Q., & Reinkensmeyer, D. J. (2024). Design and Preliminary Evaluation of a Soft Finger Exoskeleton Controlled by Isometric Grip Force. *Machines (Basel)*, *12*(4), 230. DOI: 10.3390/machines12040230

Sandin, P., Munthe, C., & Björnberg, K. E. (2021). Technology Neutrality in European Regulation of GMOs. In P. Sandin, C. Munthe, & K. E. Björnberg, Ethics Policy & Environment (Vol. 25, Issue 1, p. 52). Taylor & Francis. DOI: 10.1080/21550085.2020.1865085

Sanfilippo, F., Økter, M., Dale, J., Tuan, H. M., Zafar, M. H., & Ottestad, M. (2024). Open-Source Design of Low-Cost Sensorised Elastic Actuators for Collaborative Prosthetics and Orthotics. *HardwareX*, *19*, e00564. DOI: 10.1016/j.ohx.2024.e00564 PMID: 39176378

Santilli, G., Mangone, M., Agostini, F., Paoloni, M., Bernetti, A., Diko, A., Tognolo, L., Coraci, D., Vigevano, F., Vetrano, M., Vulpiani, M. C., Fiore, P., & Gimigliano, F. (2024). Evaluation of rehabilitation outcomes in patients with chronic neurological health conditions using a machine learning approach. *Journal of Functional Morphology and Kinesiology*, *9*(4), 176. DOI: 10.3390/jfmk9040176 PMID: 39449470

Sarkis-Onofre, R., Catalá-López, F., Aromataris, E., & Lockwood, C. (2021). How to properly use the PRISMA Statement. *Systematic Reviews*, *10*(1), 1–3. DOI: 10.1186/s13643-021-01671-z PMID: 33875004

Sartori, M., Llyod, D. G., & Farina, D. (2016). Neural data-driven musculoskeletal modeling for personalized neurorehabilitation technologies. *IEEE Transactions on Biomedical Engineering*, *63*(5), 879–893. DOI: 10.1109/TBME.2016.2538296 PMID: 27046865

Saxena, I., Kumar, M., Bharat, A. S., Verma, A., Garg, S., & Kumar, M. (2015). Effect of Age on Response to Experimental Pain in Normal Indian Males. *Journal of Clinical and Diagnostic Research : JCDR*, *9*(9), CC05–CC08. DOI: 10.7860/JCDR/2015/15385.6516 PMID: 26500901

Saxer, F., Hollinger, A., Bjurström, M. F., Conaghan, P. G., Neogi, T., Schieker, M., & Berenbaum, F. (2024). Pain-phenotyping in osteoarthritis: Current concepts, evidence, and considerations towards a comprehensive framework for assessment and treatment. *Osteoarthritis and Cartilage Open*, *6*(1), 100433. DOI: 10.1016/j.ocarto.2023.100433 PMID: 38225987

Schättin, A., Pickles, J., Flagmeier, D., Schärer, B., Riederer, Y., Niedecken, S., Villiger, S., Jurt, R., Kind, N., Scott, S. N., Stettler, C., & Martin-Niedecken, A. L. (2022). Development of a Novel Home-Based Exergame with on-Body Feedback: Usability Study. *JMIR Serious Games*, *10*(4), e38703. DOI: 10.2196/38703 PMID: 36472900

Scheier, M. F., Carver, C. S., & Bridges, M. W. (1994). Distinguishing Optimism from Neuroticism (and trait anxiety, self-mastery, and self-esteem): A re-evaluation of the Life Orientation Test. *Journal of Personality and Social Psychology*, *67*(6), 1063–1078. DOI: 10.1037/0022-3514.67.6.1063 PMID: 7815302

Schmidt, R., Schemlz, M., Forster, C., Ringcamp, M., Torebjörk, E., & Handwerker, H. (1995). Novel classes of responsive and unresponsive C nociceptors in human skin. *The Journal of Neuroscience : The Official Journal of the Society for Neuroscience*, *15*(1), 333–341. DOI: 10.1523/JNEUROSCI.15-01-00333.1995 PMID: 7823139

Schreiber, D., Yu, Z., Henderson, T., Chen, D., Norbash, A., & Yip, M. C. (2024). CRANE: A Redundant, Multi-Degree-of-Freedom Computed Tomography Robot for Heightened Needle Dexterity within a Medical Imaging Bore. *IEEE Transactions on Robotics*, (99), 1–20. DOI: 10.1109/TRO.2024.3364986

Schultz, B., Agamah, F. E., Ewuoso, C., Madden, E. B., Troyer, J., Skelton, M., & Mwaka, E. (2024). Webinar report: Stakeholder perspectives on informed consent for the use of genomic data by commercial entities. *Journal of Medical Ethics*, *50*(1), 57–61. DOI: 10.1136/jme-2022-108650 PMID: 36941048

Schulz, R.. (2018). Effects of Telemonitoring technology on the long-term care of older adults: An intervention study. *Journal of the American Geriatrics Society*, *66*(8), 1574–1579.

Schwartz, M. S. (2017). *Biofeedback: A Practitioner's Guide* (4th ed.). The Guilford Press.

Schwenk, M., Howe, C., Saleh, A., Mohler, J., Grewal, G., Armstrong, D., & Najafi, B. (2014). Frailty and technology: A systematic review of gait analysis in those with frailty. *Gerontology*, *60*(1), 79–89. DOI: 10.1159/000354211 PMID: 23949441

Schwertfeger, J. L., Beyer, C., Hung, P., Ung, N., Madigan, C., Cortes, A. R., Swaminathan, B., & Madhavan, S. (2023). A map of evidence using transcranial direct current stimulation (tDCS) to improve cognition in adults with traumatic brain injury (TBI). *Frontiers in Neuroergonomics*, *4*, 1170473. DOI: 10.3389/fnrgo.2023.1170473 PMID: 38234478

Sedda, G., Franzosi, R., Mazzone, A., Sanguineti, V., & Colombo, R. (2019). Robot Assisted Exercise: Modelling the Recovery Process to Personalise Therapy. In Converging Clinical and Engineering Research on Neurorehabilitation III: Proceedings of the 4th International Conference on NeuroRehabilitation (ICNR2018), October 16-20, 2018, Pisa, Italy 5 (pp. 236-240). Springer International Publishing.

Seiça, E. C., Mendes, D., Sousa, M. R., & Vide, J. (2024). Artificial Intelligence in Foot and Ankle Surgery. In *Artificial Intelligence in Orthopaedic Surgery Made Easy* (pp. 135–154). Springer. DOI: 10.1007/978-3-031-70310-2_14

Senadheera, I., Hettiarachchi, P., Haslam, B., Nawaratne, R., Sheehan, J., Lockwood, K. J., Alahakoon, D., & Carey, L. M. (2024). AI Applications in Adult Stroke Recovery and Rehabilitation: A Scoping Review Using AI. *Sensors (Basel)*, *24*(20), 6585. DOI: 10.3390/s24206585 PMID: 39460066

Seneviratne, S., Hu, Y., Nguyen, T., Lan, G., Khalifa, S., Thilakarathna, K., Hassan, M., & Seneviratne, A. (2017). A survey of wearable devices and challenges. *IEEE Communications Surveys and Tutorials*, *19*(4), 2573–2620. DOI: 10.1109/COMST.2017.2731979

Shan, L., Chen, Q., Yu, R., Gao, C., Liu, L., Guo, T., & Chen, H. (2023). A sensory memory processing system with multi-wavelength synaptic-polychromatic light emission for multi-modal information recognition. *Nature Communications*, *14*(1), 2648. DOI: 10.1038/s41467-023-38396-7 PMID: 37156788

Shao, Y., Li, T., Shi, W., Liu, Y., & Yang, D. (2024). *PrivacyLens: Evaluating Privacy Norm Awareness of Language Models in Action*

Sharma, R., Agarwal, P., & Mahapatra, R. P. (2020). Evolution in big data analytics on internet of things: applications and future plan. In *Multimedia Big Data Computing for IoT Applications* (pp. 453–477). Springer., DOI: 10.1007/978-981-13-8759-3_18

Shefa, F. R., Sifat, F. H., Uddin, J., Ahmad, Z., Kim, J.-M., & Kibria, M. G. (2024). Deep Learning and IoT-Based Ankle–Foot Orthosis for Enhanced Gait Optimization. [MDPI.]. *Health Care*, *12*, 2273. PMID: 39595470

Sherstinsky, A. (2020). Fundamentals of recurrent neural network (RNN) and long short-term memory (LSTM) network. *Physica D. Nonlinear Phenomena, 404*, 132306. DOI: 10.1016/j.physd.2019.132306

Shinohara, K., & Wobbrock, J. O. (2011). "In the shadow of misperception: assistive technology use and social interactions." CHI Conference on Human Factors in Computing Systems. ACM Digital Library: https://dl.acm.org/doi/10.1145/1978942.1979044

Shrestha, A. B., Taha, A. M., Siddiq, A., Shrestha, S., Thakur, P., Chapagain, S., Sharma, S., Halder, A., Rajak, K., & Shah, V. (2024). Virtual and augmented reality in cardiovascular care in low and middle income country. *Current Problems in Cardiology*, *49*(3), 102380. DOI: 10.1016/j.cpcardiol.2024.102380 PMID: 38191103

Shtar, G., Rokach, L., Shapira, B., Nissan, R., & Hershkovitz, A. (2021). Using machine learning to predict rehabilitation outcomes in postacute hip fracture patients. [Elsevier.]. *Archives of Physical Medicine and Rehabilitation*, *102*(3), 386–394. DOI: 10.1016/j.apmr.2020.08.011 PMID: 32949551

Shull, P. B., Jirattigalachote, W., Hunt, M. A., Cutkosky, M. R., & Delp, S. L. (2014). Quantified self and human movement: A review on the clinical impact of wearable sensing and feedback for gait analysis and intervention. *Gait & Posture*, *40*(1), 11–19. DOI: 10.1016/j.gaitpost.2014.03.189 PMID: 24768525

Singh, N. a. (2024). Securing Cloud-Based Internet of Things: Challenges and Mitigations. *arXiv preprint arXiv:2402.00356.*

Singh, J., Bagga, S., & Kaur, R. (2020). Software-based Prediction of Liver Disease with Feature Selection and Classification Techniques. *Procedia Computer Science*, *167*, 1970–1980. DOI: 10.1016/j.procs.2020.03.226

Singh, R., Sharma, L., & Verma, H. (2023). Natural Language Processing in Assistive Communication. *Speech and Language Technologies*, *7*(1), 75–93.

Sivakumar, C., Mone, V., & Abdumukhtor, R. (2024). Addressing privacy concerns with wearable health monitoring technology. *Wiley Interdisciplinary Reviews. Data Mining and Knowledge Discovery*, *14*(3), 1535. DOI: 10.1002/widm.1535

Smith, A. A., Li, R., & Tse, Z. T. H. (2023). Reshaping healthcare with wearable biosensors. *Scientific Reports*, *13*(1), 4998. DOI: 10.1038/s41598-022-26951-z PMID: 36973262

Smith, B. W., Dalen, J., Wiggins, K., Tooley, E., Christopher, P., & Bernard, J. (2008). The brief resilience scale: Assessing the ability to bounce back. *International Journal of Behavioral Medicine*, *15*(3), 194–200. DOI: 10.1080/10705500802222972 PMID: 18696313

Smith, T., Zhang, L., & Huang, R. (2020). Intelligent Prosthetics: A Review of AI Integration. *Biomedical Engineering Advances*, *14*(5), 234–251.

Soufineyestani, M., Dowling, D., & Khan, A. (2020). Electroencephalography (EEG) technology applications and available devices. *Applied Sciences (Basel, Switzerland)*, *10*(21), 7453. DOI: 10.3390/app10217453

Spies, N. C., Rangel, A., English, P., Morrison, M., O'Fallon, B., & Ng, D. P. (2025). Machine Learning Methods in Clinical Flow Cytometry. *Cancers (Basel)*, *17*(3), 3. Advance online publication. DOI: 10.3390/cancers17030483 PMID: 39941850

Sreejith, S., Khanna Nehemiah, H., & Kannan, A. (2020). Clinical data classification using an enhanced SMOTE and chaotic evolutionary feature selection. *Computers in Biology and Medicine*, *126*, 103991. DOI: 10.1016/j.compbiomed.2020.103991 PMID: 32987205

Srivastava, R. (2021). AI-based predictive health monitoring: A paradigm shift. *IEEE Engineering in Medicine and Biology Magazine*, *40*(5), 35–45.

Stenum, J., Cherry-Allen, K. M., Pyles, C. O., Reetzke, R. D., Vignos, M. F., & Roemmich, R. T. (2021). Applications of pose estimation in human health and performance across the lifespan. *Sensors (Basel)*, *21*(21), 7315.

Stewart-Williams, S., & Podd, J. (2004). The placebo effect: Dissolving the expectancy versus conditioning debate. *Psychological Bulletin*, *130*(2), 324–340. DOI: 10.1037/0033-2909.130.2.324 PMID: 14979775

Stinear, C. M. (2007). Functional potential in chronic stroke patients depends on corticospinal tract integrity. *Brain*, •••, 170–180. PMID: 17148468

Sturgeon, J. A., & Zautra, A. J. (2010). Resilience: A New Paradigm for Adaptation to Chronic Pain. *Current Pain and Headache Reports*, *14*(2), 105–112. DOI: 10.1007/s11916-010-0095-9 PMID: 20425199

Subramanian, N.. (2019). Social engagement through technology: Challenges and opportunities. *International Journal of Aging & Human Development*, *89*(3), 292–308.

Sullivan, M. J., Bishop, S. R., & Pivik, J. (1995). The Pain Catastrophizing Scale: Development and validation. *Psychological Assessment*, *7*(4), 524–532. https://psycnet.apa.org/doi/10.1037/1040-3590.7.4.524. DOI: 10.1037/1040-3590.7.4.524

Sun, J., Wang, Z., Zhang, S., He, X., Zhao, H., Zhang, G., & Zhou, X. (2022). "One-pose: One-Shot Object Pose Estimation without Cad Models." In *Proceedings of the IEEE/CVF Conference on Computer Vision and Pattern Recognition*, 6825–34. DOI: 10.1109/CVPR52688.2022.00670

Sun, X., & Freeman, C. T. (2024). Parameterised function ILC with application to stroke rehabilitation. *Control Engineering Practice*, *145*, 105878. DOI: 10.1016/j.conengprac.2024.105878

Surgical, I. (2013). da Vinci. Surgical System. http://www. intusurg. com/html/davinci. html

Swieboda, P., Filip, R., Prystupa, A., & Drozd, M. (2013). Assessment of pain: Types, mechanism and treatment. *Annals of Agricultural and Environmental Medicine*, *20*(1), 2–7. PMID: 25000833

Tagliaferri, S. D., Wilkin, T., Angelova, M., Fitzgibbon, B. M., Own, P. J., Miller, C. T., & Belavy, D. L. (2022). Chronic back pain sub-grouped via psychosocial, brain and physical factors using machine learning. *Scientific Reports*, *12*(1), 15194. Advance online publication. DOI: 10.1038/s41598-022-19542-5 PMID: 36071092

Takacs, B. (2006). Cognitive, mental, and physical rehabilitation using a configurable virtual reality system. [Citeseer.]. *The International Journal of Virtual Reality : a Multimedia Publication for Professionals*, *5*(4), 1–12.

Talaat, F. M. (2022). Effective Deep Q-Networks (EDQN) Strategy for Resource Allocation Based on Optimized Reinforcement Learning Algorithm. *Multimedia Tools and Applications*, *81*(28), 39945–39961. DOI: 10.1007/s11042-022-13000-0

Taleb, W. B., Snoun, A., Bouchrika, T., & Jemai, O. (2022). "Reinforcement Learning for Assistance of Alzheimer's Disease Patients." In *2022 8th International Conference on Control, Decision and Information Technologies (CoDIT)*, 1:274–79. IEEE.

Tang, C., Xu, Z., Occhipinti, E., Yi, W., Xu, M., Kumar, S., Virk, G. S., Gao, S., & Occhipinti, L. G. (2023). From brain to movement: Wearables-based motion intention prediction across the human nervous system. *Nano Energy*, *115*, 108712. DOI: 10.1016/j.nanoen.2023.108712

Tao, W., Liu, T., Zheng, R., & Feng, H. (2012). Gait analysis using wearable sensors. *Sensors (Basel)*, *12*(2), 2255–2283. DOI: 10.3390/s120202255 PMID: 22438763

Tariq, M. U. (2024). Application of blockchain and Internet of Things (IoT) in modern business. In Sinha, M., Bhandari, A., Priya, S., & Kabiraj, S. (Eds.), *Future of customer engagement through marketing intelligence* (pp. 66–94). IGI Global., DOI: 10.4018/979-8-3693-2367-0.ch004

Tariq, M. U. (2024). Emerging trends and innovations in blockchain-digital twin integration for green investments: A case study perspective. In Jafar, S., Rodriguez, R., Kannan, H., Akhtar, S., & Plugmann, P. (Eds.), *Harnessing blockchain-digital twin fusion for sustainable investments* (pp. 148–175). IGI Global., DOI: 10.4018/979-8-3693-1878-2.ch007

Tariq, M. U. (2024). Emotional intelligence in understanding and influencing consumer behavior. In Musiolik, T., Rodriguez, R., & Kannan, H. (Eds.), *AI impacts in digital consumer behavior* (pp. 56–81). IGI Global., DOI: 10.4018/979-8-3693-1918-5.ch003

Tariq, M. U. (2025). Cultivating Cultural Intelligence for the Global Workforce. In Huzooree, G., & Chandan, H. (Eds.), *Revitalizing Student Skills for Workforce Preparation* (pp. 297–332). IGI Global., DOI: 10.4018/979-8-3693-3856-8.ch010

Tariq, M. U. (2025). Leveraging Open Innovation for Sustainable Growth in the Digital Era. In Taherdoost, H. (Ed.), *Mastering Innovation in Business* (pp. 157–192). IGI Global., DOI: 10.4018/979-8-3693-3759-2.ch007

Tariq, M. U. (2025). Vision and Strategy: Steering Modern Enterprises Towards Long-Term Success. In Sedky, A. (Ed.), *Resiliency Strategies for Long-Term Business Success* (pp. 51–78). IGI Global., DOI: 10.4018/979-8-3693-9168-6.ch003

Teng, B., Zhang, X., Ge, M., Miao, M., Li, W., & Ma, J. (2024). Personalized three-year survival prediction and prognosis forecast by interpretable machine learning for pancreatic cancer patients: A population-based study and an external validation. *Frontiers in Oncology, 14*, 1488118. DOI: 10.3389/fonc.2024.1488118 PMID: 39497722

Thirunavukkarasu, K., Singh, A. S., Irfan, M., & Chowdhury, A. (2018). Prediction of Liver Disease using Classification Algorithms. *2018 4th International Conference on Computing Communication and Automation (ICCCA)*, 1–3. DOI: 10.1109/CCAA.2018.8777655

Thompson, W. G. (1989). Proctalgia Fugax. In *Gut Reactions* (pp. 259–267). Springer., DOI: 10.1007/978-1-4899-6491-5_17

Thornton, T., & Sanchez, A. (2020). The role of wearable technology in promoting physical activity among older adults. *Journal of Aging and Physical Activity, 28*(2), 241–256.

Tian, Y., Vaskov, A. K., Adidharma, W., Cederna, P. S., & Kemp, S. W. P. (2024). Merging Humans and Neuroprosthetics through Regenerative Peripheral Nerve Interfaces. *Seminars in Plastic Surgery, 38*(01), 010–018. DOI: 10.1055/s-0044-1779028

Tizi, W., & Berrado, A. (2023). Machine learning for survival analysis in cancer research: A comparative study. *Scientific African*, *21*, e01880. DOI: 10.1016/j.sciaf.2023.e01880

Topo, E. J. (2016). Technology and human interaction: Elderly individuals' perspectives. *Journal of Applied Gerontology*, *35*(5), 534–548.

Tousignant-Laflamme, Y., Houle, C., Cook, C., Naye, F., LeBlanc, A., & Décary, S. (2022). Mastering prognostic tools: An opportunity to enhance personalized care and to optimize clinical outcomes in physical therapy. *Physical Therapy*, *102*(5), pzac023. DOI: 10.1093/ptj/pzac023 PMID: 35202464

Tran, D. A., Pajaro-Blazquez, M., Daneault, J. F., Gallegos, J. G., Pons, J., Fregni, F., Bonato, P., & Zafonte, R. (2016). Combining dopaminergic facilitation with robot-assisted upper limb therapy in stroke survivors: A focused review. *American Journal of Physical Medicine & Rehabilitation*, *95*(6), 459–474. DOI: 10.1097/PHM.0000000000000438 PMID: 26829074

Triwiyanto, T., Caesarendra, W., Ahmed, A. A., & Abdullayev, V. H. (2023). How Deep Learning and Neural Networks Can Improve Prosthetics and Exoskeletons: A Review of State-of-the-Art Methods and Challenges. *Journal of Electronics, Electromedical Engineering, and Medical Informatics*, *5*(4), 277–289. DOI: 10.35882/jeeemi.v5i4.333

Turk, D. C., & Swanson, K. S. (2008). Psychological Interventions. In *Raj's Practical Management of Pain* (4th ed., pp. 739–755). Mosby., DOI: 10.1016/B978-032304184-3.50042-X

Turk, D. C., Swanson, K. S., & Tunks, E. R. (2008). Psychological Approaches in the Treatment of Chronic Pain Patients—When Pills, Scalpels, and Needles Are Not Enough. *Canadian Journal of Psychiatry*, *53*(4), 213–223. DOI: 10.1177/070674370805300402 PMID: 18478824

Ueshima, H., Sekikawa, A., Miura, K., Turin, T. C., Takashima, N., Kita, Y., Watanabe, M., Kadota, A., Okuda, N., Kadowaki, T., Nakamura, Y., & Okamura, T. (2008). Cardiovascular disease and risk factors in Asia: A selected review. *Circulation*, *118*(25), 2702–2709. DOI: 10.1161/CIRCULATIONAHA.108.790048 PMID: 19106393

Vaia, S., Iavarone, A., Moschiano, F., Strube, C., Gamboz, N., De Pietro, G., Gentile, S., Garofalo, E., Sannino, M., & Mazzi, M. C. (2022). Computer-Aided Cognitive Training in Patients with Neurocognitive Vascular Impairment: Effects on Cognition, Depression and Behavior. *JOURNAL OF GERONTOLOGY AND GERIATRICS*, *70*(2), 99–104. DOI: 10.36150/2499-6564-N357

Valero-Cuevas, F. J., Finley, J., Orsborn, A., Fung, N., Hicks, J. L., Huang, H., Reinkensmeyer, D., Schweighofer, N., Weber, D., & Steele, K. M. (2024). NSF DARE—Transforming modeling in neurorehabilitation: Four threads for catalyzing progress. *Journal of Neuroengineering and Rehabilitation*, *21*(1), 46. DOI: 10.1186/s12984-024-01324-x PMID: 38570842

Vallabh, P., & Malekian, R. (2018). Fall detection monitoring systems: A comprehensive review. *Journal of Ambient Intelligence and Humanized Computing*, *9*(6), 1809–1833. DOI: 10.1007/s12652-017-0592-3

Van Hooren, B., Goudsmit, J., Restrepo, J., & Vos, S. (2020). Real-time feedback by wearables in running: Current approaches, challenges and suggestions for improvements. *Journal of Sports Sciences*, *38*(2), 214–230. DOI: 10.1080/02640414.2019.1690960 PMID: 31795815

van Valkenhoef, G., Kuiper, J., & van Valkenhoef, M. G. (2016). Package 'gemtc'.

Vapnik, V. (1995). Support-vector networks. *Machine Learning*, *20*(3), 273–297. DOI: 10.1007/BF00994018

Vapnik, V., & Chapelle, O. (2000). Bounds on error expectation for support vector machines. *Neural Computation*, *12*(9), 2013–2036. DOI: 10.1162/089976600300015042 PMID: 10976137

Vaswani, A. (2017). Attention is all you need. *Advances in Neural Information Processing Systems*.

Vats, V., Zhang, L., Chatterjee, S., Ahmed, S., Enziama, E., & Tepe, K. (n.d.). A Comparative Analysis of Unsupervised Machine Techniques for Liver Disease Prediction. *A. K.*

Veeranki, S. R., & Varshney, M. (2022). Intelligent Techniques and Comparative Performance Analysis of Liver Disease Prediction. *International Journal of Mechanical Engineering*, *7*(1).

Vélez-Guerrero, M. A., Callejas-Cuervo, M., & Mazzoleni, S. (2021). Artificial Intelligence-Based Wearable Robotic Exoskeletons for Upper Limb Rehabilitation: A Review. *Sensors (Basel)*, *21*(6), 2146. DOI: 10.3390/s21062146 PMID: 33803911

Vergaray, A. D., Miranda, J. C. H., Cornelio, J. B., Carranza, A. R. L., & Sanchez, C. F. P. (2023). Prediction of Heart Disease Using Machine Learning: A Systematic Literature Review. *Journal of System and Management Sciences*, *13*(6), 40–60. DOI: 10.33168/JSMS.2023.0603

Villalba-Meneses, F., Guevara, C., Lojan, A. B., Gualsaqui, M. G., Arias-Serrano, I., Velásquez-López, P. A., Almeida-Galárraga, D., Tirado-Espín, A., Marín, J., & Marín, J. J. (2024). Classification of the Pathological Range of Motion in Low Back Pain Using Wearable Sensors and Machine Learning. *Sensors (Basel)*, *24*(3), 831. DOI: 10.3390/s24030831 PMID: 38339548

Visweswaran, S., Sadhu, E. M., Morris, M., & Samayamuthu, M. J. (2023). Clinical Algorithms with Race: An Online Database. In S. Visweswaran, E. M. Sadhu, M. Morris, & M. J. Samayamuthu, medRxiv (Cold Spring Harbor Laboratory). Cold Spring Harbor Laboratory. DOI: 10.1101/2023.07.04.23292231

von Baeyer, C. L., Piira, T., Chambers, C. T., Trapanotto, M., & Zeltzer, L. K. (2005). Guidelines for the cold pressor task as an experimental pain stimulus for use with children. *The Journal of Pain*, *6*(4), 218–227. DOI: 10.1016/j.jpain.2005.01.349 PMID: 15820909

Vu, P. P., Vaskov, A. K., Lee, C., Jillala, R. R., Wallace, D. M., Davis, A. J., Kung, T. A., Kemp, S. W. P., Gates, D. H., Chestek, C. A., & Cederna, P. S. (2023). Long-Term Upper-Extremity Prosthetic Control Using Regenerative Peripheral Nerve Interfaces and Implanted EMG Electrodes. *Journal of Neural Engineering*, *20*(2), 026039. DOI: 10.1088/1741-2552/accb0c PMID: 37023743

Walz, W. (2024). The Brain as an Organ. In *The Gliocentric Brain* (pp. 7–27). Phenotype Plasticity of the Damaged Brain.

Wang, S., & Zhou, G. (2015). A review on radio based activity recognition. In Digital Communications and Networks (Vol. 1, Issue 1, pp. 20–29). Elsevier BV. DOI: 10.1016/j.dcan.2015.02.006

Wang, Z., ... (2020). "Deep learning algorithms in medical prediction." Journal of Biomedical Informatics. ScienceDirect: https://www.sciencedirect.com/science/article/pii/S1532046420301203

Wang, L. (Eds.). (2010). *Machine learning for vision-based motion analysis: Theory and techniques*. Springer Science & Business Media. DOI: 10.4018/978-1-60566-900-7

Wang, P., Li, Y., & Reddy, C. K. (2019). Machine learning for survival analysis: A survey. *ACM Computing Surveys*, *51*(6), 1–36. DOI: 10.1145/3214306

Wang, Q., Markopoulos, P., Yu, B., Chen, W., & Timmermans, A. (2017). Interactive wearable systems for upper body rehabilitation: A systematic review. *Journal of Neuroengineering and Rehabilitation*, *14*(1), 20. DOI: 10.1186/s12984-017-0229-y PMID: 28284228

Wang, T., Xu, J., & Lin, H. (2021). AI for Human-Machine Interfaces in Prosthetics. *Journal of Machine Learning Applications*, *13*(5), 456–473.

Wan, M., Simonin, E. M., Johnson, M. M., Zhang, X., Lin, X., Gao, P., Patel, C. J., Yousuf, A., Snyder, M. P., Hong, X., Wang, X., Sampath, V., & Nadeau, K. C. (2025). Exposomics: A review of methodologies, applications, and future directions in molecular medicine. *EMBO Molecular Medicine*, *17*(4), 1–10. DOI: 10.1038/s44321-025-00191-w PMID: 39870881

Waqas, M., & Humphries, U. W. (2024). A critical review of RNN and LSTM variants in hydrological time series predictions. *MethodsX*, *13*, 102946. DOI: 10.1016/j.mex.2024.102946 PMID: 39324077

Watson, D., Clark, L. A., & Tellegan, A. (1988). Development and validation of brief measures of positive and negative affect: The PANAS Scales. *Journal of Personality and Social Psychology*, *54*(6), 1063–1070. DOI: 10.1037/0022-3514.54.6.1063 PMID: 3397865

Waydhas, C., Ull, C., Cruciger, O., Hamsen, U., Schildhauer, T. A., Gaschler, R., & Weckwerth, C. (2024). Behavioral pain scale may not be reliable in awake non-verbal intensive care patients: A case control study. *BMC Anesthesiology*, *24*(1), 84. DOI: 10.1186/s12871-024-02472-2 PMID: 38424502

Webber, C. M., Riberdy, A., Saha, A., Marinac-Dabić, D., Caños, D., & Tarver, M. E. (2023). Integrating Patient-Generated Health Data Throughout the Total Product Life Cycle of Medical Devices [Review of Integrating Patient-Generated Health Data Throughout the Total Product Life Cycle of Medical Devices]. Therapeutic Innovation & Regulatory Science, 57(5), 952. Springer Science+Business Media. DOI: 10.1007/s43441-023-00505-5

Weber, N. a. (2017). Unsupervised learning in human activity recognition: A first foray into clustering data gathered from wearable sensors.

White, H., & Taylor, J. (2022). NLP in Assistive Communication Devices: A Review. *Applied Artificial Intelligence*, *39*(8), 564–580.

Whitfield, M. C. (2021). Robotic caregivers: Ethics and practice. *AI & Society*, *35*(2), 413–424.

Williams, C., Vakanski, A., Lee, S., & Paul, D. (2019). Assessment of physical rehabilitation movements through dimensionality reduction and statistical modeling. *Medical Engineering & Physics*, *74*, 13–22. DOI: 10.1016/j.medengphy.2019.10.003 PMID: 31668858

Wilson, G., & Brown, C. (2023). AI Prosthetics and User-Centered Design. *Human Factors in Engineering*, *14*(3), 87–110.

Winstein, C. J., & Kay, D. B. (2015). Translating the science into practice: Shaping rehabilitation practice to enhance recovery after brain damage. *Progress in Brain Research*, *218*, 331–360. DOI: 10.1016/bs.pbr.2015.01.004 PMID: 25890145

Winstein, C. J., Stein, J., Arena, R., Bates, B., Cherney, L. R., Cramer, S. C., Deruyter, F., Eng, J. J., Fisher, B., Harvey, R. L., Lang, C. E., MacKay-Lyons, M., Ottenbacher, K. J., Pugh, S., Reeves, M. J., Richards, L. G., Stiers, W., & Zorowitz, R. D. (2016). Guidelines for Adult Stroke Rehabilitation and Recovery: A Guideline for Healthcare Professionals from the American Heart Association/American Stroke Association. *Stroke*, *47*(6), e98–e169. DOI: 10.1161/STR.0000000000000098 PMID: 27145936

World Health Organization (WHO). (2017, March 25). Cardiovascular diseases fact sheet. https://www.who.int/mediacentre/factsheets/fs317/en/

World Health Organization. "Assistive technology," 2018. [Online]; https://www.who.int/news-room/fact-sheets/detail/assistive-technology

Wu, C. C., Yeh, W. C., Hsu, W. D., Islam, M. M., Nguyen, P. A. A., Poly, T. N., & Li, Y. C. J. (2019). Prediction of fatty liver disease using machine learning algorithms. *Computer Methods and Programs in Biomedicine*, *170*, 23–29.

Xin, Y., Owen, R., Bradbury, N., Cooper, N., & Sutton, A. MetaInsight. https://crsu.shinyapps.io/MetaInsight/. Accessed 05 February 2025.

Xu, K., Ba, J., Kiros, R., Cho, K., Courville, A., Salakhudinov, R., . . . Bengio, Y. (2015, June). Show, attend and tell: Neural image caption generation with visual attention. In International conference on machine learning (pp. 2048-2057). PMLR.

Xu, S., Liu, Y., Lee, H., & Li, W. (2024). Neural interfaces: Bridging the brain to the world beyond healthcare. *Exploration*, *4*(5), 20230146. DOI: 10.1002/EXP.20230146 PMID: 39439491

Yadav, S. K., Tiwari, K., Pandey, H. M., & Akbar, S. A. (2021). A review of multimodal human activity recognition with special emphasis on classification, applications, challenges and future directions. In *Knowledge-Based Systems* (Vol. 223, p. 106970). Elsevier BV., DOI: 10.1016/j.knosys.2021.106970

Yamada, K.. (2019). Augmented reality (AR) glasses and cognitive aids for seniors with mild dementia. *Journal of Ambient Intelligence and Humanized Computing*, *10*(3), 1129–1139.

Yang, J., Nguyen, M. N., San, P. P., Li, X., & Krishnaswamy, S. (2015, July). Deep convolutional neural networks on multichannel time series for human activity recognition. In Ijcai (Vol. 15, pp. 3995-4001).

Yang, J., & Wu, Q. (2023). Optimizing NLP Algorithms for Accessibility. *Natural Language Processing Applications*, *15*(2), 340–360.

Yan, X., Wang, W., Xiao, M., Li, Y., & Gao, M. (2024, March). Survival prediction across diverse cancer types using neural networks. In *Proceedings of the 2024 7th International Conference on Machine Vision and Applications* (pp. 134-138). DOI: 10.1145/3653946.3653966

Yao, Y., Shao, D., Tarabini, M., Moezi, S. A., Li, K., & Saccomandi, P. (2024). Advancements in Sensor Technologies and Control Strategies for Lower-Limb Rehabilitation Exoskeletons: A Comprehensive Review. *Micromachines*, *15*(4), 489. DOI: 10.3390/mi15040489 PMID: 38675301

Yılmaz, H., & Özdem, M. (2024). EyeMo: A Solution for Individuals with Disabilities to Use a Computer Through Eye Movements. *Gazi University Journal of Science Part C: Design and Technology*, *12*(1), 1–1. DOI: 10.29109/gujsc.1404305

Yoo, J., & Shoaran, M. (2021). Neural Interface Systems with On-Device Computing: Machine Learning and Neuromorphic Architectures. *Current Opinion in Biotechnology*, *72*, 95–101. DOI: 10.1016/j.copbio.2021.10.012 PMID: 34735990

Young, F., Mason, R., Morris, R. E., Stuart, S., & Godfrey, A. (2023). IoT-enabled gait assessment: The next step for habitual monitoring. *Sensors (Basel)*, *23*(8), 4100.

Yu, L., Zeng, Z., Liu, A., Xie, X., Wang, H., Xu, F., & Hong, W. (2022). A Lightweight Complex-Valued DeepLabv3+ for Semantic Segmentation of PolSAR Image. *IEEE Journal of Selected Topics in Applied Earth Observations and Remote Sensing*, *15*, 930–943. DOI: 10.1109/JSTARS.2021.3140101

Yurtman, A. a. (2019). Novel noniterative orientation estimation for wearable motion sensor units acquiring accelerometer, gyroscope, and magnetometer measurements. *IEEE Transactions on Instrumentation and Measurement*, •••, 3206–3215.

Zaidan, M. A., Xie, Y., Motlagh, N. H., Wang, B., Nie, W., Nurmi, P., Tarkoma, S., Petaja, T., Ding, A., & Kulmala, M. (2022). Dense air quality sensor networks: Validation, analysis, and benefits. *IEEE Sensors Journal*, *22*(23), 23507–23520. DOI: 10.1109/JSEN.2022.3216071

Zautra, A., Smith, B., Affleck, G., & Tennen, H. (2001). Examinations of chronic pain and affect relationships: Applications of a dynamic model of affect. *Journal of Consulting and Clinical Psychology*, *69*(5), 786–795. DOI: 10.1037/0022-006X.69.5.786 PMID: 11680555

Zhang, Q., Jin, T., Cai, J., Xu, L., He, T., Wang, T., Tian, Y., Li, L., Peng, Y., & Lee, C. (2021). Wearable Triboelectric Sensors Enabled Gait Analysis and Waist Motion Capture for IoT-Based Smart Healthcare Applications. In Q. Zhang, T. Jin, J. Cai, L. Xu, T. He, T. Wang, Y. Tian, L. Li, Y. Peng, & C. Lee, Advanced Science (Vol. 9, Issue 4). Wiley. DOI: 10.1002/advs.202103694

Zhang, H., Le Jiao, S. Y., Li, H., Jiang, X., Feng, J., Zou, S., Xu, Q., Gu, J., & Wang, X. (2024). Brain–Computer Interfaces: The Innovative Key to Unlocking Neurological Conditions. *International Journal of Surgery*, *110*(9), 5745–5762. DOI: 10.1097/JS9.0000000000002022 PMID: 39166947

Zhang, L., Yu, J., Gao, Z., & Ni, Q. (2024). A multi-channel hybrid deep learning framework for multi-sensor fusion enabled human activity recognition. *Alexandria Engineering Journal*, *91*, 472–485. DOI: 10.1016/j.aej.2024.01.030

Zhang, L., & Yu, P. (2022). Gesture Recognition for NLP-Powered Devices. *Sensors and Actuators*, *34*(1), 15–30.

Zhang, Q., Zhang, Z., Huang, X., Zhou, C., & Xu, J. (2022). Application of logistic regression and decision tree models in the prediction of activities of daily living in patients with stroke. [Wiley Online Library.]. *Neural Plasticity*, *2022*(1), 9662630. DOI: 10.1155/2022/9662630 PMID: 35126507

Zhang, S., Jung, K., Langner, R., Florin, E., Eickhoff, S. B., & Popovych, O. V. (2024). Impact of data processing varieties on DCM estimates of effective connectivity from task-fMRI. *Human Brain Mapping*, *45*(8), 26751. DOI: 10.1002/hbm.26751 PMID: 38864293

Zhang, X., Rong, X., & Luo, H. (2024). Optimizing lower limb rehabilitation: The intersection of machine learning and rehabilitative robotics. *Frontiers in Rehabilitation Sciences*, *5*, 1246773. DOI: 10.3389/fresc.2024.1246773 PMID: 38343790

Zhang, X., Zhang, X., Chen, W., Li, C., & Yu, C. (2024). Improving Speech Depression Detection Using Transfer Learning with Wav2vec 2.0 in Low-Resource Environments. *Scientific Reports*, *14*(1), 9543. DOI: 10.1038/s41598-024-60278-1 PMID: 38664511

Zhang, Y., Cheng, K., & Zhang, L. (2023). 3D Model Construction System for Personalized Rehabilitation Prosthetics Based on Machine Vision. *International Journal of Biology and Life Sciences*, *2*(2), 1–7. DOI: 10.54097/ijbls.v2i2.6140

Zhang, Y., Wang, X., & Zhao, Q. (2023). Real-Time Feedback in AI Prosthetics. *International Journal of Bioinformatics Research*, *18*(2), 89–110.

Zhang, Y., Zheng, Y., Wang, M., & Guo, X. (2021). Prediction of exercise sudden death in rabbit exhaustive swimming using deep neural network. *Biomedical Engineering Online*, *20*(1), 87. DOI: 10.1186/s12938-021-00925-0 PMID: 34461905

Zhao, F., & Sun, L. (2022). Deep Learning in Assistive Technologies. *Deep Learning Applications in Healthcare*, *5*(6), 78–101.

Zhao, X., Dannenberg, K., Repsibler, D., Gerdle, B., Molander, P., & Hesser, H. (2024). Prognostic subgroups of chronic pain patients using latent variable mixture modeling within a supervised machine learning framework. *Scientific Reports*, *14*(1), 12543. Advance online publication. DOI: 10.1038/s41598-024-62542-w PMID: 38822075

Zheng, Y. L., Ding, X. R., Poon, C. C. Y., Lo, B. P. L., Zhang, H., Zhou, X. L., Yang, G.-Z., Zhao, N., & Zhang, Y. T. (2014). Unobtrusive sensing and wearable devices for health informatics. *IEEE Transactions on Biomedical Engineering*, *61*(5), 1538–1554. DOI: 10.1109/TBME.2014.2309951 PMID: 24759283

Zhetenbayev, N. a. (2023). Developing of a wearable ankle rehabilitation robotic device. *Vibroengineering Procedia*, 36--41.

Zhou, S., Ma, Q., Lou, Y., Lv, X., Tian, H., Wei, J., Zhang, K., Zhu, G., Chen, Q., Si, T., Wang, G., Wang, X., Zhang, N., Huang, Y., Liu, Q., & Yu, X. (2021). Machine Learning to Predict Clinical Remission in Depressed Patients after Acute Phase Selective Serotonin Reuptake Inhibitor Treatment. *Journal of Affective Disorders*, *287*, 372–379. DOI: 10.1016/j.jad.2021.03.079 PMID: 33836365

Zini, F., Le Piane, F., & Gaspari, M. (2022). Adaptive Cognitive Training with Reinforcement Learning. [TiiS]. *ACM Transactions on Interactive Intelligent Systems*, *12*(1), 1–29. DOI: 10.1145/3476777

Zou, J., Zhang, X., Zhang, Y., & Jin, Z. (2024). Prediction of Medial Knee Contact Force Using Multisource Fusion Recurrent Neural Network and Transfer Learning. *Medical & Biological Engineering & Computing*, *62*(5), 1333–1346. DOI: 10.1007/s11517-023-03011-w PMID: 38182944

Zwijsen, K., Niemeijer, A., & Hertogh, C. M. (2011). Ethics of using assistive technology in the care for community-dwelling elderly people: An overview of the literature. *Aging & Mental Health, 15*(4), 419–427. DOI: 10.1080/13607863.2010.543662 PMID: 21500008

About the Contributors

Rajesh Kumar K V is a distinguished academic and researcher currently serving as Chief Technological Scientist at the AI Research Centre and Associate Professor at the School of Business - Business Analytics department, Woxsen University, Hyderabad, India. Currently, he is leading an engineering team working on interdisciplinary research projects. He holds the prestigious Chair Professor of France Belanger of Information Systems and is actively involved as Co-Chairperson of the Centre of Excellence – Sports Analytics and Management. Furthermore, he is the Advertflair Chair Professor in Marketing and Advertising, specializing in AI Projects. His academic credentials include an M. Tech in Embedded Systems and a Ph.D. in Applied Artificial Intelligence in biomechanical engineering. His research specialization is Human Computer Interface-based signal Data Analytics for Bio-Medical Applications, Machine and Deep Learning, and Business Analytics. In 2022, he showcased his expertise in sports analytics at the Data Con LA+ IM Data 2022 conference in the US, California. His significant research contributions were recognized at ICRA 2023-UK in a workshop on Computer Vision for Wearable Robotics by Harvard University. He recently attended as a panel member to discuss "Digital landscape – Beyond AI" at the Digital Innovation Summit – Bucharest, Romania, and "How AI is changing the landscape of work" at the AI Tech Summit in April 2024, in Malaga, Spain. Recently he participated as a panel member to discuss "Future Cars: How Does it Looks Like" at the MOVE Conference, in June 2024 in London, UK.

Padmini Ranasinghe, MD MPH is an Assistant Professor at Johns Hopkins School of Medicine. After completing her medical education in Colombo Medical Faculty in Sri Lanka, she completed a residency in combined Internal Medicine and Preventive Medicine along with an MPH at Yale School of Public Health. She is a fellow of ACP, ACPM, and SHM. She is a clinician, educator, and researcher. Currently serving as co-director of education in the Division of Hospital Medicine.

She teachers and mentors' medical students, residents, and public health students. Her research interests are in the health and wellness of medical students, residents, and practicing physicians, disaster medicine, climates and health, global health, chronic disease prevention, health informatics/role of AI in health care, and advocacy & policy. At national level, she has been active in American Medical Association (AMA) and has served as chair of the AMA International Medical Graduate Section for 2013-14. She has been elected to serve on the Council on Science and Public Health (CSAPH) and is currently a member of its executive committee. The mission of the council is to represent the AMA's core belief that scientific evidence is the basis for improving the quality of patient care, promoting medical progress, and enhancing the health of the public. At the state level, she has been elected as the president-elect to MedChi, Maryland State Medical Society to represent physicians of Maryland.

Dorianne Feldman is an assistant professor of physical medicine and rehabilitation at the Johns Hopkins University School of Medicine. She focuses on critical care physical medicine and rehabilitation. She combines both her skills as a physical therapist and physiatrist when treating her patients. Dr. Feldman holds B.S. and M.S.P.T. degrees from Boston University, and received her M.D. from the George Washington University School of Medicine. Following medical school, she completed a preliminary year in internal medicine at Mercy Medical Center/ University of Maryland and then a residency in physical medicine and rehabilitation at the Johns Hopkins University School of Medicine. She served as chief resident from 2008-2009 for the Department of Physical Medicine and Rehabilitation, and was subsequently appointed as a clinical associate. Dr. Feldman has published extensively, including five chapters in professional books. She has received numerous awards and honors, and was twice the recipient of the Hopkins Healer Award for excellence in patient care during residency. In April 2017, Dr. Feldman was inducted into the Miller-Coulson Academy of Clinical Excellence. Inductees are honored for their professionalism, communication skills, diagnostic prowess, depth of knowledge, ability to negotiate the health care system, passion for patient care and service as a role model to medical trainees.

***

Ashwitha A is working as an Assistant Professor in the Department of Information Technology, Manipal Institute of Technology, Bengaluru. Her research Interests include data mining, machine learning and Artificial Intelligence. she has published many international articles and conference papers in reputed journals.

Pinaki Pratim Acharjya earned his doctorate in philosophy in 2016 from National Institute of Technology, Agartala, Tripura, India. He is currently employed as a professor in the department of computer science and Engineering, Haldia Institute of Technology, Haldia, West Bengal, India. In several AICTE-approved engineering institutions across India, he has more than 15 years of teaching experience and more than fourteen years of research experience. In numerous national and international journals, conferences, books (written/edited), and book chapters, he has published more than hundred research publications. He is currently conducting research in the fields of Deep Learning, Machine Learning, Data Analytics, Blockchain Technology, Digital Image Processing, Computer Vision, and Artificial Intelligence.

Bhanuprakash Ananthakumar is a Research Scholar, Department of Life Sciences Sri Sathya Sai University for Human Excellence, India. His research are Genomics, Diabetes, Assistive Technologies.

G. Shirisha is currently serving as an Associate Professor in the Department of Mathematics at Stanley College of Engineering and Technology for Women, located in Hyderabad. She has more than 16 years of teaching experience and has gained expertise in mathematics education and research. She earned her PhD from BITS-Pilani, Hyderabad, where she specialized in advanced mathematical concepts and methodologies. Her research interest is diversified across several frontier domains of mathematics, including neural networks, mathematical modelling, and dynamical systems. Through her work she has made significant contributions to these fields, with multiple research articles published in prestigious international conferences and journals.

Bhuvana GudibandaNagaraja is a Research Scholar in Department of Life Sciences, Sri Sathya Sai University for Human Excellence, India.

T. Harikala is a dedicated researcher and a passionate author. Her interested domains include Image processing and wireless Sensor Networks. Her Specialization work is MIMO Radar systems in which she completed her Ph.D. from S.V. University, Tirupati; Andhra Pradesh. She has received her M. Tech degree in LICS from S.V. University, Tirupati, Andhra Pradesh, India.And B. Tech degree in ECE from JNTUH, India. She has Publications in Scopus, National, and International Journals/conferences, she also reviewed Journal Paper as a reviewer. Currently, she is deputed to the Department of CSE and is passionate about research areas like Wireless Communications, Computer Networks, etc.

Rituraj Jain is currently working in the Department of Information Technology, Marwadi University, Rajkot, GUjarat, India. He has published many papers in

International Journals and Conferences. He has published 4 books. He is an Oracle Database SQL Certified Expert. He is also associated with professional bodies like the Indian Society of Technical Education (ISTE), Computer Science Teachers Association (CSTA), Academy & Industry Research Collaboration Center (AIRCC), International Association of Computer Science and Information Technology (IACSIT), International Association of Engineers (IAENG). His research interests include Cloud Computing, Machine Learning, Deep Learning, Fuzzy Logic, IoT, Genetic Algorithms, Big Data and Software Engineering.

J. Jeyaranjani completed her B.E in Computer Science and Engineering in the year 2009 from KLNCIT, Sivagangai and M.Tech in Computer Science and Engineering in the year 2011 from Veltech University, Chennai. She obtained her Ph.D from Kalasalingam Academy of Research and Education in the year 2023. She has guided 3 M.E thesis. She worked as a faculty in Computer Science and Engineering department of Kalasalingam Academy of Research and Academy for 12 years. Since 2023, she is working as Assistant Professor and Head in Department of Information Technology, SRM Madurai College for Engineering and Technology, Sivagangai Dt. Her Research interest include Data Science, Machine Learning, Data Analytics and Artificial Intelligence.

V.Kishen Ajay Kumar was born in Proddatur, India, in 1980. He received the B.Tech. degree in electronics and communications engineering from the University of Sri Krishnadevaraya, Anantapuram, India, in 2001, and the M. Tech degree in digital systems and computer electronics from Jawaharlal Nehru Technological University (JNTU), Hyderabad, India, in 2007. He completed his PhD from JNTUA, Anantapuram in the year 2021. During the years 2007-2015, he worked as an Assistant professor and Associate professor, and in 2015, he joined as a Full-Time Research scholar in G. PullaReddy engineering college (Autonomous), which is affiliated to JNTU, Anantapuram, India. His current research interests include optical networks, communication networks. He is a Life Member of the Indian Society for Technical Education (ISTE). He has published 12 peer reviewed research articles in the area of communication networks and signal processing

A.V.Senthil Kumar is working as a Professor and Director, PG and Research Department of Computer Applications, Hindusthan College of Arts & Science, Coimbatore, Tamilnadu. To his credit he has industrial experience for five years and teaching experience of 27 years. He has also received his Doctor of Science (D.Sc in Computer Science). He has to his credit 50 Book Chapters, 225 papers in International and National Journals 64 papers in International Conferences in International and National Conferences, and edited 14 books and 2 Text books.

He is as Associate Editor of IEEE Access. He is an Editor-in-Chief for many journals and Key Member for India, Machine Intelligence Research Lab (MIR Labs). He is an Editorial Board Member and Reviewer for various International Journals. He is also a Committee member for various International Conferences.

Achyuth Mukund is currently a pre-final year student pursuing B.Tech Computer Science and Engineering with a specialization in IoT at Shiv Nadar University Chennai. He is also a student at IIT Madras, parallelly pursuing B.S. Degree in Data Science and Applications. With hands-on experience in IoT, Machine Learning, Assistive Systems, TensorFlow, and NLP, he derives actionable insights from big data and wearable devices. His groundbreaking work integrates machine learning, biomechanical engineering, and digital health technologies to develop cutting-edge assistive systems. His previous publications include a book chapter named "Enhancing Security in Federated Learning for Healthcare Data Sharing" under upcoming publication of the book "Building Secure Ecosystems: Advances in Privacy-Preserving Machine Learning". A Guinness World Record-holding keyboardist, he performs regularly at corporate gigs and cafés. Also a fellow petrolhead, an automobile enthusiast and competitive cricketer, he balances tech innovation with creative and physical pursuits, always exploring the synergy between code, music, and machines. His current research explores the convergence of artificial intelligence, wearable sensors, and personalized medicine, with a particular emphasis on neurological rehabilitation and cardiovascular health monitoring.

Divyashree N is an Assistant Professor at Reva University, Bengaluru, with over five years of academic experience. She holds an M.Tech in Computer Science and Engineering and specializes in C programming, Python, Data Structures, Cryptography, and Machine Learning. She has published research on Opinion Mining and Sentiment Analysis. Divyashree is committed to continuous learning, regularly attending workshops in emerging technologies and AI. She is fluent in English and Kannada and is known for her adaptability, leadership, and dedication.

Umamaheswari Purushothaman holds a B.E. in Information Technology from Periyar Maniammai College of Engineering and Technology (2003), an M.B.A. from Alagappa University, Karaikudi, Tamil Nadu (2006), and an M.Tech in Computer Science from SASTRA Deemed University, Thanjavur, Tamil Nadu (2011). She earned her Ph.D. in Computer Science and Engineering from SASTRA Deemed University. With two decades of experience, Dr. Uma Purushothaman has taught both undergraduate and postgraduate courses in Computer Science. She is currently an Assistant Professor in the Department of Computer Science and Engineering at SRC Campus, SASTRA University, Kumbakonam. Her research interests focus on

Data Mining, Machine Learning, and Deep Learning. She has published numerous research papers in international conferences, SCI-indexed journals, Scopus, and book chapters.

Damodharan Palaniappan works as an Associate Professor & Head in the Department of Information Technology, Marwadi University, Rajkot, Gujarat. He completed his Ph.D. at Anna University, Chennai, M.E. in Computer Science and Engineering at C.I.E.T, Coimbatore and B.E. in Computer Science and Engineering at CSI College of Engineering, Ketty, Nilgiri. He has 19 years' experience of teaching and research. Currently, he guides 6 Ph.D. research scholars. He has authored 8 book chapters, and he has published research papers in reputed journals. His interested areas of research are Data Mining, Image Processing, Software, Machine Learning and Deep Learning.

Ramya Raghavan is a researcher with a Ph.D. from school of medicine, where the research team delved into epigenetic factors leading to intellectual disability with severe speech impairment and behavioral problems. Dr. Raghavan has published peer-reviewed articles in prestigious scientific publishers. Her recently edited book reflects her dedication to advancing cancer treatment through innovative spatial omics approaches.

Revathi Ravilisetty received her Ph.D degree in Applied Mathematics, from BITS-Pilani, Hyderabad in 2022. She works as an Assistant Professor at the School of Sciences, Woxsen University, Hyderabad. Before joining Woxsen, she was an INSPIRE Research Fellow at the Department of Mathematics, BITS-Pilani, Hyderabad. Her research interests are broadly in the field of Computational Fluid Dynamics, Statistical Analysis and Optimisation Techniques. Specifically, she explores problems in the areas of Compressible Flows and Shock Waves.

S. Abiramasundari received B.Sc., Computer Science from Government College for women at Kumbakonam in 2001. She completed M.Sc., Computer Science from Sengamala Thayaar Educational Trust at Mannargudi in 2003. She completed M.Phil., degree in Computer Science at Bharathidhasan University in 2006. She has been working as an Assistant Professor in SASTRA University, since 2006. She is pursuing Ph.D. Computer Science at SASTRA University.

Bhanu Prakash Saripalli is an Assistant Professor at the School of Technology, Woxsen University, bringing more than 13 years of valuable experience in teaching and research. He has significantly contributed to the field throughout his academic journey, publishing papers in esteemed national and international conferences and peer-reviewed journals. In 2022, he earned his Ph.D. from DIT University, India, focusing on supercapacitor-based smoothing of Solar Photovoltaic (PV) power generation fluctuations. His research interests center around Mitigating fluctuations in solar photovoltaic power generation, Energy Management, Power electronics for renewable energy, Solar PV waste management, and Supercapacitor Energy storage systems. His expertise is well-established with Six peer-reviewed publications in reputed journals, three conference papers, two patents, and Seven book chapters. Dr. Prakash's current pursuits involve Energy management and Modeling and Parameter estimation of Solar Photovoltaic Systems.

Swati Singh working as Assistant professor in IT department of Vardhaman College of Engineering Hyderabad. She has been also worked as Software Engineer in corporate world with Microsoft Technologies. She is also contributing her knowledge as blogger on www.viaresearch.in. Her Qualification is M.Tech in Computer Science and Technology in Central University of Punjab (CUP), Bathinda.

Malla Sudhakara, a seasoned Senior Computer Vision Scientist and Tech Lead at Chistats Labs Private Limited in Pune holds a Ph.D. in Computer Science and Engineering from VIT, which he received in 2024. He is a top expert in machine learning, computer vision, and deep learning, with a remarkable 11-year career in research and industry. Sudhakara's contributions to these disciplines may be seen in his publications in SCIE and Scopus-indexed journals and his active participation in conferences, where he was awarded the best paper award in 2021. His research includes underwater picture improvement tactics based on deep learning algorithms, showcasing his dedication to pushing the boundaries of computer vision applications. Notably, he also works as a resource person, sharing his machine learning, Python programming, and software engineering knowledge with various universities. Sudhakara's fascinating pastime as a YouTuber implies a passion for knowledge sharing, making him a great asset to the scholarly community and a wider audience interested in his expertise

Muhammad Usman Tariq has more than 16+ year's experience in industry and academia. He has authored more than 200+ research articles, 110+ case studies, 120+ book chapters and several books other than 4 patents. He is founder and CEO of The Case HQ, a unique repository for courses, narrative and video case studies. He has been working as a consultant and trainer for industries representing six sigma, quality, health and safety, environmental systems, project management, and information security standards. His work has encompassed sectors in aviation, manufacturing, food, hospitality, education, finance, research, software and transportation. He has diverse and significant experience working with accreditation agencies of ABET, ACBSP, AACSB, WASC, CAA, EFQM and

NCEAC. Additionally, Dr. Tariq has operational experience in incubators, research labs, government research projects, private sector startups, program creation and management at various industrial and academic levels. He is Certified Higher Education Teacher from Harvard University, USA, Certified Online Educator from HMBSU, Certified Six Sigma Master Black Belt and has been awarded PFHEA, SFSEDA, SMIEEE, and CMBE.

Sai Mahima Umesh is Research Scholar in Department of Life Science, Sri Sathya Sai University for Human Excellence, India.

Kavya Vijaysankar is a BSc Psychology (Honours) Graduate from Christ University. She is a cognitive science enthusiast with a strong interest in applying gamification and machine learning to mental health research. Her most recent project involved developing a two-player cooperative video game as a tool for couples therapy to promote interpersonal skills. She will be pursuing her masters from the University of Nottingham in computational neuroscience, cognition, and AI in September 2025. She aspires to advance research in assistive technology for learning, neurodevelopmental disorders, and other cognitive deficits.

Index

A

B

C

D

E

N

P

R

S

T

W

X

www.ingramcontent.com/pod-product-compliance
Lightning Source LLC
LaVergne TN
LVHW061532290926
849162LV00004B/761